Nanoarchitectonics for Brain Drug Delivery

This book discusses basics of brain diseases and the role of nanobiotechnology in existing treatment options for neurodegenerative disorders. It begins with an overview of brain diseases and the need for novel drug-delivery approaches. It highlights the current route for the intranasal advanced drug-delivery systems for brain diseases. It also discusses innovative categories of drug-delivery systems, including mesoporous silica nanoparticles, polymeric nanocarriers, and lipid-based nanocarriers through multi-responsive DDSs and their implications in brain disorders.

Features:

- Includes an overview of brain diseases and highlights the need for novel drug-delivery approaches.
- Focuses on theoretical aspects of advanced drug-delivery systems for brain diseases including challenges and progress in nose-to-brain delivery.
- Provides an overview of technological approaches and their implications for neurodegenerative disorders, central nervous system (CNS), and brain drug delivery in brain cancer.
- Discusses key advances in the development of polymer nanoparticles for drug delivery to the CNS.
- Reviews the role of herbal medicines and naturally derived polymeric nanoparticle for the treatment of neurodegenerative disorders.

This book is aimed at graduate students and researchers in biomedical engineering, biotechnology, drug delivery, and neurology.

Advances in Bionanotechnology

***Series Editors: Ravindra Pratap Singh**, Department of Biotechnology, Indira Gandhi National Tribal University, Anuppur, Madhya Pradesh, India; **Jay Singh**, Department of Chemistry, Institute of Science, Banaras Hindu University, Varanasi, Uttar Pradesh, India; and **Charles Oluwaseun Adetunji**, Department of Microbiology, Edo State University Uzairue, Iyamho, Edo State, Nigeria*

Bionanotechnology is a multidisciplinary field that shows immense applicability in different domains, namely chemistry, physics, material sciences, biomedicine, agriculture, environment, robotics, aeronautics, energy, electronics, and so forth. This book series explores the enormous utility of bionanotechnology for the biomedical, agricultural, environmental, food technology, space industry, and many other fields. It aims to highlight all the spheres of bionanotechnological applications and their safety and regulations for using biogenic nanomaterials that are a key focus of researchers globally.

Bionanotechnology towards Sustainable Management of Environmental Pollution
Edited by Naveen Dwivedi and Shubha Dwivedi

Natural Products and Nano-formulations in Cancer Chemoprevention
Edited by Shiv Kumar Dubey

Bionanotechnology towards Green Energy
Innovative and Sustainable Approach
Edited by Shubha Dwivedi and Naveen Dwivedi

Biotic Stress Management of Crop Plants Using Nanomaterials
Edited by Krishna Kant Mishra and Santosh Kumar

Bionanotechnology for Advanced Applications
Edited by Ajaya Kumar Singh and Bhawana Jain

Nanoarchitectonics for Brain Drug Delivery
Edited by Anurag Kumar Singh, Vivek K. Chaturvedi, and Jay Singh

For more information about this series, please visit: www.routledge.com/Advances-in-Bionanotechnology/book-series/CRCBIONAN

Nanoarchitectonics for Brain Drug Delivery

Edited by
Anurag Kumar Singh, Vivek K. Chaturvedi,
and Jay Singh

CRC Press
Taylor & Francis Group
Boca Raton London New York

CRC Press is an imprint of the
Taylor & Francis Group, an **informa** business

Designed cover image: © Shutterstock

First edition published 2024
by CRC Press
2385 NW Executive Center Drive, Suite 320, Boca Raton FL 33431

and by CRC Press
4 Park Square, Milton Park, Abingdon, Oxon, OX14 4RN

CRC Press is an imprint of Taylor & Francis Group, LLC

ISBN: 9781032555393 (hbk)
ISBN: 9781032661957 (pbk)
ISBN: 9781032661964 (ebk)

DOI: 10.1201/9781032661964

Typeset in Times
by Newgen Publishing UK

Dedicated

---

to those who care, conserve, and protect but do not destroy the beauty and unique characteristics of

Kshit (Earth)

Jal (Water)

Pawak (Fire)

Gagan (Sky)

and

Sameera (Air)

Contents

Preface

Over the past decades, the pharmaceutical industry has faced significant challenges in developing drug-delivery systems (DDSs) that efficiently treat the disease in question with minor side effects. Thus, the rapid advances in micro- and nanomaterials for biomedical applications have received tremendous experimental attention in almost every field of biosciences and are now a reality coming into practice and expected to have an enormous impact on human healthcare. The applications of these materials include, but are not limited to, brain drug delivery, brain tumour delivery, natural products delivery, central nervous system delivery, and blood–brain barrier drug delivery. These materials also hold great promise in biomedical applications for early diagnostics, non-invasive imaging, and targeting the delivery of therapeutics, as well as for combined functions, such as concurrent therapy and the monitoring of diseases (nanoarchitectonics). More than ever, there are combined efforts from many scientists worldwide with different backgrounds to develop efficient and promising DDSs. As a result, promising advanced DDSs with high payloads of therapeutic agents, specific for controlled and targeted drug delivery at effective local concentrations with the fewest side effects possible, have been developed. At the same time, the biocompatibility and biodegradability of these DDSs are imperative and are usually associated with the efficiency and safety of the DDSs. For example, inorganic porous-based biomaterials can be used as, for example, drug carriers and for locally controlling the dose and duration of the release of therapeutic agents. This is expected to significantly improve healthcare quality while reducing costs, particularly for patients with chronic illnesses. The field of drug delivery and biomaterials is rather interdisciplinary and rapidly growing. The administration of particulate systems for drug delivery has to be preceded by an extensive series of preclinical and clinical tests and critical issues such as biodistribution, circulation, immune response, toxicity, and clearance, which need to be evaluated before applying them to humans. The great advantage of these DDSs is that they are non-toxic and biodegradable in most cases, which renders them greatly promising for the future when moving from a preclinical to a clinical setting. This book is a part of *Nanoarchitectonics for Brain Drug Delivery: A Boon for Healthy Brain*. However, the book is focused on the types of central nervous system (CNS) disorders and brain drug delivery and blood–brain barrier (BBB) penetration. It is devoted to presenting various nanocarriers' recent therapeutic and diagnostic applications in brain drug delivery and CNS delivery. The book contains 14 chapters. Chapter 1 discusses nanoparticles and their types and route of administration as well as their role in drug delivery (BBB and CNS), the second chapter discussed the fundamentals of brain diseases, comprising a valuable background for the that follow. In this chapter, the book provides an overview of brain diseases and the need for novel drug delivery approaches, thereby introducing and discussing the basic concepts and their potential clinical use. Both Chapters 3 and 4 discuss the theoretical aspects of advanced drug delivery systems for brain diseases and the challenges and progress in nose-to-brain delivery. Chapters 5, 6, 7, and 8 discuss innovative categories of DDSs, including mesoporous silica nanoparticles, polymeric nanocarriers, lipid-based nanocarriers, and combination as well as multi-responsive DDSs, respectively, and discuss technological approaches and their implications for neurodegenerative disorders, CNS, and brain drug delivery. Chapter 9 discusses the applications of targeted delivery systems in brain cancer. Herbal medicine-loaded nanoparticles and natural polymeric nanoparticles are discussed in Chapters 10, 11, and 12, which include herbal medicines and naturally derived polymeric nanoparticles for the treatment of neurodegenerative disorders. The last two chapters, 13 and 14, provide a detailed overview of progressive perspectives on solid lipid nanoparticles in brain targeting, as well as the neuropharmacological potential of ayurvedic nanomedicines and their implications in a preclinical and clinical setting.

AIM AND SCOPE

Nanoscience has the potential to transform the existing treatment options for neurodegenerative disorders like Alzheimer's disease, Parkinson's disease, brain cancer, haemorrhages, and so on. In malignant brain tumours, the mainstay of care is maximal surgical resection (if possible), followed by radiation, chemotherapy, and symptomatic treatment. The brain accounts for nearly all malignant CNS tumours. Cancerous brain tumours are prone to relapse and remain unmet challenges for clinicians. Due to the high rate of intracranial metastases, new chemotherapeutics have transformed the prognosis for many forms of cancer. Multiple studies have indicated that nanomaterials can successfully be used to treat CNS disorders. Nanoparticles may act as a drug transporter that can precisely target sick brain subregions and provide better therapeutic benefits of the loaded drugs. Multifunctional nanoparticles carrying bioactive moiety which serve two basic purposes: (i) improving drug distribution, and (ii) easily enabling cell dynamics imaging and pharmacokinetic studies. Improved diagnostic and therapeutic outcomes could be achieved using nanotechnology and polymer science. Nanomedicines are also used to treat oxidative stress. Despite their potential in disease management, nanomedicines have yet to establish themselves as widely available treatment options. However, the development of nanomedicines to cure neurodegenerative and inflammatory diseases of the nervous system is critical. The utilization of nanotechnology as a therapeutic carrier and diagnostic agent has shown promising and inherent outcomes. The safety concern is a major hurdle that needs to cleared before industrial and/or clinical translation of nanomaterials. Nanotechnology-based drug delivery systems can easily cross the BBB and blood–cerebrospinal fluid barrier (BCFB), making it possible to overcome the limitations of conventional therapeutics and finally improve the therapeutic benefits of loaded active moieties. Scientists globally, both from academia and the pharmaceutical industry, are trying to produce an associative strategy to develop nanotechnology based drug products to overcome challenges associated with existing CNS therapies. In the future, nanomaterials and their complex mixtures including therapeutic substances could be an effective tool in brain drug delivery.

Anurag Kumar Singh
Vivek K. Chaturvedi
Jay Singh

Contributors

Gufran Ahmed
Department of Biochemistry, Rajendra Memorial Research Institute of Medical Sciences, Patna, India

Arshad J. Ansari
Department of Pharmacy, School of Chemical Sciences and Pharmacy, Central University of Rajasthan, Bandarsindri, Ajmer, Rajasthan, India

Aditi Bhatnagar
School of Biochemical Engineering, Indian Institute of Technology (Banaras Hindu University), Varanasi, India

Vivek K. Chaturvedi
Department of Gastroenterology, Institute of Medical Sciences, Banaras Hindu University, Varanasi, Uttar Pradesh, India

Pritee Chaudhary
Department of Medicine, Institute of Medical Sciences, Banaras Hindu University, Varanasi, Uttar Pradesh, India

Ratiram G. Choudhary
Post Graduate Department of Chemistry, Seth Kesarimal Porwal College of Arts and Science and Commerce, Kamptee, India

Kanhaiya M. Dadure
Department of Chemistry, J. B. College of Science, Wardha, Maharashtra, India

Hagera Dilnashin
Department of Biochemistry, Institute of Science, Banaras Hindu University, Varanasi (U.P.), India

Juhaina M. Abu Ershaid
Department of Applied Pharmaceutical Sciences and Clinical Pharmacy, Faculty of Pharmacy, Isra University, Amman, Jordan

Andri Frediansyah
Research Center for Food Technology and Processing, National Research and Innovation Agency (BRIN), Yogyakarta, Indonesia

Animeshchandra G. M. Haldar
Department of Applied Chemistry, Priyadarshini Bhagwati College of Engineering, Nagpur, Maharashtra, India

Achmad Himawan
Department of Pharmaceutical Science and Technology, Faculty of Pharmacy, Hasanuddin University, Tamalanrea, Makassar, Indonesia; School of Pharmacy, Queen's University Belfast, Belfast, United Kingdom

Shaliha Irfan
Department of Botany, Patna University, Patna, India

Aditya Kadam
Minnesota Dental Research Center for Biomaterials and Biomechanics, University of Minnesota, Minneapolis, MN, USA

Shradha Karande
Delhi Pharmaceutical Sciences and Research University, Delhi, India

Soumya Katiyar
School of Biochemical Engineering, Indian Institute of Technology (Banaras Hindu University), Varanasi, India.

Gábor Katona
Institute of Pharmaceutical Technology and Regulatory Affairs, Faculty of Pharmacy, University of Szeged, Eötvös, Szeged, Hungary

Shazia Kazmi
Department of Botany, Patna University, Patna, India

Iliyas Khan
Department of Pharmacy, School of Chemical Sciences and Pharmacy, Central University of Rajasthan, Bandarsindri, Ajmer, Rajasthan, India

Mukesh Kumar Yadav
Vaccine and Infectious Disease Research Center, Division of Virology, Translational Health Science and Technology Institute, Faridabad, Haryana, India

Vikash Kumar
Department of Biochemistry and Molecular Biology, Institute for Medical Research Israel-Canada, Faculty of Medicine, Hebrew University of Jerusalem, Israel

Ashish Kumar
Department of Biochemistry, Rajendra Memorial Research Institute of Medical Sciences, Patna, India

Hitesh Kumar
Department of Pharmaceutics, JSS College of Pharmacy, JSS Academy of Higher Education & Research, Shivarathreeshwara Nagara, Mysuru-570015, India; Faculty of Pharmacy, Kalinga University, Kotni, Near Mantralaya, Naya Raipur (CG) India

Pankaj Kumar
Faculty of Ayurveda, Institute of Medical Sciences, Banaras Hindu University, India

Shikha Kumari
School of Biochemical Engineering, Indian Institute of Technology (Banaras Hindu University), Varanasi, India

Eeneko Larrañeta
School of Pharmacy, Queen's University Belfast, Belfast, United Kingdom

Debarshi Kar Mahapatra
Department of Pharmaceutical Chemistry, Kamalprakash Pharmacy College and Research Centre, Washim, Maharashtra, India

Sukamto S. Mamada
Department of Pharmacy, Faculty of Pharmacy, Hasanuddin University, Tamalanrea, Makassar, Indonesia

Sandra Aulia Mardikasari
Department of Pharmaceutical Science and Technology, Faculty of Pharmacy, Hasanuddin University, Tamalanrea, Makassar, Indonesia

Anand Maurya
Institute of Medical Sciences, Faculty of Ayurveda, Department of Medicinal

Chemistry, Banaras Hindu University, Varanasi, Uttar Pradesh, India

Shardendu Kumar Mishra
Department of Pharmacology, KIET School of Pharmacy, Ghaziabad, Uttar Pradesh, India

Vishal Mishra
School of Biochemical Engineering, IIT (BHU) Varanasi, India

Abha Mishra
School of Biochemical Engineering, Indian Institute of Technology (Banaras Hindu University), Varanasi, India.

Namdev More
Sangam Health Science Pune, Maharashtra, India

Firzan Nainu
Department of Pharmacy, Faculty of Pharmacy, Hasanuddin University, Tamalanrea, Makassar, Indonesia

Gaurav K. Pandit
Department of Biochemistry, Rajendra Memorial Research Institute of Medical Sciences, Patna, India

Anjali Kiran Pandya
Department of Pharmaceutical Sciences and Technology, Institute of Chemical Technology, Mumbai, India

Vandana Patravale
Department of Pharmaceutical Sciences and Technology, Institute of Chemical Technology, Mumbai, India

Andi Dian Permana
Department of Pharmaceutical Science and Technology, Faculty of Pharmacy, Hasanuddin University, Tamalanrea, Makassar, Indonesia

Wahyu Aristyaning Putri
Department of Tropical Biology, Faculty of Biology, Gadjah Mada University. Yogyakarta, Indonesia

Winda Adipuri Ramadaningrum
National Agency of Drug and Food Control (BPOM), Jakarta, Indonesia

Mirnawati Salampe
Sekolah Tinggi Ilmu Farmasi Makassar, Tamalanrea, Makassar, Indonesia

K. Trideva Sastri
Department of Pharmaceutics, JSS College of Pharmacy, JSS Academy of Higher Education & Research, Shivarathreeshwara Nagara, Mysuru, India

Rohit Sharma
Department of Rasa Shastra and Bhaishajya Kalpana, Faculty of Ayurveda, Institute of Medical Science, Banaras Hindu University, Varanasi, Uttar Pradesh, India

Dilip Sharma
New Jersey Medical School, Rutgers University, Newark, NJ, USA.

Snigdha Singh
Centre of Experimental Medicine & Surgery, Institute of Medical Sciences, Banaras Hindu University, Varanasi, Uttar Pradesh, India

Santosh Kumar Singh
Centre of Experimental Medicine and Surgery, Institute of Medical Sciences, Banaras Hindu University, Varanasi, Uttar Pradesh, India

Richa Singh
Department of Biochemistry, Institute of Science, Banaras Hindu University, Varanasi (U.P.), India

Shekhar Singh
Department of Biochemistry, Institute of Science, Banaras Hindu University, Varanasi (U.P.), India

Surya Pratap Singh
Department of Biochemistry, Institute of Science, Banaras Hindu University, Varanasi (U.P.), India

Veer Singh
Department of Biochemistry, Rajendra Memorial Research Institute of Medical Sciences, Patna, India

Meenakshi Singh
Department of Botany, Patna University, Patna, India

Jay Singh
Department of Chemistry, Institute of Science, Banaras Hindu University, Varanasi, Uttar Pradesh, India

Anurag Kumar Singh
Department of Pharmaceutical Enginering & Technology, Indian Insitute of Technology (Banaras Hindu Uniiversity), Varanasi, Uttar Pradesh, India and Cancer Biology Research and Training, Department of Biological Sciences, Alabama State University, Montgomery, Alabama, United States

Manish Singh
Department of Pharmacology, Institute of Medical Sciences, Banaras Hindu University, Varanasi, Uttar Pradesh, India

Ritika Singh
School of Biotechnology, Institute of Science, Banaras Hindu University, Varanasi, India

Fajar Sofyantoro
Department of Tropical Biology, Faculty of Biology, Gadjah Mada University. Yogyakarta, Indonesia

Pradeep K. Srivastava
School of Biochemical Engineering, Indian Institute of Technology (Banaras Hindu University), Varanasi, India.

Shreya Thakkar
Fresenius Kabi Oncology Ltd, Gurugram, Haryana, India

Ritesh K. Tiwari
Department of Biochemistry, Rajendra Memorial Research Institute of Medical Sciences, Patna, India

Abhay Dev Tripathi
School of Biochemical Engineering, Indian Institute of Technology (Banaras Hindu University), Varanasi, India.

Lalitkumar K. Vora
School of Pharmacy, Queen's University Belfast, Belfast, United Kingdom

About the Editors

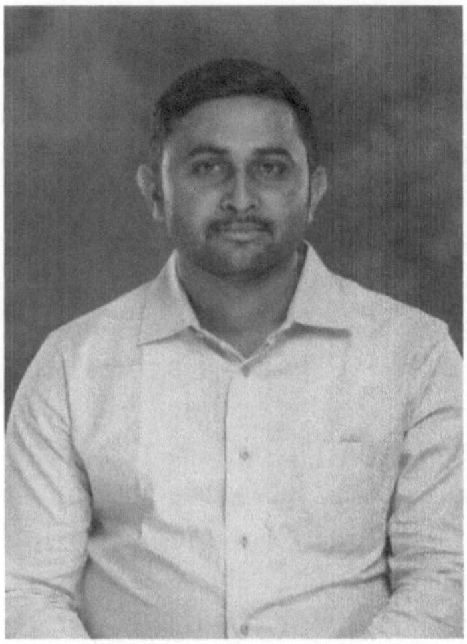

Anurag Kumar Singh is currently working as an Indian Council of Medical Research (ICMR) Research Associate (RA) fellow in the Department of Pharmaceutical Engineering & Technology, Indian Institute of Technology (Banaras Hindu University), Varanasi-21005, Uttar Pradesh, India. Prior to joining as ICMR-RA fellow in Indian Institute of Technology, he worked as a postdoctoral research assistant in Cancer Biology Research and Training at the Department of Biological Sciences, Alabama State University (USA). He completed his doctoral degree from the Centre of Experimental Medicine and Surgery, Institute of Medical Sciences, Banaras Hindu University, Varanasi, Uttar Pradesh, India. He earned a M. Pharm degree from the School of Chemical Sciences and Pharmacy, Central University of Rajasthan, Ajmer, Rajasthan, India. His scholarly interests range from developing novel nanoparticulate systems for brain-targeted drug delivery, including dendrimer, nanoporous silica/silicon materials, and polymeric nanoparticles for controlled drug delivery to diagnostics and therapy. His research interests include the development of nanoparticles/nanomedicines for biomedical and healthcare applications and the building of a bridge between engineering, pharmaceutical, and medical research. He has published several research papers, including reviews, journal editorials, and book chapters in various peer-reviewed national and international journals.

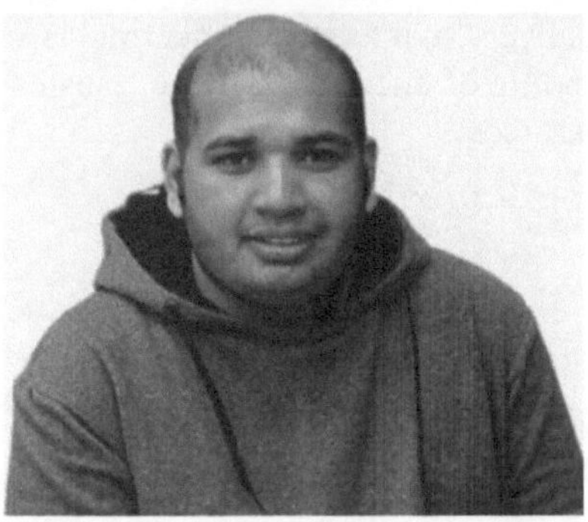

Vivek K. Chaturvedi is a Young-Scientist Fellow (Department of Health Research, Ministry of Health and Family Welfare) at the Institute of Medical Sciences, Banaras Hindu University, Varanasi, India. Before joining the laboratory as a Young-Scientist Fellow, he worked as postdoctoral research associate at the Department of Gastroenterology, IMS-BHU, Varanasi. He earned his PhD in Biotechnology from the University of Allahabad (a central university), Prayagraj, India. He has received his B.Sc. degree in Zoology and Chemistry, and his M.Sc. degree in Biochemistry from Veer Bahadur Singh Purvanchal University, Jaunpur, India. Dr. Chaturvedi's research interests include the synthesis and functionalization of nanomaterials as well as their fabrication for the development of various biosensors that may be useful for the early detection and treatment of cancer and gastrointestinal diseases. He has voluntarily served as reviewer and published a number of original articles in peer-reviewed high-impact journals along with many international books, magazine articles, and chapters.

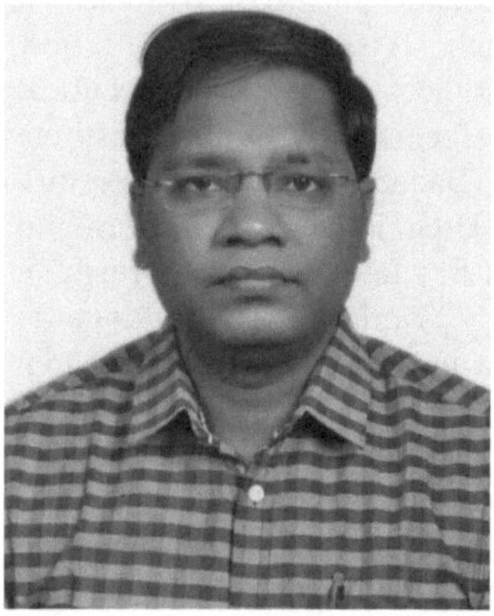

Jay Singh is currently working as an assistant professor at the Department of Chemistry, Institute of Sciences, Banaras Hindu University, Varanasi, Uttar Pradesh, since 2017. He received his PhD in Polymer Science from Motilal Nehru National Institute of Technology in 2010 and obtained his MSc and BSc from Allahabad University, Uttar Pradesh, India. He has held postdoctoral fellowships at the National Physical Laboratory, New Delhi; Chonbuk National University, South Korea; and Delhi Technological University, Delhi. Dr. Jay has been honoured with prestigious fellowships such as the CSIR (RA) DST-Young Scientist Fellowship, and the DST-INSPIRE Faculty Award. His research focuses on the development of chemically and biologically synthesized nanomaterials and their nanobiocomposites, on conducting polymers, and on self-assembled monolayers. He is dedicated to creating clinically significant biosensors and sensors for the estimation of various bioanalytes based on enzymes, antibodies, DNA, and toxic chemicals and gases. With over 100 international research papers published and a total citation count exceeding 4,000, Dr. Jay possesses an h-index of 36. He has successfully completed or is currently running various research projects funded by different agencies. Moreover, he has authored/edited more than 15 books and contributed over 40 book chapters for internationally renowned publishers. Dr. Jay has also handled special issues in esteemed journals. Currently, his active research involves the fabrication of sustainable metal oxide-based biosensors for clinical diagnosis, food packaging applications, drug delivery, and tissue engineering. His work has significantly contributed to the understanding of interfacial charge transfer processes and sensing capabilities of metal nanoparticles.

Acknowledgements

It gives us immense pleasure to acknowledge Bharat Ratna Mahamana Pt. Madan Mohan Malviya Ji, founder of the Banaras Hindu University, Varanasi, Uttar Pradesh, India. Anurag Kumar Singh would like acknowledge the Indian Council of Medical Research (ICMR), Department of Health Research, Ministry of Health and Family Welfare, Government of India, for support through the Research Associate (ICMR-RA) Award (No: 3/1/2/110Neuro/2019-NCD-I). Vivek K. Chaturvedi gratefully acknowledges the Department of Health Research (DHR), Ministry of Health and Family Welfare, Government of India, for support through the Young Scientist Fellowship Grant R.12014/56/2022-HR. Jay Singh would like to acknowledge Institutes of Eminence (IoE), Ministry of Education, India, for providing constant assistance in all possible ways. It is also our great pleasure to acknowledge and express our enormous debt to all the contributors who have provided quality material to prepare this book. We are grateful to our beloved family members, who joyfully supported and stood with us in the many hours of our absence to finish this book project. We are also grateful to our friends and colleagues who offered their support and encouragement throughout the writing process. I would also like to acknowledge the publishing team at CRC Press for their professionalism, enthusiasm, and belief in this project. Their expertise in design, production, and marketing has been essential in bringing this book to life.

Anurag Kumar Singh
Vivek K. Chaturvedi
Jay Singh

1 Nanomedicine at the Forefront

Transforming Brain Drug Delivery with Innovative Strategies

Snigdha Singh, Anurag Kumar Singh, Anand Maurya, Vivek K. Chaturvedi, Jay Singh, and Santosh Kumar Singh

1.1 INTRODUCTION

The human body's most complex and essential organ is the brain. Consequently, it is vital to safeguard it against any affronts that might perhaps prompt disease, aggravation, ill-advised initiation, and, surprisingly, the passing of cerebral cells [1]. The central nervous system (CNS) comprises the mind and the spinal string. There are two main barriers that protect these areas: the blood-cerebrospinal fluid barrier (BCFB) and the blood–brain barrier (BBB) [1]. Since these barriers of the CNS function as a selectively permeable membrane and do not completely block all incoming compounds, the use of the term "barrier" to describe these interfaces is misleading [2].

The BBB is characterized by an unmistakable construction and communication between the acellular and the cell parts in the cerebrum. The essential capability of the BBB is to ensure that there exists a reasonable climate for the communication and the working of the neurons, which is significant for keeping up with homeostasis, directing efflux and deluge, and safeguarding the mind from pathogenic specialists [1]. The BBB consists of a nonstop layer of endothelial cells associated through close intersections (TJs), follower intersections (AJs), and hole intersections (GJs). TJs are the most important component of the BBB's composition and enhance trans-endothelial resistance in the BBB [3]. By tethering the adjacent cells so tightly that they obstruct the space between them, these junctions enable the controlled passage of drugs across the BBB [2, 3]. Pericytes, astrocytes, microglia, and adjacent neurons are specialized cells that can be found in the BBB. From a physical perspective, pericytes are multifunctional painting cells that fold over endothelial cells and control TJs, AJs, and transcytosis across the BBB [4]. A nano drug delivery system (NDDS) has unique advantages in drug delivery. The appropriate physicochemical properties including solubility, particle size, potential, and morphology contribute to improving the pharmacokinetics and tissue distribution. What's more, surface modification may enhance the accumulation of drugs in the target tissue to improve the therapeutic

DOI: 10.1201/9781032661964-1

effect. In addition, the NDDS has specific drug release behaviour, which increases the concentration of drug in the target site and reduces the concentration of drugs in the non-target site, thereby reducing adverse reactions. Furthermore, a NDDS makes it easy to realize a combined treatment to achieve synergistic effects [5].

Nanostructures have several benefits, such as variable particle size, shape, and high drug-loading capacity. Drug delivery systems (DDSs) have recently become more and more necessary to diminish the drawbacks of conventional therapies, such as their lack of selectivity and poor biodistribution [6]. By precisely delivering a therapeutic molecule to the intended site while maintaining the integrity of the therapeutic molecule, a well-designed DDS can significantly improve the therapeutic efficacy of a therapeutic molecule, minimizing any unintended side effects. Due to their distinctive physicochemical and biological characteristics, nanoparticles (particles smaller than 100 nm) have also been proved to be advantageous as effective drug delivery carriers in the course of recent nanotechnology advancements [7].

Novel DDSs comprise a diverse range of materials like silica- and carbon-based porous nanoparticles [8, 9], SLNs, self-emulsifying emulsions, dendrimers [10, 11, 12], responsive liposomes, and magnetic and polymeric nanoparticles [8, 13]. DDS-based nanoparticles have been employed for brain targeting and have proven to be good candidates for enhancing the active ingredient's efficacy and reducing its undesirable effects. Furthermore, due to its physico-chemical features, such as a homogeneous pore network, a wide surface area, less toxicity, and enhanced bio-distribution of the loaded cargo [8, 13], nanoparticles have been thoroughly researched in terms of controlled drug release.

1.2 CLASSIFICATION OF NANOPARTICLES

Nanoparticles (NPs) are classified into several types based on their chemical characteristics, morphology, and size. Some well-known classes of NPs are listed below based on their chemical and physical properties (Figure.1.1).

1.2.1 Inorganic Nanoparticles

This class includes nanoparticles (NPs) that are not comprised of organic or carbon elements. Metal, ceramic, and semiconductor NPs are classic examples of inorganic NPs. Metal NPs are entirely composed of metal precursors and can be bimetallic, monometallic [14], or polymetallic [15]. Furthermore, some metal NPs have unique biological, thermal, and magnetic properties [16]. This makes them increasingly significant materials for the creation of nanodevices that can be employed in a wide range of biological, physical, biomedical, chemical, and pharmacological applications [17]. Nowadays, the shape-, size-, and facet-controlled synthesis of metal NPs is critical for developing cutting-edge materials [17].

1.2.2 Polymeric Nanoparticles

Organic-based NPs are typically known as polymeric nanoparticles (PNPs). They are generally shaped like nanocapsules or nanospheres [18, 19]. The former are matrix

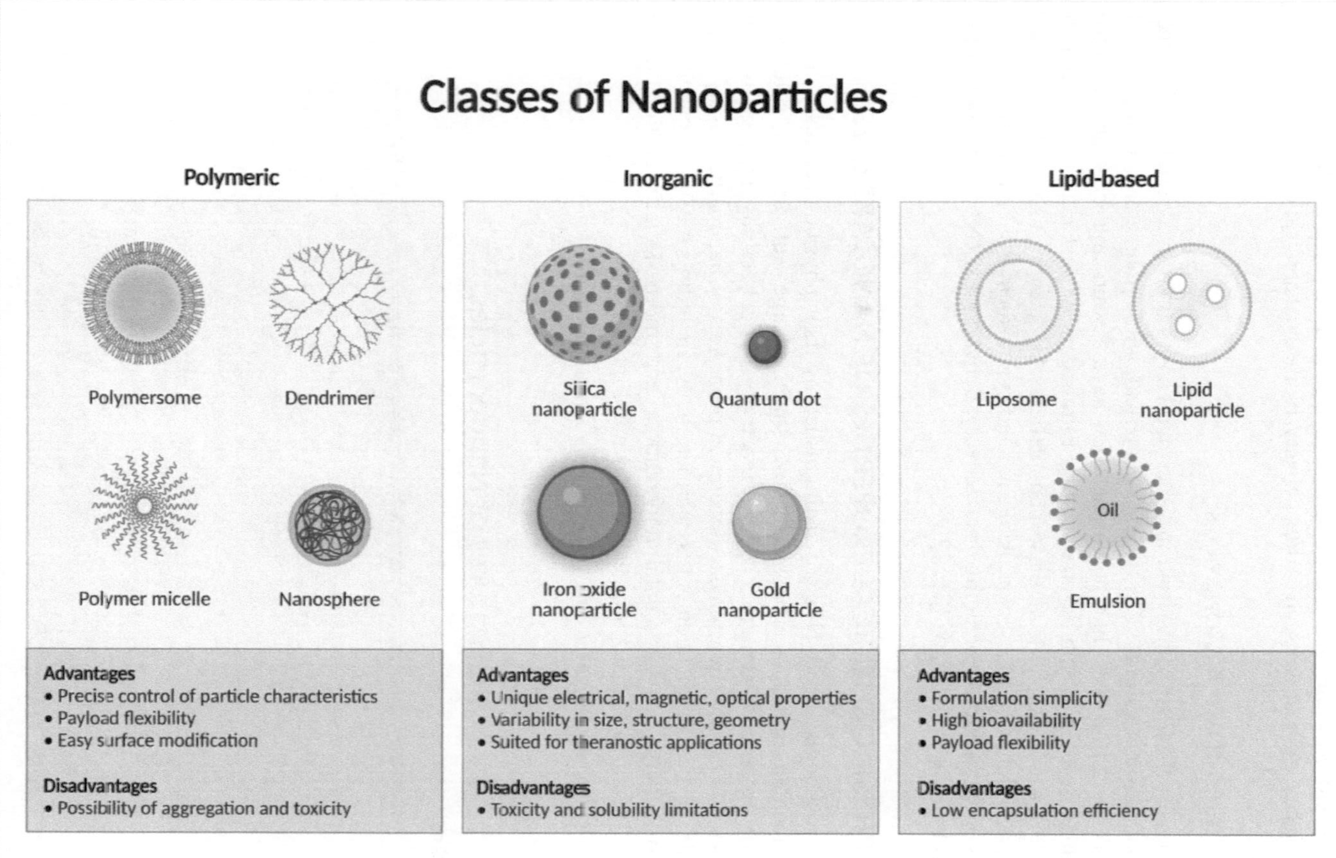

FIGURE 1.1 Different types of nanoparticles with their demerits and merits.

particles with a usually solid overall mass, whereas the other molecules are adsorbed at the spherical surface's outer edge. In the latter state of the preparation, the solid mass is entirely enclosed within the particle [19]. PNPs are easily functionalized and so have a wide range of applications such as drug delivery, biomedical application, and so on. [20].

1.2.3 Lipid-Based Nanoparticles

These types of NPs include lipid moieties and can be used in a variety of biomedical applications. A lipid NP is typically spherical, with a diameter ranging from 10 to 1000 nm. Lipid NPs, like polymeric NPs, have a solid lipid core and a matrix containing soluble lipophilic compounds. Emulsifiers or surfactants were used to stabilize the exterior core of these nanoparticles [19]. Lipid nanotechnology is a widespread field that focuses on the design and synthesis of lipid nanoparticles for a variety of applications, including drug delivery, delivery of siRNA in cancer therapy, stem cell therapy, and so on [21, 22].

1.3 PHYSICOCHEMICAL PROPERTIES OF NANOPARTICLES

As previously discussed, NPs are distinguished by their physico-chemical features, which include enormous mechanical size, shape, charge, surface area, solubility, magnetic properties, strength, chemical reactivity, optical activity, aggregation, and depression [17, 23]. These physico-chemical properties of nanoparticles play a crucial role in their application across various fields, including medicine, electronics, catalysis, energy, environmental remediation, and more. Details of the physiochemical features of nanoparticles are shown in Figure 1.2.

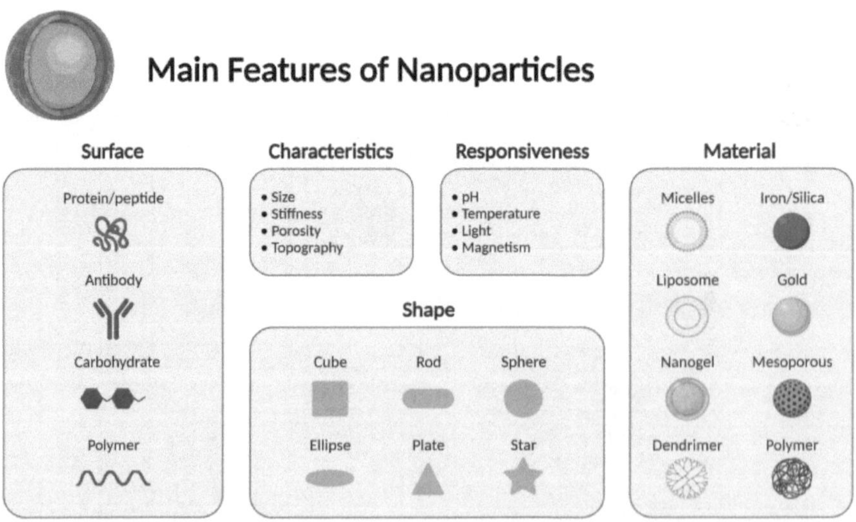

FIGURE 1.2 Basic physiochemical properties of nanoparticles.

1.4 PROMISING STRATEGIES FOR ENHANCING CENTRAL NERVOUS SYSTEM DRUG DELIVERY

To make it easier for therapeutic drugs to get to their intended location in the brain, pharmaceutical manipulation, disruption of the BBB, and other techniques involving the use of nanocarriers are currently used (Figure 1.3) [24]. Following administration, drug carriers must overcome a number of hurdles and barriers before reaching their targets. Tissue barriers, the immune system, biological hydrogels, and cellular

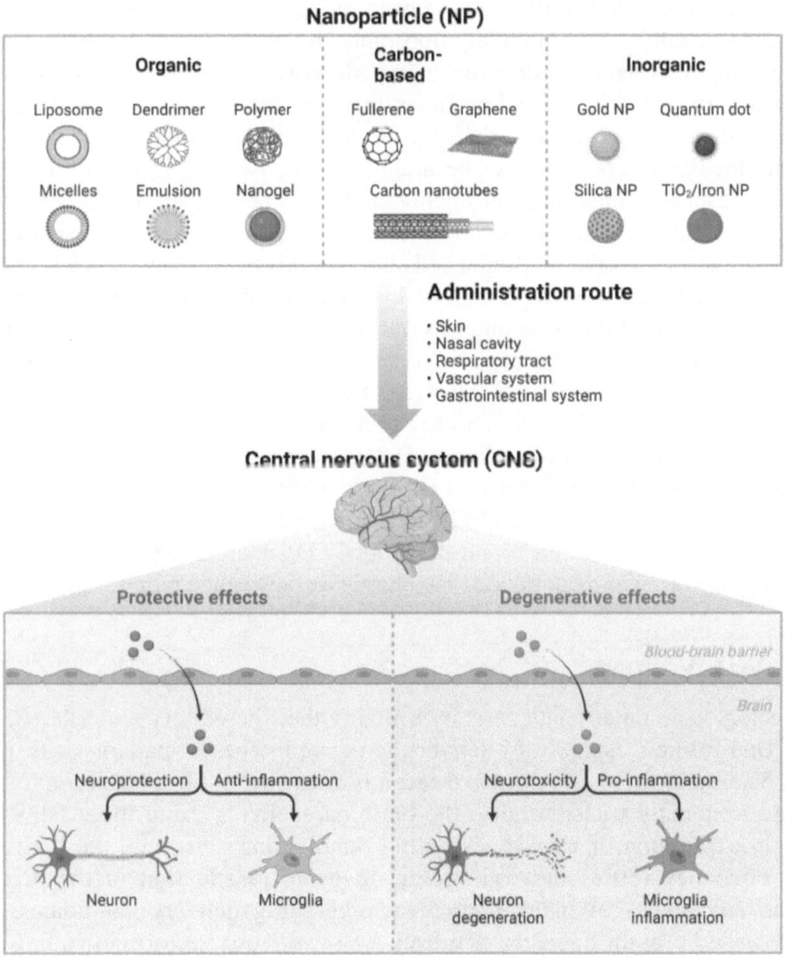

FIGURE 1.3 Illustration of impact of different types of nanoparticles in central nervous system.

trafficking routes are all active obstacles to drug delivery that the body erects. These biological barriers are critical physiological components that protect the body from invading pathogens and preserve homeostasis, but they also provide distinct hurdles to drug carrier entry and navigation to their target region. In this part, we will provide examples of new material designs that enable dynamic bio-interfacing between drug carriers and biological barriers in order to optimize drug delivery outcomes.

1.4.1 Liposomes

Liposomes with gigantic prescription stacking limit are made of no less than one phospholipid two overlay layers. Although it typically has limited freedom time and a low passage rate, joining PEG and concentrating on ligands can overcome these issues. Additionally, PEG-modified liposomes have improved auxiliary stability against the rapid arrival of medication atoms. Moreover, Pardridge and his colleagues developed a series of immune liposomes that counteract agent-joined PEGylated liposomes for receptor-mediated delivery of various therapeutics containing nucleic acids and medication particles to the brain [25–28]. Recently, Feng et al. utilized immune liposomes containing an enemy of EGFR neutralizer to deliver sodium borocaptate for the treatment of boron catch neurons [29]. Numerous boron molecules were specifically delivered to glioma cells through this novel conveyance framework during the *in vitro* and *in vivo* phases. In this step mice treated with the control liposome coming up short on the counter EGFR mAb, the level of BSH was low in both growth and regular tissues. Then, again, in resistant liposome-treated mice, BSH was perceived in the growth and enveloping regions at 24 h a short time after imbuement and remained at a critical level for another 24 h [29]. Some immune system demyelinating diseases, such as multiple sclerosis (MS) and other neurodegenerative diseases, may benefit from the inhibition of reactive oxygen species (ROS). Additionally, Grahn and colleagues used non-PEGylated liposomes to simultaneously exemplify gadodiamide (gadoCED) and topotecan (topoCED), facilitating treatment of glioblastoma multiforme and continuous nanoparticle conveyance monitoring [30].

1.4.2 Viral Vectors

Viral vectors can contaminate cells by utilizing their hereditary material (RNA or DNA). Due to their capacity to deliver the desired genes to patients with neurological disorders, these vectors have recently received a lot of attention. Nucleic acids are frequently transported to the brain parenchyma using these DDSs. The long-term expression of transgenes within nondividing cells, and the high transfection efficiency (80%) of viral vectors in gene transduction in the brain are the main advantages of using them over other drug delivery candidates. Drug delivery into the brain has been achieved by some viral vectors, including lentivirus, herpes simplex virus (HSV), adenovirus (AdV), and adeno-associated virus (AAV). However, in addition to their immunogenicity, these vectors have a number of limitations for drug delivery applications, including high production costs and manufacturing difficulties. Several administration methods, including stereotaxic injection and injection into the CSF, have been developed to circumvent the BBB because viruses cannot passively cross it. In order to move viral vectors from preclinical to clinical studies, more research needs to be done on their application, safety, and immunogenicity. In the study, the conveyance of the glutamic corrosive decarboxylase quality in the AVV2 vector was concentrated on utilizing 42 PD patients. Open-label research was used throughout the study's 12-month duration. A decrease in levodopa-prompted dyskinesias was seen at a year in a gathering infused with the AAV2-glutamic corrosive decarboxylase quality contrasted. As a result, at 12 months, patients who received the AAV2-glutamic acid decarboxylase gene injections showed clinical benefits [31].

1.4.3 Nanoemulsion

Twenty years ago, nanoemulsions with specific droplet sizes of 20–200 nm were developed [32, 33]. They are routinely alluded to as scaled-down submicron, ultrafine or around over the scattered emulsions [34, 35]. Their non-toxic and non-aggravation nature makes them non-toxic in nature [36]. Nanoemulsion oil droplets are either dispersed in an aqueous medium (O/W) or the other way around (W/O) in nanoemulsion [37, 38]. Two significant cycles might be helpful for the development of nanoemulsions, either by high-energy emulsification techniques (for example, high-pressure homogenizers) or low-energy techniques (for example, unconstrained emulsification) [39–41]. The choice of an oil component in a nanoemulsion is crucial for drug delivery to the brain. Various mind take-up examinations have outlined the particular take-up of fundamental polyunsaturated unsaturated fats and omega-6 unsaturated fats, for example, pinolenic and linoleic acids.

1.4.4 Solid Lipid Nanoparticles

These drugs can be liquefied to the core area of solid lipid nanoparticles (SLN), which are a lipid-derived nanocarrier with a solid, hydrophobic lipid shell. They are of a smaller size (40–200 nm), which enables them to leak from the reticulo-endothelial structure and cross the BBB's close-fitting endothelial layer [42]. Bio-constituent lipids like fatty acids, triglycerides, and waxes are used to construct solid lipid nanoparticles [43]. The drug and the liquefied lipid are typically distributed in the aqueous surfactant during manufacturing thanks to the increased gravity of microemulsification. The advantages of SLN are their profile circulation, drugs have higher ensnarement capability connected with other nanoparticles, and they work to give a steady arrival of the medication for a long time [44]. Improved drug delivery to the brain mediated by SLN is the subject of numerous reports. For example, SLN transport of a calcium channel blocker medication, taken intravenously into a rat, showed that the medication was more prominent delivery by the cerebrum and saved high medication stages for an additional time frame related to free medication suspension. According to Wang and colleagues, the preparation of 3,5-dioctanoyl-5-fluoro-2-deoxyuridine (DO-FUdR) was made to lessen the medication's restricted access and SLN entrapment. Researchers hypothesized that SLN could improve the drug's suitability to penetrate through the BBB and is a promising drug targeting system for the neurodegenerative disease [45], and that the results demonstrated that DO-FUdR-SLN had brain targeting efficiency *in vivo* that was approximately two times greater than that of free FUdR [46].

1.4.5 Polymeric Micelles

Poymeric micelles are made up of amphiphilic copolymers with formation in hydrophilic media continuing to shape the spheroidal construction with a hydrophilic shell and hydrophobic environmental factors. [47]. The solidness of polymeric micelles can be overhauled by the technique of cross-linking. Polymeric micelle advancements offer a promising potential to overcome rapid, stimulus-triggered responses, such as temperature, pH, ultrasound, and light. These innovations enable precise control over the release of encapsulated drugs [48]. One of the most commonly employed polymers is a block copolymer, specifically the pluronic type, derived from ethylene and propylene oxide. Pluronic polymers possess the ability to bypass host defenses and often precisely target drug delivery to specific locations [49]. Upon entering the cellular structure, these polymeric micelles disrupt various cellular functions, including mitochondrial respiration, ATP synthesis, genetic regulation, and apoptotic signal transduction. Furthermore, these micelles can influence the BBB, the gastrointestinal tract, and p-glycoprotein in drug-resistant tumors, ultimately enhancing drugs absorption in the intestines and facilitating drug entry into the brain.

The possibilities for distributing drugs to the brain using polymeric nanoparticles have been discussed. For instance, chitosan-involved pluronic nanocarriers with a specific brain target peptide (the glycoprotein of the rabies virus; RVG29) after intravenous injection into mice revealed *in vivo* brain gathering either of a protein conjugated into the nanocarrier or of a quantum dot fluorophore attached to the carrier.

1.4.6 Niosomes

Niosomes are nanoparticles with a double-layer structure made by self-linking non-ionic surfactants and cholesterol in an aqueous layer. By protecting the drug from harsh environmental conditions, it improves the therapeutic performance of implanted drugs [50]. Many chemotherapeutic agents exhibit cytotoxic limitations, often leading to significant adverse effects in normal cells. A significant number of the chemotherapeutic agents exhibit cytotoxic limitations, often leading to significant adverse effects in normal cells. However, it is anticipated that the drug's involvement in a vesicular-like noisome will spread more widely than its occurrence in the systemic pathway, resulting in increased penetration into the main site with less toxicity [51]. The nanocarrier does not just build the flow of the ensnared drug, but it additionally improves its organ appropriation and metabolic movement. For the treatment of glioblastoma, a grade IV astrocytoma, or a hostile brain tumour, temozolomide (TMZ), an oral DNA-alkylating drug, is the best option [52]. In order to selectively deliver the anticancer agent exclusively to glioblastoma cells while avoiding damage to normal brain tissue, researchers have re-evaluated encapsulated drugs within niosomes. These niosomes are equipped with a specific peptide called chlorotoxin

(CTX), composed of 36 amino acids derived from the venom of the scorpion Leiurus quinquestriatus [53]. Chlorotoxin demonstrates a strong affinity for the brain, particularly in the context of gliomas.

1.4.7 Dendrimers

Extensive research has demonstrated that nanomaterials can be successfully used to treat brain diseases. Brain drug delivery can be divided into two categories: bypassing and traversing the BBB. Based on the numerous dendritic polymer architectures and characteristics, drug molecules can be entrapped inside the internal cavities of dendritic polymers or conjugated to the terminal functional groups [54]. Tailoring the peripheral functionalities of dendrimers might be viewed as a cost-effective way to introduce new features. Surface-engineered dendrimers will have improved drug-release kinetics, biocompatibility, and the ability to target the BBB while also accelerating the transport of bioactive substances over the BBB.

Dendrimers have been shown to be effective anti-amyloidogenic agents. As a result, these are effective against the development and progression of Alzheimer's disease. [55]. Donepezil (DZ) conjugation to G4 Poly(amidoamine) (PAMAM) dendrimers nanoparticles for improved brain uptake and *in vitro* acetylcholine esterase (AChE) inhibition activity of DZ (ester)-PAMAM conjugate (PDZ) formulation was significantly higher ($p < 0.05$) than DZ alone at 1 μM dose. This research focuses on medication delivery to the brain utilizing dendrimers and the conjugation technique [10].

1.4.8 Silica Nanoparticles

Inert silica nanoparticles (SiNPs) can be easily loaded with fluorescent probes or surface functionalization [13]. For example, a report suggested that MSNs loaded with neurotrophic factor (brain-derived), were able to persist in the neurons of the ganglia and achieve sustained neurotrophic factor release for 80 days [13, 8]. Furthermore, *in vivo* investigations demonstrated that MSNs can penetrate neurons without causing cytotoxicity in drosophila. MSNs can also traverse the BBB in mice, and their transport efficiency is dependent on size rather than drug loading [13, 8].

MSNs have been shown to have a larger loading capacity, prevent drug concentration change in the blood, and reduce side effects. In theory, when a cap covers MSNs at the molecular level, the capping molecule exhibits the potential to limit drug release [8]. As a result, when exposed to appropriate conditions (enzymatic, variation in pH, light), the conjugate will be liable and released in the sustained manner [8]. Singh et al. (2021) synthesized MCM-41 using the Stöber process, loaded it with berberine, an isoquinoline alkaloid, using the "passive method," and then coated it with liposomes using the thin-film hydration method. The lipid coating on these MSNs was thought to create a physical barrier between the berberine and the physiological buffer, resulting in delayed drug release. The acetylcholinesterase inhibitory activity of synthesized Lipid-coated (L) mesoporous silica nanoparticles (MSNs) containing berberine (BBR) MSNs-BBR-Ldisplayed a significantly higher ($p < 0.05$) acetylcholine esterase (AChE) inhibitory activity in comparision with MCM-41 and pure berberine solutions. The

MSNs-BBR-Ldisplayed lowered malondialdehyde levels, and significant amyloid fibrillation inhibition in AD via down-regulating BACE1 expression [8].

1.4.9 Gold Nanoparticles

For the transport of therapeutic drugs to the CNS, gold nanoparticles have several specific benefits. Smaller nanoparticles (< 10 nm) can successfully penetrate into the brain endothelial cells effectively *in vitro* and *in vivo* via a combination of cytosolic and vesicular transport pathways. The gold core interacts with biological molecules displays nominal interaction, resulting in very low cytotoxicity and immunogenicity. The drug transportation capacity of nanoparticles varies with size, although the smallest can have up to 50% of their molecular mass as cargo molecules or surface-bound ligands. Another study using a mouse brain endothelial cell line showed that 70 nm nanoparticles had the maximal gold uptake, although nanoparticles below (20 nm) had the highest loading capacity [56]. This study emphasizes that the number of cargo molecules that enter the CNS is more crucial than the amount of gold, unless the goal is to use the gold itself for imaging. Most studies to date have examined gold uptake or entry into the CNS rather than the amount of drug/ligand distributed [57].

1.5 CONCLUSIONS AND FUTURE PROSPECTS

In conclusion, recent advancements in brain drug delivery have brought about significant progress in overcoming the challenges associated with targeting the CNS. Non-invasive techniques like focused ultrasound and magnetic nanoparticles have shown promise in breaching the BBB and delivering therapeutic agents directly into the brain. Additionally, nanotechnology-based approaches, such as nanoparticle-mediated drug carriers and implantable devices, offer precise control over drug release and extended therapeutic effects. These advancements hold tremendous potential for revolutionizing the treatment of neurological disorders and optimizing the efficacy of brain-targeted therapies. Another promising avenue is the integration of brain drug delivery with emerging technologies such as gene therapy, stem cell therapy, and optogenetics. By combining these modalities, researchers can explore novel synergistic approaches for precisely modulating brain function and promoting neural repair. Additionally, the integration of artificial intelligence and machine learning algorithms can aid in the optimization of drug delivery strategies by predicting individual responses and tailoring treatments accordingly.

In summary, recent advancements in brain drug delivery have set the stage for transformative breakthroughs in the field of neuroscience. With continued research and innovation, we can envision a future where targeted and personalized therapies for neurological disorders are not only achievable but also revolutionize patient care and improve quality of life.

REFERENCES

1. Thomas M. Barchet and Mansoor M. Amiji. 2009. "Challenges and opportunities in CNS delivery of therapeutics for neurodegenerative diseases." *Expert Opinion on Drug Delivery* 6 (3), 211–225. https://doi.org/10.1517/17425240902758188
2. Mark Habgood and Joakim Ek. 2010 "Delivering drugs into the brain: barriers and possibilities." *Therapeutic Delivery* 1 (4), 483–488. https://doi.org/10.4155/tde.10.58
3. Yiqun Zhou, Zhili Peng, Elif S. Seven, and Roger M. Leblanc. 2018. "Crossing the blood–brain barrier with nanoparticles." *Journal of Controlled Release* 270, 290–303. https://doi.org/10.1016/j.jconrel.2017.12.015
4. Quanguo He, Jun Liu, Jing Liang, Xiaopeng Liu, Wen Li, Zhi Liu, Ziyu Ding, and Du Tuo. 2018. "Towards improvements for penetrating the blood–brain barrier-recent progress from a material and pharmaceutical perspective." *Cells* 7(4), 24. https://doi.org/10.3390/cells7040024
5. Eilam Yeini, Paula Ofek, Nitzan Albeck, Daniel Rodriguez Ajamil, Lena Neufeld, Anat Eldar-Boock, Ron Kleiner, Daniella Vaskovich, Shani Koshrovski-Michael, Sahar Israeli Dangoor, Adva Krivitsky, Christian Burgos Luna, Gal Shenbach-Koltin, Miki Goldenfeld, Ori Hadad, Galia Tiram, and Ronit Satchi-Fainaro. 2021. "Targeting glioblastoma: Advances in drug delivery and novel therapeutic approaches." *Advanced Therapy* 4 (1), 2000124. https://doi.org/10.1002/adtp.202000124
6. Saurabh Bhatia. 2016. "Nanoparticles types, classification, characterization, fabrication methods and drug delivery applications." In: Natural Polymer Drug Delivery Systems. Springer, Cham. 33–93. https://doi.org/10.1007/978-3-319-41129-3_2
7. Abuzer Alp Yetisgin, Sibel Cetinel, Merve Zuvin, Ali Kosar, and Ozlem Kutlu. 2020. "Therapeutic nanoparticles and their targeted delivery applications." *Molecules* 25 (9), 2193. https://doi.org/10.3390/molecules25092193
8. Anurag Kumar Singh, Saumitra Sen Singh, Aaina Singh Rathore, Surya Pratap Singh, Gaurav Mishra, Rajendra Awasthi, Sunil Kumar Mishra, and Santosh Kumar Singh. 2021. "Lipid-coated mcm-41 mesoporous silica nanoparticles loaded with berberine improved inhibition of acetylcholine esterase and amyloid formation." *ACS Biomaterials Science & Engineering* 7 (8), 3737–3753. https://doi.org/10.1021/acsbiomaterials.1c00514
9. Anurag Kumar Singh, Sunil Kumar Mishra, Gaurav Mishra, Anand Maurya, Rajendra Awasthi, Mukesh Kumar Yadav, Neelam Atri, Pawan Kumar Pandey, and Santosh Kumar Singh. 2019. "Inorganic clay nanocomposite system for improved cholinesterase inhibition and brain pharmacokinetics of donepezil." *Drug Development and Industrial Pharmacy* 46 (1), 8–19. https://doi.org/10.1080/03639045.2019.1698594
10. Anurag Kumar Singh, Avinash Gothwal, Sarita Rani, Monika Rana, Anuj Kumar Sharma, Awesh Kumar Yadav, and Umesh Gupta. 2019. "Dendrimer donepezil conjugates for improved brain delivery and better in vivo pharmacokinetics." *ACS Omega* 4 (3), 4519–4529. https://doi.org/10.1021/acsomega.8b03445
11. Anurag Kumar Singh, Sonam Choudhary, Sarita Rani, Ashok Kumar Sharma, Lokesh Gupta, and Umesh Gupta. 2015. "Dendrimer-drug conjugates in drug delivery and targeting." *Pharmaceutical Nanotechnology* 3 (4), 239–260. https://doi.org/10.2174/2211738504666160213000307
12. Anurag Kumar Singh, Ashok Kumar Sharma, Iliyas Khan, Avinash Gothwal, Lokesh Gupta, and Umesh Gupta. 2017. "Oral drug delivery potential of dendrimers." In: *Nanostructures for Oral Medicine. Elsevier,* 231–261. https://doi.org/10.1016/B978-0-323-47720-8.00010-9

13. Mohamed S. Attia, Ahmed Yahya, Nada Abdel Monaem, and Shereen A. Sabry. 2023. "Mesoporous silica nanoparticles: Their potential as drug delivery carriers and nanoscavengers in Alzheimer's and Parkinson's diseases." 31 (3), 417–432. https://doi.org/10.1016/j.jsps.2023.01.009
14. Naoki Toshima and Tetsu Yonezawa. "Bimetallic nanoparticles-novel materials for chemical and physical applications." *New Journal of Chemistry* 22 (11), 1179–1201. https://doi.org/10.1039/A805753B
15. Mayra A. Nascimento, Jean C. Cruz, Guilherme D. Rodrigues, André F. de Oliveira, and Renata P. Lopes. 2018. "Synthesis of polymetallic nanoparticles from spent lithium-ion batteries and application in the removal of reactive blue 4 dye." *Journal of Cleaner Production* 202, 264–272. https://doi.org/10.1016/j.jclepro.2018.08.118
16. S. Anu Mary Ealia and M. P. Saravanakumar. 2017. "A review on the classification, characterisation, synthesis of nanoparticles and their application." In *IOP Conference Series: Materials Science and Engineering* 263 (3), 032019. https://doi.org/10.1088/1757-899X/263/3/032019
17. Nadeem Joudeh and Dirk Linke. 2022. "Nanoparticle classification, physicochemical properties, characterization, and applications: A comprehensive review for biologists." *Journal of Nanobiotechnology* 20 (1), 262. https://doi.org/10.1186/s12951-022-01477-8
18. Muhammad Mansha, Ibrahim Khan, Nisar Ullah, and Ahsanulhaq Qurashi. 2017. "Synthesis, characterization and visible-light-driven photoelectrochemical hydrogen evolution reaction of carbazole-containing conjugated polymers." *International Journal of Hydrogen Energy* 42 (16), 10952–10961. https://doi.org/10.1016/j.ijhydene.2017.02.053
19. Ibrahim Khan, Khalid Saeed, and Idrees Khan. 2017. "Nanoparticles: Properties, applications and toxicities." *Arabian Journal of Chemistry* 12 (7), 908–931. https://doi.org/10.1016/j.arabjc.2017.05.011
20. Noura H. Abd Ellah and Sara A. Abouelmagd. 2017. "Surface functionalization of polymeric nanoparticles for tumor drug delivery: Approaches and challenges." *Expert Opinion on Drug Delivery* 14 (2), 201–214. https://doi.org/10.1080/17425247.2016.1213238
21. Maneesh Gujrati, Anthony Malamas, Tesia Shin, Erlei Jin, Yunlu Sun, and Zheng-Rong Lu. 2014. "Multifunctional cationic lipid-based nanoparticles facilitate endosomal escape and reduction-triggered cytosolic siRNA release." *Molecular Pharmaceutics* 11 (8), 2734–2744. https://doi.org/10.1021/mp400787s
22. Nilesh Rai, Anurag Kumar Singh, Santosh Kumar Singh, Bhaskar Gaurishankar, Swapnil C. Kamble, Pradeep Mishra, Deepak Kotiya, Suvakanta Barik, and Vibhav Gautam. 2020. "Recent technological advancements in stem cell research for targeted therapeutics." *Drug Delivery and Translational Research* 10 (4), 1147–1169. https://doi.org/10.1007/s13346-020-00766-9
23. Anand Maurya, Anurag Kumar Singh, Gaurav Mishra, Komal Kumari, Arati Rai, Bhupesh Sharma, Giriraj T Kulkarni, and Rajendra Awasthi. 2018. "Strategic use of nanotechnology in drug targeting and its consequences on human health: A focused review." *Interventional Medicine and Applied Science* 11 (1), 38–54. https://doi.org/10.1556/1646.11.2019.04
24. Gaurav Mishra, Rajendra Awasthi, Anurag Kumar Singh, Snigdha Singh, Sunil Kumar Mishra, Santosh Kumar Singh, and Manmath K. Nandi. 2022. "Intranasally co-administered berberine and curcumin loaded in transfersomal vesicles improved inhibition of amyloid formation and BACE-1." *ACS Omega* 7 (47), 43290–43305. https://doi.org/10.1021/acsomega.2c06215

25. Yun Zhang and William M. Pardridge. 2001. "Conjugation of brain-derived neurotrophic factor to a blood–brain barrier drug targeting system enables neuroprotection in regional brain ischemia following intravenous injection of the neurotrophin." *Brain Research* 889 (1–2), 49–56. https://doi.org/10.1016/S0006-8993(00)03108-5
26. Hwa Jeong Lee, Britta Engelhardt, Jayne Lesley, Ulrich Bickel, and William M. Pardridge. 2000. "Targeting rat anti-mouse transferrin receptor monoclonal antibodies through blood–brain barrier in mouse." *Journal of Pharmacology and Experimental Therapeutics* 292 (3), 1048–1052.
27. Ruben J. Boado, Yufeng Zhang, Yun Zhang, and William M. Pardridge. 2007 "Humanization of anti-human insulin receptor antibody for drug targeting across the human blood–brain barrier." *Biotechnology and Bioengineering* 96 (2), 381–391. https://doi.org/10.1002/bit.21120
28. Jean-Christophe Olivier, Ramon Huertas, Hwa Jeong Lee, Frederic Calon, and William M. Pardridge. 2002. "Synthesis of pegylated immunonanoparticles." *Pharmaceutical Research* 8, 1137–1143. https://doi.org/10.1023/a:1019842024814
29. Bin Feng, Kazuhito Tomizawa, Hiroyuki Michiue, Shin-ichi Miyatake, Xiao-Jian Han, Atsushi Fujimura, Masaharu Seno, Mitsunori Kirihata, and Hideki Matsui. 2009. "Delivery of sodium borocaptate to glioma cells using immunoliposome conjugated with anti-EGFR antibodies by ZZ-His." *Biomaterials* 30 (9), 1746–1755. https://doi.org/10.1016/j.biomaterials.2008.12.010
30. Amy Y. Grahn, Krystof S. Bankiewicz, Millicent Dugich-Djordjevic, John R. Bringas, Piotr Hadaczek, Greg A. Johnson, Simon Eastman, and Matthias Luz. 2009. "Non-PEGylated liposomes for convection-enhanced delivery of topotecan and gadodiamide in malignant glioma: initial experience." *Journal of Neuro-Oncology* 95, 185–197. https://doi.org/10.1007/s11060-009-9917-1
31. Martin Niethammer, Chris C. Tang, Peter A. LeWitt, Ali R. Rezai, Maureen A. Leehey, Steven G. Ojemann, Alice W. Flaherty, Emad N. Eskandar, Sandra K. Kostyk, Atom Sarkar, Mustafa S. Siddiqui, Stephen B. Tatter, Jason M. Schwalb, Kathleen L. Poston Jaimie M. Henderson, Roger M. Kurlan, Irene H. Richard, Christine V. Sapan, David Eidelberg, Matthew J. During, Michael G. Kaplitt, and Andrew Feigin. 2017. "Long-term follow-up of a randomized AAV2-GAD gene therapy trial for Parkinson's disease." *JCI Insight* 2 (7), e90133. https://doi.org/10.1172/jci.insight.90133
32. T. G. Mason, S. M. Graves, J. N. Wilking, and M. Y. Lin. 2006. "Extreme emulsification: Formation and structure of nanoemulsions." *Condensed Matter Physics 9*. 1(45), 193–199.
33. J. M. Gutiérrez, C. González, A. Maestro, I. Solè, C. M. Pey, and J. Nolla. 2008 "Nano-emulsions: New applications and optimization of their preparation." *Current Opinion in Colloid & Interface Science* 13 (4), 245–251. https://doi.org/10.1016/j.cocis.2008.01.005
34. Maytal Bivas-Benita, Marion Oudshoorn, Stefan Romeijn, Krista van Meijgaarden, Henk Koerten, Hans van der Meulen, Gregory Lambert, Tom Ottenhoff, Simon Benita, Hans Junginger, and Gerrit Borchard. 2004. "Cationic submicron emulsions for pulmonary DNA immunization." *Journal of Controlled Release* 100 (1), 145–155. https://doi.org/10.1016/j.jconrel.2004.08.008.100, 145-155
35. Hideo Nakajima. 1997. "Microemulsions in cosmetics." *Surfactant Science Series* 66, 175–197.
36. Reza Aboofazeli. 2010. "Nanometric-scaled emulsions (nanoemulsions)." *Iranian Journal of Pharmaceutical Research: IJPR* 9 (4), 325.
37. M. Wulff-Pérez, A. Torcello-Gómez, M. J. Gálvez-Ruíz, and A. Martín-Rodríguez. 2009. "Stability of emulsions for parenteral feeding: Preparation and characterization of o/w

nanoemulsions with natural oils and pluronic f68 as surfactant." *Food Hydrocolloids* 23 (4), 1096–1102. https://doi.org/10.1016/j.foodhyd.2008.09.017

38. Faiyaz Shakeel and Wafa Ramadan. 2010. "Transdermal delivery of anticancer drug caffeine from water-in-oil nanoemulsions." *Colloids and Surfaces B: Biointerfaces* 75 (1), 356–362. https://doi.org/10.1016/j.colsurfb.2009.09.010
39. Kawthar Bouchemal, S. Briançon, E. Perrier, and H. Fessi. 2004. "Nano-emulsion formulation using spontaneous emulsification: Solvent, oil and surfactant optimisation." *International Journal of Pharmaceutics* 280 (1–2), 241–251. https://doi.org/10.1016/j.ijpharm.2004.05.016
40. Nicolas Anton, Pascal Gayet, Jean-Pierre Benoit, and Patrick Saulnier. 2007. "Nano-emulsions and nanocapsules by the PIT method: An investigation on the role of the temperature cycling on the emulsion phase inversion." *International Journal of Pharmaceutics* 344 (1–2), 44–52. https://doi.org/10.1016/j.ijpharm.2007.04.027
41. Ngoc Trinh Huynh, C. Passirani, Patrick Saulnier, and Jean-Pierre Benoît. 2009. "Lipid nanocapsules: A new platform for nanomedicine." *International Journal of Pharmaceutics* 379 (2), 201–209. https://doi.org/10.1016/j.ijpharm.2009.04.026
42. Indu Pal Kaur, Rohit Bhandari, Swati Bhandari, and Vandita Kakkar. 2008. "Potential of solid lipid nanoparticles in brain targeting." *Journal of Controlled Release* 127 (2), 97–109. https://doi.org/10.1016/j.jconrel.2007.12.018
43. Chandrakantsing Pardeshi, Pravin Rajput, Veena Belgamwar, Avinash Tekade, Ganesh Patil, Kapil Chaudhary, and Abhijeet Sonje. 2012 "Solid lipid based nanocarriers: An overview/Nanonosači na bazi čvrstih lipida: Pregled." *Acta Pharmaceutica* 62 (4), 433–472.
44. B. Mishra, Bhavesh B. Patel, and Sanjay Tiwari. 2010. "Colloidal nanocarriers: A review on formulation technology, types and applications toward targeted drug delivery." *Nanomedicine: Nanotechnology, Biology and Medicine* 6 (1), 9–24. https://doi.org/10.1016/j.nano.2009.04.008
45. Jian-Xin Wang, Xun Sun, and Zhi-Rong Zhang. 2002. "Enhanced brain targeting by synthesis of 3′, 5′-dioctanoyl-5-fluoro-2′-deoxyuridine and incorporation into solid lipid nanoparticles." *European Journal of Pharmaceutics and Biopharmaceutics* 54 (3), 285–290. https://doi.org/10.1016/s0939-6411(02)00083-8
46. Susana Martins, Ingunn Tho, Isolde Reimold, Gert Fricker, Eliana Souto, Domingos Ferreira, and Martin Brandl. 2012 "Brain delivery of camptothecin by means of solid lipid nanoparticles: Formulation design, in vitro and in vivo studies." *International Journal of Pharmaceutics* 439 (1–2), 49–62. https://doi.org/ 10.1016/j.ijpharm.2012.09.054
47. Alexander V. Kabanov, Elena V. Batrakova, Nikolai S. Melik-Nubarov, Nikolai A. Fedoseev, Tatiyana Yu. Dorodnich, Valery Yu. Alakhov, Vladimir P. Chekhonin, Irina R. Nazarova, and Victor A. Kabanov. 1992. "A new class of drug carriers: Micelles of poly(oxyethylene)-poly(oxypropylene) block copolymers as microcontainers for drug targeting from blood in brain." *Journal of Controlled Release* 22 (2), 141–157. https://doi.org/10.1016/0168-3659(92)90199-2
48. Glen S. Kwon. 2003. "Polymeric micelles for delivery of poorly water-soluble compounds." *Critical Reviews™ in Therapeutic Drug Carrier Systems* 20 (5). https://doi.org/10.1615/CritRevTherDrugCarrierSyst.v20.i5.20
49. Ja-Young Kim, Won Il Choi, Young Ha Kim, and Giyoong Tae. 2013. "Brain-targeted delivery of protein using chitosan- and RVG peptide-conjugated, pluronic-based nano-carrier." *Biomaterials* 34 (4), 1170–1178. https://doi.org/10.1016/j.biomaterials.2012.09.047

50. A. J. Baillie, A. T. Florence, L. R. Hume, G. T. Muirhead, and A. Rogerson. 1985. "The preparation and properties of niosomes-non-ionic surfactant vesicles." *Journal of Pharmacy and Pharmacology* 37 (12), 863–868. https://doi.org/10.1111/j.2042-7158.1985.tb04990.x
51. P. Workman, E. O. Aboagye, F. Balkwill, A. Balmain, G. Bruder, D. J. Chaplin, J. A. Double, J. Everitt, D. A. H. Farningham, M. J. Glennie, L. R. Kelland, V. Robinson, I. J. Stratford, G. M. Tozer, S. Watson, S. R. Wedge, S. A. Eccles, and an ad hoc committee of the National Cancer Research Institute. 2010. "Guidelines for the welfare and use of animals in cancer research." *British Journal of Cancer* 102 (11), 1555–1577. https://doi.org/10.1038/sj.bjc.6605642
52. H. S. Friedman, T. Kerby, and H. Calvert. 2000. "Temozolomide and treatment of malignant glioma." *Clinical Cancer Research* 6 (7), 2585–2597.
53. Adam N. Mamelak and Douglas B. Jacoby. 2007. "Targeted delivery of antitumoral therapy to glioma and other malignancies with synthetic chlorotoxin (TM-601)." *Expert Opinion on Drug Delivery* 4 (2), 175–186. https://doi.org/10.1517/17425247.4.2.175
54. Yuefei Zhu, Chunying Liu, and Zhiqing Pang. 2019. "Dendrimer-based drug delivery systems for brain targeting." *Biomolecules* 9 (12), 790. https://doi.org/10.3390/biom9120790
55. Forum Palan and Bappaditya Chatterjee. 2022. "Dendrimers in the context of targeting central nervous system disorders." *Journal of Drug Delivery Science and Technology* 73, 103474. https://doi.org/10.1016/j.jddst.2022.103474
56. Malka Shilo, Anat Sharon, Koby Baranes, Menachem Motiei, Jean-Paul M. Lellouche, and Rachela Popovtzer. 2015. "The effect of nanoparticle size on the probability to cross the blood–brain barrier: An in-vitro endothelial cell model." *Journal of Nanobiotechnology* 13 (1), 1–7. https://doi.org/10.1186/s12951-015-0075-7
57. D. Male, R. Gromnicova, and C. McQuaid. 2016. "Gold nanoparticles for imaging and drug transport to the CNS." *International Review of Neurobiology* 130, 155–198. https://doi.org/10.1016/bs.irn.2016.05.003

2 Brain Diseases

An Introduction and the Need for Novel Drug-Delivery Approaches

Sukamto S. Mamada, Mirnawati Salampe, Rohit Sharma, Achmad Himawan, and Firzan Nainu

2.1 INTRODUCTION

The brain has a vital function in coordinating numerous bodily processes through a complex network of billions of neurons, glial cells, and other supporting cells. Therefore, it is crucial to shield this organ from factors that may compromise its functions by disrupting its homeostatic balance.

The blood–brain barrier (BBB) is the interface where systemic circulation and brain tissue intersect, serving as the protector of central nervous system (CNS) homeostasis. The BBB functions to prevent harmful molecules from entering the CNS while permitting the selective transport of nutrients and ions necessary for the proper functioning of the brain. Knowing the structure and function of the BBB is crucial to delivering medication to the brain at the right pharmacological level without disrupting the barrier's natural functions.

It is noteworthy that there are several barriers responsible for limiting the brain environment and the periphery. In addition to the BBB, the other barriers are the arachnoid barrier, the blood-cerebrospinal fluid barrier, the circumventricular organs barrier, and the glia barrier [1]. Due to space limitations, the following section will only focus on the BBB as this barrier is the most challenging barrier faced by drugs to penetrate the brain. However, anatomical, physiological, and molecular understandings of the other barriers are important as this might provide new insights into the efforts for developing the drug delivery system in the brain.

2.2 THE BLOOD–BRAIN BARRIER

The BBB (Figure 2.1) is formed by microvessels in the brain's capillaries, which comprise a layer of endothelial cells, basement membrane, pericytes, and astrocyte end-foot processes. The combination of these cells forms a structure known as the neurovascular unit.

DOI: 10.1201/9781032661964-2

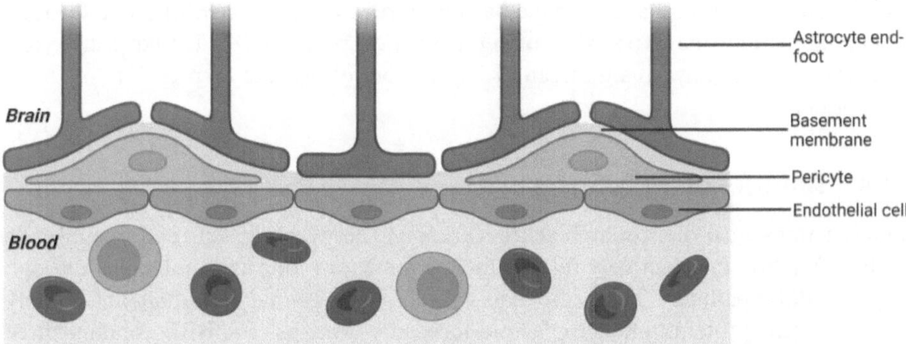

FIGURE 2.1 The structure of the blood–brain barrier (created with BioRender.com).

2.2.1 Brain Microvascular Endothelial Cells

The microvasculature spaces are lined by endothelial cells, which form a physical barrier between the blood and tissues. Brain microvascular endothelial cells (BMECs) differ morphologically from peripheral endothelial cells in several ways, including being 39% thinner [2].

Adjacent BMECs are connected by tight junctions that carefully regulate the movement of molecules and ions through the paracellular pathway, by high levels of ABC efflux transporters that regulate the movement of compounds through the transcellular pathway, by a lack of fenestrations and pinocytotic vesicles, and by more mitochondria than peripheral endothelial cells [2–5]. These unique properties work in tandem to protect the brain from harmful compounds while allowing nutrients and ions to enter the brain.

2.2.2 Astrocytes

Astrocytes, which are glial cells in the CNS with a star-like shape, create a complex network through their end feet that surround and connect endothelial cells, microglia, and neurons. This intricate network is essential for maintaining the correct characteristics and functions of the BBB. Research has demonstrated that astrocytes are essential for preserving the BBB's integrity, as seen in studies where brain endothelial cells cultured with astrocytes exhibit greater resistance to various pathogenic conditions. Astrocytes facilitate the maintenance of the BBB's selective permeability by promoting the expression of tight junction proteins and impeding the development of pericytes. Additionally, astrocytes safeguard the BBB from oxidative stress. Besides their role in developing the BBB, astrocytes also participate in scaffolding, protecting against damage, maintaining homeostasis, and clearing synapses [6, 7].

2.2.3 Pericytes

Pericytes are cells that are connected to the basement membrane and work together with endothelial cells and astrocytes. They play a key role in maintaining the integrity of the neurovascular unit and help the barrier by regulating the flow of blood through the capillaries and the expression of tight junction proteins [8]. Unlike astrocytes, pericytes do not play a significant role in controlling the expression of ABC transporters [9].

2.2.4 Tight Junction Proteins

Tight junctions are protein complexes that are found between adjacent endothelial cells and that function to selectively restrict the movement of ions and molecules through the paracellular pathway. The complexes consist of two primary components, namely transmembrane proteins and cytoplasmic accessory proteins. The BBB contains three key transmembrane proteins known as tight junction-associated MARVEL proteins (occludin, tricellulin, and MARVELD3), claudins, and junctional adhesion molecules (JAMs) [10].

Occludin is a 65 kDa phosphoprotein that was the first transmembrane protein identified [11] as tight junction and is expressed in various tissues, including the BBB, where it plays a critical role in its function [12]. Hirase and co-workers demonstrated that occludin was expressed more highly in brain endothelial cells than those in non-neural tissue [13].

Claudin-5 is one of the 26 members (claudin 1–26) of the claudin family [10], expressed ubiquitously in brain microvascular endothelial cells [14]. Proteins listed as a member of the claudins family share several characteristics including having molecular mass ranging from 20 to 24 kDa and possessing four transmembrane domains [15].

The JAM family of proteins consists of JAM-1 (JAM-A), JAM-2 (JAM-B), JAM-3 (JAM-C), and the recently identified JAM-4, all of which belong to the immunoglobulin superfamily and have a single transmembrane domain. JAM-A is the most expressed JAM in brain endothelial cells [16].

The cytoplasmic accessory proteins associated with transmembrane proteins allow the junction to seal by binding to the actin-based cytoskeleton. *Zonula occludens* (ZO; ZO-1, ZO-2, ZO-3) are the primary accessory proteins that have been identified to date [15]. While ZO-1 and ZO-2 are expressed in brain endothelial cells, ZO-3 is not expressed in these cells [17]. ZO-1 directly binds to claudins, occludin, and junctional adhesion molecules (JAMs) through its three domains, namely PDZ domains (consisting of PDZ1, PDZ2, and PDZ3), one SH3 domain, and a guanylyl-kinase (GK) domain [15]. The PDZ1 domain links claudins to ZO-1, the PDZ3 domain links JAMs and occludin to ZO-1, and the GK domain links occludin to ZO-1 [18].

Various approaches have been studied to transiently open the tight junction proteins, targeting either transmembrane proteins or cytoplasmic accessory proteins or both. By opening this junction, the transport of substances through the paracellular gap can be enhanced. However, this action has a risk in terms of the penetration of harmful substances into the gap and their eventually reaching the brain.

2.2.5 ABC Transporters

Efflux transporters, known as ATP-binding cassette (ABC) transporters, use energy from ATP hydrolysis to transport substances against the concentration gradient [19]. This class of transporters is essential because they limit the penetration of harmful xenobiotics and pollutants into the brain, and can also affect the delivery of therapeutic drugs across the BBB.

Humans have 48 genes that encode ABC transporters, divided into seven subfamilies labelled from ABCA to ABCG [20]. While members of the ABCA, ABCB, ABCC, ABCD, and ABCG subfamilies consist of two functional domains, namely transmembrane domains (TMDs) containing the substrate-binding site and cytoplasmic nucleotide-binding domains (NBDs) involved in ATP hydrolysis, members of the ABCE and ABCF subfamilies only have NBD [20].

The luminal membrane of human BBB capillary endothelial cells primarily expresses major ABC transporters, including ABCB1, ABCC5, and ABCG2 [21]. According to studies, the expression of ABCB1 and ABCG2 is more than 20 times greater in microvessels compared to the brain cortex (Figure 2.2) [22].

Several compounds have been used for inhibiting the activity of ABC transporters. For example, elacridar is an inhibitor of ABCB1. The use of this drug can inhibit the functional activity of ABCB1, leading to the enhanced entry of a drug that is also an ABCB1 substrate [23]. A study reported that the level of paclitaxel in the CNS increased five-fold when elacridar was also given [24]. This is a promising approach because the expression of ABC transporters in brain cancer is relatively overexpressed [25]. It is hypothesized that inhibition of ABC transporters could open a pathway for chemotherapy drugs to achieve effective concentration in the cancerous environment.

2.3 VARIABLES IMPACTING DELIVERY TO THE BRAIN

Some variables play essential roles in determining the transport of drugs into the brain and consequently affect the concentration of the drugs within the brain. These factors can be divided into two main aspects, that is, physico-chemical properties of the drugs and properties associated with the host's biology and physiology (Table 2.1) [7].

This section will not discuss further the details of each factor. Instead, we will focus on the pathological conditions affecting the integrity of the BBB. It is noteworthy that conditions can start from inside the brain, such as neurodegenerative diseases, or from outside the brain, for example, a systemic bacterial infection. Discussion of these issues is provided in the next section.

2.4 DISRUPTION OF THE BLOOD–BRAIN BARRIER IN CERTAIN PATHOLOGICAL CONDITIONS

2.4.1 Neurodegenerative Diseases

Various neurodegenerative diseases have different pathological mechanisms, but they all involve the formation of insoluble aggregates from the build-up of specific

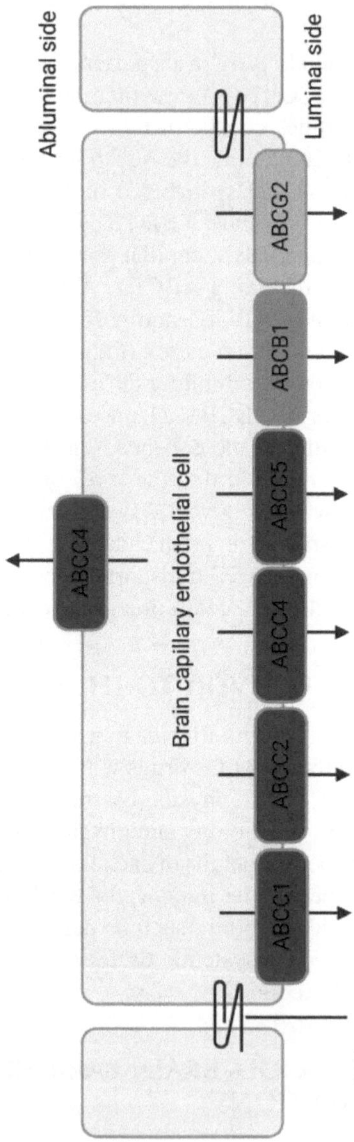

FIGURE 2.2 Distribution of the ATP-binding cassette efflux transporters in capillary endothelial cells of the blood–brain barrier.

TABLE 2.1
Variables That Are Responsible for Determining Levels of Drug Delivery and Distribution in the Brain

Physicochemical properties of drugs	Biological and physiological aspects
Partition coefficient	The states of pathological conditions in the BBB
The substrate of ABC transporters (e.g., ABCB1 and ABCG2)	Blood flow in the brain
Acid dissociation constant (pKa)	Presence and functionality of efflux transporters (e.g., ABC transporters)
Hydrogen bonding	Presence and functionality of influx transporters (e.g., SLC transporters)
Size of drug molecules	Presence and distribution of receptors and enzymes
The polarity of the surface area	pH status in blood and tissue
The affinity of the drug to the receptor	Volumes of intra- and extra-cellular fluid
Bound vs. unbound drugs	Homeostatic regulation

TABLE 2.2
Several Neurodegenerative Diseases and Their Related Pathogenic Proteins Accumulation

Neurodegenerative diseases	Protein deposition
Alzheimer's disease (AD)	Amyloid beta, tau
Parkinson's disease (PD)	α-synuclein
Huntington's disease (HD)	Huntingtin
Amyotrophic lateral sclerosis (ALS)	TDP-43, SOD1

proteins in the CNS (Table 2.2) [26, 27]. Two main factors contribute to the accumulation of pathologic proteins: excessive production of the proteins and impairment of the clearance mechanism. These factors can work independently or together. Interestingly, there is mounting evidence that abnormal proteins can be transmitted between cells through pathways that are currently under intensive investigation.

The accumulation of pathogenic proteins in the CNS usually affects neurons first. Neurons are particularly vulnerable to damage because of their long axons, postmitotic nature, poor regeneration capacity, and complex synaptic connections [27]. When neurons are damaged, it can lead to problems with the connections between glial cells and synapses, affecting physiological processes [28]. Although it is well established that neurons are affected by the accumulation of proteins, recent evidence suggests that glial cells, such as astrocytes and oligodendrocytes, may also be affected [29].

This paragraph discusses the alterations that can occur in the BBB during BBB breakdown. The functional constituents of the BBB can break down naturally with aging, even if no underlying conditions are causing declining cognition and dementia. [30]. However, when healthy aging is combined with a secondary factor like inflammation, the disruption that occurs can become more damaging [31]. This natural disturbance is influenced by multiple factors, such as an imbalance in the level of antioxidants and oxidants, epigenetic modifications, disruption in the genome stability, malfunction of the telomere, and abnormal regulation of inflammatory cascades and cellular signaling [32]. Deterioration of the BBB typically relates to the disruption of endothelial cells, down-regulated expression of tight junction proteins, and imbalanced molecular transport. Furthermore, BBB breakdown may also be attributed to the detachment of astrocytic end feet from the vascular basement membrane, pericyte degeneration, and disruptions to the basement membrane [33–35].

The BBB can become more permeable under pathological conditions due to increased expression of leukocyte adhesion molecules, resulting in increased movement and migration of leukocytes into the brain [36, 37]. This interaction can release various mediators of barrier disruption, such as reactive oxygen species and cytokines, leading to further BBB permeability [38]. On the other hand, this barrier can also be restored endogenously, but the mechanisms involved in regulating BBB repair are not well understood. It has also been shown that astrocytes and microglia contribute to the restoration of the BBB following injury, and microglia are especially crucial for preserving the integrity of the BBB [38]. Microglia can collaborate with brain endothelial cells where their contribution to BBB modulation can vary depending on the type of insult [39]. In response to stroke, microglia initially contribute to BBB disruption by secreting several molecules, especially proinflammatory cytokines. It has been demonstrated that these secreted cytokines play a pivotal function in repairing the disrupted BBB in the later stage [39]. However, in the case of a sustained condition of inflammation, astrocytes can be phagocytosed by microglia leading to BBB disruption [40].

Inflammation causes various changes in the functioning and physiology of BBB, such as the activation of glial cells, recruitment of leukocytes, and disruption of BBB leading to changes in tight junction protein expression and paracellular and transcellular transport [41]. To study the effect of inflammation on BBB, the model can be treated with lipopolysaccharide (LPS). It has been demonstrated that this treatment leads to the activation of the immune system and induction of proinflammatory cytokines release [42, 43]. Further, LPS has also been shown to reduce trans-endothelial electrical resistance (TEER) and increase permeability, disrupting tight junction proteins both in their expression and distribution [44, 45]. BBB disruption caused by inflammation also results in features, for example, apoptotic events on endothelial cells, damage of mitochondria, and disruption of membrane function [44, 46].

Oxidative stress marked by an imbalance condition between oxidants and antioxidant defense can also lead to the disruption of the BBB [47]. The excessive level of oxidants, for example, nitric oxide, hydrogen peroxide, and hydroxyl radicals, has been known to have noxious effects on the BBB. It is noteworthy that the brain is highly susceptible to oxidative stress, and the endothelial cells are the most vulnerable sites. Several mechanisms have been proposed to explain the way by which oxidative stress disrupts the BBB, that is, disruption of cellular organelles, activation of matrix metalloproteinases, cytoskeleton reorganization, tight junction protein modulation, and upregulation of inflammatory mediators [33, 47, 48]. Ultimately, these events disturb the structural integrity of the cells, leading to the interference of some crucial cellular processes, for example, cellular traffic, ATP production, and ionic equilibrium. Several signaling pathways (RhoA, PI3, and PKB/Akt) that are crucially involved in the maintenance, regulation, and distribution of actin cytoskeleton and junctional proteins (e.g., occludin, claudin-5, *zonula occludens*) are also attacked by the radical oxygen species, leading to altered BBB permeability [49].

The breakdown of the BBB is a distinctive feature linked to various disorders, including neurodegenerative illnesses, and it is commonly found in higher levels of disease than in normal aging. Numerous studies have explored the phenomenon of BBB breakdown in a range of conditions, including Alzheimer's disease, Parkinson's disease, amyotrophic lateral sclerosis, multiple sclerosis, and Huntington's disease. The precise cause and pathology of many of these diseases remain unclear, resulting in difficulty in determining whether BBB dysfunction acts as an initial pathogenic cause, an effect, or a combinative event. Research indicates that the excessive level of the pathogenic proteins in the brains of deceased Alzheimer's disease patients could be associated with a reduced expression of junctional proteins leading to increased BBB permeability [50, 51]. Another study indicates that alterations in BBB integrity are the result of changes in functional activity and the expression of BBB transporters and receptors, such as GLUT1 and ABCB1 [41]. Disintegrated BBB breakdown is also characterized by the dysfunctionality of both endothelial cells and pericytes [51].

2.4.2 Brain Tumor

Typically, the BBB controls the flow of materials between the brain and the bloodstream, maintaining a balance in the CNS. Despite being slightly more permeable around tumor microvessels, the BBB does not permit adequate amounts of drugs or therapeutic agents to enter the innermost part of the tumor tissues. The BBB is a complicated and detailed structure with the primary location being the continuous endothelial cells linked by tight junctions. These cells are mostly covered by astrocytic end feet and pericytes are associated with them [52].

In the early stages of glioma development, the tumor cells mimic the BBB, which is responsible for regulating the passage of materials between the blood and the brain to maintain CNS homeostasis. However, as the gliomas grow and achieve a specified level, the BBB is disrupted and substituted by a new barrier called the blood–brain tumor barrier (BBTB), formed by the newly created blood vessels within the capillaries of the brain tumor. This barrier is distinct from the BBB. While glioblastomas have great permeability in tumor zones, the BBB and BBTB combination presents a significant challenge for drug delivery to brain tumors, especially in peripheral regions where permeability is low or non-existent. Strategies such as opening tight junctions with hyperosmotic solutions, inhibiting efflux transporters, and using receptor-mediated delivery strategies can improve drug delivery to brain tumors selectively. Additionally, nanoparticles with cell-permeable peptides on their surface can be used to target glioma cells. Despite the heterogeneous permeability of the blood-tumor barrier (BTB) to various molecules, this barrier is still the primary factor that restricts the effective treatment of brain tumors, as it does not allow the accumulation of high drug concentrations from the surrounding area within the tumor tissue due to its limited permeability. [52–54].

2.4.3 Infection

As described in the previous section, inflammation is one of the key factors responsible for disrupting the integrity of the BBB. Overactivation of the immune system as a response to an infection followed by excessive release of pro-inflammatory cytokines is strongly associated with BBB damage.

Any infection that occurs within the body will turn the immune system on as this can develop a defense mechanism system. One of the components of the bacteria that has been known as the activator of the immune system is lipopolysaccharide (LPS). This component is mainly found in the cell wall of gram-negative bacteria.

As mentioned in the earlier section, LPS can have a seriously harmful impact on the integrity of the BBB. This impact of LPS can be generated by both direct and indirect mechanisms. While the former mechanism involves the effects of LPS directly on the systems expressed in the layer of microvessel (e.g., junctional proteins and paracellular pathways, endothelial cells, and transcellular transport systems) and its accessories, the latter is linked to the action of LPS on the supporting cells of the BBB, such as microglia, astrocytes, and pericytes [45].

It has been reported in several studies that LPS increases the permeability of the BBB by damaging the functionality of junctional proteins (i.e., tight junction and adherens junction) [55–57]. LPS not only disturbs the activity of junctional proteins but also lowers the expression and changes the distribution of the proteins [56]. Consequently, noxious compounds can easily find entry into the brain via the paracellular pathway of the damaged BBB.

LPS also disturbs transcellular transport mechanisms, such as diffusion, transport assisted by carriers, and transcytosis. For example, as mentioned earlier, ABC transporters are essential for maintaining the homeostasis of the brain. They play a major role, especially in pumping harmful compounds out of the cells. It has been reported that LPS can impair the activity of ABC transporters, leading to the accumulation of toxic compounds in the brain [44, 58]. This action eventually weakens the permeability of the BBB.

Infection also influences the functionality of endothelial cells. Several studies have confirmed that LPS can induce apoptosis and reduce the proliferation of endothelial cells. LPS's harmful effect is also linked to its ability to disturb the physiological functions of mitochondria. Damage in mitochondria leads to bioenergetic abnormality and eventually disturbs all processes in the endothelial cells, including proliferation [59]. In addition, LPS exposure can result in disturbances in regulating processes of inflammation and oxidative stress leading to increased permeability of the BBB [45].

As many components of the BBB are attached to the basement membrane, any damage or disruption of this matrix will lead to BBB impairment. Several studies reported that LPS treatment increases the expression of matrix metalloproteinases (MMPs) acting as degrading enzymes for the basement membrane matrix, resulting in the destruction of BBB [60, 61]. One example showed that LPS treatment in the tested animal increases the level of MMP-2 and MMP-9, causing increased BBB permeability [62].

An infection can also attack BBB via indirect mechanisms by disturbing the functions of astrocytes, pericytes, microglia, and other BBB-supporting cells. Several mechanisms have been proposed to explain the role of those cells in impairing BBB physiological functions. However, of those putative mechanisms, inflammation-related BBB disruptions mediated by the action of those cells have attracted more interest. For example, upon exposing LPS to the model used in the study, it was found that astrocytes are activated followed by the activation of microglia as a response to cytokines released from the astrocytes [63, 64]. Another study reported that LPS exposure can induce the release of proinflammatory cytokines from the activated pericytes [65]. An excessive level of these cytokines leads to a harmful effect on BBB functionality.

2.5 CURRENT STRATEGIES FOR BRAIN DRUG DELIVERY

2.5.1 Transport of Substances across the Blood–Brain Barrier

The transportation of substances across the BBB and the BCSF is a complicated and discriminating activity that occurs through various mechanisms, as explained in the following sections.

2.5.1.1 Simple and Facilitated Diffusion

Paracellular diffusion is a process by which molecules pass through the space between two adjoining endothelial cells. This form of nonspecific transport is facilitated by a negative concentration gradient from the bloodstream to the brain and can only facilitate small, water-soluble molecules that weigh up to 500 Da [7]. In the context of drug delivery, a modification in the tight junctions can be utilized to enhance the paracellular diffusion of a certain molecule or drug.

On the other hand, transcellular diffusion involves the transfer of particles (e.g., alcohol and steroid hormones) through an endothelium. This pathway is merely suitable for small molecules having optimal lipophilicity and that are not ionized to pass through and achieve the BBB [66]. Similar to paracellular diffusion, a negative concentration gradient drives transcellular diffusion. Highly lipophilic molecules with a hydrogen bonding capacity of less than eight to ten bonds and a molecular weight of less than 400–500 Da could easily go across the BBB via this pathway [66, 67]. The characteristics of a substance are significant in the delivery process to target the CNS, and the gas molecules have been demonstrated to diffuse across the BBB following the concentration gradients [67].

2.5.1.2 Carrier-Mediated Transport

The BBB utilizes solute carrier (SLC) transporters, for example, SLC2, SLC7, and SLC16, to actively transport low-molecular-weight drugs, amino acids, ions, neuropeptides, and endogenous biomolecules like vitamins and carbohydrates across the barrier [68]. The technique works by altering the conformation of the transporters following their interaction with glucose or amino acids, allowing them to pass through the BBB. However, this technique has limitations as some transporters are only capable of transporting specific molecules to cross the BBB, thereby reducing its utility in drug administration [7].

The existence of efflux pumps on the apical part of the BBB adds another layer of complexity to the drug delivery process through the BBB [7]. Examples of efflux pumps include ABCB1 and ABCG2. These efflux pumps act in concert to avoid the accumulation of various lipophilic molecules and noxious compounds in the brain. Additionally, these pumps impede drugs from moving into the endothelial cells in the initial stage and expel a number of anti-cancer drugs such as daunorubicin, vinblastine, and doxorubicin from the brain in the later stage. [69]. Therefore, these efflux pumps play a double-edged-sword role in the BBB. On one edge, the pumps have the potential to decrease the neurotoxic side effects of medications, while on the other edge, limiting the delivery of effective therapies given to patients suffering from pathogenic conditions in the CNS, for example, neurodegenerative diseases. Consequently, adjusting efflux pumps has the potential to be a beneficial approach in improving the availability of therapeutics to the brain, creating new possibilities for treating brain-related disorders [7].

2.5.1.3 Receptor-Mediated Transport

This transcytosis utilizes receptors found in the luminal areas of the endothelial cells of the BBB. This mechanism allows the delivery of several molecules, particularly those having high molecular weight. Also, nanoparticles can be transported through this mechanism. This process employs endocytosis involving the ligand binding to the receptor, which in turn creates an intracellular vesicle via the invagination of the membrane. Several receptors are commonly targeted to mediate the transport, for example, receptors of lactoferrin, insulin, transferrin, and others [7].

Furthermore, the clathrin or caveolae-mediated mechanisms cause membrane invagination in receptor-mediated transport (RMT). Mechanistically, there is a different process of vesicle formation between these two mechanisms. While the former mechanism involves the formation of a clathrin-coated pit in the cytoplasmic areas of the endothelia, the latter mechanism, the caveolae-mediated RMT, involves caveolae that create lipid rafts leading to the formation of endocytic vesicles [70]. Following this formation, the vesicles are then released and distributed to various sites, where they release their contents or are degraded through the process of maturation involving the endosome-lysosome [71, 72].

2.5.1.4 Adsorptive-Mediated Transcytosis

The method of adsorptive-mediated transcytosis (AMT) facilitates the transportation of a number of molecules with specific characteristics, such as macromolecules and charged nanoparticles, to penetrate the BBB using electrostatic interactions [73, 74]. Mechanistically, the transport occurs because of the interaction between drug carriers and several membrane domains on the endothelial cells (e.g., cytoplasmic membrane and basement membrane) having positive and negative charges, respectively. AMT does not require specialized surface receptors, so a large number of molecules can attach to the surface of the cell surface with a weak affinity. However, this method requires that drugs or their carriers undergo cationic changes, which can influence the effectiveness of the given drugs. Additionally, the non-specificity of the AMT drug delivery mechanism may lead to drug accumulation in some other tissues or organs, as noted in the related references [7, 73].

2.5.1.5 Cell-Mediated Transport

The transportation of drugs or drug-loaded nanocarriers across the BBB can be achieved through the utilization of the host's cells such as lymphocytes and monocytes [75]. These cells are attracted to sites of inflammation in the brain due to their unique abilities to cross the BBB through diapedesis and chemotaxis. During the inflammatory response phase of a brain disorder, these cells can act as "cellular Trojan horses," transporting drugs or drug-loaded nanocarriers across the BBB to inflammatory sites in the brain [76].

2.5.1.6 Peptide-Vector-Mediated Transport

A different strategy that is being researched involves the use of peptides with cell-penetrating properties in combination with the RMT approach. It has been proposed that peptides, including the B6 peptide, could function as carriers to deliver drugs. Nonetheless, the precise mechanisms of how they function are not yet fully understood [74, 77, 78].

2.5.2 Recent Strategies for Delivering Drugs into the Brain

Studies have shown that the BBB significantly reduces the movement of many drugs into the brain with no entry detected for large-molecule drugs, while small-molecule drugs are mostly prevented from crossing the BBB [79]. To cross the BBB effectively, a small-molecule drug must have two key features, including a molecular mass of less than 400 Da and high lipid solubility [80]. These factors make it challenging for pharmaceutical industries to target drugs to the brain. Various techniques and strategies have been explored to achieve successful clinical outcomes for different CNS disorders.

Due to space limitations, this section will not cover all delivery strategies. Instead, we only focus on several strategies that have attracted more interest from the related parties (Table 2.3). Nevertheless, we provide all strategies as presented in Figure 2.3, Figure 2.4, and Figure 2.5 based on the classification made by Rawal and colleagues [7].

TABLE 2.3
Strategies for Delivering Drugs to the Brain

Strategies/ Formulation	Advantages	Disadvantages	References
Direct systemic delivery	• Could avoid first-pass metabolism • As the brain has a vast network of capillaries, this approach is effective in targeting drugs into the brain	• Except for the trans-nasal route, other known routes of administration are considered invasive techniques. • The BBB is still a big hurdle in preventing a sufficient level of drugs from reaching the brain	[81]
Direct CNS delivery	• The drug directly reaches the brain • As each route in this approach (intracerebral, intraventricular, intrathecal routes) indicates a different site of injection, this provides an option based on the disorder that the patient suffers from.	• The administration is invasive. • Could induce reactivity from other cells in the brain, e.g., astrocytes. • Could cause damage in other parts of the brain following this invasive technique. • In the intracerebral route, the dose given is relatively higher as the movement of the drugs in the densely packed cells of both gray and white matter is slow.	[81, 82, 83]
BBB disruption strategies	• Could transiently increase the permeability of BBB • This strategy is used to assist other drugs to cross the BBB and reach the brain.	• Opening the BBB could increase the risk of the entry of harmful entities. • As several studies conducted in animals and humans still reported contradiction regarding the effectivity, this strategy needs to be further elucidated.	[54]
Chemistry- and biotechnology-based approach	• Except for viral vectors, the use of antibodies and other endogenous peptides could find a way to reach the brain via a certain transport mechanism, e.g., transcytosis. • For viral vectors, the efficiency of gene transfection has been tested with satisfying outcomes.	• The route utilized is mostly invasive surgery. • As the vectors are typically peptides or viruses, the risk of excessive immune responses could not be ignored.	[54, 81, 84, 85]

TABLE 2.3 (Continued)
Strategies for Delivering Drugs to the Brain

Strategies/ Formulation	Advantages	Disadvantages	References
Delivery via the autonomous nervous system	• This approach shows a promising future as this could be used for transporting viral vectors to the CNS.	• The effectiveness of this route is still questionable. • Along with this, the safety aspect of this route also still needs further studies.	[86]
Nanoparticles	• Nanoparticles show a better possibility to interact with various systems which could assist their entry into the brain. • Several drugs have been successfully formulated in the nanoparticle dosage form. • Nanoparticles have been reported to reach the tumor tissue.	• Due to the minute size of nanoparticles along with their large surface area, the toxicology aspect should be paid close attention to. • The nano size does not necessarily mean they could easily cross the BBB.	[87, 88]
Exosomes	• Non-immunogenic property • Can be loaded with various types of molecules (e.g., hydrophilic and lipophilic molecules, small molecules, proteins, nucleic acids, and lipids)	• Data regarding safety and efficiency are still being awaited. • Isolation and loading procedures need to be optimized • It is also important to decide from which cells the exosomes should be isolated.	[54, 89]
Microspheres	• They can be administered non-invasively via the intranasal route. • Various polymers can be used for coating the structure of the microspheres.	• The selection of the polymeric matrix used in the formulation is pivotal for mediating the release of the drug. • To date, no microsphere-based drug formulation has been available in the market.	[7, 90]
Hydrogels	• The properties resemble the physicochemical properties of many soft tissues. • Despite hydrogels being able to be administered via various routes, e.g., intranasal and injection, their administration via implant is recommended.	• As with other invasive techniques, the uncomfortable procedure of the injection has also been complained about. • Some reported the emergence of inflammation, immune-related response, and systemic adverse effects.	[91, 92]

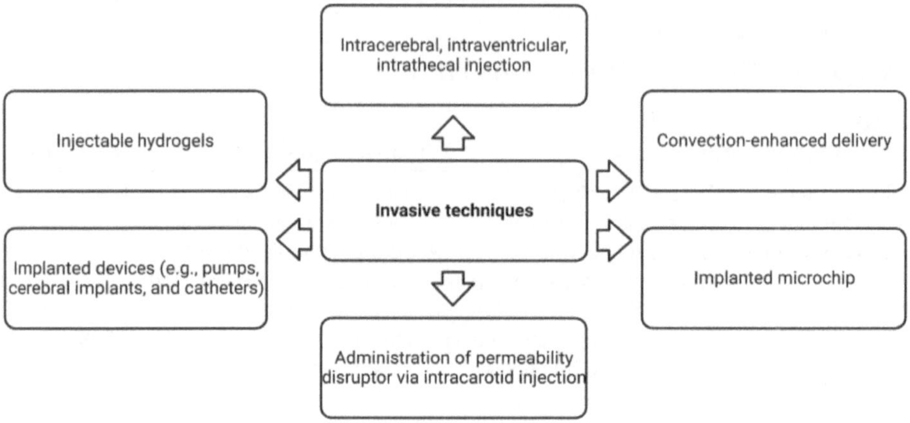

FIGURE 2.3 Invasive techniques commonly used for brain drug delivery.

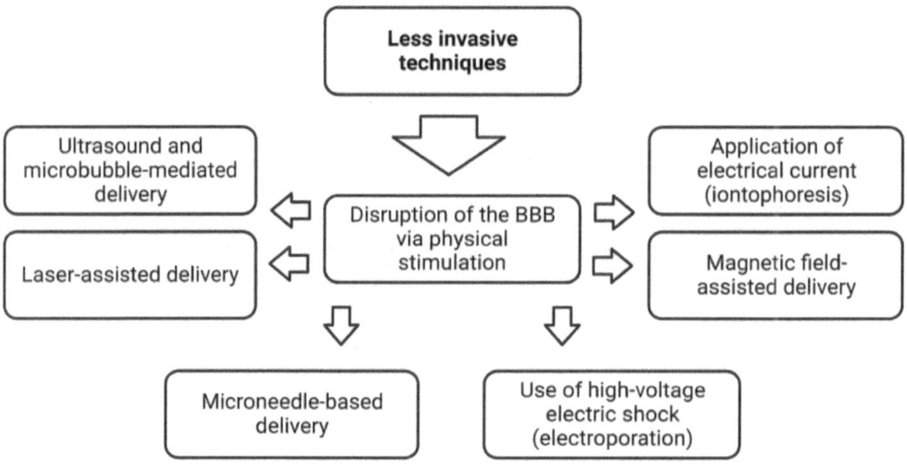

FIGURE 2.4 Techniques considered as less invasive ways for brain drug delivery.

2.5.2.1 Administration Aiming for Systemic Delivery

Three main routes are usually utilized to deliver the drug to the brain through systemic delivery, that is, the intravenous, intra-arterial, and intranasal routes [81]. However, we also add brief information about injectable hydrogels, which have attracted more attention recently.

2.5.2.1.1 Intravenous Route

The intravenous (IV) route is commonly used to administer large doses of drugs because it avoids first-pass metabolism and has the potential to deliver drugs to the brain through general circulation [93]. As the brain contains a vast network of

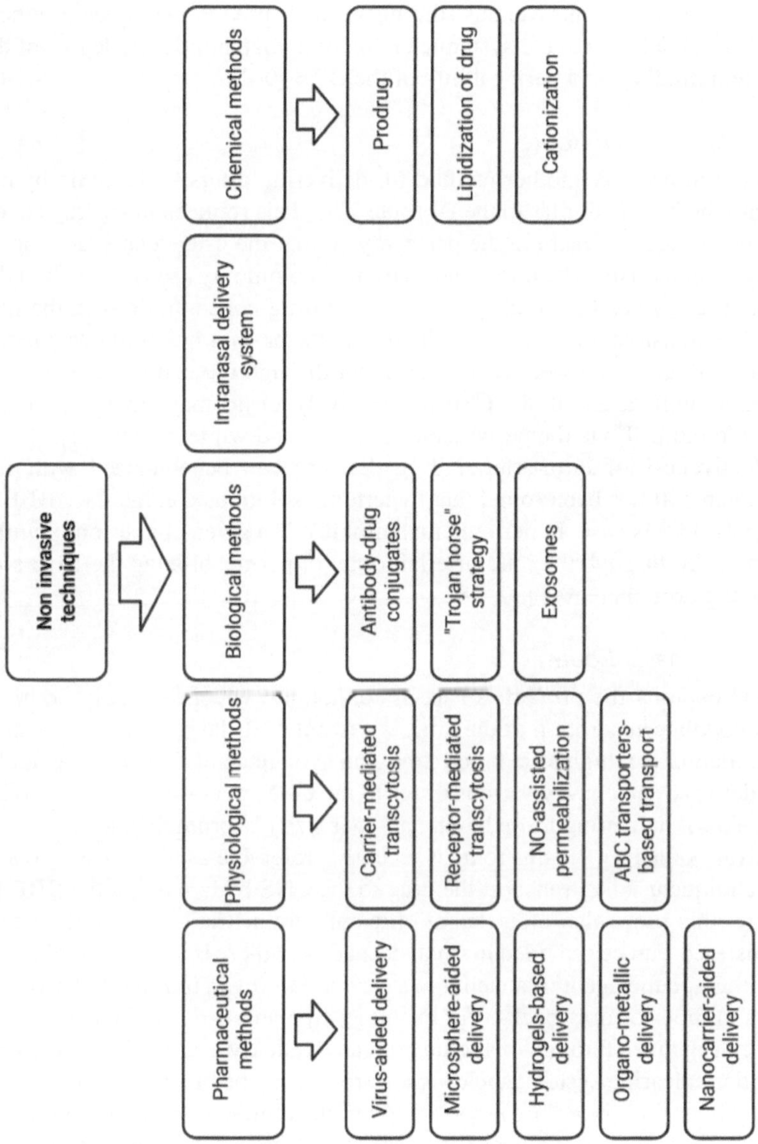

FIGURE 2.5 Non-invasive techniques used to deliver drugs into the brain.

capillaries with a surface area of around $20m^2$, the transvascular approach is effective in targeting drugs into the brain [79]. The high potential of this approach to deliver drugs to most neurons in the brain is due to the neurons' strong connection with blood vessels. However, drug accumulation in the brain is limited due to the BBB and rapid clearance of drugs from the extracellular fluid (ECF). The drug's accessibility in the brain subsequent to intravenous administration is predominantly determined by factors such as its half-life in the systemic circulation, metabolic rate, degree of drug-plasma protein binding, and permeability of the BBB [94].

2.5.2.1.2 Intra-arterial Route

The intra-arterial route is another method for delivering drugs to the brain by direct injection into the blood, similar to the IV route [79]. This route enables drugs to enter the brain vessels before reaching the periphery so that the drugs can evade the first-pass effect of metabolism. The intra-arterial route is commonly used to transport drugs treating brain tumors as this method can increase drug concentrations in the tumor. The process responsible for drug bioavailability in the brain is believed to entail transport across capillaries followed by its movement through the choroid plexus epithelium, culminating in access to the CSF. Alternatively, drugs may enter arterial blood and journey to the CSF via the perivascular pathway and white matter [95].

The effectiveness of intra-arterial drug delivery can be enhanced with BBB-disrupting agents. It has been found that hypertonic solutions can increase BBB permeability [96]. In this case, hypertonic mannitol is often given concurrently with the drug administered through the intra-arterial route for permeabilizing the BBB so that the entry of the drug increases [97, 98].

2.5.2.1.3 Intranasal Route

This method exploits the property of nasal epithelium, which is highly permeable, allowing immediate absorption of the drug as a result of its large surface area, porous endothelial membrane, high total blood flow, and avoidance of first-pass metabolism. Intranasal delivery can convey various drugs to the CNS, not only for small molecule drugs but also for delivering those having a larger size (macromolecules).

The delivery of a drug via this route is recently preferable as this is a less to a non-invasive technique used to transport the drug to the CNS by bypassing the BBB [99]. Furthermore, this route also offers more efficient administration as the drug can be self-administered, can be provided in small dosages and there is an absence of the need to alter the therapeutic agent or attach it to a carrier. However, intranasal delivery also possesses a number of drawbacks. For example, frequent use can damage the nasal mucosa; the drug given through this route is cleared quickly as a result of the action of the mucociliary clearing system; and drug absorption can be blocked because of nasal congestion. Other limitations are associated with the elimination of the drug via both local degradation in the nasal mucosa and systemic clearance mechanisms [100, 101].

2.5.2.1.4 Injectable Hydrogels

Several invasive routes can be applied to inject the injectable hydrogels into the body, for example, intravenous injection, given as an implant, and local injection [91, 92].

Hydrogels can be defined as networks of polymers arranged three-dimensionally that have the ability to absorb a large portion of water (70%–99%), causing hydrogels' physical properties to mimic living tissues [91]. At this point, hydrogels are seriously considered a promising formulation for drug delivery to the brain.

Several reports have demonstrated that hydrogel-based drug delivery had potency as a carrier for drugs used to treat brain-related diseases, including neurodegenerative diseases. For example, Wang and colleagues reported success in formulating L-dopa delivered from hydrogel structure as a treatment for PD [102]. This strategy has changed the previous properties of L-dopa to be released faster. Moreover, this formulation increases the residence time in the nasal cavity. Ultimately, the hydrogels-based L-dopa formulation increases the level of the drug in the brain [102].

2.5.2.2 Direct Central Nervous System Delivery

Various methods have been applied for delivering drugs directly into the CNS. These include the administration of drugs directly into the brain parenchyma (intracerebral delivery), through cerebral ventricles (transcranial delivery), and through intrathecal injection. Other methods are delivery of drugs via cerebrospinal fluid, formulation of polymer depot, and via the technique of BBB disruption [81].

2.5.2.2.1 Intracerebral Delivery

Direct administration of drugs into the brain parenchyma can be achieved through intracerebral delivery methods [103]. This technique can be carried out in several ways, for example, through injection of either bolus or infusion via intrathecal catheters, through the use of the membrane, which could control the release of the drugs from matrices, through microencapsulation, and through the development of recombinant cells. However, the movement of drugs is hindered by the restricted diffusion coefficient of molecules in the densely packed cells of both gray and white matter in the brain. This results in the slow movement of the drugs, necessitating a high dosage for achieving a suitable drug concentration in the parenchyma. [82].

Intracerebral implants are designed to control the release of drugs at the targeted site in the brain. These devices are composed of biodegradable or non-biodegradable polymeric materials that contain the drugs. The drugs are released from the implants through diffusion. These implants are surgically implanted in the brain and release the drugs over a specific period of time [81].

2.5.2.2.2 Transcranial/ Intraventricular Drug Delivery

The intraventricular route is another method to bypass the BBB by directly instilling therapeutic agents into the cerebral ventricles. This is especially effective in treating meningiomas and metastatic cells of CSF since it spreads drugs primarily to the brain's ventricles and subarachnoid space [104]. One key benefit of this approach is that it does not connect with the brain's interstitial fluid, as opposed to intracerebral delivery. As a result, the drug can reach higher concentrations in the brain compared to its distribution outside of blood vessels [105]. Nonetheless, the primary drawback is the potential for inducing astrocyte reactivity in the subependymal site because of the elevated drug exposure at the brain's ependymal area [81].

2.5.2.2.3 *Intrathecal Delivery*

This approach is applied by delivering drugs through the intrathecal route. This can be done by administering the drug through a space in the brain filled with CSF, called the cisterna magna. While this approach is less invasive compared to intraventricular administration, it does not lead to drug accumulation in the deep structures of the brain parenchyma, which is essential for maintaining drug release over time [104]. The primary drawback inherently linked to this method is the potential for the drug to spread throughout the distal region of the spinal canal [106]. This route is suitable for treating spinal-related diseases as well as disseminated meningeal diseases. However, research has proposed that intrathecal delivery cannot provide an effective outcome when applied to treating glioblastoma or other large parenchymal diseases [107].

2.5.2.3 BBB Disruption Approach

The use of chemical substances or energy like ultrasound or electromagnetic radiation externally can directly deliver drug substances to the CNS, enabling drugs to enter the brain by opening tight junctions [79]. Several major techniques have been developed to disrupt the BBB. The first technique is carried out by using chemical substances with a hyperosmolar nature that have higher osmotic pressure or hypertonicity, leading to the disruption of tight junctions caused by increased osmotic pressure and ultimately allowing drug entry paracellularly [108].

The second technique is associated with the utilization of ultrasound and electromagnetic radiation, showing benefits in targeting specific areas in the brain [109]. At least three mechanisms have been provided for explaining the process of drug entry via the use of this technique. First, the applied ultrasonic waves can induce lesions because of the temperature of the waves. This will in turn cause a generalized opening of the BBB [110]. Second, the injected fluid's cavitation effect results in the formation of cavities filled by the air. These cavities mainly occur in the luminal area of the membrane, making drug entry more efficient and easier [111]. Finally, micro-bubbles can be formed by an ultrasound contrast agent, resulting in disruption of tight junctions, making the permeability on the BBB higher. Recently, this technique has been regarded as a significant non-invasive strategy for delivering drugs to the brain [112].

The opening of the BBB can also be induced by using the microneedles-based method. This method uses very tiny needles that have a length of less than 1 mm. As the administration of microneedles produces a less painful sensation, this method has gained popularity in drug delivery systems, including delivery to the brain [113]. Among the several types of microneedles, dissolving microneedles are promising as once they are injected, the polymer contents are readily dissolved [7, 113]. The use of microneedles for drug delivery into the brain is commonly applied in concert with convection-based delivery as this combination can assist the direct movement of drugs into the brain. This was demonstrated by an experiment carried out to study the entry of drugs loaded into microneedles in hydrocephalus conditions. It was found that the use of microneedles gave advantages in terms of reducing the duration of drug infusion as well as the number of catheters applied to the brain [114].

2.5.2.4 Chemistry-Based Approach

Chemical substances delivering drugs across the BBB are considered promising agents for delivery. Numerous research efforts have focused on developing innovative strategies for transporting neurotherapeutics across the BBB. Among these strategies, the utilization of chimeric peptides has attracted attention. In addition, the use of proteins that have positive charges (cationic proteins) for assisting the entry of drugs has also gained popularity.

2.5.2.4.1 Chimeric Peptides

In Greek, chimeric is a term used to describe a creature possessing a human head and the body of a lion. This analogy is relevant to drug compounds that cannot cross the BBB and are therefore combined with a transport vector to form a molecule that is more easily transportable. Several vectors have been recognized, for example, antibodies, endogenous peptides, and various types of peptidomimetics [115]. Chimeric peptides are generated by covalently linking the neuropeptide with the appropriate vector. These peptides are then trafficked via several pathways, for example, receptor-mediated transport, to the brain. In this case, insulin and transferrin are the most known peptides that are transported across the BBB by their corresponding insulin and transferrin receptors [81].

Two important principles are considered before selecting a peptide for drug delivery. The first principle is that the vector used for delivery should have its pharmacological activity, such as insulin, which has its transport mechanism. The second principle states that for targeted drug delivery to the brain, the bond between the peptide vector and its binding receptor site should be extremely specific.

2.5.2.4.2 Cationic Proteins

The process of cationization alters the unbound carboxyl groups of acid amino acids in a polypeptide, leading to an increase in the overall positive charge of the peptide. This technique is ideal for transporting proteins and peptides to the brain, especially those having a basic isoelectric point [81].

Typically, due to their high molecular weight, protein molecules are too large to penetrate the BBB [79]. The method of cationic proteins offers a strategy to transport the protein across the BBB by modifying the charges of the proteins and peptides into cationic charges, allowing them to be transported into the brain more easily. This is explained by their interaction with the appropriate anionic functional moieties expressed on the cell surface [81].

2.5.2.4.3 Prodrug Formulation

Prodrugs are formulated to facilitate the delivery of hydrophilic drugs to the brain. They are chemically altered versions of the original active pharmaceutical ingredient, which results in a bulkier structure without any biological toxicity or activity. Unlike chimeric peptides, due to their specificity toward certain enzymes, prodrugs containing amino acids as pro-moiety are not biologically active. However, upon reaching the brain through the bloodstream, the enzymes present on the surface of the

BBB metabolize the prodrugs to generate active agents, which can then penetrate the BBB and accumulate in the brain [80].

2.5.2.5 Biotechnology-based Approach

Biotechnology concepts have been applied in various fields, with no exception in the field of drug delivery systems. A biotechnology-based technique, for example, protein engineering and recombinant DNA, have attracted attention to be applied for effectively targeting neuro-pharmaceuticals to the brain, including brain tumors

2.5.2.5.1 Monoclonal Antibodies

This section discusses the preparation of monoclonal antibodies (mAbs) using hybridoma technology. The tumor cells of melanoma are combined with anti-tumor antibodies that target specific antigens present on malignant cells in animals such as rats. However, these mAbs are not used directly for brain targeting. Instead, the antibodies undergo structural modification to produce monoclonal antibodies that are modified genetically. As an example, a study developed chimeric HIR mAb by engineering the human insulin receptor (HIR). This approach demonstrated the vectors penetrate at a better level into the brain, as evidenced by a primate-based study [116].

2.5.2.5.2 Genomics Application

It has been recognized that the use of small molecules has failed to provide effective therapy for brain-related diseases such as stroke, brain cancer, and neurodegenerative diseases. At this point, large-molecule pharmaceuticals can potentially treat these conditions, but they do not typically cross the BBB. However, gene technologies can be used to transport these drugs across the BBB.

For this purpose, the efforts for identifying novel proteins expressed in the BBB that can act as vectors or carriers are crucial. These vectors potentially assist the movement of drugs with large molecular weight, such as peptides, which can find an entry into the brain and release their pharmacological actions [115]. One of the efforts is related to the production of monoclonal antibodies through an engineered genetic process. The antibodies are then aimed at targeting the transporters expressed in the BBB. Another effort is to conjugate certain radiopharmaceuticals to the drug-targeted vectors. This conjugate can be used to image the expression of a gene in the brain. Genomics programs can also be applied for identifying new systems that can be utilized for transporting drugs into the CNS [117].

2.5.2.5.3 Exosomes

As exosomes are generated and secreted by cells, the use of these extracellular vesicles for delivering drugs into the brain brings a certain benefit in terms of their non-immunogenic property [54]. Physiologically, exosomes are produced by all cells and play certain roles, mainly in mediating cell-cell communication and regulating several vital functions, for example, immune response, transcription, translation, and reproduction [118]. To conduct these functions appropriately, exosomes carry proteins, lipids, amino acids, metabolites, and nucleic acids in their structure

[118]. It has been shown that these contents can be transported into the targeted cells efficiently.

Haqqani and colleagues have successfully extracted exosomes secreted by brain endothelial cells and they demonstrated the pivotal functions of these vesicles in modulating the traffic of various molecules across the BBB [119]. Based on these properties, exosomes have been becoming a promising system for delivering drugs into the brain. For example, Yang and colleagues reported the ability of exosomes isolated from brain endothelial cells to transport siRNA into the brain by penetrating the BBB [120].

However, a number of obstacles have been reported when using exosomes as carriers. As this approach has been newly introduced, studies focusing on the safety or toxicology aspect of exosomes are relatively limited. In line with that, studies that attempt to elaborate the pharmacokinetics of exosomes upon administration are also awaited. Another major drawback is associated with exosomes' capacity to load drugs. Not only that issue, but the optimization of protocols used to load drugs into the structure of exosomes is also pivotal [54, 101].

2.5.2.5. 4 "Trojan Horse" for Brain Targeting

Monocytes are blood cells that lack granules. They can serve as Trojan Horses for drug delivery to the brain by trapping the drug inside them. This method involves loading the drug molecules into the monocytes through receptor-mediated endocytosis, which occurs when they bind to appropriate ligands. The human insulin receptor (HIR) is a highly potent monoclonal antibody that is particularly effective at the BBB, making it a popular choice for use in Trojan Horse drug delivery [115, 121].

2.5.2.6 Delivery through the Autonomous Nervous System

The autonomic nervous system has become a promising avenue for delivering drugs to the brain, in addition to CNS drug delivery methods. This approach was first identified by Prusiner during a study of prion diseases. It was discovered that the pathogen responsible for this disease enters the CNS through a distinct pathway other than the BBB. It finds its way to the CNS by utilizing the pathway called retrograde axonal transport [122]. This transport moves a compound from the axon to the cell body of sensory neurons, which is located in the CNS. It has been demonstrated that drugs administered via enteral and lymphoid routes can find entry to the CNS via sensory fibers and ultimately reach the CNS [123].

2.5.2.7 Recent Pharmaceutical Formulations for Delivering Drugs

The concept of drug delivery through novel methods has emerged as a favorable approach for targeting drugs to the brain. This approach involves the use of small colloidal particles, which have been widely accepted due to their controlled release and targeted delivery mechanism.

2.5.2.7.1 *Viral Vectors*

Instead of using peptides as the vector, the virus has gained popularity as the vector for delivering neurotherapeutics into the brain. Several viruses have been identified as useful vectors, that is, the lentivirus, the adenovirus, and the adeno-associated virus [54, 96]. Of these viruses, the latter is more used in the effort to test gene therapy on patients suffering from brain diseases. This prominence is supported by the safety profiles that have been shown by the virus. Nevertheless, as with other viral vectors, surveillance of immunogenicity that can emerge after using the adeno-associated virus as the vector has to be strictly controlled [85].

Furthermore, as viruses cannot cross the BBB passively, efforts to design the appropriate route for transporting the vectors into the brain are still on the way [54]. Although several routes of administration have been proposed, it seems that each approach possesses drawbacks that cannot be neglected. For example, injection of the dosage form into the cerebrospinal fluid brings some benefits, but problems can emerge during invasive surgery carried out on patients. It has been reported that severe adverse events appeared following a clinical trial on a patient receiving a viral vector-based treatment administered through neurosurgery [124]. Although the role of the vector in those events was not clearly stated, the invasive surgery undertaken played a role that could not have been negligible.

2.5.2.7.2 *Liposomes*

Liposomes are a type of biocompatible and biodegradable carrier formulated from animal lipids (e.g., phospholipids). They have become increasingly popular in drug delivery technology, particularly for targeting the brain, due to their non-invasive and non-toxic properties, their ability to carry various molecules (i.e., hydrophilic, lipophilic, or amphoteric drug molecules), and their flexibility to carry a molecule either by trapping it inside their structure or by attaching them on their surface. Lipids such as phospholipids can be formed into a bilayered structure that can further form different sizes of liposomes, including unilamellar and multilamellar vesicles [81, 125, 126].

2.5.2.7.3 *Nanocarrier-aided Delivery*

In recent years, there has been increasing interest in using nanoparticles to deliver drugs to the brain. Nanoparticles have the potential to overcome BBB and improve drug delivery to the CNS. Various types of nanosystems have been developed for this purpose, including polymeric nanoparticles, nanospheres, nanosuspensions, and nanoemulsions, among others. Although the exact mechanism of how nanoparticles open the BBB is still not clear, it is believed that they can enter the brain by various endocytic mechanisms. Some of the mechanisms that have been reported to increase nanoparticle concentration in the brain include increased retention of drugs in brain blood capillaries, adsorption to capillary walls, the opening of tight junctions between endothelial cells, inhibition of the ABCB1 efflux system, the endocytic mechanism, and the permeabilization of the BBB endothelial cells [10, 127, 128].

2.5.2.7.4 Microspheres Technology

The use of microspheres as a drug carrier has attracted attention recently. This is a technique used to increase the delivery of a drug into the targeted locations, including the brain. As its name, microspheres are particles in polymeric and spheric form with sizes ranging from 1–1,000 μm containing the entrapped drugs distributed uniformly within their matrix [74].

In addition to their ability to release the drugs in controlled and sustained release modes, microspheres show an optimal absorption level, leading to their great bioavailability due to their tiny size with a large surface area [129]. Several drugs have been formulated via this platform to optimize their entry into the brain, for example, rivastigmine [130], zolmitriptan [131], clonazepam [132], and methotrexate [133]. All of these drugs showed the capacity to get into the brain via intranasal administration.

However, several drawbacks should be considered. For optimal drug absorption and efficacy, the release of the encapsulated drugs from the polymer is pivotal. Therefore, the composition of the polymer used in the formulation of microspheres is critical for that issue. Also, the data about safety and effectiveness have not been sufficient for making microspheres for targeted delivery available in the market as of today [90].

2.6 CONCLUSION AND FUTURE INSIGHTS

Despite its crucial function in protecting the brain from the attack of dangerous substances, the BBB has become a big hurdle for drugs trying to get into the brain. Many strategies have been developed to overcome this problem as described in the body sections of this chapter. However, each strategy has shown limitations. Therefore, the efforts undertaken to design or develop other means for drugs to target the brain are crucial.

In principle, the use of any strategy for transporting drugs into the brain should fulfill two main requirements, effectivity and safety. The strategy of choice has to ensure that the drugs remain stable and effective in treating the diseases. At the same time, it has to demonstrate satisfying safety aspects for the patients. In this context, the brain drug delivery system is not solely about finding new techniques or strategies. The efforts can also focus on how to optimize the two aspects above.

Of course, a better understanding of the anatomy and physiology of the BBB will provide valuable information in the efforts to develop a new strategy in brain drug delivery. At this point, studies about the molecular mechanism of how the barrier experiences a disruption are also essential.

As mentioned in the introductory section, the existence of other barriers protecting the brain from substances coming from the periphery also has to be studied in depth. Further understanding concerning these barriers might provide valuable insights into designing or developing an appropriate drug delivery system for the brain.

Supported by advanced progress in the field of pharmaceutical technology in the last two decades, these efforts will soon offer a better strategy for delivering drugs to treat brain-related disorders without disturbing the physiological roles of the BBB.

REFERENCES

1. Islam, Yamir, Andrew G Leach, Jayden Smith, Stefano Pluchino, Christopher R Coxon, Muttuswamy Sivakumaran, James Downing, Amos A Fatokun, Meritxell Teixidò, and Touraj Ehtezazi. "Physiological and Pathological Factors Affecting Drug Delivery to the Brain by Nanoparticles." *Advanced Science* 8, no. 11 (2021): 2002085.
2. Coomber, BL, and PA Stewart. "Morphometric Analysis of Cns Microvascular Endothelium." *Microvascular Research* 30, no. 1 (1985): 99–115.
3. Cantrill, Carina A, Robert A Skinner, Nancy J Rothwell, and Jeffrey I Penny. "An Immortalised Astrocyte Cell Line Maintains the in Vivo Phenotype of a Primary Porcine in Vitro Blood–Brain Barrier Model." *Brain Research* 1479 (2012): 17–30.
4. Daneman, Richard, and Alexandre Prat. "The Blood–Brain Barrier." *Cold Spring Harbor Perspectives in Biology* 7, no. 1 (2015): a020412.
5. Oldendorf, William H, Marcia E Cornford, and W Jann Brown. "The Large Apparent Work Capability of the Blood-Brain Barrier: A Study of the Mitochondrial Content of Capillary Endothelial Cells in Brain and Other Tissues of the Rat." *Annals of Neurology: Official Journal of the American Neurological Association and the Child Neurology Society* 1, no. 5 (1977): 409–17.
6. Kondo, T., H. Kinouchi, M. Kawase, and T. Yoshimoto. "Astroglial Cells Inhibit the Increasing Permeability of Brain Endothelial Cell Monolayer Following Hypoxia/Reoxygenation." *Neuroscience Letters* 208, no. 2 (1996): 101–04.
7. Rawal, Shruti U, Bhoomika M Patel, and Mayur M Patel. "New Drug Delivery Systems Developed for Brain Targeting." *Drugs* 82, no. 7 (2022): 749–92.
8. Armulik, Annika, Guillem Genové, Maarja Mäe, Maya H Nisancioglu, Elisabet Wallgard, Colin Niaudet, Liqun He, Jenny Norlin, Per Lindblom, and Karin Strittmatter. "Pericytes Regulate the Blood–Brain Barrier." *Nature* 468, no. 7323 (2010): 557–61.
9. Berezowski, Vincent, Christophe Landry, Marie-Pierre Dehouck, Roméo Cecchelli, and Laurence Fenart. "Contribution of Glial Cells and Pericytes to the mRNA Profiles of P-Glycoprotein and Multidrug Resistance-Associated Proteins in an in Vitro Model of the Blood–Brain Barrier." *Brain Research* 1018, no. 1 (2004): 1–9.
10. Zihni, Ceniz, Clare Mills, Karl Matter, and Maria S Balda. "Tight Junctions: From Simple Barriers to Multifunctional Molecular Gates." *Nature Reviews Molecular Cell Biology* 17, no. 9 (2016): 564–80.
11. Furuse, Mikio, Tetsuaki Hirase, Masahiko Itoh, Akira Nagafuchi, Shigenobu Yonemura, Sachiko Tsukita, and Shoichiro Tsukita. "Occludin: A Novel Integral Membrane Protein Localizing at Tight Junctions." *The Journal of Cell Biology* 123, no. 6 (1993): 1777–88.
12. Feldman, Gemma J, James M Mullin, and Michael P Ryan. "Occludin: Structure, Function and Regulation." *Advanced Drug Delivery Reviews* 57, no. 6 (2005): 883–917.
13. Hirase, Tetsuaki, James M Staddon, Mitinori Saitou, Yuhko Ando-Akatsuka, Masahiko Itoh, Mikio Furuse, Kazushi Fujimoto, Shoichiro Tsukita, and Lee L Rubin. "Occludin as a Possible Determinant of Tight Junction Permeability in Endothelial Cells." *Journal of Cell Science* 110, no. 14 (1997): 1603–13.
14. Morita, Kazumasa, Hiroyuki Sasaki, Mikio Furuse, and Shoichiro Tsukita. "Endothelial Claudin: Claudin-5/Tmvcf Constitutes Tight Junction Strands in Endothelial Cells." *The Journal of Cell Biology* 147, no. 1 (1999): 185–94.
15. Liu, Wei-Ye, Zhi-Bin Wang, Li-Chao Zhang, Xin Wei, and Ling Li. "Tight Junction in Blood-Brain Barrier: An Overview of Structure, Regulation, and Regulator Substances." *CNS Neuroscience & Therapeutics* 18, no. 8 (2012): 609–15.

16. Wilhelm, Imola, and István A Krizbai. "In Vitro Models of the Blood–Brain Barrier for the Study of Drug Delivery to the Brain." *Molecular Pharmaceutics* 11, no. 7 (2014): 1949–63.
17. Inoko, Akihito, Masahiko Itoh, Atsushi Tamura, Miho Matsuda, Mikio Furuse, and Shoichiro Tsukita. "Expression and Distribution of Zo-3, a Tight Junction Maguk Protein, in Mouse Tissues." *Genes to Cells* 8, no. 11 (2003): 837–45.
18. Furuse, Mikio, Masahiko Itoh, Tetsuaki Hirase, Akira Nagafuchi, Shigenobu Yonemura, Sachiko Tsukita, and Shoichiro Tsukita. "Direct Association of Occludin with Zo-1 and Its Possible Involvement in the Localization of Occludin at Tight Junctions." *Journal of Cell Biology* 127, no. 6 (1994): 1617–26.
19. Tarling, Elizabeth J, Thomas Q de Aguiar Vallim, and Peter A Edwards. "Role of Abc Transporters in Lipid Transport and Human Disease." *Trends in Endocrinology & Metabolism* 24, no. 7 (2013): 342–50.
20. Neumann, Jennifer, Dania Rose-Sperling, and Ute A Hellmich. "Diverse Relations between ABC Transporters and Lipids: An Overview." *Biochimica et Biophysica Acta (BBA)-Biomembranes* 1859, no. 4 (2017): 605–18.
21. Kubo, Yoshiyuki, Sumio Ohtsuki, Yasuo Uchida, and Tetsuya Terasaki. "Quantitative Determination of Luminal and Abluminal Membrane Distributions of Transporters in Porcine Brain Capillaries by Plasma Membrane Fractionation and Quantitative Targeted Proteomics." *Journal of Pharmaceutical Sciences* 104, no. 9 (2015): 3060–68.
22. Dauchy, Sandrine, Fabien Dutheil, Richard J Weaver, Francine Chassoux, Catherine Daumas-Duport, Pierre-Olivier Couraud, Jean-Michel Scherrmann, Isabelle De Waziers, and Xavier Declèves. "ABC Transporters, Cytochromes P450 and Their Main Transcription Factors: Expression at the Human Blood–Brain Barrier." *Journal of Neurochemistry* 107, no. 6 (2008): 1518–28.
23. Amin, ML "P-Glycoprotein Inhibition for Optimal Drug Delivery." *Drug Target Insights* 7 (2013): 27–34.
24. Kemper, EM., AE van Zandbergen, C Cleypool, HA Mos, W Boogerd, JH Beijnen, and O van Tellingen, "Increased Penetration of Paclitaxel into the Brain by Inhibition of P-Glycoprotein." *Clinical Cancer Research* 9, no. 7 (2003): 2849–55.
25. Sun, YL, A Patel, P Kumar, and ZS Chen. "Role of ABC Transporters in Cancer Chemotherapy." *Chinese Journal of Cancer* 31, no. 2 (2012): 51–7.
26. Brettschneider, J, K Del Tredici, VM Lee, and JQ Trojanowski. "Spreading of Pathology in Neurodegenerative Diseases: A Focus on Human Studies." *Nature Reviews Neuroscience* 16, no. 2 (2015): 109–20.
27. Wolfe, Michael S. "Chapter 1 – Solving the Puzzle of Neurodegeneration." In *The Molecular and Cellular Basis of Neurodegenerative Diseases*, edited by Michael S Wolfe, 1–22: Academic Press, 2018.
28. Kovacs, GG "Molecular Pathology of Neurodegenerative Diseases: Principles and Practice." *Journal of Clinical Pathology* 72, no. 11 (2019): 725–35.
29. Dugger, BN, and DW Dickson. "Pathology of Neurodegenerative Diseases." *Cold Spring Harbor Perspectives in Biology* 9, no. 7 (2017).
30. Erdő, Franciska, László Denes, and Elizabeth de Lange. "Age-Associated Physiological and Pathological Changes at the Blood–Brain Barrier: A Review." *Journal of Cerebral Blood Flow & Metabolism* 37, no. 1 (2017): 4–24.
31. Wen, Jian, Yan Ding, Le Wang, and Ying Xiao. "Gut Microbiome Improves Postoperative Cognitive Function by Decreasing Permeability of the Blood–Brain Barrier in Aged Mice." *Brain Research Bulletin* 164 (2020): 249–56.

32. Banks, William A, May J Reed, Aric F Logsdon, Elizabeth M Rhea, and Michelle A Erickson. "Healthy Aging and the Blood–Brain Barrier." *Nature Aging* 1, no. 3 (2021): 243–54.
33. Obermeier, Birgit, Richard Daneman, and Richard M Ransohoff. "Development, Maintenance and Disruption of the Blood–Brain Barrier." *Nature Medicine* 19, no. 12 (2013): 1584–96.
34. Sweeney, Melanie D, Zhen Zhao, Axel Montagne, Amy R Nelson, and Berislav V Zlokovic. "Blood–Brain Barrier: From Physiology to Disease and Back." *Physiological Reviews* (2018).
35. Yang, Andrew C, Marc Y Stevens, Michelle B Chen, Davis P Lee, Daniel Stähli, David Gate, Kévin Contrepois, Winnie Chen, Tal Iram, and Lichao Zhang. "Physiological Blood–Brain Transport Is Impaired with Age by a Shift in Transcytosis." *Nature* 583, no. 7816 (2020): 425–30.
36. Brochard, Vanessa, Béhazine Combadière, Annick Prigent, Yasmina Laouar, Aline Perrin, Virginie Beray-Berthat, Olivia Bonduelle, Daniel Alvarez-Fischer, Jacques Callebert, and Jean-Marie Launay. "Infiltration of Cd4+ Lymphocytes into the Brain Contributes to Neurodegeneration in a Mouse Model of Parkinson Disease." *Journal of Clinical Investigation* 119, no. 1 (2008).
37. Gerwien, Hanna, Sven Hermann, Xueli Zhang, Eva Korpos, Jian Song, Klaus Kopka, Andreas Faust, Christian Wenning, Catharina C Gross, and Lisa Honold. "Imaging Matrix Metalloproteinase Activity in Multiple Sclerosis as a Specific Marker of Leukocyte Penetration of the Blood–Brain Barrier." *Science Translational Medicine* 8, no. 364 (2016): 364ra152.
38. Profaci, Caterina P, Roeben N Munji, Robert S Pulido, and Richard Daneman. "The Blood–Brain Barrier in Health and Disease: Important Unanswered Questions." *Journal of Experimental Medicine* 217, no. 4 (2020).
39. Kang, Ruiqing, Marcin Gamdzyk, Cameron Lenahan, Jiping Tang, Sheng Tan, and John H Zhang. "The Dual Role of Microglia in Blood–Brain Barrier Dysfunction after Stroke." *Current Neuropharmacology* 18, no. 12 (2020): 1237–49.
40. Haruwaka, Koichiro, Ako Ikegami, Yoshihisa Tachibana, Nobuhiko Ohno, Hiroyuki Konishi, Akari Hashimoto, Mami Matsumoto, Daisuke Kato, Riho Ono, and Hiroshi Kiyama. "Dual Microglia Effects on Blood Brain Barrier Permeability Induced by Systemic Inflammation." *Nature Communications* 10, no. 1 (2019): 5816.
41. Knox, Emily G, Maria R Aburto, Gerard Clarke, John F Cryan, and Caitriona M O'Driscoll. "The Blood–Brain Barrier in Aging and Neurodegeneration." *Molecular Psychiatry* 27, no. 6 (2022): 2659–73.
42. Muroi, Masashi, and Ken-ichi Tanamoto. "The Polysaccharide Portion Plays an Indispensable Role in Salmonella Lipopolysaccharide-Induced Activation of Nf-Kb through Human Toll-Like Receptor 4." *Infection and Immunity* 70, no. 11 (2002): 6043–47.
43. Pålsson-McDermott, Eva M, and Luke AJ O'Neill. "Signal Transduction by the Lipopolysaccharide Receptor, Toll-Like Receptor-4." *Immunology* 113, no. 2 (2004): 153–62.
44. Cardoso, Filipa L, Agnes Kittel, Szilvia Veszelka, Ines Palmela, Andrea Tóth, Dora Brites, Mária A Deli, and Maria A Brito. "Exposure to Lipopolysaccharide and/or Unconjugated Bilirubin Impair the Integrity and Function of Brain Microvascular Endothelial Cells." *PLOS One* 7, no. 5 (2012): e35919.
45. Peng, X, Z Luo, S He, L Zhang, and Y Li. "Blood–Brain Barrier Disruption by Lipopolysaccharide and Sepsis-Associated Encephalopathy." *Frontiers in Cellular and Infection Microbiology* 11 (2021): 768108.

46. Varatharaj, Aravinthan, and Ian Galea. "The Blood–Brain Barrier in Systemic Inflammation." *Brain, Behavior, and Immunity* 60 (2017): 1–12.
47. Pun, Pamela BL, JIA Lu, and Shabbir Moochhala. "Involvement of ROS in BBB Dysfunction." *Free Radical Research* 43, no. 4 (2009): 348–64.
48. Olmez, Inan, and Huseyin Ozyurt. "Reactive Oxygen Species and Ischemic Cerebrovascular Disease." *Neurochemistry International* 60, no. 2 (2012): 208–12.
49. Spindler, Katherine R, and Tien-Huei Hsu. "Viral Disruption of the Blood–Brain Barrier." *Trends in microbiology* 20, no. 6 (2012): 282–90.
50. Pan, Yijun, and Joseph A Nicolazzo. "Impact of Aging, Alzheimer's Disease and Parkinson's Disease on the Blood–Brain Barrier Transport of Therapeutics." *Advanced Drug Delivery Reviews* 135 (2018): 62–74.
51. Sweeney, Melanie D, Abhay P Sagare, and Berislav V Zlokovic. "Blood–Brain Barrier Breakdown in Alzheimer Disease and Other Neurodegenerative Disorders." *Nature Reviews Neurology* 14, no. 3 (2018): 133–50.
52. Arvanitis, Costas D, Gino B Ferraro, and Rakesh K Jain. "The Blood–Brain Barrier and Blood–Tumour Barrier in Brain Tumours and Metastases." *Nature Reviews Cancer* 20, no. 1 (2020): 26–41.
53. Sharma, Hari Shanker, Dafin F Muresanu, Rudy J Castellani, Ala Nozari, José Vicente Lafuente, Z Ryan Tian, Seaab Sahib, Igor Bryukhovetskiy, Andrey Bryukhovetskiy, and Anca D Buzoianu. "Pathophysiology of Blood–Brain Barrier in Brain Tumor. Novel Therapeutic Advances Using Nanomedicine." *International Review of Neurobiology* 151 (2020): 1–66.
54. Dong, X. "Current Strategies for Brain Drug Delivery." *Theranostics* 8, no. 6 (2018): 1481–93.
55. Alexandrov, PN, JM Hill, Y Zhao, T Bond, CM Taylor, ME Percy, W Li, and WJ Lukiw. "Aluminum-Induced Generation of Lipopolysaccharide (Lps) from the Human Gastrointestinal (Gi)-Tract Microbiome-Resident Bacteroides Fragilis." *Journal of Inorganic Biochemistry* 203 (2020): 110886.
56. Cheng, Xiao, Ying-Lin Yang, Huan Yang, Yue-Hua Wang, and Guan-Hua Du. "Kaempferol Alleviates Lps-Induced Neuroinflammation and BBB Dysfunction in Mice Via Inhibiting Hmgb1 Release and Down-Regulating Tlr4/Myd88 Pathway." *International Immunopharmacology* 56 (2018): 29–35.
57. Seok, Sun Mi, Jae Mi Kim, Tae Yeop Park, Eun Joo Baik, and Soo Hwan Lee. "Fructose-1, 6-Bisphosphate Ameliorates Lipopolysaccharide-Induced Dysfunction of Blood–Brain Barrier." *Archives of Pharmacal Research* 36 (2013): 1149–59.
58. Veszelka, Szilvia, Mária Pásztói, Attila E Farkas, István Krizbai, Ngo Thi Khue Dung, Masami Niwa, Csongor S Ábrahám, and Mária A Deli. "Pentosan Polysulfate Protects Brain Endothelial Cells against Bacterial Lipopolysaccharide-Induced Damages." *Neurochemistry International* 50, no. 1 (2007): 219–28.
59. Tang, Xiaoqiang, Yu-Xuan Luo, Hou-Zao Chen, and De-Pei Liu. "Mitochondria, Endothelial Cell Function, and Vascular Diseases." *Frontiers in Physiology* 5 (2014): 175.
60. Lee, Sae-Won, Kyung Hee Jung, Chul Ho Jeong, Ji Hae Seo, Dae-Kwann Yoon, Jun-Kyu Suh, Kyu-Won Kim, and Woo Jean Kim. "Inhibition of Endothelial Cell Migration through the Down-Regulation of Mmp-9 by a-Kinase Anchoring Protein 12." *Molecular Medicine Reports* 4, no. 1 (2011): 145–49.
61. Qin, Lan-hui, Wen Huang, Xue-an Mo, Yan-lan Chen, and Xiang-hong Wu. "LPS Induces Occludin Dysregulation in Cerebral Microvascular Endothelial Cells via MAPK Signaling and Augmenting MMP-2 Levels." *Oxidative Medicine and Cellular Longevity* 2015 (2015): 120641.

62. Dal-Pizzol, Felipe, Hugo Alberto Rojas, Emilia Marcelina Dos Santos, Francieli Vuolo, Larissa Constantino, Gustavo Feier, Matheus Pasquali, Clarissa M Comim, Fabrícia Petronilho, and Daniel Pens Gelain. "Matrix Metalloproteinase-2 and Metalloproteinase-9 Activities Are Associated with Blood–Brain Barrier Dysfunction in an Animal Model of Severe Sepsis." *Molecular Neurobiology* 48 (2013): 62–70.
63. Bowyer, John F, Sumit Sarkar, Susan M Burks, Jade N Hess, Serena Tolani, James P O'Callaghan, and Joseph P Hanig. "Microglial Activation and Responses to Vasculature That Result from an Acute LPS Exposure." *Neurotoxicology* 77 (2020): 181–92.
64. Vutukuri, Rajkumar, Robert Brunkhorst, Roxane-Isabelle Kestner, Lena Hansen, Nerea Ferreiros Bouzas, Josef Pfeilschifter, Kavi Devraj, and Waltraud Pfeilschifter. "Alteration of Sphingolipid Metabolism as a Putative Mechanism Underlying LPS-Induced BBB Disruption." *Journal of Neurochemistry* 144, no. 2 (2018): 172–85.
65. Kovac, Andrej, Michelle A Erickson, and William A Banks. "Brain Microvascular Pericytes Are Immunoactive in Culture: Cytokine, Chemokine, Nitric Oxide, and LRP-1 Expression in Response to Lipopolysaccharide." *Journal of Neuroinflammation* 8, no. 1 (2011): 1–9.
66. Burek, Malgorzata, and Carola Y Förster. "Culturing of Rodent Brain Microvascular Endothelial Cells for in vitro Modeling of the Blood–Brain Barrier." In *Blood–Brain Barrier*, edited by Tatiana Barichello, 45–54. New York, NY: Springer New York, 2019.
67. Abbott, NJ. "Evidence for Bulk Flow of Brain Interstitial Fluid: Significance for Physiology and Pathology." *Neurochemistry International* 45, no. 4 (2004): 545–52.
68. Azarmi, M, H Maleki, N Nikkam, and H Malekinejad. "Transcellular Brain Drug Delivery: A Review on Recent Advancements." *International Journal of Pharmaceutics* 586 (2020): 119582.
69. Chen, Y, and L Liu. "Modern Methods for Delivery of Drugs across the Blood–Brain Barrier." *Advanced Drug Delivery Reviews* 64, no. 7 (2012): 640–65.
70. Ye, D, T Zimmermann, V Demina, S Sotnikov, CL Ried, H Rahn, M Stapf, C Untucht, M Rohe, GC Terstappen, K Wicke, M Mezler, H Manninga, and AH Meyer. "Trafficking of JC Virus-Like Particles across the Blood–Brain Barrier." *Nanoscale Advances* 3, no. 9 (2021): 2488–500.
71. Ding, S., AI Khan, X Cai, Y Song, Z Lyu, D Du, P Dutta, and Y Lin. "Overcoming Blood–Brain Barrier Transport: Advances in Nanoparticle-Based Drug Delivery Strategies." *Mater Today (Kidlington)* 37 (2020): 112–25.
72. Lajoie, JM, and EV Shusta. "Targeting Receptor-Mediated Transport for Delivery of Biologics across the Blood–Brain Barrier." *Annual Review of Pharmacology and Toxicology* 55 (2015): 613–31.
73. Lu, W. "Adsorptive-Mediated Brain Delivery Systems." *Current Pharmaceutical Biotechnology* 13, no. 12 (2012): 2340–48.
74. Patel, MM, and BM Patel. "Crossing the Blood–Brain Barrier: Recent Advances in Drug Delivery to the Brain." *CNS Drugs* 31, no. 2 (2017): 109–33.
75. Patel, MM, BR Goyal, SV Bhadada, JS Bhatt, and AF Amin. "Getting into the Brain: Approaches to Enhance Brain Drug Delivery." *CNS Drugs* 23, no. 1 (2009): 35–58.
76. Jain, S, V Mishra, P Singh, PK Dubey, DK Saraf, and SP Vyas. "RGD-Anchored Magnetic Liposomes for Monocytes/Neutrophils-Mediated Brain Targeting." *International Journal of Pharmaceutics* 261, no. 1–2 (2003): 43–55.
77. Stalmans, S, N Bracke, E Wynendaele, B Gevaert, K Peremans, C Burvenich, I Polis, and B De Spiegeleer. "Cell-Penetrating Peptides Selectively Cross the Blood–Brain Barrier in vivo." *PLOS one* 10, no. 10 (2015): e0139652.

78. Zhou, X, QR Smith, and X Liu. "Brain Penetrating Peptides and Peptide-Drug Conjugates to Overcome the Blood–brain Barrier and Target CNS Diseases." *Wiley Interdisciplinary Reviews Nanomedicine Nanobiotechnology* 13, no. 4 (2021): e1695.
79. Pardridge, WM "Blood–Brain Barrier Delivery." *Drug Discovery Today* 12, no. 1–2 (2007): 54–61.
80. ———. "The Blood–Brain Barrier and Neurotherapeutics." *NeuroRx* 2, no. 1 (2005): 1–2.
81. Alam, MI, S Beg, A Samad, S Baboota, K Kohli, J Ali, A Ahuja, and M Akbar. "Strategy for Effective Brain Drug Delivery." *European Journal of Pharmaceutical Sciences* 40, no. 5 (2010): 385–403.
82. Kawakami, K, M Kawakami, M Kioi, SR Husain, and RK Puri. "Distribution Kinetics of Targeted Cytotoxin in Glioma by Bolus or Convection-Enhanced Delivery in a Murine Model." *Journal of Neurosurgery* 101, no. 6 (2004): 1004–11.
83. Nicholson, C, and E Syková. "Extracellular Space Structure Revealed by Diffusion Analysis." *Trends in Neurosciences* 21, no. 5 (1998): 207–15.
84. Gray, SJ, KT Woodard, and RJ Samulski. "Viral Vectors and Delivery Strategies for Cns Gene Therapy." *Therapeutic Delivery* 1, no. 4 (2010): 517–34.
85. Mingozzi, F, and KA High. "Immune Responses to AAV Vectors: Overcoming Barriers to Successful Gene Therapy." *Blood* 122, no. 1 (2013): 23–36.
86. Wang, Jingjing, and Liqin Zhang. "Retrograde Axonal Transport Property of Adeno-Associated Virus and Its Possible Application in Future." *Microbes and Infection* 23, no. 8 (2021): 104829.
87. Zielińska, A, B Costa, MV Ferreira, D Miguéis, JMS Louros, A Durazzo, M Lucarini, P Eder, MV Chaud, M Morsink, N Willemen, P Severino, A Santini, and EB Souto. "Nanotoxicology and Nanosafety: Safety-by-Design and Testing at a Glance." *International Journal of Environmental Research and Public Health* 17, no. 13 (2020).
88. Huang, L, and Y Liu. "In Vivo Delivery of RNAI with Lipid-Based Nanoparticles." *Annual Review of Biomedical Engineering* 13 (2011): 507–30.
89. Wang, Jin, Derek Chen, and Emmanuel A Ho. "Challenges in the Development and Establishment of Exosome-Based Drug Delivery Systems." *Journal of Controlled Release* 329 (2021): 894–906.
90. Yawalkar, Ankita N, Manoj A Pawar, and Pradeep R Vavia. "Microspheres for Targeted Drug Delivery – a Review on Recent Applications." *Journal of Drug Delivery Science and Technology* 75 (2022): 103659.
91. Li, J, and DJ Mooney. "Designing Hydrogels for Controlled Drug Delivery." *Natural Reviews Materials* 1, no. 12 (2016).
92. Alonso, JM, J Andrade Del Olmo, R Perez Gonzalez, and V Saez-Martinez. "Injectable Hydrogels: From Laboratory to Industrialization." *Polymers (Basel)* 13, no. 4 (2021).
93. Huynh, GH, DF Deen, and FC Szoka Jr. "Barriers to Carrier Mediated Drug and Gene Delivery to Brain Tumors." *Journal of Controlled Release* 110, no. 2 (2006): 236–59.
94. Patel, M, C McCully, K Godwin, and FM Balis. "Plasma and Cerebrospinal Fluid Pharmacokinetics of Intravenous Temozolomide in Non-Human Primates." *Journal of Neurooncology* 61, no. 3 (2003): 203–7.
95. Rautioa, J, and PJ Chikhale. "Drug Delivery Systems for Brain Tumor Therapy." *Current Pharmaceutical Design* 10, no. 12 (2004): 1341–53.
96. Bellavance, MA, M Blanchette, and D Fortin. "Recent Advances in Blood–Brain Barrier Disruption as a CNS Delivery Strategy." *AAPS Journal* 10, no. 1 (2008): 166–77.
97. Borlongan, CV, and DF Emerich. "Facilitation of Drug Entry into the CNS via Transient Permeation of Blood Brain Barrier: Laboratory and Preliminary Clinical Evidence from Bradykinin Receptor Agonist, Cereport." *Brain Research Bulletin* 60, no. 3 (2003): 297–306.

98. Chu, C, A Jablonska, Y Gao, X Lan, WG Lesniak, Y Liang, G Liu, S Li, T Magnus, M Pearl, M Janowski, and P Walczak. "Hyperosmolar Blood–Brain Barrier Opening Using Intra-Arterial Injection of Hyperosmotic Mannitol in Mice under Real-Time Mri Guidance." *Nature Protocols* 17, no. 1 (2022): 76–94.
99. Costantino, HR, L Illum, G Brandt, PH Johnson, and SC Quay. "Intranasal Delivery: Physicochemical and Therapeutic Aspects." *International Journal of Pharmaceutics* 337, no. 1–2 (2007): 1–24.
100. Ali, J, M Ali, S Baboota, JK Sahani, C Ramassamy, L Dao, and Bhavna. "Potential of Nanoparticulate Drug Delivery Systems by Intranasal Administration." *Current Pharmaceutical Design* 16, no. 14 (2010): 1644–53.
101. Illum, L. "Transport of Drugs from the Nasal Cavity to the Central Nervous System." *European Journal of Pharmaceutical Sciences* 11, no. 1 (2000): 1–18.
102. Li, Qing, Xinxin Shao, Xianglin Dai, Qiong Guo, Bolei Yuan, Ying Liu, and Wei Jiang. "Recent Trends in the Development of Hydrogel Therapeutics for the Treatment of Central Nervous System Disorders." *NPG Asia Materials* 14, no. 1 (2022): 14.
103. MacKay, JA, DF Deen, and FC Szoka Jr. "Distribution in Brain of Liposomes after Convection Enhanced Delivery; Modulation by Particle Charge, Particle Diameter, and Presence of Steric Coating." *Brain Research* 1035, no. 2 (2005): 139–53.
104. Groothuis, DR, H Benalcazar, CV Allen, RM Wise, C Dills, C Dobrescu, V Rothholtz, and RM Levy. "Comparison of Cytosine Arabinoside Delivery to Rat Brain by Intravenous, Intrathecal, Intraventricular and Intraparenchymal Routes of Administration." *Brain Research* 856, no. 1–2 (2000): 281–90.
105. Lo, EH, AB Singhal, VP Torchilin, and NJ Abbott. "Drug Delivery to Damaged Brain." *Brain Research Reviews* 38, no. 1–2 (2001): 140–8.
106. Savaraj, N., L. G. Feun, K. Lu, K. Gray, C. Wang, and T. L. Loo. "Pharmacology of Intrathecal Vp-1s 6–213 in Dogs." *J Neurooncol* 13, no. 3 (1992): 211–5.
107. Kerr, J. Z., S. Berg, and S. M. Blaney. "Intrathecal Chemotherapy." *Crit Rev Oncol Hematol* 37, no. 3 (2001): 227–36.
108. Rapoport, SI. "Osmotic Opening of the Blood–Brain Barrier: Principles, Mechanism, and Therapeutic Applications." *Cellular and Molecular Neurobiology* 20, no. 2 (2000): 217–30.
109. Fritze, K, C Sommer, B Schmitz, G Mies, KA Hossmann, M Kiessling, and C Wiessner. "Effect of Global System for Mobile Communication (GSM) Microwave Exposure on Blood–Brain Barrier Permeability in Rat." *Acta Neuropathologica* 94, no. 5 (1997): 465–70.
110. McDannold, N, N Vykhodtseva, and K Hynynen. "Use of Ultrasound Pulses Combined with Definity for Targeted Blood–Brain Barrier Disruption: A Feasibility Study." *Ultrasound in Medicine and Biology* 33, no. 4 (2007): 584–90.
111. Vykhodtseva, NI, K Hynynen, and C Damianou. "Histologic Effects of High Intensity Pulsed Ultrasound Exposure with Subharmonic Emission in Rabbit Brain in Vivo." *Ultrasound in Medicine and Biology* 21, no. 7 (1995): 969–79.
112. Unger, EC, T Porter, W Culp, R Labell, T Matsunaga, and R Zutshi. "Therapeutic Applications of Lipid-Coated Microbubbles." *Advanced Drug Delivery Reviews* 56, no. 9 (2004): 1291–314.
113. Muresan, Paula, Phoebe McCrorie, Fiona Smith, Catherine Vasey, Vincenzo Taresco, David J Scurr, Stefanie Kern, Stuart Smith, Pavel Gershkovich, Ruman Rahman, and Maria Marlow. "Development of Nanoparticle Loaded Microneedles for Drug Delivery to a Brain Tumour Resection Site." *European Journal of Pharmaceutics and Biopharmaceutics* 182 (2023): 53–61.

114. Hood, RL, RT Andriani Jr., S Emch, JL Robertson, CG Rylander, and JH Rossmeisl Jr. "Fiberoptic Microneedle Device Facilitates Volumetric Infusate Dispersion during Convection-Enhanced Delivery in the Brain." *Lasers in Surgery and Medicine* 45, no. 7 (2013): 418–26.
115. Pardridge, WM. "Brain Drug Targeting and Gene Technologies." *Japanese Journal of Pharmacology* 87, no. 2 (2001): 97–103.
116. Pardridge, WM, YS Kang, JL Buciak, and J Yang. "Human Insulin Receptor Monoclonal Antibody Undergoes High Affinity Binding to Human Brain Capillaries in vitro and Rapid Transcytosis through the Blood–Brain Barrier in vivo in the Primate." *Pharmaceutical Research* 12, no. 6 (1995): 807–16.
117. Li, JY, RJ Boado, and WM Pardridge. "Blood–Brain Barrier Genomics." *Journal of Cerebral Blood Flow and Metabolism* 21, no. 1 (2001): 61–8.
118. Kalluri, R, and VS LeBleu. "The Biology, Function, and Biomedical Applications of Exosomes." *Science* 367, no. 6478 (2020).
119. Haqqani, AS, CE Delaney, TL Tremblay, C Sodja, JK Sandhu, and D B. Stanimirovic. "Method for Isolation and Molecular Characterization of Extracellular Microvesicles Released from Brain Endothelial Cells." *Fluids Barriers of the CNS* 10, no. 1 (2013): 4.
120. Yang, T, B Fogarty, B LaForge, S Aziz, T Pham, L Lai, and S Bai. "Delivery of Small Interfering RNA to Inhibit Vascular Endothelial Growth Factor in Zebrafish Using Natural Brain Endothelia Cell-Secreted Exosome Nanovesicles for the Treatment of Brain Cancer." *AAPS Journal* 19, no. 2 (2017): 475–86.
121. Molema, G, RW Jansen, R Pauwels, E de Clercq, and DK Meijer. "Targeting of Antiviral Drugs to T4-Lymphocytes. Anti-HIV Activity of Neoglycoprotein-Aztmp Conjugates in Vitro." *Biochemical Pharmacology* 40, no. 12 (1990): 2603–10.
122. Prusiner, SB "Prions." *Proceedings of the National Academy of Sciences of the United States of America* 95, no. 23 (1998): 13363–83.
123. Prinz, M, M Heikenwalder, T Junt, P Schwarz, M Glatzel, FL Heppner, YX Fu, M Lipp, and A Aguzzi. "Positioning of Follicular Dendritic Cells within the Spleen Controls Prion Neuroinvasion." *Nature* 425, no. 6961 (2003): 957–62.
124. Vagner, T, A Dvorzhak, AM Wójtowicz, C Harms, and R Grantyn. "Systemic Application of AAV Vectors Targeting GFAP-Expressing Astrocytes in Z-Q175-Ki Huntington's Disease Mice." *Molecular and Cellular Neuroscience* 77 (2016): 76–86.
125. Samad, A, Y Sultana, and M Aqil. "Liposomal Drug Delivery Systems: An Update Review." *Current Drug Delivery* 4, no. 4 (2007): 297–305.
126. Duong, Van-An, Thi-Thao-Linh Nguyen, and Han-Joo Maeng. "Recent Advances in Intranasal Liposomes for Drug, Gene, and Vaccine Delivery." *Pharmaceutics* 15, no. 1 (2023): 207.
127. Barbu, E, E Molnàr, J Tsibouklis, and DC Górecki. "The Potential for Nanoparticle-Based Drug Delivery to the Brain: Overcoming the Blood–Brain Barrier." *Expert Opinion on Drug Delivery* 6, no. 6 (2009): 553–65.
128. Mistry, A, S Stolnik, and L Illum. "Nanoparticles for Direct Nose-to-Brain Delivery of Drugs." *International Journal of Pharmaceutics* 379, no. 1 (2009): 146–57.
129. Alli, Swapna, Sateesh Kumar Vemula, and Prabhakar Reddy Veerareddy. "Role of Microspheres in Drug Delivery-an Overview." *Drug Delivery Letters* 3, no. 3 (2013): 191–99.
130. Gao, Yang, Waleed H Almalki, Obaid Afzal, Sunil K Panda, Imran Kazmi, Majed Alrobaian, Hanadi A Katouah, Abdulmalik Saleh Alfawaz Altamimi, Fahad A Al-Abbasi, and Sultan Alshehri. "Systematic Development of Lectin Conjugated

Microspheres for Nose-to-Brain Delivery of Rivastigmine for the Treatment of Alzheimer's Disease." *Biomedicine & Pharmacotherapy* 141 (2021): 111829.

131. Gavini, Elisabetta, Giovanna Rassu, Luca Ferraro, Sarah Beggiato, Amjad Alhalaweh, Sitaram Velaga, Nicola Marchetti, Pasquale Bandiera, Paolo Giunchedi, and Alessandro Dalpiaz. "Influence of Polymeric Microcarriers on the in vivo Intranasal Uptake of an Anti-Migraine Drug for Brain Targeting." *European Journal of Pharmaceutics and Biopharmaceutics* 83, no. 2 (2013): 174–83.
132. Shaji, J, A Poddar, and S Iyer. "Brain-Targeted Nasal Clonazepam Microspheres." *Indian Journal of Pharmaceutical Sciences* 71, no. 6 (2009): 715.
133. Sun, Yu, Kai Shi, and Feng Wan. "Methotrexate-Loaded Microspheres for Nose to Brain Delivery: in vitro/in vivo Evaluation." *Journal of Drug Delivery Science and Technology* 22, no. 2 (2012): 167–74.

3 Advanced Drug-Delivery Systems for Brain Diseases across the Blood–Brain Barrier

K. Trideva Sastri, Hitesh Kumar, Arshad J. Ansari, Anurag Kumar Singh, and Iliyas Khan

3.1 INTRODUCTION

3.1.1 Targeting Concepts for Drug Delivery

3.1.1.1 Passive Targeting

Passive targeting exploits the natural properties of the drug delivery system to passively accumulate at the site of action, which offers several advantages over active targeting mechanisms [1]. Nanoparticles can be engineered to be small enough to surpass the blood–brain barrier (BBB) and attain high concentrations in the brain. The modified surface of these nanoparticles with molecules can increase their affinity for the BBB, such as polyethylene glycol (PEG), which can enhance their circulation time in the bloodstream and reduce their clearance by the immune system. Several studies have demonstrated the potential of the nanoparticles for their passive targeting ability for managing innumerable brain diseases and other disorders [2].

Liposomes are another drug delivery system that passively accumulates at sites of inflammation due to the increased permeability of blood vessels in inflamed tissue. This accumulation can be further enhanced by modifying the surface of the liposome with suitable targeting ligands that recognize specific receptors on inflammatory cells. Liposomes have great potential for treating various inflammatory disorders, such as rheumatoid arthritis and Crohn's disease [3]. Solid lipid nanoparticles (SLNs) are a type of nanoparticle that can passively accumulate at sites of infection or inflammation due to augmented permeation and retention. In addition, SLNs can be designed to release therapeutic molecules as a reaction to explicit triggers, such as alterations in pH or temperature, which can further enhance their therapeutic efficacy. SLNs have shown potential for treating various infectious diseases, such as tuberculosis and leishmaniasis [4]. Passive targeting is a promising drug delivery strategy with several advantages over active targeting mechanisms. By utilizing the natural properties of the drug delivery system, passive targeting can improve drug delivery efficiency and reduce toxicity, improving the therapeutic efficacy of drugs and enhancing patient outcomes. One of the significant advantages of passive targeting for crossing the

DOI: 10.1201/9781032661964-3

BBB is the ease of manufacturing and scalability. Passive targeting does not require targeting ligands or complex drug delivery systems, making it a more straightforward and cost-effective approach [5].

3.1.1.2 Active Targeting

Active targeting is a promising strategy for delivering drugs through the BBB to manage brain disorders. Active targeting can enhance drug delivery efficiency and specificity by targeting ligands to recognize and bind to receptors on the surface of brain cells. One approach for actively targeting the BBB is to use antibodies or peptides as targeting ligands. The transferrin receptor is significantly expressed on the surface of brain capillary endothelial cells comprising the BBB. Targeting the transferrin receptor with transferrin or antibodies against the transferrin receptor has been shown to enhance drug delivery across the BBB in animal models of brain diseases. Similarly, peptides targeting the BBB, such as the rabies virus glycoprotein (RVG) peptide, also exhibits their affinity towards the brain, which is quite impressive [6]. Liposomes and nanoparticles can be modified to transport the drug molecules across the BBB. These drug delivery systems facilitate functionalization by targeting ligands, like antibodies or peptides, to enhance their specificity for brain cells. Additionally, the surface can be modified so that it can trigger the release of drugs in response to specific stimuli, such as enzymes or pH changes, to enhance their therapeutic efficacy [7]. Therefore, the significant advantages of active targeting for crossing the BBB is the ability to enhance drug delivery efficiency through targeting moieties [8, 9].

3.1.1.3 Intracellular Targeting

Intracellular targeting can be achieved through several mechanisms, including receptor-mediated endocytosis, macropinocytosis, and caveolae-mediated endocytosis. Receptor-mediated endocytosis involves binding a ligand to a specific receptor on the target cell's surface, followed by internalization of the ligand-receptor complex into the cell through endocytosis. Macropinocytosis involves the cell's nonspecific uptake of fluid and solutes by forming large intracellular vesicles. Caveolae-mediated endocytosis involves the internalization of cargo by forming small vesicles that bud off from invaginated caveolae on the cell membrane [10]. To facilitate drug delivery across the BBB for brain diseases, intracellular targeting mechanisms can be explored by functionalizing drug delivery systems, such as nanoparticles or liposomes, with targeting molecules that can interact with specific receptors or antigens on the surface of brain cells, such as neurons or glia cells. These targeting molecules can be designed to specifically bind to receptors or antigens expressed at higher levels in the BBB or brain tissue, allowing for increased uptake of the drug delivery system by brain cells. Nanoparticles' positive surface charges, facilitate their interaction with negatively charged cell membranes and their internalization into cells through endocytosis [11]. Intracellular targeting for delivering therapeutic molecules via the BBB can revolutionize the treatment of brain diseases by enabling more effective and targeted drug delivery to the site of action [12].

Biocompatibility is crucial as the drug delivery system must be designed not to cause an immune response or any toxicity issues. Additionally, stability during storage and transportation is essential to maintain the therapeutic efficacy of the drug delivery system. Targeting efficiency is another critical factor, as the drug delivery system must reach the intended site of action while minimizing uptake by non-target tissues or organs. One approach to enhance targeting efficiency is optimizing the delivery system's physicochemical properties, like size and shape, besides surface charge [13]. Controlled release is another significant factor to consider in designing drug delivery systems. Biodegradable polymers can also enhance biocompatibility and allow for sustained drug release. Quality control measures can also be employed to ensure the consistency and stability of drug delivery systems during manufacturing [14]. Despite the challenges associated with designing drug delivery systems for brain diseases, continued research and development can help overcome these challenges, producing safe and effective drug-delivery strategies for treating brain diseases [15,16].

3.2 FUNCTIONALIZATION CONCEPTS FOR ENHANCED BRAIN TARGETING

3.2.1 Ligand-Mediated Targeting

Ligand-mediated targeting involves attaching a ligand to a drug molecule, which allows it to attach receptors in the BBB. The ligand-receptor interaction triggers receptor-mediated endocytosis, which enables the transportation of therapeutic molecules through the BBB and to reach the brain [15]. There are several factors to consider in designing a ligand targeting the BBB. The ligand must possess a high affinity for the receptor to ensure efficient and specific binding. Another critical factor is the size and shape of the ligand. The ligand should be small enough to penetrate the BBB but large enough to provide stable binding to the receptor. The shape of the ligand can also play a role in receptor binding, as receptors often have specific binding sites that require a particular shape or conformation. The chemical properties of the ligand can also impact its effectiveness in targeting the BBB. Lipophilic ligands are often more effective at penetrating the BBB than hydrophilic ligands. However, lipophilic ligands can also have higher toxicity and be more difficult to remove from the body [17]. During receptor-mediated endocytosis, the cell membrane invaginates around the ligand-bound drug, forming a vesicle. The vesicle is then transported through the BBB and released into the brain's extracellular fluid. The drug can then diffuse into nearby neurons or glial cells, where it can exert its therapeutic effects. By choosing a ligand that binds to a receptor which is only expressed in some brain regions, the drug can be delivered directly to those areas while minimizing exposure to other regions. This can reduce the risk of side effects and improve the drug's efficacy [18].

3.2.2 Antibody-Mediated Targeting

This technique involves using antibodies to specifically target and bind to proteins or receptors in the BBB. Attaching a drug molecule to an antibody can allow the antibody to be transported across the BBB and into the brain [19]. Antibodies are large molecules that can recognize and bind to specific proteins or receptors with high specificity and affinity. This property makes them an attractive tool for selectively delivering drugs to the brain. This is achieved through a process known as antibody engineering, which involves modifying the structure of antibodies to increase their specificity and binding affinity [20]. Once the antibody has been designed and produced, it is conjugated into a drug molecule. The conjugation process involves attaching the drug molecule to the antibody using a linker molecule. This linker molecule can be designed to be stable in the bloodstream but can also be cleaved once the antibody-drug conjugate reaches its target in the brain. The internalized antibody-drug conjugate is then moved through the BBB and into the brain's extracellular fluid, where the drug can exert its therapeutic effects [21]. By selecting an antibody that binds to a protein or receptor which is only expressed in some brain regions, the drug can be delivered directly to those areas while minimizing exposure to other regions. This can reduce the risk of side effects and improve the drug's efficacy. Another advantage of antibody-mediated targeting is its potential for increased drug penetration into the brain [22]. However, antibody-mediated targeting also has some limitations, namely, immunogenicity, as the immune system may recognize the antibody-drug conjugate as a foreign substance and mount an immune response [23].

3.2.3 pH-Sensitive Functionalization

The pH-sensitive functionalization technique for enhanced uptake and brain targeting involves designing drug delivery systems that respond to the lower pH environment at the BBB and release the drug payload [24]. One approach is to use pH-sensitive nanoparticles or liposomes. These particles can be functionalized with pH-sensitive groups such as poly(ethylene glycol) (PEG) or poly(L-histidine). PEG is a hydrophilic polymer that can prevent particle aggregation and clearance by the immune system. Poly(L-histidine) is a pH-sensitive polymer that can protonate at lower pH values, causing the nanoparticles to release their cargo. When these particles reach the lower pH environment at the BBB, the poly(L-histidine)'s protonation triggers the drug payload's release. Another approach is using pH-sensitive chemical modifications to functionalize the drug molecule. Prodrug formulations activated by the lower pH at the BBB can be designed to release the active drug molecule. A prodrug approach was designed in which 5-fluorouracil (5-FU) contained a pH-sensitive hydrazone bond between the drug molecule and a targeting moiety. The hydrazone bond is stable at neutral pH but is hydrolyzed at lower pH values, releasing the active drug molecule [25]. The pH-sensitive linker molecules can connect the drug molecule to a targeting moiety, such as a peptide or antibody. These linker molecules contain pH-sensitive bonds that can be cleaved at the lower pH environment at the BBB, releasing the drug payload. pH-sensitive functionalization can also be used to target specific cell types in the brain. When the peptide-conjugated drug reaches the target cell, the lower pH in the endosomal compartment can trigger drug release. A pH-sensitive peptide conjugated to a doxorubicin molecule was designed to target glioblastoma cells. The peptide-conjugate was shown to release the doxorubicin in response to the lower pH in the endosomal compartment, resulting in improved cytotoxicity against the cancer cells [26]. The pH-sensitive functionalization technique for enhanced uptake and brain targeting involves designing drug delivery systems that respond to the BBB's lower pH environment and release the drug payload [27,28].

3.3 ADVANCED TECHNOLOGIES FOR ENHANCING DRUG DELIVERY THROUGH BBB

3.3.1 Ultrasound-Mediated BBB Disruption

Ultrasound-mediated BBB disruption technology is a cutting-edge approach for improving drug delivery to the brain [29]. Ultrasound-mediated BBB disruption is a non-invasive and targeted technique that has shown the potential to overcome the limitations of traditional drug delivery methods. This technique involves applying focused ultrasound waves to the targeted brain region at 500 kHz to 1.5 MHz frequency. These frequencies enable the waves to penetrate the skull and reach the brain tissue. The application of ultrasound waves leads to microbubbles within the blood vessels of the BBB. The microbubbles expand and contract, creating small gaps in the tight junctions between the endothelial cells of the BBB. The disruption of these tight junctions leads to increased permeability of the BBB, allowing therapeutic agents to pass through and reach the brain parenchyma. This process is reversible, and the BBB returns to its normal state within a few hours [30]. Moreover, this technique has shown promise for treating various neurological disorders, including Alzheimer's disease, Parkinson's disease, and brain tumours [31].

3.3.2 Microbubble-Mediated

Microbubble-mediated drug delivery technology is an innovative approach that harnesses the physical properties of microbubbles and ultrasound waves to enhance drug delivery across the BBB [32]. Microbubble-mediated drug delivery technology involves using microbubbles, which are small gas-filled particles combined with ultrasound waves to disrupt the BBB and allow drugs to pass through temporarily. The microbubbles are injected intravenously and targeted to specific areas of the brain using focused ultrasound waves. The ultrasound waves create microscopic vibrations in the microbubbles, which cause them to oscillate and temporarily open gaps in the BBB, allowing drugs to pass through and reach the brain [33]. The microbubbles are designed to be small enough to pass through the capillaries of the BBB and stable enough to withstand the ultrasound waves. The ultrasound waves are targeted to specific brain areas, and the disruption is precise and localized. Unlike traditional drug delivery methods to the brain, such as direct injection or implantation of drug delivery devices, this technique does not require surgery. As a result, patients have a safer and less invasive option with a lower chance of consequences [34]. Moreover, this technique has been shown to have a high level of selectivity towards specific brain areas [35].

3.3.3 Magnetophoretic Mediated

The BBB is essential for maintaining a stable and consistent environment for the brain, but it also prevents most substances, including many drugs, from entering the brain tissue. Researchers have been developing various strategies to enhance drug delivery across the BBB to overcome this obstacle. One of the most promising approaches is magnetophoresis, which uses magnetic fields to guide drug-loaded magnetic particles across the BBB and into the brain tissue [36]. The size and surface properties of the magnetic particles are carefully optimized to ensure efficient and safe drug delivery [37]. The magnetic particles are then injected into the bloodstream, where they circulate and are attracted to the targeted area of the brain by an external magnet. The external magnet is typically positioned outside the body. Its strength and direction are adjusted to ensure the magnetic particles are guided to the desired location in the brain tissue. Once the magnetic particles reach the target area, they can be dissociated from the drug molecules, releasing the drug and enabling it to exert its therapeutic effect. Several technicalities must be considered when using magnetophoresis for drug delivery across the BBB. Firstly, the size of the magnetic particles is critical, as they should be small enough to pass through the narrow gaps between the endothelial cells of the BBB but not too small that the body's immune system rapidly clears them [38]. Secondly, the strength and direction of the magnetic field are important factors that affect the efficiency and specificity of drug delivery [39]. Thirdly, the coating of the magnetic particles should be carefully chosen to minimize any immunogenicity and toxicity [40].

3.3.4 Laser-Guided Technology

Laser-guided technology relies on focused laser energy to create transient and reversible openings in the BBB, allowing drugs to pass through and into the brain. The mechanism of action for laser-guided technology involves using a laser to create localized heating of a targeted area of the BBB [41]. To achieve this, a laser system is used to focus laser light onto a specific area of the skull, penetrating through the skull and brain tissue to create a small, precise, and controlled opening in the BBB. The size and duration of the opening can be controlled by adjusting the laser parameters, such as the laser's energy, duration, and wavelength. Laser-guided technology has several advantages over other drug delivery methods, such as being non-invasive and not requiring invasive surgical procedures. It also offers a high degree of precision and control over the location and size of the opening in the BBB, allowing targeted therapeutic molecules to reach certain brain regions [42]. Despite the promising potential of laser-guided technology for drug delivery, several technical challenges still need to be addressed before it can become a reliable and effective method for enhancing drug delivery across the BBB. Further research is required in order to evaluate fully the safety and efficacy of this approach. The potential benefits of a non-invasive, precise, and targeted drug delivery method to the brain make laser-guided technology an exciting area of research in neuroscience and pharmacology [43,44].

3.3.5 Transcranial Magnetic Stimulation (TMS)

TMS has promising prospects as a non-invasive and targeted method for delivering drugs to the brain. One possible mechanism for TMS-mediated enhancement of drug delivery across the BBB is the disruption of the tight junctions between endothelial cells forming the BBB. TMS has been shown to transiently alter the electrical properties of the BBB, potentially increasing its permeability. This effect has been observed in animal models, where TMS has been shown to increase the uptake of small molecules into the brain. Another possible mechanism is the induction of a transient increase in blood flow to the targeted area of the brain. TMS has been shown to induce changes in regional cerebral blood flow, which could potentially increase and facilitate drugs to the targeted area of the brain. This effect has been observed in human studies, where TMS has been shown to increase blood flow to specific brain regions, as measured by functional magnetic resonance imaging (fMRI). A third possible mechanism is the modulation of endogenous substances, such as growth factors or cytokines, that can modify the BBB and enhance drug delivery. TMS has been shown to stimulate the release of various substances, including brain-derived neurotrophic factor (BDNF), which has been shown to increase the permeability of the BBB [45]. TMS may alter the pharmacokinetics and pharmacodynamics of the drugs themselves, potentially leading to unintended effects or toxicity [46]. The promising advantages of a non-invasive and precisely targeted drug delivery approach to the brain render TMS a captivating field of investigation in the realms of neuroscience and pharmacology [47]. A schematicrepresentation of various technologies for enhancing drug delivery via the BBB is shown in Figure 3.1.

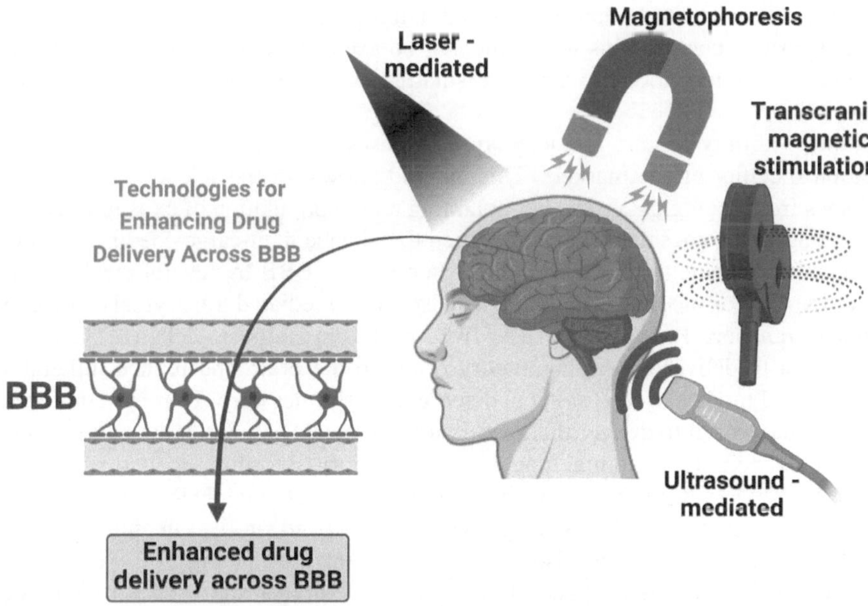

FIGURE 3.1 Various technologies for enhancing drug delivery via BBB.

3.4 ADVANCED DRUG DELIVERY SYSTEMS FOR BRAIN DISEASE

3.4.1 Exosomes

Exosomes are small membrane-bound vesicles ranging in size from 30 to 150 nm and comprising a lipid bilayer that encapsulates a cargo of proteins, lipids, and nucleic acids. Exosomes play a vital role in intercellular communication by transferring their cargo from one cell to another, allowing for the exchange of information between cells in different tissues and organs throughout the body. They have been implicated in various biological processes, including immune response, tissue regeneration, and cancer progression. In recent years, exosomes have gained significant attention as potential drug delivery vehicles due to their unique characteristics, such as biocompatibility, stability, and low immunogenicity [48]. Exosomes naturally target specific cells and tissues in the body, making them ideal candidates for delivering therapeutic drugs directly to the site of action. Exosomes can be engineered to carry specific cargo, such as drugs, proteins, or nucleic acids, by modifying the donor cells or directly loading them into the exosomes. Various techniques, such as electroporation, sonication, and chemical treatment, can load drugs into exosomes [49].

Exosomes also have a long half-life in circulation, which allows them to deliver drugs over an extended period, increasing their therapeutic efficacy [50]. Exosomes can be prepared from various sources, including cell culture supernatants, blood plasma, urine, and other bodily fluids. Differential ultracentrifugation is the most commonly used technique for exosome isolation. It involves a series of centrifugation steps at increasing speeds to separate the different types of extracellular vesicles based on their size and density. This technique can yield a pure population of exosomes, but it is time-consuming and requires specialized equipment. Size-exclusion chromatography is another method for exosome isolation that separates exosomes based on their size and surface charge. This technique can be used to isolate pure populations of exosomes, but it may not be suitable for isolating exosomes from complex biological fluids [51].

Immuno-affinity capture is a technique that uses antibodies to capture exosomes based on specific surface markers. This method allows for the selective isolation of exosomes from biological fluids, but obtaining a pure population of exosomes can be challenging. Exosomes can also be modified to enhance their cargo-loading capacity and targeting specificity [52]. Exosomes can cross the BBB by several mechanisms, including receptor-mediated transcytosis, adsorptive-mediated transcytosis, and cell-mediated transport. Exosomes derived from mesenchymal stem cells (MSCs) have been shown to deliver anti-inflammatory drugs to the brain and reduce inflammation in animal models of neurological disorders. Exosomes derived from neural stem cells have been used to deliver therapeutic RNA molecules to the brain and promote neuronal regeneration in animal models of brain injury. Exosomes loaded with small interfering RNA (siRNA) have also been shown to target and silence genes in brain tumours, leading to reduced tumour growth and improved survival in animal models [53]. Lipid modifications can also be used to enhance the binding of exosomes to the BBB and improve their uptake into brain cells. Another approach is to engineer the exosomes to express specific proteins or RNA molecules that can enhance their uptake into brain cells or target specific cell types in the brain [54].

3.4.2 Biomimetic Nanoparticles

Biomimetic nanoparticles are drug-delivery systems designed to mimic the properties and functions of natural biomolecules, such as proteins, lipids, and carbohydrates. These nanoparticles can be engineered to carry and deliver drugs to specific target sites in the body, including cancer cells and diseased tissues, while minimizing damage to healthy cells and tissues. Biomimetic nanoparticles can be produced from various natural and synthetic materials, including lipids, polymers, and metals. These materials can be modified with specific functional groups, such as peptides or antibodies, to enhance their targeting and delivery properties [55].

One of the advantages of biomimetic nanoparticles is their ability to mimic the natural biological processes involved in drug delivery. Some nanoparticles are designed to mimic the behavior of lipoproteins, which are natural transporters of cholesterol and other lipids in the body. These nanoparticles can be used to carry drugs that are insoluble in water, such as anticancer drugs, and deliver them to cancer cells. Many nanoparticles are coated with a layer of polyethylene glycol (PEG), which can prevent recognition and clearance by immune cells in the body. This can improve the circulation time of the nanoparticles and increase their accumulation at target sites [56].

Nanoparticles are designed to release their cargo in response to changes in pH, such as in tumour cells. It can improve the efficiency and specificity of drug delivery and reduce side effects. In addition to their potential for drug delivery, biomimetic nanoparticles have applications in diagnostic imaging and therapeutic monitoring. Some nanoparticles are designed to carry contrast agents for imaging modalities such as MRI or CT scans, allowing for improved visualization of target tissues. Others can be designed to respond to specific disease biomarkers, such as elevated levels of certain enzymes or proteins, and release therapeutic agents in response to these biomarkers [57].

The transferrin receptor (TfR) is highly expressed on the BBB, and nanoparticles functionalized with transferrin or antibodies that target TfR can effectively cross the BBB and deliver drugs to brain tissue. Other receptors, such as insulin and low-density lipoprotein, have also been targeted with biomimetic nanoparticles for brain delivery [58]. Another approach is to use stimuli-responsive nanoparticles that can cross the BBB in response to specific environmental cues in the brain. In one study, pH-sensitive nanoparticles composed of lipids and polymers were designed to release their cargo in response to the lower pH in the brain compared to the blood, allowing for more targeted and efficient drug delivery. In addition to their targeting properties, biomimetic nanoparticles can also be designed to carry a variety of drugs for neurological disorders, including small molecules, peptides, and nucleic acids [59]. Ongoing research is focused on developing and optimizing these systems for various applications, including drug delivery to specific brain regions and treatment of complex neurological disorders [60].

3.4.3 Magnetic-Targeting Delivery Systems

The principle of magnetic targeting delivery systems (MTDS) involves using a magnetic field to guide magnetic nanoparticles (MNPs) loaded with therapeutic agents across the BBB and to specific brain regions. The MNPs used in MTDS are typically composed of iron oxide or cobalt ferrite and are coated with biocompatible materials such as polymers, lipids, or proteins. The MNPs are designed to be stable and biocompatible and can be functionalized with targeting ligands to enhance their BBB penetration and target specific brain regions. To enhance the BBB penetration and targeting of MNPs, they can be functionalized with specific ligands such as antibodies, peptides, or aptamers that recognize and bind to receptors on the BBB or target cells within the brain tissue. This can increase the efficiency and specificity of MTDS, reducing off-target effects and improving therapeutic efficacy [61]. The magnetic field used in MTDS can be generated using an external magnetic source, such as a magnetic coil or an implanted magnetic device that can be remotely controlled. The strength and duration of the magnetic field can be optimized to achieve the desired drug delivery efficiency and reduce the potential for adverse effects. MTDS has shown promising results in preclinical studies for treating various neurological disorders such as brain tumours, Alzheimer's disease, and Parkinson's disease. In a study on the treatment of glioblastoma, MNPs loaded with the chemotherapy drug doxorubicin were combined with an external magnetic field to achieve targeted drug delivery to the tumour site, resulting in improved therapeutic efficacy and reduced systemic toxicity [62]. The most commonly used techniques are chemical precipitation, co-precipitation, solvothermal synthesis, and thermal decomposition [63]. In the chemical precipitation method, iron salts such as iron chloride or iron nitrate are reacted with a base such as ammonium hydroxide in the presence of a stabilizer to form MNPs. The co-precipitation method involves the simultaneous precipitation of iron salts and a dopant such as cobalt, manganese, or nickel to form MNPs with improved magnetic properties. This method can produce MNPs with a high magnetic moment and good crystallinity, but the resulting MNPs may have a broad size distribution. They may require additional processing steps to achieve a narrow size distribution. Solvothermal synthesis involves the reaction of iron salts with a reducing agent such as hydrazine or sodium borohydride in a high-pressure and high-temperature environment in the presence of a surfactant to form MNPs. This method can produce MNPs with high crystallinity and a narrow size distribution, but it is more complex and expensive than other methods. Thermal decomposition involves heating an iron precursor in the presence of a surfactant at a high temperature to form MNPs. This method can produce MNPs with a narrow size distribution and high crystallinity, but it can also result in MNPs with low yield and poor reproducibility [64]. Once the MNPs are synthesized, they can be coated with biocompatible polymers, lipids, or proteins to improve their stability, biocompatibility, and targeting efficiency. The coating material can also be functionalized with targeting ligands such as antibodies, peptides, or aptamers to enhance BBB penetration and the brain targeting of MNPs. Despite their promising potential for brain drug delivery, MTDS-using MNPs face several challenges. One of the significant challenges is the specificity and efficiency of targeting the MNPs to the brain across the BBB. While the magnetic field can direct the MNPs towards the brain, the BBB presents a significant barrier that limits their penetration. The size and surface chemistry of the MNPs can affect their interaction with the BBB and their ability to cross it. Additionally, the complex and heterogeneous nature of the brain tissue can further complicate their targeting and distribution. Another challenge is the potential toxicity and biocompatibility of the MNPs. MNPs in the body may induce inflammation, oxidative stress, and immune responses. The surface coating and functionalization of the MNPs can mitigate some of these effects. However, their long-term safety and potential accumulation in the brain tissue must be thoroughly investigated. Furthermore, the magnetic field required for the MTDS may cause heat generation and tissue damage, particularly at high field strengths or prolonged exposure times. The choice of MNP size, concentration, and coating can affect the magnetic properties and heat generation of the MNPs [65]. Finally, the cost and scalability of producing MNPs with the required properties for brain drug delivery can be challenging. Some synthesis methods may be too complex or expensive for large-scale production, and specific targeting ligands or coatings may further increase the cost. In summary, while MTDS using MNPs holds excellent promise for brain drug delivery, several challenges need to be addressed, including BBB penetration, biocompatibility, heat generation, and production cost. Addressing these challenges will require further research and development in the field [66,67].

3.4.4 CRISPR-Cas9 Gene Editing Technology

CRISPR-Cas9 is a revolutionary gene-editing tool that has revolutionized the field of genetic engineering. The first part of the term stands for Clustered Regularly Interspaced Short Palindromic Repeats, and Cas9 is the protein that acts as the molecular "scissors" to cut the DNA strands at precise locations. Recently, a new gene-editing technology called CRISPR-Cas13 was developed, commonly known as CRISPR-CasRx or CRISPR-CasRxn. This new system is based on the same principles as CRISPR-Cas9, but instead of cutting DNA, it targets and cleaves RNA. CRISPR-Cas13 uses a guide RNA (gRNA) to direct the Cas13 protein to a specific RNA sequence, which cleaves the RNA. This can be used to target and destroy specific RNA sequences, which can be helpful in various applications, including gene expression regulation, RNA virus detection, and diagnostics. One of the most exciting potential applications of CRISPR-Cas13 is in the field of cancer therapy. Cancer cells often overexpress specific RNA sequences that are not present in healthy cells. Targeting these sequences with CRISPR-Cas13 could provide a targeted and specific way to kill cancer cells while leaving healthy cells unharmed. Another potential application of CRISPR-Cas13 is treating genetic diseases caused by RNA mutations. Targeting and cleaving the mutant RNA may be possible in order to correct the disease-causing mutation and restore normal function. Despite its potential, CRISPR-Cas13 is still a relatively new technology, and much research is needed to fully understand its capabilities and limitations. Additionally, as with any gene-editing technology, there are ethical considerations to be taken into account, particularly in the case of editing germline cells, which could have permanent and heritable effects on future generations [68]. CRISPR-Cas9 gene editing has the potential to revolutionize the treatment of brain diseases by enabling precise and targeted modifications of disease-causing genes in the brain. One promising approach for using CRISPR-Cas9 in the brain is to deliver the gene-editing machinery directly to the affected brain cells using viral vectors. These vectors can target specific types of brain cells, such as neurons or glial cells, and deliver the CRISPR-Cas9 system to them. Once inside the cells, the system can target and modify disease-causing genes, such as those responsible for producing abnormal proteins in Alzheimer's disease. Another approach is using CRISPR-Cas9 to modify genes outside the brain that indirectly affect brain function. For example, mutations in the C9orf72 gene have been linked to both amyotrophic lateral sclerosis (ALS) and frontotemporal dementia, two neurodegenerative diseases that affect the brain. By using CRISPR-Cas9 to modify the C9orf72 gene in other parts of the body, such as the liver, it may be possible to indirectly modify its effects on the brain and slow the progression of these diseases. Despite the promising potential of CRISPR-Cas9 for treating brain diseases, many challenges still need to be overcome. One major challenge is developing safe and effective delivery methods targeting specific types of brain cells without causing damage or inflammation. Nonetheless, with ongoing research and development, CRISPR-Cas9 gene editing holds great promise for treating brain diseases [69]. Advanced drug delivery systems offer several promising approaches for delivering CRISPR-Cas9 to the brain. Several types of nanoparticles have been developed for this purpose, including lipid nanoparticles, polymeric nanoparticles, and dendrimers [70]. Lipid nanoparticles have been shown to deliver CRISPR-Cas9 to the brain when efficiently administered intravenously. These nanoparticles can be designed to target specific types of brain cells, such as neurons or glial cells, and can be loaded with the CRISPR-Cas9 system to enable precise gene editing. Polymeric nanoparticles, conversely, offer the advantage of being highly customizable. They can be engineered to have specific sizes, shapes, and surface properties, which can be tailored to optimize their delivery to the brain. Polymeric nanoparticles can also be functionalized with targeting moieties, such as antibodies or peptides, to improve their specificity and efficiency. Dendrimers are another type of nanoparticle investigated for delivering CRISPR-Cas9 to the brain. These nanoparticles have a highly branched structure and can be synthesized with a high degree of control over their size and surface properties. They can also be functionalized by targeting moieties or other molecules, such as siRNA or drug molecules, to enhance their therapeutic potential [71]. Viral vectors, such as an adeno-associated virus (AAV) and lentivirus, have been widely used for gene therapy applications and offer several advantages for delivering CRISPR-Cas9 to the brain. These vectors can be engineered to target specific types of brain cells and deliver large DNA payloads. However, they can also elicit immune responses and may have limitations regarding their safety and specificity. Cell-penetrating peptides (CPPs) are another strategy for delivering CRISPR-Cas9 to the brain. These short peptides can cross the BBB and enter cells, including neurons and glial cells. CPPs can be conjugated to the CRISPR-Cas9 system to enable targeted gene editing [72]. In addition to nanoparticles, other advanced drug delivery systems investigated for delivering CRISPR-Cas9 to the brain include viral vectors, cell-penetrating peptides, and exosomes. Each approach has advantages and limitations, and ongoing research is needed to optimize their effectiveness and safety for clinical use. Overall, advanced drug delivery systems offer promising approaches for delivering CRISPR-Cas9 to the brain to treat neurological diseases [73].

3.4.5 Green Synthesis and Nanotechnology-Based Drug Delivery Systems

These approaches use naturally occurring materials and eco-friendly synthesis techniques to develop drug delivery systems that effectively target the brain while minimizing toxicity and adverse effects [74]. Green synthesis involves using plant extracts, microbes, and other natural sources to synthesize nanoparticles for drug delivery. This approach offers several advantages, including low cost, biodegradability, and biocompatibility. Plant extracts, in particular, have been shown to contain various natural compounds that can be used to synthesize nanoparticles with specific properties for drug delivery. Green nanotechnology involves using sustainable and environmentally friendly approaches to design and manufacture nanomaterials for drug delivery. This includes the use of biodegradable and biocompatible materials, as well as the development of eco-friendly manufacturing processes that minimize waste and energy consumption. Several green syntheses and nanotechnology-based drug delivery systems have been developed for brain targeting across the BBB. Gold nanoparticles synthesized using green tea extract have been shown to effectively cross the BBB and deliver therapeutic molecules to the brain. Similarly, chitosan nanoparticles derived from crustacean shells effectively deliver drugs to the brain [75]. These drug-delivery systems can be engineered to target specific cell types in the brain. They can be loaded with therapeutic molecules to treat various brain disorders, including Alzheimer's disease, Parkinson's disease, and brain tumours. Despite the potential benefits of green synthesis and nanotechnology-based drug delivery systems, several challenges must be addressed. These include optimizing the synthesis and manufacturing processes, improving the stability and efficiency of the drug delivery systems, and ensuring safety and biocompatibility [76]. Overall, green synthesis and nanotechnology-based drug delivery systems offer a promising approach for targeting the brain across the BBB in a sustainable and environmentally friendly manner. Ongoing research and development are needed to further refine these approaches and enable their translation into clinical practice for treating brain disorders [77]. Preparation techniques for green synthesis and nanotechnology-based drug delivery systems vary depending on the material used and the specific application.

The plant extracts contain phytochemicals such as flavonoids, terpenoids, and phenolic compounds that act as reducing agents to convert metal ions into nanoparticles. The resulting nanoparticles can then be coated with polymers to improve their stability and biocompatibility. Solvent evaporation involves using organic solvents to dissolve a polymer and a drug, followed by the evaporation of the solvent to produce nanoparticles, while emulsion methods involve forming an emulsion of a polymer and a drug in an aqueous phase, followed by adding a cross-linking agent to form nanoparticles. Supercritical fluid methods involve using supercritical carbon dioxide as a solvent to dissolve a polymer and a drug, followed by the expansion of the carbon dioxide to produce nanoparticles [78]. By utilizing natural materials and eco-friendly manufacturing techniques, these systems can reduce the environmental impact of drug delivery while also providing effective and safe treatment options for brain disorders. Developing green synthesis and nanotechnology-based drug delivery systems for brain targeting across the BBB is challenging and requires overcoming several obstacles. One of the main challenges is the lack of standardization in the preparation techniques, which can lead to variability in the performance of different systems. To overcome this challenge, researchers can work towards developing standardized protocols that can be used to prepare green synthesis and green nanotechnology-based drug delivery systems. This will help increase the results' reproducibility and enable comparison between different systems. Another challenge is the limited scalability of some preparation techniques. Many techniques used to prepare green synthesis and nanotechnology-based drug delivery systems are still in the research and development stage. They may not be easily scaled up for large-scale production. To overcome this challenge, researchers can focus on developing scalable preparation techniques that can be easily adapted for large-scale production [79]. In addition, the limited stability of some green synthesis and nanotechnology-based drug delivery systems is also a significant challenge. These systems may degrade over time, impacting their efficacy and safety. To overcome this challenge, researchers can explore different coating and surface modification techniques to improve the stability of these systems and increase their shelf life. Limited biocompatibility is another challenge in developing green synthesis and green nanotechnology-based drug delivery systems for brain targeting across the BBB. Some of these systems may not be compatible with the human body, which can lead to adverse effects. To overcome this challenge, researchers can explore different materials and surface modifications to improve the biocompatibility of these systems. Researchers can work towards optimizing these systems' size and surface properties using techniques such as surface modification, functionalization, and engineering. In summary, developing green synthesis and nanotechnology-based drug delivery systems for brain targeting across the BBB faces several challenges. However, these can be overcome by developing standardized preparation techniques, scalability, stability, biocompatibility, and optimizing the size and surface properties of the systems [80].

3.4.6 Photo-Stimulated Drug Delivery Systems

These systems utilize photosensitizers that generate reactive oxygen species upon activation by specific wavelengths of light. The reactive oxygen species can trigger the release of a drug from a drug carrier, such as a liposome or nanoparticle. The use of light allows for precise control over drug release and can target specific cells or tissues in the brain while minimizing damage to surrounding healthy tissue [81]. One standard method for creating light-activated drug delivery systems involves using gold nanoparticles. Gold nanoparticles can be conjugated into a drug and a photosensitizer and targeted to specific cells or tissues in the brain using antibodies or other targeting agents. Once the nanoparticles reach their target site, they can be activated by a particular wavelength of light, which causes the photosensitizer to generate reactive oxygen species and release the drug. Another approach for creating light-activated drug delivery systems involves using light-sensitive polymers. These polymers can be designed to respond to specific wavelengths of light and trigger the release of a drug. The polymer can then be conjugated into a drug and targeted to specific cells or tissues in the brain using various targeting agents [82]. One significant advantage of photo-stimulated drug delivery systems is their ability to provide spatiotemporal control over drug release, which can reduce the risk of off-target effects and increase the drug's therapeutic index [83]. These nano-carriers can be engineered to target specific cells or tissues in the brain, such as tumour cells or neurons, using surface ligands or antibodies [84]. The photosensitizer molecule must generate ROS efficiently and selectively to avoid off-target damage to healthy tissue [85]. Photo-stimulated drug delivery systems for brain diseases could be a promising area of research with potential applications in treating brain tumours, neurodegenerative diseases, and other brain disorders [86].

3.5 CONCLUSIONS

Advanced drug delivery systems have shown promising results in treating brain diseases. Despite the challenges associated with the clinical translation of these systems, such as safety, regulatory approval, scalability, and cost-effectiveness, the potential benefits of using these systems are enormous. Future research should focus on overcoming these challenges by optimizing the safety and efficacy of these systems, reducing their cost, and expanding the scope of their applications to target various neurological disorders. Additionally, developing personalized medicine approaches based on genomics and proteomics can further improve treatment outcomes and reduce side effects. Therefore, with continued research and development, advanced drug delivery systems have the potential to revolutionize the treatment of brain diseases and enhance the quality of life for millions of patients worldwide.

REFERENCES

1. Tewabe, Ashagrachew, Atlaw Abate, Manaye Tamrie, Abyou Seyfu, and Ebrahim Abdela Siraj. 2021. "Targeted Drug Delivery – From Magic Bullet to Nanomedicine: Principles, Challenges, and Future Perspectives." *Journal of Multidisciplinary Healthcare* 14. Dove Press: 1711. doi:10.2147/JMDH.S313968
2. Teleanu, Daniel Mihai, Cristina Chircov, Alexandru Mihai Grumezescu, Adrian Volceanov, and Raluca Ioana Teleanu. 2018. "Blood–Brain Delivery Methods Using Nanotechnology." *Pharmaceutics* 10 (4). Multidisciplinary Digital Publishing Institute (MDPI). doi:10.3390/PHARMACEUTICS10040269
3. Juhairiyah, Firda, and Elizabeth C.M. de Lange. 2021. "Understanding Drug Delivery to the Brain Using Liposome-Based Strategies: Studies That Provide Mechanistic Insights Are Essential." *AAPS Journal* 23 (6). Springer. doi:10.1208/S12248-021-00648-Z
4. Sastri, Koduru Trideva, Gadela Venkata Radha, Sruthi Pidikiti, and Priya Vajjhala. 2020. "Solid Lipid Nanoparticles: Preparation Techniques, Their Characterization,

and an Update on Recent Studies." *Journal of Applied Pharmaceutical Science* 10 (6). Open Science Publishers: 126–41. doi:10.7324/JAPS.2020.10617

5. Alexander, Amit, Mukta Agrawal, Ajaz Uddin, Sabahuddin Siddique, Ahmed M. Shehata, Mahmoud A. Shaker, Syed Ata Ur Rahman, Mohi Iqbal M. Abdul, and Mohamed A. Shaker. 2019. "Recent Expansions of Novel Strategies towards the Drug Targeting into the Brain." *International Journal of Nanomedicine* 14. Dove Press: 5895. doi:10.2147/IJN.S210876
6. Yoo, Jihye, Changhee Park, Gawon Yi, Donghyun Lee, and Heebeom Koo. 2019. "Active Targeting Strategies Using Biological Ligands for Nanoparticle Drug Delivery Systems." *Cancers* 11 (5). MDPI AG. doi:10.3390/CANCERS11050640
7. Mohapatra, Adityanarayan, Saji Uthaman, and In Kyu Park. 2021. "External and Internal Stimuli-Responsive Metallic Nanotherapeutics for Enhanced Anticancer Therapy." *Frontiers in Molecular Biosciences* 7 (January). Frontiers Media S.A.: 437. doi:10.3389/FMOLB.2020.597634/BIBTEX
8. Rana, Abhilash, Meheli Adhikary, Praveen Kumar Singh, Bhudev C. Das, and Seema Bhatnagar. 2023. "'Smart' Drug Delivery: A Window to Future of Translational Medicine." *Frontiers in Chemistry* 10 (January). Frontiers Media S.A. doi:10.3389/FCHEM.2022.1095598/FULL
9. Dong, Xiaowei. 2018. "Current Strategies for Brain Drug Delivery." *Theranostics* 8 (6). Ivyspring International Publisher: 1481. doi:10.7150/THNO.21254
10. Harisa, Gamaleldin I., and Tarek M. Faris. 2019. "Direct Drug Targeting into Intracellular Compartments: Issues, Limitations, and Future Outlook." *Journal of Membrane Biology* 252 (6). Springer New York: 527–39. doi:10.1007/S00232-019-00082-5/METRICS
11. Upadhyay, Ravi Kant. 2014. "Drug Delivery Systems, CNS Protection, and the Blood Brain Barrier." *BioMed Research International* 2014. Hindawi Limited. doi:10.1155/2014/869269
12. Ruan, Shaobo, Yang Zhou, Xinguo Jiang, and Huile Gao. 2021. "Rethinking CRITID Procedure of Brain Targeting Drug Delivery: Circulation, Blood Brain Barrier Recognition, Intracellular Transport, Diseased Cell Targeting, Internalization, and Drug Release." *Advanced Science* 8 (9). John Wiley & Sons: 2004025. doi:10.1002/ADVS.202004025
13. Patra, Jayanta Kumar, Gitishree Das, Leonardo Fernandes Fraceto, Estefania Vangelie Ramos Campos, Maria Del Pilar Rodriguez-Torres, Laura Susana Acosta-Torres, Luis Armando Diaz-Torres et al. 2018. "Nano Based Drug Delivery Systems: Recent Developments and Future Prospects." *Journal of Nanobiotechnology* 16 (1). BioMed Central: 71. doi:10.1186/S12951-018-0392-8
14. Sheng, Yan, Jiaming Hu, Junfeng Shi, and Ly James Lee. 2019. "Stimuli-Responsive Carriers for Controlled Intracellular Drug Release." *Current Medicinal Chemistry* 26 (13): 2377–88. doi:10.2174/0929867324666170830102409
15. Pardridge, William M., and William H. Oldendorf. 1977. "Transport of Metabolic Substrates through the Blood–Brain Barrier." *Journal of Neurochemistry* 28 (1): 5–12. doi:10.1111/j.1471-4159.1977.tb07702.x
16. Puris, Elena, Gert Fricker, and Mikko Gynther. 2022. "Targeting Transporters for Drug Delivery to the Brain: Can We Do Better?" *Pharmaceutical Research* 39 (7). Springer: 1415–55. doi:10.1007/S11095-022-03241-X
17. Lingineni, Karthik, Vilas Belekar, Sujit R. Tangadpalliwar, and Prabha Garg. 2017. "The Role of Multidrug Resistance Protein (MRP-1) as an Active Efflux Transporter on Blood–Brain Barrier (BBB) Permeability." *Molecular Diversity* 21 (2). Springer International Publishing: 355–65. doi:10.1007/s11030-016-9715-6

18. Ndemazie, Nkafu Bechem, Andriana Inkoom, Ellis Fualefeh Morfaw, Taylor Smith, Monica Aghimien, Dexter Ebesoh, and Edward Agyare. 2021. "Multi-Disciplinary Approach for Drug and Gene Delivery Systems to the Brain." *AAPS PharmSciTech 2021 23:1* 23 (1). Springer: 1–21. doi:10.1208/S12249-021-02144-1
19. Kouhi, Aida, Vyshnavi Pachipulusu, Talya Kapenstein, Peisheng Hu, Alan L. Epstein, and Leslie A. Khawli. 2021. "Brain Disposition of Antibody-Based Therapeutics: Dogma, Approaches and Perspectives." *International Journal of Molecular Sciences* 22 (12). Multidisciplinary Digital Publishing Institute (MDPI): 22. doi:10.3390/IJMS22126442
20. Grabrucker, Andreas M., Barbara Ruozi, Daniela Belletti, Francesca Pederzoli, Flavio Forni, Maria Angela Vandelli, and Giovanni Tosi. 2016. "Nanoparticle Transport across the Blood Brain Barrier." *Tissue Barriers* 4 (1). Taylor and Francis. doi:10.1080/21688370.2016.1153568
21. Ribecco-Lutkiewicz, Maria, Caroline Sodja, Julie Haukenfrers, Arsalan S. Haqqani, Dao Ly, Peter Zachar, Ewa Baumann et al. 2018. "A Novel Human Induced Pluripotent Stem Cell Blood–Brain Barrier Model: Applicability to Study Antibody-Triggered Receptor-Mediated Transcytosis." *Scientific Reports* 8 (1). Nature Publishing Group: 1873. doi:10.1038/s41598-018-19522-8
22. Alavijeh, Mohammad S., Mansoor Chishty, M. Zeeshan Qaiser, and Alan M. Palmer. 2005. "Drug Metabolism and Pharmacokinetics, the Blood–Brain Barrier, and Central Nervous System Drug Discovery." *NeuroRx* 2 (4). American Society for Experimental Neurotherapeutics: 554–71. doi:10.1602/NEURORX.2.4.554
23. Yu, Y. Joy, and Ryan J. Watts. 2013. "Developing Therapeutic Antibodies for Neurodegenerative Disease." *Neurotherapeutics* 10 (3): 459–72. doi:10.1007/S13311-013-0187-4
24. Yang, Hang, Yan Luo, Hang Hu, Sibo Yang, Yanan Li, Huijuan Jin, Shengcai Chen et al. 2021. "PH-Sensitive, Cerebral Vasculature-Targeting Hydroxyethyl Starch Functionalized Nanoparticles for Improved Angiogenesis and Neurological Function Recovery in Ischemic Stroke." *Advanced Healthcare Materials* 10 (12). Adv Healthc Mater. doi:10.1002/ADHM.202100028
25. Hughes, Krystal A., Bishal Misra, Maryam Maghareh, and Sharan Bobbala. 2023. "Use of Stimulatory Responsive Soft Nanoparticles for Intracellular Drug Delivery." *Nano Research.* Nano Res. doi:10.1007/S12274-022-5267-5
26. Cheng, Ru, Fenghua Meng, Chao Deng, Harm Anton Klok, and Zhiyuan Zhong. 2013. "Dual and Multi-Stimuli Responsive Polymeric Nanoparticles for Programmed Site-Specific Drug Delivery." *Biomaterials* 34 (14): 3647–57. doi:10.1016/j.biomaterials.2013.01.084
27. Wells, Carlos M., Michael Harris, Landon Choi, Vishnu Priya Murali, Fernanda Delbuque Guerra, and J. Amber Jennings. 2019. "Stimuli-Responsive Drug Release from Smart Polymers." *Journal of Functional Biomaterials* 10 (3). MDPI AG. doi:10.3390/jfb10030034
28. He, Wenxiu, Zhiwen Zhang, and Xianyi Sha. 2021. "Nanoparticles-Mediated Emerging Approaches for Effective Treatment of Ischemic Stroke." *Biomaterials* 277 (October). Elsevier. doi:10.1016/j.biomaterials.2021.121111
29. Kovacsa, Zsofia I., Saejeong Kima, Neekita Jikariaa, Farhan Qureshia, Blerta Miloa, Bobbi K. Lewisa, Michele Breslera, Scott R. Burksa, and Joseph A. Franka. 2017. "Disrupting the Blood–Brain Barrier by Focused Ultrasound Induces Sterile Inflammation." *Proceedings of the National Academy of Sciences of the United States of America* 114 (1). National Academy of Sciences: E75–84. doi:10.1073/PNAS.1614777114/SUPPL_FILE/PNAS.201614777SI.PDF

30. Arvanitis, Costas D., Margaret S. Livingstone, Natalia Vykhodtseva, and Nathan McDannold. 2012. "Controlled Ultrasound-Induced Blood–Brain Barrier Disruption Using Passive Acoustic Emissions Monitoring." *PLOS One* 7 (9). doi:10.1371/JOURNAL.PONE.0045783
31. Aryal, Muna, Costas D. Arvanitis, Phillip M. Alexander, and Nathan McDannold. 2014. "Ultrasound-Mediated Blood–Brain Barrier Disruption for Targeted Drug Delivery in the Central Nervous System." *Advanced Drug Delivery Reviews* 0 (June). NIH Public Access: 94. doi:10.1016/J.ADDR.2014.01.008
32. Upadhyay, Awaneesh, Bhrugu Yagnik, Priti Desai, and Sameer V. Dalvi. 2018. "Microbubble-Mediated Enhanced Delivery of Curcumin to Cervical Cancer Cells." *ACS Omega* 3 (10). American Chemical Society: 12824–31. doi:10.1021/ACSOMEGA.8B01737/ASSET/IMAGES/LARGE/AO-2018-01737X_0001.JPEG
33. Lee, Seunghyun, Hoyoon Jeon, Shinyong Shim, Maesoon Im, Jinsik Kim, Jung Hoon Kim, and Byung Chul Lee. 2021. "Preclinical Study to Improve Microbubble-Mediated Drug Delivery in Cancer Using an Ultrasonic Probe with an Interchangeable Acoustic Lens." *Scientific Reports 2021 11:1* 11 (1). Nature Publishing Group: 1–10. doi:10.1038/s41598-021-92097-z
34. Ibsen, Stuart, Carolyn E. Schutt, and Sadik Esener. 2013. "Microbubble-Mediated Ultrasound Therapy: A Review of Its Potential in Cancer Treatment." *Drug Design, Development and Therapy* 7 (May). Dove Press: 375. doi:10.2147/DDDT.S31564
35. Chowdhury, Sayan Mullick, Lotfi Abou-Elkacem, Taehwa Lee, Jeremy Dahl, and Amelie M. Lutz. 2020. "Ultrasound and Microbubble Mediated Therapeutic Delivery: Underlying Mechanisms and Future Outlook." *Journal of Controlled Release* 326 (October). Elsevier: 75–90. doi:10.1016/J.JCONREL.2020.06.008
36. Price, Paige M., Waleed E. Mahmoud, Ahmed A. Al-Ghamdi, and Lyudmila M. Bronstein. 2018. "Magnetic Drug Delivery: Where the Field Is Going." *Frontiers in Chemistry* 6 (Dec). Frontiers Media S.A.: 619. doi:10.3389/FCHEM.2018.00619/BIBTEX
37. Al-Jamal, Khuloud T., Jie Bai, Julie Tzu Wen Wang, Andrea Protti, Paul Southern, Lara Bogart, Hamed Heidari, et al. 2016. "Magnetic Drug Targeting: Preclinical in vivo Studies, Mathematical Modeling, and Extrapolation to Humans." *Nano Letters* 16 (9). American Chemical Society: 5652–60. doi:10.1021/ACS.NANOLETT.6B02261
38. Altanerova, U., M. Babincova, P. Babinec, K. Benejova, J. Jakubechova, V. Altanerova, M. Zduriencikova, V. Repiska, and C. Altaner. 2017. "Human Mesenchymal Stem Cell-Derived Iron Oxide Exosomes Allow Targeted Ablation of Tumor Cells via Magnetic Hyperthermia." *International Journal of Nanomedicine* 12 (October). Dove Medical Press: 7923–36. doi:10.2147/IJN.S145096
39. Arami, Hamed, Amit Khandhar, Denny Liggitt, and Kannan M. Krishnan. 2015. "In vivo Delivery, Pharmacokinetics, Biodistribution and Toxicity of Iron Oxide Nanoparticles." *Chemical Society Reviews* 44 (23). Royal Society of Chemistry: 8576–8607. doi:10.1039/C5CS00541H
40. Liu, Jessica F., Bian Jang, David Issadore, and Andrew Tsourkas. 2019. "Use of Magnetic Fields and Nanoparticles to Trigger Drug Release and Improve Tumor Targeting." *Wiley Interdisciplinary Reviews. Nanomedicine and Nanobiotechnology* 11 (6). NIH Public Access: e1571. doi:10.1002/WNAN.1571
41. Hædersdal, Merete, Fernanda H. Sakamoto, William A. Farinelli, Apostolos G. Doukas, Josh Tam, and R. Rox Anderson. 2010. "Fractional CO2 Laser-Assisted Drug Delivery." *Lasers in Surgery and Medicine* 42 (2): 113–22. doi:10.1002/LSM.20860

42. Alegre-Sánchez, A., N. Jiménez-Gómez, and P. Boixeda. 2018. "Laser-Assisted Drug Delivery." *Actas Dermo-Sifiliograficas* 109 (10). Elsevier Doyma: 858–67. doi:10.1016/J.AD.2018.07.008
43. Wenande, Emily, R. Rox Anderson, and Merete Haedersdal. 2020. "Fundamentals of Fractional Laser-Assisted Drug Delivery: An in-Depth Guide to Experimental Methodology and Data Interpretation." *Advanced Drug Delivery Reviews* 153 (January). Elsevier B.V.: 169–84. doi:10.1016/J.ADDR.2019.10.003
44. Ng, William Hao Syuen, and Saxon D. Smith. 2022. "Laser-Assisted Drug Delivery: A Systematic Review of Safety and Adverse Events." *Pharmaceutics* 14 (12). Multidisciplinary Digital Publishing Institute (MDPI). doi:10.3390/PHARMACEUTICS14122738
45. Steele, Vaughn R. 2020. "Transcranial Magnetic Stimulation as an Interventional Tool for Addiction." *Frontiers in Neuroscience* 14 (October). Frontiers Media S.A.: 1073. doi:10.3389/FNINS.2020.592343/BIBTEX
46. Vazana, Udi, Lior Schori, Uri Monsonego, Evyatar Swissa, Gabriel S. Pell, Yiftach Roth, Pnina Brodt, Alon Friedman, and Ofer Prager. 2020. "TMS-Induced Controlled BBB Opening: Preclinical Characterization and Implications for Treatment of Brain Cancer." *Pharmaceutics* 12 (10). Pharmaceutics: 1–16. doi:10.3390/PHARMACEUTICS12100946
47. Chail, Amit, Rajiv Kumar Saini, P. S. Bhat, Kalpana Srivastava, and Vinay Chauhan. 2018. "Transcranial Magnetic Stimulation: A Review of Its Evolution and Current Applications." *Industrial Psychiatry Journal* 27 (2). Wolters Kluwer – Medknow Publications: 172. doi:10.4103/IPJ.IPJ_88_18
48. Druzhkova, T. A., and A. A. Yakovlev. 2018. "Exosome Drug Delivery through the Blood–Brain Barrier: Experimental Approaches and Potential Applications." *Neurochemical Journal* 12 (3). Springer: 195–204. doi:10.1134/S1819712418030030
49. Pardridge, William M. 2015. "Blood–Brain Barrier Endogenous Transporters as Therapeutic Targets: A New Model for Small Molecule CNS Drug Discovery." *Expert Opinion of Therapeutic Targets* 19 (8). Taylor and Francis: 1059–72. doi:10.1517/14728222.2015.1042364
50. Rehman, Fawad Ur, Yang Liu, Meng Zheng, and Bingyang Shi. 2023. "Exosomes Based Strategies for Brain Drug Delivery." *Biomaterials* 293 (February). Elsevier: 121949. doi:10.1016/J.BIOMATERIALS.2022.121949
51. Jiang, Yuan, Fengbo Wang, Ke Wang, Yongqiang Zhong, Xiaofei Wei, Qiongfen Wang, and Hong Zhang. 2022. "Engineered Exosomes: A Promising Drug Delivery Strategy for Brain Diseases." *Current Medicinal Chemistry* 29 (17). Curr Med Chem: 3111–24. doi:10.2174/0929867328666210902142015
52. Yuan, Lin, and Jia Yi Li. 2019. "Exosomes in Parkinson's Disease: Current Perspectives and Future Challenges." *ACS Chemical Neuroscience* 10 (2). American Chemical Society: 964–72. doi:10.1021/acschemneuro.8b00469
53. Heidarzadeh, Morteza, Yasemin Gürsoy-Özdemir, Mehmet Kaya, Aysan Eslami Abriz, Amir Zarebkohan, Reza Rahbarghazi, and Emel Sokullu. 2021. "Exosomal Delivery of Therapeutic Modulators through the Blood–Brain Barrier: Promise and Pitfalls." *Cell & Bioscience* 11 (1). BioMed Central: 1–28. doi:10.1186/S13578-021-00650-0
54. Armstrong, James P.K., Margaret N. Holme, and Molly M. Stevens. 2017. "Re-Engineering Extracellular Vesicles as Smart Nanoscale Therapeutics." *ACS Nano* 11 (1). American Chemical Society: 69–83. doi:10.1021/acsnano.6b07607
55. Wu, Hao, Yanhong Liu, Liqing Chen, Shuangqing Wang, Chao Liu, Heming Zhao, Mingji Jin et al. 2022. "Combined Biomimetic MOF-RVG15 Nanoformulation Efficient over BBB for Effective Anti-Glioblastoma in Mice Model." *International*

Journal of Nanomedicine 17 (December). Dove Press: 6377–98. doi:10.2147/IJN.S387715
56. Yang, Yue, Na Yin, Zichen Gu, Yuzhen Zhao, Changhua Liu, Tonghai Zhou, Kaixiang Zhang, Zhenzhong Zhang, Junjie Liu, and Jinjin Shi. 2022. "Engineered Biomimetic Drug-Delivery Systems for Ischemic Stroke Therapy." *Medicine in Drug Discovery* 15 (September). Elsevier: 100129. doi:10.1016/J.MEDIDD.2022.100129
57. Zhang, Meilin, Ying Du, Shujun Wang, and Baoan Chen. 2020. "A Review of Biomimetic Nanoparticle Drug Delivery Systems Based on Cell Membranes." *Drug Design, Development and Therapy* 14. Dove Press: 5495. doi:10.2147/DDDT.S282368
58. Nowak, Maksymilian, Matthew E. Helgeson, and Samir Mitragotri. 2020. "Delivery of Nanoparticles and Macromolecules across the Blood–Brain Barrier." *Advanced Therapeutics* 3 (1). Wiley: 1900073. doi:10.1002/ADTP.201900073
59. Li, Congwen, Jiawen Qian, and Yiwei Chu. 2022. "Advances in Brain Delivery Systems Based on Biomimetic Nanoparticles." *ChemNanoMat* 8 (6). John Wiley & Sons: e202200066. doi:10.1002/CNMA.202200066
60. Dellacherie, Maxence O., Bo Ri Seo, and David J. Mooney. 2019. "Macroscale Biomaterials Strategies for Local Immunomodulation." *Nature Reviews Materials* 4 (6). Nature Publishing Group: 379–97. doi:10.1038/s41578-019-0106-3
61. Chen, Jingfan, Muzhaozi Yuan, Caitlin A. Madison, Shoshana Eitan, and Ya Wang. 2022. "Blood–Brain Barrier Crossing Using Magnetic Stimulated Nanoparticles." *Journal of Controlled Release* 345 (May). Elsevier: 557–71. doi:10.1016/J.JCONREL.2022.03.007
62. Sánchez-Dengra, Bárbara, Isabel González-Álvarez, Marival Bermejo, and Marta González-Álvarez. 2023. "Access to the CNS: Strategies to Overcome the BBB." *International Journal of Pharmaceutics* 636 (April). Elsevier BV: 122759. doi:10.1016/J.IJPHARM.2023.122759
63. Thomsen, Louiza Bohn, Maj Schneider Thomsen, and Torben Moos. 2015. "Targeted Drug Delivery to the Brain Using Magnetic Nanoparticles." *Therapeutic Delivery* 6 (10). Future Science: 1145–55. doi:10.4155/TDE.15.56/ASSET/IMAGES/LARGE/FIGURE5.JPEG
64. Caraglia, M., G. De Rosa, G. Salzano, D. Santini, M. Lamberti, P. Sperlongano, A. Lombardi, A. Abbruzzese, and R. Addeo. 2012. "Nanotech Revolution for the Anti-Cancer Drug Delivery through Blood- Brain-Barrier." *Current Cancer Drug Targets* 12 (3). Bentham Science Publishers: 186–96. doi:10.2174/156800912799277421
65. Gabathuler, Reinhard. 2010. "Approaches to Transport Therapeutic Drugs across the Blood–Brain Barrier to Treat Brain Diseases." *Neurobiology of Disease* 37 (1): 48–57. doi:10.1016/J.NBD.2009.07.028
66. Rosa, Giuseppe De, Giuseppina Salzano, Michele Caraglia, and Alberto Abbruzzese. 2011. "Nanotechnologies: A Strategy to Overcome Blood–Brain Barrier." *Current Drug Metabolism* 13 (1). Bentham Science Publishers: 61–69. doi:10.2174/138920012798356943
67. Thomsen, Louiza Bohn, Thomas Linemann, Svend Birkelund, Gitte Abildgaard Tarp, and Torben Moos. 2019. "Evaluation of Targeted Delivery to the Brain Using Magnetic Immunoliposomes and Magnetic Force." *Materials* 12 (21). Multidisciplinary Digital Publishing Institute (MDPI). doi:10.3390/MA12213576
68. Bhardwaj, Shanu, Kavindra Kumar Kesari, Mahesh Rachamalla, Shalini Mani, Ghulam Md Ashraf, Saurabh Kumar Jha, Pravir Kumar et al. 2022. "CRISPR/Cas9 Gene Editing: New Hope for Alzheimer's Disease Therapeutics." *Journal of Advanced Research* 40 (September). Elsevier: 207–21. doi:10.1016/J.JARE.2021.07.001

69. Zou, Yan, Xinhong Sun, Qingshan Yang, Meng Zheng, Olga Shimoni, Weimin Ruan, Yibin Wang et al. 2022. "Blood–Brain Barrier – Penetrating Single CRISPR-Cas9 Nanocapsules for Effective and Safe Glioblastoma Gene Therapy." *Science Advances* 8 (16). American Association for the Advancement of Science: 8011. doi:10.1126/SCIADV.ABM8011
70. Duan, Li, Kan Ouyang, Xiao Xu, Limei Xu, Caining Wen, Xiaoying Zhou, Zhuan Qin, Zhiyi Xu, Wei Sun, and Yujie Liang. 2021. "Nanoparticle Delivery of CRISPR/Cas9 for Genome Editing." *Frontiers in Genetics* 12 (May). Frontiers Media S.A.: 788. doi:10.3389/FGENE.2021.673286/BIBTEX
71. Yang, Yue, Jin Xu, Shuyu Ge, and Liqin Lai. 2021. "CRISPR/Cas: Advances, Limitations, and Applications for Precision Cancer Research." *Frontiers in Medicine* 8 (March). Frontiers Media S.A. doi:10.3389/FMED.2021.649896/FULL
72. Xu, Christine L., Merry Z.C. Ruan, Vinit B. Mahajan, and Stephen H. Tsang. 2019. "Viral Delivery Systems for CRISPR." *Viruses* 11 (1). Multidisciplinary Digital Publishing Institute (MDPI). doi:10.3390/V11010028
73. Uddin, Fathema, Charles M. Rudin, and Triparna Sen. 2020. "CRISPR Gene Therapy: Applications, Limitations, and Implications for the Future." *Frontiers in Oncology* 10 (August). Frontiers Media S.A. doi:10.3389/FONC.2020.01387/FULL
74. Sastri, K. Trideva, N. Vishal Gupta, Sharadha M, Souvik Chakraborty, Hitesh Kumar, Pallavi Chand, V. Balamuralidhara, and D. V. Gowda. 2022. "Nanocarrier Facilitated Drug Delivery to the Brain through Intranasal Route: A Promising Approach to Transcend Bio-Obstacles and Alleviate Neurodegenerative Conditions." *Journal of Drug Delivery Science and Technology* 75 (September). Elsevier: 103656. doi:10.1016/J.JDDST.2022.103656
75. Arokiyaraj, Selvaraj, Savariar Vincent, Muthupandian Saravanan, Yoonseok Lee, Young Kyoon Oh, and Kyoung Hoon Kim. 2017. "Green Synthesis of Silver Nanoparticles Using Rheum Palmatum Root Extract and Their Antibacterial Activity against Staphylococcus Aureus and Pseudomonas Aeruginosa." *Artificial Cells, Nanomedicine and Biotechnology* 45 (2). Taylor and Francis: 372–79. doi:10.3109/21691401.2016.1160403
76. Benakashani, F., A. R. Allafchian, and S. A. H. Jalali. 2016. "Biosynthesis of Silver Nanoparticles Using Capparis Spinosa L. Leaf Extract and Their Antibacterial Activity." *Karbala International Journal of Modern Science* 2 (4). University of Kerbala: 251–58. doi:10.1016/j.kijoms.2016.08.004
77. Can, Mustafa. 2020. "Green Gold Nanoparticles from Plant-Derived Materials: An Overview of the Reaction Synthesis Types, Conditions, and Applications." *Reviews in Chemical Engineering* 36 (7). De Gruyter Open: 859–77. doi:10.1515/REVCE-2018-0051
78. Ying, Shuaixuan, Zhenru Guan, Polycarp C. Ofoegbu, Preston Clubb, Cyren Rico, Feng He, and Jie Hong. 2022. "Green Synthesis of Nanoparticles: Current Developments and Limitations." *Environmental Technology & Innovation* 26 (May). Elsevier: 102336. doi:10.1016/J.ETI.2022.102336
79. Cuevas, R., N. Durán, M. C. Diez, G. R. Tortella, and O. Rubilar. 2015. "Extracellular Biosynthesis of Copper and Copper Oxide Nanoparticles by Stereum Hirsutum, a Native White-Rot Fungus from Chilean Forests." *Journal of Nanomaterials* 2015. Hindawi Publishing. doi:10.1155/2015/789089
80. Devi, Henam Sylvia, Muzaffar Ahmad Boda, Mohammad Ashraf Shah, Shazia Parveen, and Abdul Hamid Wani. 2019. "Green Synthesis of Iron Oxide Nanoparticles Using Platanus Orientalis Leaf Extract for Antifungal Activity." *Green Processing and Synthesis* 8 (1). De Gruyter Open: 38–45. doi:10.1515/GPS-2017-0145

81. Kolarikova, Marketa, Barbora Hosikova, Hanna Dilenko, Katerina Barton-Tomankova, Lucie Valkova, Robert Bajgar, Lukas Malina, and Hana Kolarova. 2023. “Photodynamic Therapy: Innovative Approaches for Antibacterial and Anticancer Treatments.” *Medicinal Research Reviews*. John Wiley & Sons. doi:10.1002/MED.21935
82. Robertson, C. A., D. Hawkins Evans, and H. Abrahamse. 2009. “Photodynamic Therapy (PDT): A Short Review on Cellular Mechanisms and Cancer Research Applications for PDT.” *Journal of Photochemistry and Photobiology B: Biology* 96 (1): 1–8. doi:10.1016/J.JPHOTOBIOL.2009.04.001
83. Shang, Liang, Xinglu Zhou, Jiarui Zhang, Yujie Shi, and Lei Zhong. 2021. “Metal Nanoparticles for Photodynamic Therapy: A Potential Treatment for Breast Cancer.” *Molecules* 26 (21). Multidisciplinary Digital Publishing Institute: 6532. doi:10.3390/MOLECULES26216532
84. Kwiatkowski, Stanisław, Bartosz Knap, Dawid Przystupski, Jolanta Saczko, Ewa Kędzierska, Karolina Knap-Czop, Jolanta Kotlińska, Olga Michel, Krzysztof Kotowski, and Julita Kulbacka. 2018. “Photodynamic Therapy – Mechanisms, Photosensitizers and Combinations.” *Biomedicine & Pharmacotherapy* 106 (October). Elsevier Masson: 1098–1107. doi:10.1016/J.BIOPHA.2018.07.049
85. Sarı, Ceren, İsmail Değirmencioğlu, and Figen Celep Eyüpoğlu. 2023. “Synthesis and Characterization of Novel Schiff Base-Silicon (IV) Phthalocyanine Complex for Photodynamic Therapy of Breast Cancer Cell Lines.” *Photodiagnosis and Photodynamic Therapy* 42 (June). Elsevier BV: 103504. doi:10.1016/J.PDPDT.2023.103504
86. Donnelly, Ryan, Paul McCarron, and David Woolfson. 2009. “Drug Delivery Systems for Photodynamic Therapy.” *Recent Patents on Drug Delivery & Formulation* 3 (1). Recent Pat Drug Deliv Formul: 1–7. doi:10.2174/187221109787158319

4 Challenges and Progress in Nose-to-Brain Drug Delivery

Achmad Himawan, Sandra Aulia Mardikasari, Gábor Katona, Lalitkumar K. Vora, Anjali Kiran Pandya, Andi Dian Permana, Juhaina M. Abu Ershaid, Eeneko Larrañeta, and Vandana Patravale

4.1 INTRODUCTION

The intranasal (IN) route of drug administration can be utilized to deliver medications for both topical and systemic targeting [1], [2]. The IN route is a minimally invasive pathway that offers a quick onset and first-pass effect on metabolism avoidance [3]. The olfactory and respiratory regions of the nasal cavity are highly vascularized, which provides a good absorption area for administered drugs [4]. The olfactory region is located close to cerebrospinal fluid and has direct neuronal contact with the brain, making the nasal route an appealing alternative for delivering medication directly to the brain [5]. This means of delivery is known as the nose-to-brain (NtB) delivery route. Direct drug administration to the brain via this route can avoid the blood–brain barrier (BBB) and minimize drug distribution to its nontarget organ [6]. Recently, NtB has been used in many studies to improve the brain delivery of drugs for central nervous system (CNS) disorder treatment, such as schizophrenia, migraine, epilepsy, and depression. In addition, the NtB route for treating brain infections, cancer, and neuroinflammation has also been studied.

In addition to the several advantages mentioned above, the IN route can be utilized in some cases of CNS emergencies, such as seizures [7]. Because the oral route is not accessible during seizure episodes, a fast-acting nasal delivery route may be an alternative since may be easily administered by the surrounding people or caregivers of the patient [8], [9]. Another situation where the NtB route can be beneficial is delivering the neurohormone thyrotropin releasing hormone (TRH). TRH can be used to treat suicidal patients (due to suicidal depression) as well as brain injury, acute spinal trauma, and schizophrenia. NtB preparation of TRH has the potential to be used in suicidal emergency cases [10]

Furthermore, to the other routes, IN administration, to the extent of the NtB route, has limitations and challenges in delivering drug substances. Problems such as poor physicochemical properties of the drug, low permeability of the nasal membrane, nasal enzymatic degradation, and mucociliary clearance are the primary problems [11], [12]. Because of these challenges, increasing drug permeability through the

DOI: 10.1201/9781032661964-4

nasal mucous membrane, increasing drug residence time, reducing or protecting the drug substance from degradation caused by enzymatic activity, inhibiting nasal enzymes, and overcoming rapid mucociliary clearance should be the main considerations in IN formulation development to the extent of NtB.

The NtB route continues to attract researcher attention due to its versatility and uniqueness. An assessment of the current research on NtB targeting makes it abundantly evident that intranasal use frequently serves as an alternative to oral medication. In reality, several medications can have issues with oral administration if the substance is meant to reach the brain. In some cases, CNS distribution via the nasal mucosa outperforms parenteral administration [13]. In an effort to address the challenges of targeted brain delivery through the nasal passage, new formulations are introduced every year and tested on a variety of drug candidates. These innovative formulation techniques can be divided into a number of groups, including mucopenetrating systems, mucoadhesive/retentive systems, *in situ* gelling formulations, and carrier systems. This section will examine the constraints of formulation, and regulatory requirements as well as the current understanding of the anatomical and physiological barrier for the NtB route. The role of the illusive 3D printing process in aiding the development of NtB drug delivery will then be discussed, along with each formulation strategy, recent advancements in the sector, and related developments.

4.2 INTRANASAL NOSE-TO-BRAIN DRUG-DELIVERY SYSTEM: ROUTES AND BARRIERS

4.2.1 Transport Routes

The nasal cavity and the nose are intricate anatomical systems. The vestibule, respiratory, and olfactory areas make up the three divisions of the nose cavity. The anterior exterior area of the vestibule, which opens to the nasal cavity, is not involved in drug absorption after nasal administration. In humans, the respiratory epithelium is made up of basal cells, ciliated and nonciliated columnar cells, mucus-secreting goblet cells, and other cells with a total surface area of approximately 160 cm^2. The majority of medication absorption occurs in this area. The third section is the olfactory region, which is made up of basal and sustentacular cells as well as olfactory receptor cells. The surface area of this area is 10 cm^2. Bipolar neurons called olfactory receptors are involved in sensory transduction from the olfactory epithelium to the olfactory bulb [12], [14].

The nasal cavity affects how air is conditioned when it is inhaled. Before it enters the lungs, inhaled air is exposed to heating, humidification, and filtration while traveling through the cavity. This procedure reduces lung tissue damage and bronchial heat loss. Heat transfer from arterial blood to the inhaled air is mediated by the arteriovenous anastomoses (AVAs). Additionally, the nasal cavity's narrow breadth encourages contact between the nasal mucosa and the air. As a result, the nasal cavity modifies ambient air, which has a temperature range of 23°C to 32°C and a relative humidity of 40% to 98% [15]–[17].

Scientists have thus far identified three ways that intranasal medication administration can enter the brain, as illustrated in Figure 4.1. The olfactory nerves, trigeminal

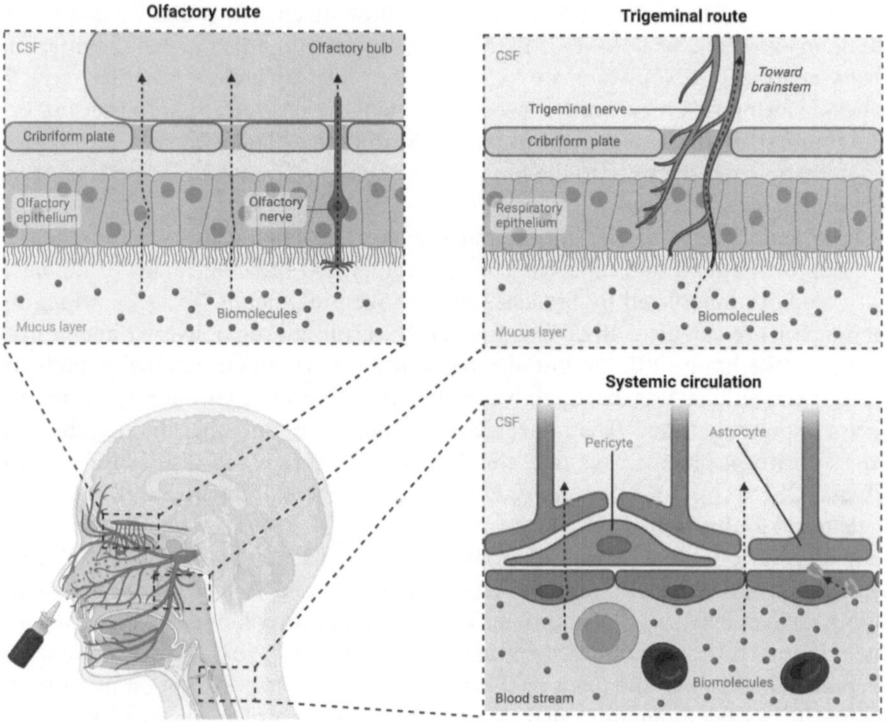

FIGURE 4.1 Nose-to-brain drug delivery transport pathway (Created with BioRender.com).

nerves, and systemic circulation are the routes. The latter is regarded as indirect since the molecules must first enter the bloodstream before passing through the BBB. Because of the anatomical and physiological barriers that are present along the routes, each transport pathway is distinct; hence, special approaches may be required to reach the delivery routes.

The olfactory neuron axons extend to the mucous layer of olfactory epithelial cells, pass through the space containing cerebrospinal fluid (CSF), and end in the mitral valve cells of the olfactory bulb. They also extend to the olfactory bundle, anterior olfactory nucleus, piriform cortex, hypothalamus, and other brain regions [18]. Direct drug delivery from the nose to the brain is likely to be most dependent on the olfactory nerve. There are two ways for drugs given intranasally to enter the olfactory pathway and then travel to the CNS. First, medications may permeate the olfactory nerve bundles' extracellular spaces. It is likely that both bulk movement and action potential transmission along olfactory neurons are necessary for later transport to the olfactory bulb. Second, intracellular mechanisms like passive diffusion, receptor-mediated endocytosis, and adsorptive endocytosis can also transport drug molecules. Comparing the two mechanisms, the speed of extracellular transport is greater than the intracellular route with a difference that can vary between minutes to an hour for the extracellular and hours to days for the intracellular pathway. Drugs that have already reached the olfactory bulb as well as cerebrospinal fluid (CSF) can enter different parts of the CNS through bulk flow mechanisms and by combining with brain extracellular fluid (ECF) [15]. Another intriguing fact is that the olfactory sensory neurons (OSNs) which are located in the olfactory area, regenerate every 3–4 weeks. During this regeneration process, proteolytic enzymes, efflux transporters, and tight junction proteins may be impaired, leading to a "leaky barrier" [19]. Direct drug delivery from the nose to the brain can be achieved by taking advantage of the decreased barrier function.

The trigeminal nerve, the largest cranial nerve, transmits sensory information to the nasal, ocular, and oral mucosa. The respiratory and olfactory areas of the nasal cavity are both innervated by branches of the trigeminal nerve. Transport along the trigeminal nerve can also, albeit less frequently, result in drug delivery directly from the nose to the brain [20]. Drug molecules can travel via the trigeminal neurons by intra or extracellular transport pathways after traveling through the respiratory and olfactory epithelial tissue. The molecules can enter the brain either through the pons or the cribriform plate. Drugs that are already in the brain can diffuse through the ECF and CSF to other CNS regions. However, it is unclear how much transport can be attributed to this route [15].

Finally, various small molecules and, to some extent, some macromolecules administered to the nasal cavity have been demonstrated to enter the CNS by the indirect route due to drugs' absorption into the systemic circulation and the lymphatic system before subsequent movement across the BBB [21], [22]. The nasal mucosa, the epithelial cells, and the junctional barrier restrict the first absorption into the circulation. It has been demonstrated that the first diffusion of medicines into mucus is highly reliant on lipophilicity. Drug molecules then pass the nasal epithelium via paracellular or transcellular transport. Lipophilic compounds partition into the lipid bilayers of the cells to cross this barrier by the transcellular route. Furthermore, receptor-mediated or vesicular transport can also result in transcellular transfer. This is different if the molecules are hydrophilic. Because hydrophilic molecules must passively diffuse through tight junctions, their weight severely restricts their ability to move within the cell. In general, medicines with a molecular weight of less than 1,000 Da do not often undergo paracellular transport. Drugs that manage to overcome these barriers will then enter the circulation. Finally, drugs must traverse the BBB to reach the CNS [15].

4.2.2 Anatomical and Physiological Barriers

The anatomical and physiological barrier present in the nasal cavity is a form of protection from harmful material. The respiratory region is vital; hence, the body develops this barrier to protect the organs from the unfavorable condition of the surrounding atmosphere as well as prevent the macro and micro particulates, living or not, that could disrupt the respiratory system. These protections come in both physical and biochemical form.

Physical protection is provided by the filtration that occurs during air inhalation. As harmful particles move through the nasal cavity, they are deposited onto the mucosal membrane that lines its surface epithelium. Furthermore, the motile cilia on ciliated cells constantly push mucus in the direction of the nasopharynx. Finally, the fate of mucus is that it is either excreted through expectoration or enters the gastrointestinal tract if swallowed [23]. This whole mechanism is known as mucociliary clearance (MCC), and in humans, the normal MCC time is between 15 and 20 minutes, with anything beyond 20 minutes considered abnormal [24]–[26]. Intriguingly, the lack of cilia mobility in the olfactory epithelium reduces mucociliary clearance. Nevertheless, the respiratory epithelium comprises ciliated cells, which in turn enhance the mucociliary clearance [15]. MCC is a major physiological aspect that significantly impacts the NtB system. This protection mechanism of the respiratory system efficiently and rapidly eliminates noxious substances, foreign particles, and microorganisms trapped in the mucus layer after air inhalation. Nonetheless, this system significantly reduces the residence time of the IN preparation [27], [28].

Mucus is secreted by goblet cells of the epithelium and submucosal glands present in the lamina propria, with the latter producing the majority of it. It is composed of approximately 95% water, 2% mucin proteins, 1% salts, 1% immunoglobulins, and 1% lipids [29]. A recent lipomic investigation revealed that human nasal mucosa is rich in n-6 PUFA species, which may have implications for olfactory function. Many kinds of ceramides implicated in cell death and proliferation have also been discovered [30]. Mucins that are heavily glycosylated (10–40 MDa) are primarily responsible for the characteristics of mucus. These glycoproteins are responsible for the viscosity and flexibility of nasal secretions. In addition, mucins include large concentrations of sialic acid and sulfate residues, which rise the distinct negative charge to the mucosal layer and contribute to the stiffness of their polymeric networks [15].

When formulating NtB dosage forms, drug transporters and mucosal metabolizing activity present in the nasal cavity must also be considered. Enzymatic metabolism may be regard as a chemical barrier for this route. To date, it has been determined that the nasal mucosal layer contains several xenobiotic-metabolizing enzymes, including the P450 enzymes (such as P450 monooxygenase), Phase-I enzymes (such as flavin monooxygenases, aldehyde dehydrogenases, epoxide hydrolases, carboxylesterases), and Phase-II enzymes (such as glucuronyl and sulfate transferases, glutathione transferase) [1]. The epithelial tissue and the lumen part of the nasal passage contain enzymes such as exopeptidase (mono aminopeptidase and diamino peptidase) and endopeptidase (cysteine, serine), which are responsible for the breakdown of numerous proteins and peptides, making it difficult to deliver protein/peptide drugs via the NtB route [31].

4.3 STRATEGIES TO INCREASE BRAIN BIOAVAILABILITY

4.3.1 Mucoadhesive Systems

As mentioned previously, this defense mechanism of the respiratory system eliminates hazardous chemicals, particle debris, and pathogens trapped in the mucus layer after air inhalation. However, this phenomenon drastically reduces the residence time of nasally administered drugs. Typical nasal formulations include hydrophilic polymers that can increase viscosity and/or provide bioadhesion to counteract MCC, extend formulation residence time, improve systemic bioavailability, and decrease variation in nasal absorption. Mucoadhesive is the term used to describe the bioadhesion characteristics of substances on mucus-coated surfaces.

Mucoadhesion is a series of several different processes that lead up to the adhesion itself. Those steps include hydration of polymeric chains, close contact with mucosal layer, diffusion and entanglement with mucin polymeric strands, dynamic generation and breakdown of labile bonds (for example, hydrogen bonds, Van der Waals connections, disulfide bridges, electrostatic attractive forces, and hydrophobic interactions). Several natural, semisynthetic, and synthetic polymers have been explored to enhance nasal drug delivery. These polymers may be included in the vehicle or used to modify the surface of drug particles/carriers.

4.3.1.1 Mucoadhesive Vehicle

Typically, mucoadhesive polymers are utilized to impart mucoadhesive properties to the vehicle of an NtB dosage form. Some polymers, including hyaluronic acid (and its sodium salt), chitosan, and a number of cellulose polymers, can be incorporated into a liquid formulation to impart mucoadhesive properties. These polymers also serve as viscosifiers in the formulation, thereby further enhancing the retention time of the dosage form after administration [32]–[34]. While the exact mechanism of this effect is not known, it is well documented that mucoadhesive additives can reduce the mucociliary clearance rate, increase the residence time of the drug formulation in the nasal cavity, and hence prolong the period of contact with the nasal mucosa, which may improve drug absorption [32]. The mucoadhesive action of the polymer comes from the interaction between the functional group in the polymeric chains and the mucous constituents either through noncovalent or covalent bonding [35]–[38]. Some popular polymer choices include hyaluronic acid (and its derivates), chitosan, and cellulose derivates.

Hyaluronic acid and its derivate have favorable characteristics, are naturally biocompatible, possess good bioadhesiveness, and are nonimmunogenic. It can be incorporated into water-based or emulsion-based formulations and has been shown to increase mucosal retention of such formulations [32], [39], [40]. Chitosan is a popular choice for NtB delivery. Chitosan has been known for decades for its excellent mucoadhesive properties and can be incorporated into aqueous solutions, suspensions, and emulsions [41], [42]. However, currently, chitosan is more popularly used as a particle coater or matrix [42], [43]. Cellulose derivates can be other alternatives. Polymers such as methylcellulose, hydroxypropyl methylcellulose, sodium carboxymethylcellulose, and cationic-hydroxyethyl cellulose have been explored for their application in nasal drug delivery [34]. Recent research on the usage of mucoadhesive vehicles always includes some type of penetration enhancer/carrier in their formulation, as the primary function of these excipients is to improve mucosal retention of the preparation. The compatibility between mucoadhesive polymers and the enhancer/carrier should be carefully considered, as the majority of them are ionic and can alter the characteristics of the drug carrier, particularly at the nanoscale level.

4.3.1.2 Mucoadhesive Particles and Carriers

Several readily available mucoadhesive polymers can be utilized to create nanoparticles/carriers or to change the surface of nanoparticles/carriers such that they possess mucoadhesive properties. Among the great variety of polymers, chitosan and its derivatives are among the most thoroughly researched. Chitosan can function as either a particle matrix or a coater. Chitosan can be used alone or in combination with other polymers as a matrix [44], [45]. As a coating material, chitosan can be coupled with various systems, including nanoemulsions, solid lipid carriers, and albumin nanoparticles [46]–[48]. Other polymers, such as pectin and HPMC, could also be utilized to create mucoadhesive particles and carriers [49]. Nanoparticles with mucoadhesive characteristics can enhance drug absorption via the process described in the previous section.

4.3.2 Penetration Enhancers

The absorption of polar drugs in nasal area can be improved by using suitable absorption enhancers, which include phospholipids (dipalmitoyl phosphatidyl choline, soybean lecithin, phosphatidylcholine), bile salts (sodium taurocholate, sodium deoxycholate, sodium glycolate), anionic surfactants (SLS24, SDS25, Laureth-9), cationic compounds (chitosan, poly-L-lysine, poly-L-arginine), cyclodextrins, fatty acids and their derivatives (palmitic acid, palmitoleic acid, stearic acid, oleyl alcohol, oleic acid, capric acid), and tight junction modulators (*Clostridium perfringens* endotoxin, *Zonula occludens* toxin) [50].

Penetration enhancers can amplify drug permeation through several mechanisms. Surfactants can enhance absorption with more than one mechanism; these include perturbing the cell membrane by leaching membrane proteins, opening tight junctions, or preventing enzymatic degradation of the drugs [51]. Cationic polymers interact with the mucosal barriers and enhance the absorption of water-soluble macromolecules via tight junction modification [50]. Tight junction modifiers are potent substances that can modulate tight junctions, a seal that fills the adjacent space between the epithelial cells, allowing compounds with higher hydrophilicity and molecular weight to pass [52]. Chitosan is one of the most intriguing polysaccharides due to its capacity not only to boost the penetration of pharmaceuticals by opening the tight junction barrier, but also to increase drug residence time in the mucosal layer to further increase the penetration of active pharmaceutical ingredients (APIs) [53].

4.3.3 In situ Gel Forming Formulations

In situ gelations appear to be a promising approach that increases drug retention time in the nasal cavity, reduces administered dose outflow via MCC, extends drug release, and increases drug absorption. Stimuli-responsive in situ gels are a novel dosage form that exhibits sol-gel transition after administration into the body cavity in response to physiological changes. It begins as a clear polymer(s) solution or low viscosity liquid that is transformed into a viscous gel by any external stimulus such as temperature, ionic change, pH, magnetic field, light, electrical signal, or biological environment [31], [54]. In situ gels can be integrated with other preparations such as microparticles and nanoparticles. The combined preparation allows an increase in nasal retention time because of the in situ gelling property of the dosage form, as well as the gaining of advantages from the microparticles and nanoparticles formulation [55]. Different in situ gelling polymers can be grouped into several categories depending on what stimuli cause the gelling of the system. The most common stimuli used in NtB delivery include thermal, pH, and ionic stimuli.

4.3.3.1 Thermal Stimulus

The thermoreversible in situ gel is a system that responds to temperature changes and, within a narrow temperature range, transforms from solution to gel [56]. It consists of thermosensitive polymers that demonstrate sol-gel transformation in a temperature range of 25°–37°C. The polymer demonstrating sol-gel transition at a temperature range between 28° and 37°C is considered ideal for nasal in situ gel formation because it prevents the transition at room temperature during storage and transportation and facilitates rapid sol-gel transition after administration in the body [31].

Poloxamers are one of the most valuable groups of thermoresponsive polymers and are often used for the formulations of nasal in situ gels. Among many poloxamers, a combination of both P407 and P108 in varying ratios is used to obtain a desirable gelling property that suits IN administration [31]. In response to a thermal stimulus, the temperature-triggered sol-gel transformation involves the micellization of thermoresponsive polymers or polymeric blends. As the temperature rises, the polymer units are arranged into micellar packing, resulting in gel formation. Due to a conformational change in the side chain, the change in temperature initially causes desolvation of the polymer. Moreover, the displacement of water molecules results in the orientation of micelles [57].

4.3.3.2 pH Stimulus

Polymers that undergo a phase shift in response to a pH change are used to achieve pH-stimulated gelation in the formulations. Carbopol (Carbopol 934 and Carbopol 940) is the most commonly used pH-responsive chemical that exhibits a sol-gel transition in response to a large pH gradient. The carbopol-based formulations are kept at a pH between 4 and 5.5, which will retain their liquid property. Upon instillation into the nasal cavity with a pH of approximately 6.2, the formulation undergoes conformational changes and forms a three-dimensional network, resulting in the sol-gel transition [31].

4.3.3.3 Ion Stimulus

Ionic-stimulated in situ gel formulations contain an ion-sensitive polymer that form a gel in the nasal environment. The mucosal layer in the nasal passage is ample with cations such as Ca^{2+}, which can react with several anionic polymers. Gellan gum, an anionic polysaccharide, is the most used ion-sensitive gelling agent for this type of preparation. When the gellan gum-based formulation is administered to the nostrils, polymeric interaction and cationic complexation occur, resulting in the sol-gel transition [57]. Pectin is a naturally occurring ion-sensitive polysaccharide that has been documented in the literature for the development of in situ nasal gel. Similar to gellan gum, pectin undergoes phase transition through cationic complexation with its functional groups, resulting in the formation of a three-dimensional network gel [31].

4.3.4 Carrier Systems

4.3.4.1 Liposomes

Liposomes are bilayer spherical vesicles consisting primarily of phospholipids from natural and synthetic origin [58]. They are characterized by the presence of a hydrophobic tail and a hydrophilic head that impart to them versatility as a carrier system capable of delivering all molecule types. Along with this, liposomes possess exceptional biocompatibility and can be easily modified to achieve targeting potential, which can be used to enhance their nasal retention in the case of NtB delivery [59]. Liposomes have been widely explored as nanocarriers to improve NtB delivery for the treatment of CNS disorders such as Alzheimer's disease, Parkinson's disease, and ischemic stroke. Hence, liposomes have been established as essential lipid nanocarriers for the successful treatment of CNS diseases [60]. Hydrophilic substances can be encapsulated in the aqueous core of liposomes, whereas lipophilic drugs are encapsulated in the phospholipid bilayer that surrounds the core. Some of the reported lipids used in NtB liposomes include cholesterol, egg-phosphatidylcholine, stearylamine, 1,2-dioleoyl-sn-glycero-3-phosphocholine, N-(carbonyl-methoxypolyethyleneglycol 2000)-1,2-distearoyl-sn-glycero-3-phosphoethanolamine, dihexadecylmethylhydroxyethylammonium bromide, and hydrogenated soy phosphatidylcholine [59].

4.3.4.2 Niosomes

Niosomes are vesicular structures composed of nonionic surfactants and cholesterol that self-assemble in aqueous conditions. Although liposomes and niosomes share a similar structure, niosomes are more stable and cost-effective; as a result, a substantial amount of research has been devoted to the creation of niosomal systems. They exhibit the ability to improve drug solubility, and impart stability, permeability, and systemic bioavailability, making them a promising NtB carrier [61]. According to their size or number of lamellar layers, niosomes can be divided into several categories: tiny unilamellar vesicles (SUVs) and large unilamellar vesicles (LUVs). Multilamellar vesicles (MLVs) and unilamellar vesicles are distinguished by the number of bilayers [62]. Niosomes have numerous advantages, including lower toxicity due to their nonionic nature, the ability to transport both hydrophilic and lipophilic medicines due to their core–shell structure, high penetration through biological membranes, and the capacity to prolong the circulation of entrapped medications. Relative to phospholipid-based vesicles, niosomes are more physically stable and less expensive to handle and store [63]. Inclusion of the medication into niosomes improved brain uptake via the direct NtB pathway, as well as brain bioavailability, drug targeting efficiency, and direct transport percentage, hence demonstrating improved central nervous system targeting via the direct olfactory pathway [64].

4.4 PROGRESS IN NOSE-TO-BRAIN DRUG-DELIVERY SYSTEMS

4.4.1 Novel Functional Excipients

Functional excipients such as polymers and lipids play a great role in NtB delivery. Although the conventional option still serves its purpose, chemical functionalization could enhance its efficiency and safety. Functionalization can be used to modulate its existing characteristics or give the material new properties. Functionalization is generally achieved through chemical reactions [65]. One primary strategy involved in developing novel functional materials for NtB delivery revolves around improving their mucoadhesiveness. Due to the anionic nature of mucin glycoproteins, electrostatic interactions with cationic materials (such as chitosan, aminated cellulose, and other amine-containing polymers) were identified as one of the initial primary bonding strategies utilized in the design of new mucoadhesive systems. Counterintuitively, anionic polymers (such as carboxymethyl cellulose, alginate, and pectin) also exhibit mucoadhesive properties. Both cationic and anionic polymers are regarded as first-generation mucoadhesive polymers [38]. Some recently reported modifications of the first-generation polymers used in NtB delivery systems include transferrin-modified chitosan [66], N,O-carboxymethyl chitosan [67], N,N,N-trimethyl chitosan [68], and oxidized alginate [69].

Second-generation mucoadhesive polymers cover a wide range of materials, each with its unique polymer-mucin interaction mechanism. This generation includes acrylated and methacrylated, maleimide-functionalized, thiolated, catechol-bearing, boronate-bearing, and N-hydroxy(sulfo)succinimide ester-functionalized materials [38]. Acrylated polymers are a novel class of mucoadhesive materials with the ability to covalently bind with cysteine residues present in mucin glycoproteins via a Michael-type addition reaction [36]. Maleimide-bearing compounds covalently react with the free thiol groups of mucin glycoproteins through a maleimide-thiol "click-like" reaction [35]. Thiolated materials form disulfide bonds with mucin [37]. Catechol compounds can form covalent bonds as a result of o-quinone formation via partial deprotonation of the catechols in physiological condition, and subsequent reaction with amine and thiol residues in mucosal polymeric chain [70]. Boronate-bearing materials' mucoadhesive properties come from their interactions with saccharide residues present in the mucus layer [71]. Another new class of polymers capable of covalently binding to mucus components was N-hydroxy(sulfo)succinimide ester-functionalized substances. These materials specifically target the lysine and arginine amino groups found in mucin glycoproteins [72]. Some of the mentioned polymers have been used in NtB delivery, such as thiolated chitosan [43], [73], thiolated polyethylene glycol-poly(lactic-co-glycolic acid) [74], acrylated Eudragit® E PO [75], and maleimide-conjugated N,N,N-trimethyl chitosan [76].

4.4.2 Advanced Vesicle Systems

Traditional carriers such as liposomes and niosomes can be decorated to further increase their brain targeting/uptake efficiency. The molecular probe can be attached to the polymer used in the formulation. For example, antibodies and/or any targeting ligands can be chemically conjugated onto a PEG lipid polymer and used to form liposomes [77], [78]. In a similar manner, functional groups, such as maleimide, can be attached to the PEGylated polymer to enhance its brain-targeting efficiency [79]. Decoration using targeting ligands such as anti-transferrin monoclonal antibody (Mab) (known to target TfR) or a peptide derivative of apolipoprotein E3 (APOe) was meant to utilize the active transport of therapeutics across the BBB. Transcytosis mediated by membrane protein carriers of small molecules and transcytosis mediated by adsorption of positively charged peptides are two active transport mechanisms. BBB (and blood-brain tumor barrier [BBTB]) cells have a diverse set of receptors on their membranes. The most abundantly expressed receptors on the BBB cell membrane are low-density lipoprotein, transferrin, and insulin receptors. The binding of macromolecules to a specific cell receptor induces endocytosis and subsequent transcytosis during receptor-mediated transcytosis. These targeted strategies boost drug delivery across these barriers, thereby increasing medication biodistribution in the brain [78], [80], [81].

Emulsomes, vesicle-like systems that combine the properties of liposomes and emulsions, can be used to deliver drugs through the NtB route. In combination with PLGA-PEG-PLGA triblock copolymer thermogel, the system was able to extend the presence of oxcarbazepine in the rat brain up to 48 hours after nasal instillation [82]. The emulsome surface can be modified by introducing cationic charge inducers (such as stearylamine) or PEGylated phospholipids into the formulation. A study using vinpocetine-loaded emulsomes showed that PEGylated-modified vesicles perform better than stearylamine-modified formulations in terms of increasing brain localization of the drug. Both formulations perform better than do bare emulsomes [68].

Other vesicular systems that have recently been studied for NtB delivery include transfersome, bilosomes, and extracellular vesicles. Transfersomes are ultradeformable vesicles that are capable of penetrating the intranasal mucosa. Each transfersome consists of an interior aqueous compartment that is surrounded by lipid bilayers. By incorporating an edge activator (such as sodium deoxycholate) into the vesicular membrane of transfersomes, their properties can be precisely modified [83]. Macromolecules such as insulin can be loaded into transfersomes [84].

Bilosomes (bile salts containing niosomes) are nanovesicular carriers made up of bile salts and a nonionic surfactant bilayer (similar to niosomes). In this instance, bile salts serve as edge activators that distinguish between niosomes and bilosomes. Edge activators reduce the surface tension of the vesicular bilayer, causing its instability and the production of deformable vesicles with improved tissue penetration [85]. Bilosomes, like other vesicular systems, can be modified to tailor specific qualities to the system. One intriguing technique is to use superparamagnetic iron oxide nanoparticles (SPIONs) as a magnetic probe that can be manipulated externally to enhance brain localization using an external magnetic field [86]

Extracellular vesicles (EVs) are quite different from the previously mentioned vesicular systems. EVs are naturally secreted cell vesicles in the nanometer to micrometer size range, that are formed by the outward budding of plasma membrane domains. EVs, including exosomes and microvesicles, are derived from different cell sources and are generally limited by their quantity, size heterogeneity, and loading efficiency [87]. EVs have recently been explored for their application in NtB delivery. While stem cell EVs share the same size and surface features as lipid nanoparticles, a similar mechanism of transport across the epithelium may be adapted to EVs. The ability of EVs to target inflammation is also essential for transepithelial migration. EVs can interact with epithelial cells and induce a cytoskeletal remodeling in epithelial cells, rendering them capable of breaching the barrier. This mechanism is mediated by chemokine gradients and could be exacerbated by inflammatory conditions. EVs can be loaded with small molecules or macromolecules [88], [89].

4.4.3 Tailored Nanoparticles

NtB nanoparticles are tiny particles that can be inhaled or instilled through the nose and transported to the brain. These nanoparticles are designed to pass through the BBB, which is a protective layer of cells that surrounds the brain and prevents most substances from entering it. Nanoparticles are superior for nasal delivery compared to larger particles. Nanoparticles (NPs) possess higher surface area, which translates into a broader interface for more prolonged residence time. Particle size lower than 500 nm allows nanoparticles to squeeze into the nonviscous aqueous pores within the entangled mucin network [28]. The mucoadhesive/penetrating ability of Nanoparticles (NPs) can be further tailored to suit NtB transport. There are three ways to modulate the uptake of intranasally administered nanoparticles. The first is to enhance mucoadhesion to prolong the interaction time of nanoparticles with the mucosa. This will increase the likelihood of the drug passing through the epithelium and ultimately reaching the brain. The second is the ability of various materials used in particle formulations to reduce the barrier function of tight junctions. These specialized particles would be capable of momentarily opening tight junctions, allowing the drug to enter the nasal mucosa. Enhancing the likelihood of nanoparticle endocytosis represents the final option. After endocytosis, the nanoparticles could release the drug, which would then be transported to the brain [27]. Certain traditional and functionalized polymers can be used to increase mucoadhesion, and this strategy has been discussed in the previous sections as well as the permeation enhancers commonly used as excipients in NtB formulations. For example, coating the surface of nanostructured lipid carriers (NLCs), a good BBB-penetrating nanoparticle system with chitosan derivates, gives it mucoadhesive properties. This approach was able to achieve higher ropinirole HCl in the brain after nasal administration of drug-dextran sulfate nanoplex loaded mucoadhesive NLC suspension in a mouse model [68].

Nanoparticle formulations can be further tailored to suit NtB delivery through an optimization process. The process aims to give the preparation certain attributes that are desired for IN NtB delivery from both pharmaceuticals and physiological points of view. For example, tailoring the BBB/BBTB properties of docetaxel-loaded NLCs can be achieved through the incorporation of liquid lipid excipients into the formulation [90]. A similar approach was able to achieve up to a 6.15-fold increase in the brain concentration of clozapine in mice after IN administration of drug-loaded NLCs. The formulation uses oleic acid and Tween® to tailor the BBB properties of the nanoparticles [91]. Furthermore, attaching molecular probes such as folate to polymeric carriers can further improve solid tumor targeting. Folate can be attached using simple EDC-NHS chemistry. Erlotinib and doxorubicin-loaded cinnamon biopolymers showed superior brain localization and enhanced antitumor efficacy after folate functionalization [92]. The extent of tailored formulation encompasses the ability to modify the dosage forms, rather than just the nanoparticles. For example, tailoring clozapine nanosuspensions intended for NtB delivery through an optimization process to achieve desired properties by changing process parameters and formulation composition is possible [93]

4.4.4 Micro- and Nanoemulsions

Microemulsion (ME) and nanoemulsion (NE) are two separate preparations that can both be included in NtB preparations. There is substantial uncertainty in the current literature regarding the distinction between ME and NE, due to the similarity in their formulation and the overlap in droplets size range. MEs spontaneously form thermodynamically stable systems, whereas NEs do not. Thus, NEs (and conventional macroemulsions) can be prepared using both high- and low-energy techniques, but MEs can only be prepared with low-energy techniques. Significant variations exist between traditional macroemulsions, NEs, and MEs in terms of droplet size range and stability characteristics [13].

ME is a transparent, thermodynamically stable, and optically isotropic system of two non-miscible phases (such as water and oil), stabilized by an interfacial coating of surfactant or a surfactant-cosurfactant mixture. It is a spontaneous pseudoternary system that arises with minimum energy input during the fabrication process, which produces nano-sized droplets, ranging in size from 1 to 400 nm. In addition to its small size, negligible interfacial tension, and good stability, the ME possesses desirable physicochemical qualities, such as its lipophilic nature and low viscosity. ME has evolved as a new colloidal delivery technology that enhances site-specific drug release for the intranasal route and lowers exposure to undesired therapeutics. The small droplet size and low interfacial tension of ME give greater membrane adhesion, enhanced penetration, and regulated drug transport [94].

ME can be used to deliver a wide range of therapeutics to the brain. Intranasal drug delivery of lipophilic ME modified with mucoadhesive agents was found to bypass the BBB and successfully deliver drugs to the brain. ME nanocarriers reduce systemic exposure and the associated toxicities. This advantage helps deliver therapeutics at effective levels to the targeted sites. In previously reported research, the bio-distribution study demonstrated rapid drug delivery to the brain; moreover, an *in vivo* safety evaluation study revealed the safety and effectiveness of the developed ME against glioblastoma with reduced risk of liver and kidney toxicity [95], [96]. A combination of drug/prodrug mixture formulated in an aqueous ME was able to achieve faster absorption and higher brain and blood drug levels after intranasal administration compared to a prodrug-only preparation [97]. A unique ME preparation that is able to spontaneously form a gel upon contact with mucosal water can be prepared by carefully selecting the composition of the ME. This system is called aqua-triggered in-situ (ATIS) gel and it can be loaded with a drug to achieve better brain delivery than the drug solution. This formulation achieved a higher brain-ECF:plasma ratio of the drug compared to diazepam solution given intranasally or intravenously [98].

NEs are dispersions of two immiscible liquids stabilized by an appropriate surfactant(s) and/or cosurfactants, with an average droplet size of approximately 100 nm and upper size limitations of up to 300 nm. In comparison to other formulations, NEs feature smaller droplets and a greater surface area. Small droplet size inhibits destabilizing events such as coalescence, creaming, and sedimentation. These characteristics give NEs long-term physical stability. Typically, the lipids used for the preparation of NEs are fractions of oils of natural origin, either alone or in combination. The lipidic phase can be grouped into long-, medium-, or short-chain triglycerides and can take up to 20% of formulation composition in a typical oil-in-water formulation [13].

NEs can be manufactured using either high-energy or low-energy processes. In high-energy methods, the formation of small droplets requires a mechanical device that generates disruptive forces which break up internal phases to produce small droplets. This process, such as ultrasonication and high-pressure homogenization, requires a significant amount of energy. The low-energy methods involve specific physicochemical processes, such as phase inversion temperature and emulsion inversion points, to reduce the size of droplets without requiring a substantial amount of energy. In low-energy methods, droplets are formed when the system undergoes a phase inversion to enters a state of low interfacial tension [13]. NEs can be loaded with neuroactive steroid, antineoplastics, or other CNS drugs. In addition, formulation of NEs in combination with mucoadhesive or in situ gel systems might enhance the brain delivery of the APIs [99]–[102].

4.4.5 Nasal Powders

Liquid nasal preparations are popular choices due to the simplicity of their formulation and the convenience of their distribution. On the other hand, instability (both chemical and microbiological), relatively large volume administration, quick evacuation from the nasal cavity, and the necessity for additives and stabilizing agents limit their use for a broader range of drugs and applications. If the medicine is manufactured as a dry powder, these issues are mostly eliminated. Dry powders are thought to be more stable than liquids [103], [104]. Powders have a simpler excipient composition (if any), allowing for the administration of larger doses of medication. In addition, powders enable the production of compounds with poor water solubility. Nasal powders have also been reported to increase drug bioavailability at the site of action in comparison to liquid formulations [105].

Notwithstanding the benefits of powder formulation, nasal powders continue to face market challenges. There are only a few approved nasal powders, such as Onzetra Xsail® (Avanir Pharmaceuticals Inc., USA), containing sumatriptan; Rhinocort® Turbuhaler® (AstraZeneca, UK), containing budesonide; Teijin Rhinocort® (Teijin, Japan), containing beclomethasone dipropionate and Erizas® (Nippon Shnyaku, Japan), containing dexamethasone cipecilate. One major reason for this small number is the lack of data on the short- and long-term local acceptability of nasal powders, which may raise concerns about toxicity to nasal physiological functions [105].

For highly potent active substances that can be easily administered in low doses via liquid formulations, it may not be necessary to develop powder formulations for nasal administration. In addition, as was observed, the administration of such medications in powder form would require dilution with an inert carrier. Without the addition of mucoadhesive excipients and/or absorption enhancers, drug absorption from the powder may not be sufficient for the desired effect with less potent systemically acting APIs. The absence of safety data and concerns over these excipients may prevent the commercialization of medication powders containing absorption enhancers [105].

Attempts to use dry powder formulations as another option for NtB delivery were explored by scientists. A proof-of-concept study showed that flurbiprofen possesses greater nasal mucosal transport when formulated into spray-dried microparticles using lecithin as the excipient in *ex vivo* conditions, and a later *in vivo* study demonstrated a superior brain localization compared to the IV group [106], [107]. Similarly, quercetin-loaded mannitol/lecithin microparticles showed better *ex vivo* nasal mucosa permeation [108], and another study demonstrated good stability, *in vitro* compatibility, and *in vitro* mucosal permeation of donezepil hydrochloride-loaded mannitol/chitosan microparticles [104]. Another work demonstrated that dexamethasone sodium phosphate combined with polymeric excipients in the form of pectin/HPMC microspheres and inert sugar carriers can provide good sprayability that can be deposited onto the olfactory region of the modeled nasal cavity [49]. The versatility of nasal powder was further demonstrated by incorporating geraniol, an oily substance, into a cyclodextrin complex that resulted in a dry powder product. An *in vivo* study reported that geraniol was able to reach the CNS after IN administration (as an aqueous suspension) [109].

It is acknowledged that further development of nasal powder formulations will necessitate powder manufacturing optimization, characterization of the powder-device combination, and a better understanding of the local effects of powder insufflation in the nasal cavity. Nonetheless, evidence regarding stability, shelf life, bioavailability, and efficient administration by newly designed devices is important in order to push the number of nasal powder products on the market. The research on this path will be worthwhile, as administering pharmaceutical and biotech products through nasal delivery will be a viable and interesting alternative in the future [105].

4.4.6 Updates in Packaging and Dosing Contraption

NtB nasal sprays are a type of drug-delivery system that transmits drugs directly to the brain via the olfactory region in the nose. The packaging for these nasal sprays is designed to ensure that the drug is delivered safely and effectively. One important consideration in the packaging of NtB nasal sprays is the material used for the bottle and the nozzle. These materials must be compatible with the drug being delivered and must not degrade or react with the drug. Typically, these nasal sprays are packaged in small, plastic bottles with a fine nozzle that can deliver a precise dose of the drug. Another important consideration is the design of the spray nozzle. The nozzle should be designed to deliver the drug in a fine mist or aerosol that can easily penetrate the nasal cavity and reach the olfactory region of the brain. The nozzle should also be designed to prevent leakage or clogging. In addition to the bottle and nozzle design, the packaging for NtB nasal sprays should also include clear instructions for use, including dosage and frequency of use. The packaging should also include any necessary warnings or precautions for the safe use of the drug [2], [110]–[112].

All current efforts to deliver medications to the brain through the NtB route provide an overview of this delivery method's potential efficacy. Despite all the benefits of the novel formulations introduced for this route of administration, the proper dosage of intranasally delivered drugs remains a significant challenge. Each of the different dosage form alternatives presents a unique problem due to their varied features. Moreover, the structure of each person's nasal cavity differs considerably. Hence, administration procedures are highly variable and must be tailored to the anatomical characteristics of each patient. Additionally, it must be ensured that the nasal mucosal surface is not affected by regular usage of these devices [27].

Deposition of formulation in the olfactory region is crucial for optimizing the direct transport of medications to the brain, which can only be achieved with an effective dosing system. In light of the current market for nasal products, nasal droppers, squeeze bottles, and spray pumps are extensively employed devices [94]. Instillation of a nasal preparation to a patient in a supine position with a dropper deposits more medication in the olfactory area compared to nasal sprays. When mixed with mucoadhesive agents, the formulation can remain in the area for a longer period. The patient's delivery technique can influence the effectiveness of nasal drops and nasal sprays, which is a significant constraint to NtB delivery. Correct administration of nasal drops necessitates sophisticated maneuvers on the part of the patient [3]. Nasal drug deposition using a spray device is based on human factors such as actuation force, actuation angle, and nasal anatomy, in addition to those imposed by the combination of device and formulation, such as droplet size, plume angle, and plume area [113].

Droppers are unpleasant for patients, whereas squeeze bottles are highly comfortable, yet unsafe, as nasal secretions can contaminate the remaining volume. A more advanced dosing contraption such as atomizer and nebulizer delivery is also unable to reach the posterior area of the nasal cavity. Targeting the olfactory region with these devices is impractical due to the mismatch between the uneven plumes produced by conventional devices and the complex dimensions of the nasal vestibule and the narrow barrier region of the nasal valve. Although the olfactory epithelium is only 7 cm from the nostril, its location in the olfactory cleft behind the small nasal valve frequently makes it difficult to access [94].

The vast majority of liquid nasal products are available with dosing pumps. They deliver liquid dosage forms in precise doses ranging from 25 to 200 μL per dose. These devices prevent contamination from entering the container, hence allowing a preservative-free formulation to be used. However, metered pump delivery is influenced by formulation properties such as variation in viscosity as well as patient handling, which introduce another source of variability. In addition, metered spray pumps require priming for accurate dosing. Several commercially available spray pumps, including Valtoco®, Nascobal®, Narcan®, Imitrex®, and Zomig® fall under the category of unit dose nasal spray pumps (UDNS), which is different from the previously described mechanism. In UDNS, an aliquot of formulation equivalent for a single dose is placed in a small vial, which is then put in a holder where a top actuator is installed. Upon activation, the dose is released into the nasal cavity. These metered dosage spray pumps are incapable of targeting the olfactory region as $< 5\%$ of the delivered amount is reported to reach the olfactory region [94].

Several new dosing devices that are more suitable for NtB delivery have been developed. Breath-Powered Bidirectional (such as OptiNose®, OptiMist™, and Onzetra® Xsail®) and Precision Olfactory Delivery (POD) devices have demonstrated their capability to deposit medications into the upper nasal cavity. Breath-Powered technology (originally presented by OptiNose®) uses the patient's own exhaled air to trigger dose release from the contraption. OptiMist™ technology is more versatile as both powder and liquid formulations can be dosed. To operate this mechanism, the user needs to insert the device's short tip into one of their nostrils and blow into the mouthpiece. A closed soft palate prevents drug deposition into the lungs, while air is expelled from the other nostril to maintain pressure. Similarly, POD was also able to deliver liquid and powder formulations. The POD device emits the dose using compressed gas as the driving force. The majority of the medication can be deposited in the olfactory region. Human studies revealed much higher deposition in the olfactory region compared to the anterior region, where deposition was extremely low. The POD device deposits nearly fourfold more drugs in the olfactory region compared to the standard nasal pump [94]. The newly designed insufflation devices can improve the pace and efficiency of medication absorption, leading to a faster and larger therapeutic effect in patients [105].

4.5 ROLE OF 3D PRINTING TECHNIQUES IN NOSE-TO-BRAIN DRUG-DELIVERY SYSTEMS

4.5.1 3D Printing for Prototyping Nasal Implants

Drug-eluting implants have recently received interest from scientists thanks to their ability to provide sustained drug delivery. For nasal administration, drugs can be incorporated into stents or implants. Chronic rhinosinusitis (CRS) is the most common medical illness treated with drug-eluting nasal implants. Clinically, nasal implants may be utilized as adjuncts to endoscopic sinus surgery. In addition to controlling bleeding, nasal implants can reduce adhesion formation and enhance drainage of the sinus mucosa that will help with the wound healing process. Incorporating antibiotics, corticosteroids, or anticancer drugs into nasal implants can improve their efficacy; consequently, this is the primary focus of drug-eluting nasal implant development at present. It has been shown that drug-eluting implants can minimize the incidence of synechiae and stenosis development. Drug-eluting sinus implants can be used very effectively to deliver drug to the sinus mucosa in a controlled manner [114]. However, these implants are designed to provide localized drug delivery. Therefore, there is a clear opportunity to develop intranasal implants to provide NtB drug delivery.

Drug-eluting nasal implants for NtB delivery have been relatively unexplored and few reports can be found on them. Intranasal implants offer the advantages of implantable devices combined with the advantages of NtB delivery. To start, they are capable of providing sustained and unattended drug delivery [115]–[117]. This can be used to treat chronic conditions affecting the CNS, such as schizophrenia. This is an extremely important feature as implantable drug-delivery systems have the potential to improve patients' adherence to treatment [118]. This is a recurrent problem in the treatment of chronic conditions. It has been reported that up to 75% of patients suffering from schizophrenia discontinue their treatment within the first year and a half [119]. Moreover, combining the advantages of implantable devices with NtB drug delivery will make it possible to reduce drug dosage, thereby minimizing side effects.

As mentioned previously, only a few examples of intranasal implants have been described in the literature. One study reported the use of core-shell nasal depot as a means to sustain the delivery of BDNF AntagoNATs, stranded short synthetic oligonucleotide-based compounds possessing the ability to inhibit brain-derived neurotrophic factor antisense (BDNF-AS) that can be used to treat neurodegenerative diseases. Driven by osmotic pressure, oligonucleotides can be released from the depot and reach the brain, where they upregulate the expression of BDNF in different areas of the brain [120]. An implantable device loaded with risperidone intended for NtB delivery was proposed in another study, in which 3D printing was involved in designing custom molds to cast PCL/PLGA-based biodegradable implants. The implants were reported to be biocompatible based on *in vitro* cell study results and able to sustain the release of the loaded drugs over 7 days, with some formulations reaching > 100 days of release [121]. Alternatively, this drug-delivery system was tested *in vivo* using a rat animal model. PLGA implants loaded with risperidone were capable of provide sustained drug delivery for at least 1 month post implantation [122].

4.5.2 3D Printing of Nasal Cast

Using 3D-printed nasal casts is one method for evaluating NtB formulations. They permit examination of the efficacy of NtB formulation in a more practical manner than normal tests and at a lower cost and with less difficulty than clinical studies. They enable determining whether the distribution of particle size is appropriate for NtB delivery and/or whether the dosing mechanism is compatible. It is important to note, however, that nasal cast experiments only evaluate the transport of the formulation from the instillation device to the olfactory zone and do not provide information about drug diffusion through nasal mucosa or brain bioavailability. The transition between numerical and physical models, on the other hand, can have an impact on the fidelity of *in vitro* geometries. As a result, selecting an appropriate 3D printing technology appears to be critical for effective *in vitro* experiments. According to the literature review, the experimental campaign with a nasal cast is typically prepared in the four stages outlined below: (1) defining the overall layout of the study while keeping constraints in mind; (2) adapting the design to the purpose of the study; (3) selecting a 3D printer appropriate for the needs; and (4) determining the type of mucus to be added to the cast [123].

4.6 FORMULATION LIMITATIONS, TESTING CHALLENGES, TOXICOLOGICAL CHALLENGES, AND REGULATORY REQUIREMENTS

4.6.1 Formulation Limitations

The nasal cavity is lined with a 10–15 μm thin layer of mucus consisting of two layers, a lower 6 μm thick liquid layer (also called: periciliary liquid), which is covered by the more viscous gel phase embedded mucin [124]. Although the nasal mucosa contains 90% water and glycoproteins as well as ions, it appears that this mucosa is primarily lipophilic in nature [125]. In addition, the fundamental brain uptake of medication after NtB administration is cellular transport, which permits the penetration of only tiny lipophilic molecules. Consequently, transcellular nasal transport is more typical for lipophilic molecules of smaller size (< 1000 Da), as the nasal membrane has pores with dimensions of 3.9 to 8.4 Å. While the permeability of polar medicines is limited, it can be realized mainly through paracellular transport [124]. According to studies, the bioavailability of hydrophilic drugs with a smaller molecular size is roughly 10%, while that of peptide drugs, such as insulin, calcitonin, and so on, is just around 1% [31]. Thus, there is a need to utilize different formulation strategies in order to improve drug permeability and the absorption of drugs that have a less lipophilic character. Scientists are currently employing a variety of permeation enhancers, colloidal drug carriers, controlled drug-delivery systems, and other innovative methods. Moreover, using appropriate mucoadhesive systems (such as mucoadhesive polymers, viscous formulations, hydrogels, or *in situ* gelling matrices) can result in increased retention time and increased resistance against mucociliary clearance. In addition, protective measures (such as encapsulation in a nanocarrier system) are required to prevent enzymatic degradation of the drug. These formulation techniques are intended to improve IN drug delivery and bioavailability. Unfortunately, due to the formulation's frequent and high dose, which may irritate the nasal mucosa, the clinical success of NtB administration remains limited. Furthermore, the protective nasal mucosa barriers reduce the efficacy of IN therapy, as only 1% or less of the administered medicine reaches the brain following IN administration [126].

In addition to this, the nature of the formulation, its excipients, and its strength should be evaluated. The human nasal cavity has a relatively small volume (approximately 15–16 cm^3) [127], [128], which when compared to the other administration routes, can only accommodate a modest amount of liquid (100–200 μl) or dry powder (up to 25 mg/dose for each nostril) formulation to be administered at one time [49], [105]. Considering this, only potent medications are appropriate for NtB delivery. Moreover, the excipients must be biocompatible and generate no offensive odor, to improve patient comfort when applying the nasal formulation. In addition, the pH, tonicity, and viscosity of the formulation need to be carefully considered during NtB dosage form development. The pH of nasal formulation should be within the range of nasal mucosa pH value (5.5–6.5) to ensure the non-irritating properties of the formulation as well as patient compliance. However, nasal mucosa pH can vary, influenced by physiological conditions. For example, slight changes in pH values can be found in illness conditions. In this case, patients with rhinosinusitis typically have nasal pH values between 5.3 and 7.6 [129]. Afterward, the particle size of the formulation should also take into consideration, as it can significantly affect drug absorption. A particle size of < 200 nm is considered optimal to promote absorption through the epithelium [130]. Meanwhile, for nasal spray formulation, the device's maximum allowable droplet size should be 10 μm or greater to avoid diffusion into the lower respiratory tract and to guarantee nasal drug deposition [131], [132].

It is imperative to note that the anterior area of the nasal cavity, especially the respiratory region adjacent to the inferior turbinates, is responsible for drug migration into the systemic circulation due to its large surface area (around 120–150 cm^2) and highly vascularized mucosa, whereas the posterior and higher regions of the nasal cavity (olfactory region) are responsible for drug absorption into the brain through its neuronal and epithelial pathways [1]. Hence, a proper delivery device is required to transport the formulation to the correct region of the nasal cavity, adding to the complexity of NtB products [126], [133]. It is essential to avoid utilizing substances with mucosal toxicity or those that cause irritation or allergic reactions. In individuals with allergies or a cold, intranasal drug delivery devices may not perform properly [27].

Many variables impact whether or not the medicine reaches the brain, resulting in diverse, even contradictory findings in NtB formulation studies. These differences suggest that a comprehensive understanding of formulation-related components is required to elucidate a successful clinical strategy to consistently deliver drug to the brain. Despite a great amount of good research data, the clinical application of NtB delivery requires significant improvement before this delivery system can be made available on the market. This is mainly because the current research focuses solely on a particular issue while the development of a good formulation must take into account all the aforementioned characteristics [126].

4.6.2 Testing Challenges

Appropriate *in vivo* models are required for the efficient development of nasal preparation. When selecting an acceptable animal model for *in vivo* studies, it is crucial to examine the architecture of the nasal cavity of the animal. The rat model was the first model used in the late 1970s, followed by the mouse, rabbit, dog, sheep, and monkey when nasal absorption studies were developed. Although mouse and rat models are particularly useful for basic NtB drug absorption studies, rabbit, dog, monkey, and sheep models are more commonly used for pharmacokinetic and pharmacodynamic studies due to their larger nose opening, which facilitates intranasal administration [134]. Due to the anatomical and physiological variations between animal and human nasal canals, there is not necessarily a correlation between the outcomes of animal studies and those of human studies [3], [135].

It is worth mentioning that MCC and cilia beating frequency (CBF) effects are usually evaluated *in vitro*. These *in vitro* tests cannot predict the ultimate effects *in vivo* because *in vitro* tests show effects on MCC and CBF, whereas in *in vivo* tests, the same compounds frequently do not cause detectable side effects. In general, many compounds have been shown to have a dose- and time-dependent inhibitory effect on mucosal clearance and CBF. The α-adrenergic receptor agonists oxymetazoline and xylometazoline, for example, inhibited human nasal mucosa *in vitro* in a dose-dependent manner. Some corticosteroids, decongestants, antimicrobial, antiviral, and antihistamine medications, as well as some intranasal drug excipients and nasal irrigation, influence MCC and CBF *in vitro* but have no adverse effects *in vivo* [1], [136].

In vitro investigations can provide a clearer understanding of the mechanistic features of nasal absorption and medication transport. RPMI 2650, Calu-3, and CaCo-2 cell lines are commonly used to assess nasal absorption and permeability. It should be noted that while these cellular models provide information on transport between cells or paracellularly, concomitant factors such as mucus, mucins, clearance, and anatomical and physiological aspects involved in nose functionality may also influence absorption. Furthermore, in the cellular models, the receiving lumen does not accurately represent the required transport from the mucosa to the receiving neurons [3].

Typically, the animal nasal mucosa is used *ex vivo* to assess the toxicity of excipients and the transmucosal transport of medications. *Ex vivo* excised animal tissue models are commonly obtained from rats, rabbits, sheep, dogs, primates, and humans. Extracted tissue studies are useful for learning about permeability, efflux, metabolism, and toxicity. *Ex vivo* models for nasal medication administration have obvious advantages, but they also have significant limitations. The most significant limiting factors in animal species are thick nasal epithelial tissues and a lack of interstitial flow rate beneath the mucosa. It becomes difficult to extend results to *in vivo* models when collecting data on permeability [3].

4.6.3 Toxicological Considerations

Safety is of the utmost importance when developing an effective and safe pharmacological formulation for IN delivery. Safety considerations must be applied not only to the medicine itself, but also to the formulation's active ingredients and excipients during the development process ("TRS 1010 - Annex 10: WHO Guidelines on Stability Testing of Active Pharmaceutical Ingredients and Finished Pharmaceutical Products" 2023). Excipients can significantly reduce the safety of the final drug product due to their own safety profile and the increased local exposure time of the drug. Furthermore, MCC is an important defensive mechanism that can be stimulated or inhibited by a variety of chemicals. Inhibitory effects, rather than stimulating effects, are primarily responsible for undesirable side effects such as nasal dryness, irritation, sneezing, nasal itching, rhinitis medicamentosa, and congestion [1].

Environmental cues (temperature and humidity), psychological factors, and individual physiological factors (infections, preexisting disease, or allergies) all influence the local interactions between medication products and nasal mucosa, as well as the drug's local tolerance. These factors influence drug absorption in the nasal mucosa and, as a result, the final product's toxicologic profile. When a drug is administered intranasally, the underlying physiological function of an organ may be altered. As a result, impairment of these functions may result in longer formulation contact times, which is advantageous, but it also causes physiological impairment and injury to the mucosa and nasal epithelium [1].

Excipients are used to protect medications from microbial contamination and degradation as well as to improve medication transport and bioavailability across the nasal mucosa and epithelial tissues. These enhancers and preservatives must be studied and tested for toxicity. For example, benzalkonium chloride (BKC), which is capable of inhibiting the frequency of ciliary beating and mucociliary clearance, is used as a preservative agent in a variety of liquid nasal formulations. Its effect, however, is dose and duration dependent, with the end result being ciliostasis and ciliotoxicity. *In vivo* histological tests on rats revealed that BKC can also cause nasal lesions (epithelial degeneration, desquamation, edema, or neutrophilic cellular infiltration) [1].

In addition to preservatives, nasal formulations also utilize penetration enhancers. These substances function to increase the transport and bioavailability of drugs across the nasal mucosa and epithelial tissue. Penetration enhancers have the desired effects of opening the tight junction of the cell to facilitate paracellular transport to the brain region, modifying the mucosal layer and inhibiting proteolytic enzymes. As a result, these disruptive functions can have more negative side effects, even though many chemicals and compounds can irritate the nasal mucosa without damaging it. Obviously, there is always a relationship between the drug and excipients in the local effects of a formulation. Furthermore, before drawing any conclusions about safety issues, the testing process, including dose, timing, and *in vitro* investigation system, as well as animal species, must be thoroughly evaluated [1].

4.6.4 Regulatory Requirements

The majority of nano-system-based formulations, as well as the use of neuropeptides and cellular-based therapies, are still in the preclinical, non-clinical phase of the pharmaceutical product development pipeline. To facilitate commercialization, numerous obstacles, such as regulatory concerns, the addressing of safety and quality aspects, as well as strict quality criteria, must be addressed. Even though nano-system formation is regarded as a promising technique for crossing the BBB, the precise mechanisms and variables associated with efficient brain targeting via the intranasal route are still unknown [137]. Acquiring regulatory approval to commercialize a proposed drug is the culmination of a lengthy drug development process, but regulatory considerations have to be taken into account from the outset. Furthermore, in order to obtain approval for a new drug, the aspects of safety, effectiveness, and quality must be considered. All required documentation must be submitted to the authorized body. For example, the regulation of new drugs in the United States is based on Food and Drug Administration approval through the new drug application (NDA) [138].

On the other hand, orally inhaled and/or nasal drug products (OINDP) are most frequently addressed for repurposing an already approved medicine, as previously reported for a number of examples, such as inhaled insulin (Exubera®), although this preparation was subsequently withdrawn from the marker. The OINDP guideline was developed by European Medicines Agency and became effective in 2006 for the European Union [139]. This guideline concerns documentation regarding the expected quality aspect of a human medicinal product delivered through the pulmonary or nasal route [131]. In line with this, drugs intended for nasal route administration include pressurized metered dose nasal sprays, liquids, and powders. Furthermore, this regulation focuses on specific safety, effectiveness, and quality considerations for respiratory delivery (inhalation and nasal products) in relation to the standards. The authorities may permit the use of some efficacy and safety data from previously approved medications for repurposed products. Yet, even while preclinical studies and systemic safety can be vindicated by evidence from prior studies of licensed medications, new preclinical and clinical research is still required to provide further information [1].

The pharmaceutical industry is currently under increased pressure to provide an innovative and efficient manufacturing process for active therapeutic products, including delivery devices. More complex and automated delivery systems will be required in the coming years to ensure accurate and reproducible intranasal dosing. The complex architecture of the nasal cavity creates a significant barrier to drug passage past the nasal valve. As a result, more efforts are needed to make this method of noninvasive medication delivery more effective and widespread [140].

4.7 CONCLUSION AND PROSPECTS

NtB drug delivery is a promising approach for the treatment of neurological disorders as it allows for direct delivery of drugs to the brain, bypassing the BBB. However, there are several challenges associated with this approach, including: nasal mucosa absorption, rapid clearance, safety concerns. Despite these challenges, significant progress has been made in NtB drug delivery. NtB nanoparticles have the potential to be used in the treatment of neurological disorders, such as Alzheimer's disease, Parkinson's disease, and brain tumors. By delivering drugs directly to the brain, these nanoparticles can bypass the BBB and provide more targeted and effective treatments. NtB mucoadhesive delivery systems are also being investigated widely for the treatment of a range of neurological disorders. Combining 3D printing technologies, researchers have explored the possibility of using 3D printing to create specialized drug delivery devices for NtB delivery. Additionally, 3D printing has been used to create personalized nasal inserts that can fit an individual's unique nasal anatomy, potentially improving drug delivery efficacy. Overall, NtB drug delivery is a rapidly evolving field with significant potential for the treatment of neurological disorders. While challenges remain, progress in drug design and delivery technologies is advancing the field.

REFERENCES

[1] Keller, Lea Adriana, Olivia Merkel, and Andreas Popp. 2021. "Intranasal drug delivery: opportunities and toxicologic challenges during drug development." *Drug Delivery and Translational Research.* 12. 4. 735–757. doi: 10.1007/S13346-020-00891-5

[2] Khatri, Dharmendra Kumar, Kumari Preeti, Shivraj Tonape, Sheoshree Bhattacharjee, Monica Patel, Saurabh Shah, Pankaj Kumar Singh, Saurabh Srivastav, Dalapathi Gugulothu, Lalit Vora, and Shashi Bala Singh. 2022. "Nanotechnological advances

for nose to brain delivery of therapeutics to improve the Parkinson therapy." *Current Neuropharmacology*. 20. doi: 10.2174/1570159X20666220507022701

[3] Erdő, Franciska, Luca Anna Bors, Dániel Farkas, Ágnes Bajza, and Sveinbjörn Gizurarson. 2018. "Evaluation of intranasal delivery route of drug administration for brain targeting." *Brain Research Bulletin*. 143. 155–170. doi: 10.1016/J.BRAINRESBULL.2018.10.009

[4] Lobaina Mato, Yadira. 2019. "Nasal route for vaccine and drug delivery: Features and current opportunities." *International Journal of Pharmaceutics*. 572. 118813. doi: 10.1016/J.IJPHARM.2019.118813

[5] Mittal, Deepti, Asgar Ali, Shadab Md, Sanjula Baboota, Jasjeet K. Sahni, and Javed Ali. 2014. "Insights into direct nose to brain delivery: current status and future perspective." *Drug Delivery*. 21. 75–86. doi: 10.3109/10717544.2013.838713

[6] Hanson, Leah R., and William H Frey II. 2008. "Intranasal delivery bypasses the blood-brain barrier to target therapeutic agents to the central nervous system and treat neurodegenerative disease." *BMC Neuroscience*. 9. S5. doi: 10.1186/1471-2202-9-S3-S5

[7] Musumeci, Teresa, Angela Bonaccorso, and Giovanni Puglisi. 2019. "Epilepsy disease and nose-to-brain delivery of polymeric nanoparticles: An overview." *Pharmaceutics*. 11. 118. doi: 10.3390/pharmaceutics11030118

[8] Chung, Steve, Jurriaan M. Peters, Kamil Detyniecki, William Tatum, Adrian L. Rabinowicz, and Enrique Carrazana. 2023. "The nose has it: Opportunities and challenges for intranasal drug administration for neurologic conditions including seizure clusters." *Epilepsy & Behavior Reports*. 21. 100581. doi: 10.1016/J.EBR.2022.100581

[9] Gonçalves, Joana, Joana Bicker, Filipa Gouveia, Joana Liberal, Rui Caetano Oliveira, Gilberto Alves, Amílcar Falcão, and Ana Fortuna. 2019. "Nose-to-brain delivery of levetiracetam after intranasal administration to mice." *International Journal of Pharmaceutics*. 564. 329–339. doi: 10.1016/J.IJPHARM.2019.04.047

[10] Zada, Moran Haim, Michael Kubek, Wahid Khan, Awanish Kumar, and Abraham Domb. 2019. "Dispersible hydrolytically sensitive nanoparticles for nasal delivery of thyrotropin releasing hormone (TRH)." *Journal of Controlled Release*. 295. 278–289. doi: 10.1016/J.JCONREL.2018.12.050

[11] Chatterjee, Bappaditya, Bapi Gorain, Keithanchali Mohananaidu, Pinaki Sengupta, Uttam Kumar Mandal, and Hira Choudhury. 2019. "Targeted drug delivery to the brain via intranasal nanoemulsion: Available proof of concept and existing challenges." *International Journal of Pharmaceutics*. 565. 258–268. doi: 10.1016/J.IJPHARM.2019.05.032

[12] Ozsoy, Yıldız, Sevgi Gungor, and Erdal Cevher. 2009. "Nasal delivery of high molecular weight drugs." *Molecules*. 14. 3754–3779. doi: 10.3390/molecules14093754

[13] Bonferoni, Maria, Silvia Rossi, Giuseppina Sandri, Franca Ferrari, Elisabetta Gavini, Giovanna Rassu, and Paolo Giunchedi. 2019. "Nanoemulsions for 'Nose-to-Brain' Drug Delivery." *Pharmaceutics*. 11. 84. doi: 10.3390/pharmaceutics11020084

[14] Selvaraj, Kousalya, Kuppusamy Gowthamarajan, and Veera Venkata Satyanarayana Reddy Karri. 2017. "Nose to brain transport pathways an overview: potential of nanostructured lipid carriers in nose to brain targeting." *Artificial Cells, Nanomedicine, and Biotechnology*. 46. 8. 1–8. doi: 10.1080/21691401.2017.1420073

[15] Ruigrok, Mitchel J. R. and Elizabeth C. M. de Lange. 2015. "Emerging insights for translational pharmacokinetic and pharmacokinetic-pharmacodynamic studies: Towards prediction of nose-to-brain transport in humans." *AAPS Journal*. 17. 493–505. doi: 10.1208/s12248-015-9724-x

[16] Hazeri, Mohammad, Zahra Farshidfar, Mohammad Faramarzi, Sasan Sadrizadeh, and Omid Abouali. 2020. "Details of the physiology of the aerodynamic and heat and moisture transfer in the normal nasal cavity." *Respiratory Physiology & Neurobiology*. 280. 103480. doi: 10.1016/J.RESP.2020.103480

[17] Na, Yang, Seung Kyu Chung, and Seongsu Byun. 2020. "Numerical study on the heat-recovery capacity of the human nasal cavity during expiration." *Computers in Biology and Medicine*. 126. 103992. doi: 10.1016/J.COMPBIOMED.2020.103992

[18] Long, Yu, Qiyue Yang, Yan Xiang, Yulu Zhang, Jinyan Wan, Songyu Liu, Nan Li, and Wei Peng. 2020. "Nose to brain drug delivery – A promising strategy for active components from herbal medicine for treating cerebral ischemia reperfusion." *Pharmacological Research*. 159. 104795. doi: 10.1016/J.PHRS.2020.104795

[19] Battaglia, Luigi, Pier Paolo Panciani, Elisabetta Muntoni, Maria Teresa Capucchio, Elena Biasibetti, Pasquale De Bonis, Silvia Mioletti, Marco Fontanella, and Shankar Swaminathan. 2018. "Lipid nanoparticles for intranasal administration: application to nose-to-brain delivery." *Expert Opinion on Drug Delivery*. 15. 369–378. doi: 10.1080/17425247.2018.1429401

[20] Sarma, Anupam, and Malay K. Das. 2020. "Nose to brain delivery of antiretroviral drugs in the treatment of neuroAIDS." *Molecular Biomedicine*. 1. 15. doi: 10.1186/s43556-020-00019-8

[21] Bourganis, Vassilis, Olga Kammona, Aleck Alexopoulos, and Costas Kiparissides. 2018. "Recent advances in carrier mediated nose-to-brain delivery of pharmaceutics." *European Journal of Pharmaceutics and Biopharmaceutics*. 128. 337–362. doi: 10.1016/J.EJPB.2018.05.009

[22] Lee, David and Tamara Minko. 2021. "Nanotherapeutics for nose-to-brain drug delivery: An approach to bypass the blood brain barrier." *Pharmaceutics*. 13. 2049. doi: 10.3390/pharmaceutics13122049

[23] Newsome, Hillary, Emily L. Lin, David M. Poetker, and Guilherme J. M. Garcia. 2019. "Clinical importance of nasal air conditioning: A review of the literature." *American Journal of Rhinology & Allergy*. 33. 763–769. doi: 10.1177/1945892419863033

[24] Koparal, Mehtap, Ercan Kurt, Emine Elif Altuntas, and Fatih Dogan. 2021. "Assessment of mucociliary clearance as an indicator of nasal function in patients with COVID-19: A cross-sectional study." *European Archives of Oto-Rhino-Laryngology*. 278. 1863–1868. doi: 10.1007/s00405-020-06457-y

[25] Shang, Yidan, Kiao Inthavong, and Jiyuan Tu. 2019. "Development of a computational fluid dynamics model for mucociliary clearance in the nasal cavity." *Journal of Biomechanics*. 85. 74–83. doi: 10.1016/J.JBIOMECH.2019.01.015

[26] Sauvalle, Marcel and Andrés Alvo. 2018. "Effect of the temperature of nasal lavages on mucociliary clearance: a randomised controlled trial." *European Archives of Oto-Rhino-Laryngology*. 275. 2403–2406. doi: 10.1007/s00405-018-5060-y

[27] Gänger, Stella and Katharina Schindowski. 2018. "Tailoring formulations for intranasal nose-to-brain delivery: A review on architecture, physico-chemical characteristics and mucociliary clearance of the nasal olfactory mucosa." *Pharmaceutics*. 10. 116. doi: 10.3390/pharmaceutics10030116

[28] Sabir, Fakhara, Qurrat Ul Ain, Abbas Rahdar, Zhugen Yang, Mahmood Barani, Mauhammad Bilal, and Nikhil Bhalla. "Functionalized nanoparticles in drug delivery: strategies to enhance direct nose-to-brain drug delivery via integrated nerve pathways," in *Synthesis and Applications of Nanoparticles*, Singapore: Springer Nature Singapore, 2022, 455–485. doi: 10.1007/978-981-16-6819-7_21

[29] Zhang, N., K. van Crombruggen, E. Gevaert, and C. Bachert. 2016. "Barrier function of the nasal mucosa in health and type-2 biased airway diseases." *Allergy*. 71. 295–307. doi: 10.1111/ALL.12809

[30] Khoury, Spiro, Volker Gudziol, Stéphane Grégoire, Stéphanie Cabaret, Susanne Menzel, Lucy Martine, Esther Mézière, Vanessa Soubeyre, Thierry Thomas-Danguin, Xavier Grosmaitre, Lionel Bretillon, Olivier Berdeaux, Niyazi Acar, Thomas Hummel, and Anne Marie Le Bon. 2021. "Lipidomic profile of human nasal mucosa and associations with circulating fatty acids and olfactory deficiency." *Scientific Reports*. 11. 16771. doi: 10.1038/s41598-021-93817-1

[31] Agrawal, Mukta, Shailendra Saraf, Swarnlata Saraf, Sunil K. Dubey, Anu Puri, Umesh Gupta, Prashant Kesharwani, V. Ravichandiran, Pramod Kumar, V. G. M. Naidu, Upadhyayula Suryanarayana Murty, Ajazuddin, and Amit Alexander. 2020. "Stimuli-responsive in situ gelling system for nose-to-brain drug delivery." *Journal of Controlled Release*. 327. 235–265. doi: 10.1016/J.JCONREL.2020.07.044

[32] Horvát, Sándor, András Fehér, Hartwig Wolburg, Péter Sipos, Szilvia Veszelka, Andrea Tóth, Lóránd Kis, Anita Kurunczi, Gábor Balogh, Levente Kürti, István Eros, Piroska Szabó-Révész, and Mária A. Deli. 2009. "Sodium hyaluronate as a mucoadhesive component in nasal formulation enhances delivery of molecules to brain tissue." *European Journal of Pharmaceutics and Biopharmaceutics*. 72. 252–259. doi: 10.1016/J.EJPB.2008.10.009

[33] Sarkar, Sanjib, Dibyendu Das, Prachurjya Dutta, Jatin Kalita, Sawlang Borsingh Wann, and Prasenjit Manna. 2020. "Chitosan: A promising therapeutic agent and effective drug delivery system in managing diabetes mellitus." *Carbohydrate Polymers*. 247. 116594. doi: 10.1016/J.CARBPOL.2020.116594

[34] Hansen, Kellisa, Gwangseong Kim, Kashappa-Goud H. Desai, Hiren Patel, Karl F. Olsen, Jaime Curtis-Fisk, Elizabeth Tocce, Susan Jordan, and Steven P. Schwendeman. 2015. "Feasibility investigation of cellulose polymers for mucoadhesive nasal drug delivery applications." *Molecular Pharmaceutics*. 12. 2732–2741. doi: 10.1021/acs.molpharmaceut.5b00264

[35] Tonglairoum, Prasopchai, Ruairí P. Brannigan, Praneet Opanasopit, and Vitaliy v. Khutoryanskiy. 2016. "Maleimide-bearing nanogels as novel mucoadhesive materials for drug delivery." *Journal of Materials Chemistry B*. 4. 6581–6587. doi: 10.1039/C6TB02124G

[36] Davidovich-Pinhas, Maya and Havazelet Bianco-Peled. 2010. "Novel mucoadhesive system based on sulfhydryl-acrylate interactions." *Journal of Materials Science: Materials in Medicine*. 21. 2027–2034. doi: 10.1007/s10856-010-4069-6

[37] Puri, Vivek, Ameya Sharma, Pradeep Kumar, and Inderbir Singh. 2020. "Thiolation of biopolymers for developing drug delivery systems with enhanced mechanical and mucoadhesive properties: A review." *Polymers*. 12. 1803. doi: 10.3390/polym12081803

[38] Brannigan, Ruairí P. and Vitaliy v. Khutoryanskiy. 2019. "Progress and current trends in the synthesis of novel polymers with enhanced mucoadhesive properties." *Macromolecular Bioscience*. 19. 1900194. doi: 10.1002/mabi.201900194

[39] Nasr, Maha. 2016. "Development of an optimized hyaluronic acid-based lipidic nanoemulsion co-encapsulating two polyphenols for nose to brain delivery." *Drug Delivery*. 23. 1444–1452. doi: 10.3109/10717544.2015.1092619

[40] Vasvani, Shyam, Pratik Kulkarni, and Deepak Rawtani. 2020. "Hyaluronic acid: A review on its biology, aspects of drug delivery, route of administrations and a special emphasis on its approved marketed products and recent clinical studies." *International Journal of Biological Macromolecules*. 151. 1012–1029. doi: 10.1016/j.ijbiomac.2019.11.066

[41] Rinaldi, Federica, Alessandra Oliva, Manuela Sabatino, Anna Imbriano, Patrizia N. Hanieh, Stefania Garzoli, Claudio M. Mastroianni, Massimiliano De Angelis, Maria Claudia Miele, Marcela Arnaut, Federica Di Timoteo, Carlotta Marianecci, Rino Ragno, and Maria Carafa. 2020. "Antimicrobial essential oil formulation: chitosan coated nanoemulsions for nose to brain delivery." *Pharmaceutics*. 12. 678. doi: 10.3390/pharmaceutics12070678

[42] Casettari, Luca and Lisbeth Illum. 2014. "Chitosan in nasal delivery systems for therapeutic drugs." *Journal of Controlled Release*. 190. 189–200. doi: 10.1016/j.jconrel.2014.05.003

[43] Sunena, Shailendra K. Singh, and Dina Nath Mishra. 2018. "Nose to brain delivery of galantamine loaded nanoparticles: In-vivo pharmacodynamic and biochemical study in mice." *Current Drug Delivery*. 16. 51–58. doi: 10.2174/1567201815666181004094707

[44] Yang, Feipeng, Maleen Cabe, Hope A. Nowak, and Kelly A. Langert. 2022. "Chitosan/poly(lactic-co-glycolic)acid nanoparticle formulations with finely-tuned size distributions for enhanced mucoadhesion." *Pharmaceutics*. 14. 95. doi: 10.3390/pharmaceutics14010095

[45] Tzeyung, Angeline, Shadab Md, Subrat Bhattamisra, Thiagarajan Madheswaran, Nabil Alhakamy, Hibah Aldawsari, and Ammu Radhakrishnan. 2019. "Fabrication, optimization, and evaluation of rotigotine-loaded chitosan nanoparticles for nose-to-brain delivery." *Pharmaceutics*. 11. 26. doi: 10.3390/pharmaceutics11010026

[46] Saini, Sumant, Teenu Sharma, Atul Jain, Harmanjot Kaur, O. P. Katare, and Bhupinder Singh. 2021. "Systematically designed chitosan-coated solid lipid nanoparticles of ferulic acid for effective management of Alzheimer's disease: A preclinical evidence." *Colloids and Surfaces B: Biointerfaces*. 205. 111838. doi: 10.1016/j.colsurfb.2021.111838

[47] Piazzini, Vieri, Elisa Landucci, Mario D'Ambrosio, Laura Tiozzo Fasiolo, Lorenzo Cinci, Gaia Colombo, Domenico E. Pellegrini-Giampietro, Anna Rita Bilia, Cristina Luceri, and Maria Camilla Bergonzi. 2019. "Chitosan coated human serum albumin nanoparticles: A promising strategy for nose-to-brain drug delivery." *International Journal of Biological Macromolecules*. 129. 267–280. doi: 10.1016/J.IJBIOMAC.2019.02.005

[48] Sipos, Bence, Ildikó Csóka, Nimród Szivacski, Mária Budai-Szűcs, Zsuzsanna Schelcz, István Zupkó, Piroska Szabó-Révész, Balázs Volk, and Gábor Katona. 2022. "Mucoadhesive meloxicam-loaded nanoemulsions: Development, characterization and nasal applicability studies." *European Journal of Pharmaceutical Sciences*. 175. 106229. doi: 10.1016/J.EJPS.2022.106229

[49] Nižić Nodilo, Laura, Ivo Ugrina, Drago Špoljarić, Daniela Amidžić Klarić, Cvijeta Jakobušić Brala, Mirna Perkušić, Ivan Pepić, Jasmina Lovrić, Vesna Saršon, Maša Safundžić Kučuk, Dijana Zadravec, Livije Kalogjera, and Anita Hafner. 2021. "A dry powder platform for nose-to-brain delivery of dexamethasone: Formulation development and nasal deposition studies." *Pharmaceutics*. 13. 795. doi: 10.3390/pharmaceutics13060795

[50] Ghadiri, Maliheh, Paul Young, and Daniela Traini. 2019. "Strategies to enhance drug absorption via nasal and pulmonary routes." *Pharmaceutics*. 11. 113. doi: 10.3390/pharmaceutics11030113

[51] Li, Ying, Jinfeng Li, Xin Zhang, Jiaojiao Ding, and Shirui Mao. 2016. "Non-ionic surfactants as novel intranasal absorption enhancers: *in vitro* and *in vivo* characterization." *Drug Delivery*. 23. 2272–2279. doi: 10.3109/10717544.2014.971196

[52] Brunner, Joël, Sakthikumar Ragupathy, and Gerrit Borchard. 2021. "Target specific tight junction modulators." *Advanced Drug Delivery Reviews*. 171. 266–288. doi: 10.1016/J.ADDR.2021.02.008

[53] Rassu, Giovanna, Luca Ferraro, Barbara Pavan, Paolo Giunchedi, Elisabetta Gavini, and Alessandro Dalpiaz. 2018. "The role of combined penetration enhancers in nasal microspheres on in vivo drug bioavailability." *Pharmaceutics*. 10. 206. doi: 10.3390/pharmaceutics10040206

[54] Kumar, Amresh, Pradeep Kumar Naik, Deepak Pradhan, Goutam Ghosh, and Goutam Rath. 2020. "Mucoadhesive formulations: innovations, merits, drawbacks, and future outlook." *Pharmaceutical Development and Technology*. 25. 797–814. doi: 10.1080/10837450.2020.1753771

[55] Gadhave, Dnyandev, Nishant Rasal, Rahul Sonawane, Mahendran Sekar, and Chandrakant Kokare. 2021. "Nose-to-brain delivery of teriflunomide-loaded lipid-based carbopol-gellan gum nanogel for glioma: Pharmacological and in vitro cytotoxicity studies." *International Journal of Biological Macromolecules*. 167. 906–920. doi: 10.1016/J.IJBIOMAC.2020.11.047

[56] Mardikasari, Sandra Aulia, Mária Budai-Szűcs, László Orosz, Katalin Burián, Ildikó Csóka, and Gábor Katona. 2022. "Development of thermoresponsive-gel-matrix-embedded amoxicillin trihydrate-loaded bovine serum albumin nanoparticles for local intranasal therapy." *Gels*. 8. 750. doi: 10.3390/gels8110750

[57] Karavasili, Christina and Dimitrios G. Fatouros. 2016. "Smart materials: In situ gel-forming systems for nasal delivery." *Drug Discovery Today*. 21. 157–166. doi: 10.1016/J.DRUDIS.2015.10.016

[58] Nagalingam, Arunkumar. 2017. "Drug delivery aspects of herbal medicines." *Japanese Kampo Medicines for the Treatment of Common Diseases: Focus on Inflammation*. 143–164. doi: 10.1016/B978-0-12-809398-6.00015-9

[59] Hong, Soon-Seok, Kyung Taek Oh, Han-Gon Choi, and Soo-Jeong Lim. 2019. "Liposomal formulations for nose-to-brain delivery: Recent advances and future perspectives." *Pharmaceutics*. 11. 540. doi: 10.3390/pharmaceutics11100540

[60] Kurano, Takumi, Takanori Kanazawa, Aoi Ooba, Yudai Masuyama, Nao Maruhana, Mayu Yamada, Shingo Iioka, Hisako Ibaraki, Yasuhiro Kosuge, Hiromu Kondo, and Toyofumi Suzuki. 2022. "Nose-to-brain/spinal cord delivery kinetics of liposomes with different surface properties." *Journal of Controlled Release*. 344. 225–234. doi: 10.1016/J.JCONREL.2022.03.017

[61] Sita, V. G., Dhananjay Jadhav, and Pradeep Vavia. 2020. "Niosomes for nose-to-brain delivery of bromocriptine: Formulation development, efficacy evaluation and toxicity profiling." *Journal of Drug Delivery Science and Technology*. 58. 101791. doi: 10.1016/J.JDDST.2020.101791

[62] Chen, Shuo, Sara Hanning, James Falconer, Michelle Locke, and Jingyuan Wen. 2019. "Recent advances in non-ionic surfactant vesicles (niosomes): Fabrication, characterization, pharmaceutical and cosmetic applications." *European Journal of Pharmaceutics and Biopharmaceutics*. 144. 18–39. doi: 10.1016/J.EJPB.2019.08.015

[63] Fahmy, Usama A., Shaimaa M. Badr-Eldin, Osama A. A. Ahmed, Hibah M. Aldawsari, Singkome Tima, Hani Z. Asfour, Mohammed W. Al-Rabia, Aya A. Negm, Muhammad H. Sultan, Osama A. A. Madkhali, and Nabil A. Alhakamy. 2020. "Intranasal niosomal in situ gel as a promising approach for enhancing flibanserin bioavailability and brain delivery: In vitro optimization and ex vivo/in vivo evaluation." *Pharmaceutics*. 12. 485. doi: 10.3390/pharmaceutics12060485

[64] Thabet, Yasmeena, Mahmoud Elsabahy, and Noura G. Eissa. 2022. "Methods for preparation of niosomes: A focus on thin-film hydration method." *Methods*. 199. 9–15. doi: 10.1016/J.YMETH.2021.05.004

[65] Ojeda-Hernández, Doddy Denise, Alejandro A. Canales-Aguirre, Jorge Matias-Guiu, Ulises Gomez-Pinedo, and Juan C. Mateos-Díaz. 2020. "Potential of chitosan and its derivatives for biomedical applications in the central nervous system." *Frontiers in Bioengineering and Biotechnology*. 8. 389. doi: 10.3389/fbioe.2020.00389

[66] Gabold, Bettina, Friederike Adams, Sophie Brameyer, Kirsten Jung, Christian L. Ried, Thomas Merdan, and Olivia M. Merkel. 2023. "Transferrin-modified chitosan nanoparticles for targeted nose-to-brain delivery of proteins." *Drug Delivery and Translational Research*. 13. 822–838. doi: 10.1007/s13346-022-01245-z

[67] Trapani, Adriana, Stefania Cometa, Elvira De Giglio, Filomena Corbo, Roberta Cassano, Maria Luisa Di Gioia, Sonia Trombino, Md Niamat Hossain, Sante Di Gioia, Giuseppe Trapani, and Massimo Conese. 2022. "Novel nanoparticles based on n,o-carboxymethyl chitosan-dopamine amide conjugate for nose-to-brain delivery." *Pharmaceutics*. 14. 147. doi: 10.3390/pharmaceutics14010147

[68] Pardeshi, Chandrakantsing V. and Veena S. Belgamwar. 2020. "Improved brain pharmacokinetics following intranasal administration of *N,N,N* -trimethyl chitosan tailored mucoadhesive NLCs." *Materials Technology*. 35. 249–266. doi: 10.1080/10667857.2019.1674522

[69] Trapani, Adriana, Filomena Corbo, Gennaro Agrimi, Nicoletta Ditaranto, Nicola Cioffi, Filippo Perna, Andrea Quivelli, Erika Stefàno, Paola Lunetti, Antonella Muscella, Santo Marsigliante, Antonio Cricenti, Marco Luce, Cristina Mormile, Antonino Cataldo, and Stefano Bellucci. 2021. "Oxidized Alginate Dopamine Conjugate: In vitro Characterization for Nose-to-Brain Delivery Application." *Materials*. 14. 3495. doi: 10.3390/ma14133495

[70] Hu, Shanshan, Xibo Pei, Lunliang Duan, Zhou Zhu, Yanhua Liu, Junyu Chen, Tao Chen, Ping Ji, Qianbing Wan, and Jian Wang. 2021. "A mussel-inspired film for adhesion to wet buccal tissue and efficient buccal drug delivery." *Nature Communications*. 12. 1689. doi: 10.1038/s41467-021-21989-5

[71] Surendranath, Medha, M. R. Rekha, and Ramesh Parameswaran. 2022. "Recent advances in functionally modified polymers for mucoadhesive drug delivery." *Journal of Materials Chemistry B*. 10. 5913–5924. doi: 10.1039/D2TB00856D

[72] Leichner, Christina, Patrizia Wulz, Randi Angela Baus, Claudia Menzel, Sina Katharina Götzfried, Ronald Gust, and Andreas Bernkop-Schnürch. 2019. "*N*-Hydroxysulfosuccinimide esters versus thiomers: A comparative study regarding mucoadhesiveness." *Molecular Pharmaceutics*. 16. 1211–1219. doi: 10.1021/acs.molpharmaceut.8b01183

[73] Haroon, Hajira Banu, Dhrubojyoti Mukherjee, Jayaraman Anbu, and Banala Venkatesh Teja. 2021. "Thiolated chitosan-centella asiatica nanocomposite: a potential brain targeting strategy through nasal route." *AAPS PharmSciTech*. 22. 251. doi: 10.1208/s12249-021-02131-6

[74] Patil, Dilip, Sopan Nangare, Gaurav Patil, Kalpesh Nerkar, and Ganesh Patil. 2022. "Development of thiolated polyethylene glycol-poly (lactic-co-glycolic acid) copolymeric nanoparticles for intranasal delivery of quetiapine: *In vitro – ex vivo* characterization." *International Journal of Polymeric Materials and Polymeric Biomaterials*. 1–11. doi: 10.1080/00914037.2022.2052728

[75] Porfiryeva, Natalia N., Shamil F. Nasibullin, Svetlana G. Abdullina, Irina K. Tukhbatullina, Rouslan I. Moustafine, and Vitaliy v. Khutoryanskiy. 2019. "Acrylated Eudragit® E PO as a novel polymeric excipient with enhanced mucoadhesive properties

for application in nasal drug delivery." *International Journal of Pharmaceutics*. 562. 241–248. doi: 10.1016/J.IJPHARM.2019.03.027

[76] Chu, Liuxiang, Aiping Wang, Ling Ni, Xiuju Yan, Yina Song, Mingyu Zhao, Kaoxiang Sun, Hongjie Mu, Sha Liu, Zimei Wu, and Chunyan Zhang. 2018. "Nose-to-brain delivery of temozolomide-loaded PLGA nanoparticles functionalized with anti-EPHA3 for glioblastoma targeting." *Drug Delivery*. 25. 1634–1641. doi: 10.1080/10717544.2018.1494226

[77] Zong, Taili, Ling Mei, Huile Gao, Wei Cai, Pengjin Zhu, Kairong Shi, Jiantao Chen, Yang Wang, Fabao Gao, and Qin He. 2014. "Synergistic dual-ligand doxorubicin liposomes improve targeting and therapeutic efficacy of brain glioma in animals." *Molecular Pharmaceutics*. 11. 2346–2357. doi: 10.1021/mp500057n

[78] Markoutsa, E., K. Papadia, A. D. Giannou, M. Spella, A. Cagnotto, M. Salmona, G. T. Stathopoulos, and S. G. Antimisiaris. 2014. "Mono and dually decorated nanoliposomes for brain targeting, in vitro and in vivo studies." *Pharmaceutical Research*. 31. 1275–1289. doi: 10.1007/s11095-013-1249-3

[79] Qu, Mengke, Qing Lin, Shanshan He, Luyao Wang, Yao Fu, Zhirong Zhang, and Ling Zhang. 2018. "A brain targeting functionalized liposomes of the dopamine derivative N-3,4-bis(pivaloyloxy)-dopamine for treatment of Parkinson's disease." *Journal of Controlled Release*. 277. 173–182. doi: 10.1016/J.JCONREL.2018.03.019

[80] Ramalho, Maria João, Joana Angélica Loureiro, Manuel A. N. Coelho, and Maria Carmo Pereira. 2022. "Transferrin receptor-targeted nanocarriers: Overcoming barriers to treat glioblastoma." *Pharmaceutics*. 14. 279. doi: 10.3390/pharmaceutics14020279

[81] Wang, Zi Ying, Sravan Gopalkrishnashetty Sreenivasmurthy, Ju Xian Song, Jing Yi Liu, and Min Li. 2019. "Strategies for brain-targeting liposomal delivery of small hydrophobic molecules in the treatment of neurodegenerative diseases." *Drug Discovery Today*. 24. 595–605. doi: 10.1016/J.DRUDIS.2018.11.001

[82] El-Zaafarany, Ghada, Mahmoud Soliman, Samar Mansour, Marco Cespi, Giovanni Palmieri, Lisbeth Illum, Luca Casettari, and Gehanne Awad. 2018. "A tailored thermosensitive PLGA-PEG-PLGA/emulsomes composite for enhanced oxcarbazepine brain delivery via the nasal route." *Pharmaceutics*. 10. 217. doi: 10.3390/pharmaceutics10040217

[83] Eid, Hussein M., Mohammed H. Elkomy, Shahira F. el Menshawe, and Heba F. Salem. 2019. "Transfersomal nanovesicles for nose-to-brain delivery of ofloxacin for better management of bacterial meningitis: Formulation, optimization by Box-Behnken design, characterization and in vivo pharmacokinetic study." *Journal of Drug Delivery Science and Technology*. 54. 101304. doi: 10.1016/J.JDDST.2019.101304

[84] Nojoki, Fahimeh, Bahman Ebrahimi-Hosseinzadeh, Ashrafalsadat Hatamian-Zarmi, Fariba Khodagholi, and Khadijeh Khezri. 2022. "Design and development of chitosan-insulin-transfersomes (Transfersulin) as effective intranasal nanovesicles for the treatment of Alzheimer's disease: In vitro, in vivo, and ex vivo evaluations." *Biomedicine & Pharmacotherapy*. 153. 113450. doi: 10.1016/J.BIOPHA.2022.113450

[85] Taweel, Mai M. El, Mona H. Aboul-Einien, Mohammed A. Kassem, and Nermeen A. Elkasabgy. 2021. "Intranasal zolmitriptan-loaded bilosomes with extended nasal mucociliary transit time for direct nose to brain delivery." *Pharmaceutics*. 13. 1828. doi: 10.3390/PHARMACEUTICS13111828/S1

[86] Abbas, Haidy, Hanan Refai, Nesrine el Sayed, Laila Ahmed Rashed, Mohamed R. Mousa, and Mariam Zewail. 2021. "Superparamagnetic iron oxide loaded chitosan coated bilosomes for magnetic nose to brain targeting of resveratrol." *International Journal of Pharmaceutics*. 610. 121244. doi: 10.1016/J.IJPHARM.2021.121244

[87] Wang, Kai, Uday S. Kumar, Negar Sadeghipour, Tarik F. Massoud, and Ramasamy Paulmurugan. 2021. "A microfluidics-based scalable approach to generate extracellular vesicles with enhanced therapeutic microRNA loading for intranasal delivery to mouse glioblastomas." *ACS Nano*. 15. 18327–18346. doi: 10.1021/acsnano.1c07587

[88] Li, Yaosheng, Honghui Wu, Xinchi Jiang, Yunfei Dong, Juanjuan Zheng, and Jianqing Gao. 2022. "New idea to promote the clinical applications of stem cells or their extracellular vesicles in central nervous system disorders: Combining with intranasal delivery." *Acta Pharmaceutica Sinica B*. 12. 3215–3232. doi: 10.1016/J.APSB.2022.04.001

[89] Pusic, Kae M., Richard P. Kraig, and Aya D. Pusic. 2021. "IFNγ-stimulated dendritic cell extracellular vesicles can be nasally administered to the brain and enter oligodendrocytes." *PLOS One*. 16. e0255778. doi: 10.1371/JOURNAL.PONE.0255778

[90] Zwain, Tamara, Jane Elizabeth Alder, Bassem Sabagh, Andrew Shaw, Andrea J. Burrow, and Kamalinder K. Singh. 2021. "Tailoring functional nanostructured lipid carriers for glioblastoma treatment with enhanced permeability through in-vitro 3D BBB/BBTB models." *Materials Science and Engineering: C*. 121. 111774. doi: 10.1016/J.MSEC.2020.111774

[91] Patel, Hetal P., Priyanshi A. Gandhi, Priyanka S. Chaudhari, Bhargavi v. Desai, Ditixa T. Desai, Praful P. Dedhiya, Furqan A. Maulvi, and Bhavin A. Vyas. 2021. "Clozapine loaded nanostructured lipid carriers engineered for brain targeting via nose-to-brain delivery: Optimization and in vivo pharmacokinetic studies." *Journal of Drug Delivery Science and Technology*. 64. 102533. doi: 10.1016/J.JDDST.2021.102533

[92] Farheen, Ms, Md Habban Akhter, Havagiray Chitme, Md Sayeed Akhter, Fauzia Tabassum, Mariusz Jaremko, and Abdul-Hamid Emwas. 2023. "Harnessing folate-functionalized nasal delivery of dox–erlo-loaded biopolymeric nanoparticles in cancer treatment: development, optimization, characterization, and biodistribution analysis." *Pharmaceuticals*. 16. 207. doi: 10.3390/ph16020207

[93] Patel, Hetal P., Priyanka S. Chaudhari, Priyanshi A. Gandhi, Bhargavi v. Desai, Ditixa T. Desai, Praful P. Dedhiya, Bhavin A. Vyas, and Furqan A. Maulvi. 2021. "Nose to brain delivery of tailored clozapine nanosuspension stabilized using (+)-alpha-tocopherol polyethylene glycol 1000 succinate: Optimization and in vivo pharmacokinetic studies." *International Journal of Pharmaceutics*. 600. 120474. doi: 10.1016/J.IJPHARM.2021.120474

[94] Shah, Brijesh. 2021. "Microemulsion as a promising carrier for nose to brain delivery: journey since last decade." *Journal of Pharmaceutical Investigation 2021 51:6*. 51. 611–634. doi: 10.1007/S40005-021-00528-W

[95] Gadhave, Dnyandev, Bapi Gorain, Amol Tagalpallewar, and Chandrakant Kokare. 2019. "Intranasal teriflunomide microemulsion: An improved chemotherapeutic approach in glioblastoma." *Journal of Drug Delivery Science and Technology*. 51. 276–289. doi: 10.1016/J.JDDST.2019.02.013

[96] Ramreddy, Srividya and Krishnaveni Janapareddi. 2019. "Brain targeting of chitosan-based diazepam mucoadhesive microemulsions via nasal route: formulation optimization, characterization, pharmacokinetic and pharmacodynamic evaluation." *Drug Development and Industrial Pharmacy*. 45. 147–158. doi: 10.1080/03639045.2018.1526186

[97] Pires, Patrícia C., Ana C. Fazendeiro, Márcio Rodrigues, Gilberto Alves, and Adriana O. Santos. 2021. "Nose-to-brain delivery of phenytoin and its hydrophilic prodrug fosphenytoin combined in a microemulsion – formulation development and in vivo pharmacokinetics." *European Journal of Pharmaceutical Sciences*. 164. 105918. doi: 10.1016/J.EJPS.2021.105918

[98] Bachhav, Sagar S., Vikas Dighe, Nitin Mali, Nithya J. Gogtay, Urmila M. Thatte, and Padma V. Devarajan. 2020. "Nose-to-brain delivery of diazepam from an intranasal aqua-triggered in-situ (ATIS) gelling microemulsion: Monitoring brain uptake by microdialysis." *European Journal of Drug Metabolism and Pharmacokinetics*. 45. 785–799. doi: 10.1007/s13318-020-00641-5

[99] Kumbhar, Santosh Ashok, Chandrakant R. Kokare, Birendra Shrivastava, Bapi Gorain, and Hira Choudhury. 2021. "Antipsychotic potential and safety profile of TPGS-based mucoadhesive aripiprazole nanoemulsion: Development and optimization for nose-to-brain delivery." *Journal of Pharmaceutical Sciences*. 110. 1761–1778. doi: 10.1016/J.XPHS.2021.01.021

[100] Bayanati, Masoumeh, Abolfazl Ghafouri Khosroshahi, Maryam Alvandi, and Mohammad Mehdi Mahboobian. 2021. "Fabrication of a thermosensitive in situ gel nanoemulsion for nose to brain delivery of temozolomide." *Journal of Nanomaterials*. 2021. doi: 10.1155/2021/1546798

[101] Kannavou, Maria, Kanelina Karali, Theodora Katsila, Eleni Siapi, Antonia Marazioti, Pavlos Klepetsanis, Theodora Calogeropoulou, Ioannis Charalampopoulos, and Sophia G. Antimisiaris. 2023. "Development and comparative in vitro and in vivo study of BNN27 mucoadhesive liposomes and nanoemulsions for nose-to-brain delivery." *Pharmaceutics*. 15. 419. doi: 10.3390/pharmaceutics15020419

[102] Kaur, Atinderpal, Kuldeep Nigam, Sukriti Srivastava, Amit Tyagi, and Shweta Dang. 2020. "Memantine nanoemulsion: A new approach to treat Alzheimer's disease." *Journal of Microencapsulation*. 37. 355–365. doi: 10.1080/02652048.2020.1756971

[103] Giuliani, Alessandro, Anna Giulia Balducci, Elisa Zironi, Gaia Colombo, Fabrizio Bortolotti, Luca Lorenzini, Viola Galligioni, Giampiero Pagliuca, Alessandra Scagliarini, Laura Calzà, and Fabio Sonvico. 2018. "*In vivo* nose-to-brain delivery of the hydrophilic antiviral ribavirin by microparticle agglomerates." *Drug Delivery*. 25. 376–387. doi: 10.1080/10717544.2018.1428242

[104] Perkušić, Mirna, Laura Nižić Nodilo, Ivo Ugrina, Drago Špoljarić, Cvijeta Jakobušić Brala, Ivan Pepić, Jasmina Lovrić, Gordana Matijašić, Matija Gretić, Dijana Zadravec, Livije Kalogjera, and Anita Hafner. 2022. "Tailoring functional spray-dried powder platform for efficient donepezil nose-to-brain delivery." *International Journal of Pharmaceutics*. 624. 122038. doi: 10.1016/J.IJPHARM.2022.122038

[105] Tiozzo Fasiolo, Laura, Michele Dario Manniello, Elena Tratta, Francesca Buttini, Alessandra Rossi, Fabio Sonvico, Fabrizio Bortolotti, Paola Russo, and Gaia Colombo. 2018. "Opportunity and challenges of nasal powders: Drug formulation and delivery." *European Journal of Pharmaceutical Sciences*. 113. 2–17. doi: 10.1016/j.ejps.2017.09.027

[106] Tiozzo Fasiolo, Laura, Michele Dario Manniello, Fabrizio Bortolotti, Francesca Buttini, Alessandra Rossi, Fabio Sonvico, Paolo Colombo, Georgia Valsami, Gaia Colombo, and Paola Russo. 2019. "Anti-inflammatory flurbiprofen nasal powders for nose-to-brain delivery in Alzheimer's disease." *Journal of Drug Targeting*. 27. 984–994. doi: 10.1080/1061186X.2019.1574300

[107] Tiozzo Fasiolo, Laura, Michele Dario Manniello, Sabrina Banella, Laura Napoli, Fabrizio Bortolotti, Eride Quarta, Paolo Colombo, Evangelos Balafas, Nikolaos Kostomitsopoulos, Dimitrios M. Rekkas, Georgia Valsami, Paraskevi Papakyriakopoulou, Gaia Colombo, and Paola Russo. 2021. "Flurbiprofen sodium microparticles and soft pellets for nose-to-brain delivery: Serum and brain levels in rats after nasal insufflation." *International Journal of Pharmaceutics*. 605. 120827. doi: 10.1016/J.IJPHARM.2021.120827

[108] Papakyriakopoulou, Paraskevi, Konstantina Manta, Christina Kostantini, Stefanos Kikionis, Sabrina Banella, Efstathia Ioannou, Eirini Christodoulou, Dimitrios M. Rekkas, Paraskevas Dallas, Maria Vertzoni, Georgia Valsami, and Gaia Colombo. 2021. "Nasal powders of quercetin-β-cyclodextrin derivatives complexes with mannitol/lecithin microparticles for Nose-to-Brain delivery: In vitro and ex vivo evaluation." *International Journal of Pharmaceutics*. 607. 121016. doi: 10.1016/J.IJPHARM.2021.121016

[109] Truzzi, Eleonora, Cecilia Rustichelli, Edilson Ribeiro de Oliveira Junior, Luca Ferraro, Eleonora Maretti, Daniel Graziani, Giada Botti, Sarah Beggiato, Valentina Iannuccelli, Eliana Martins Lima, Alessandro Dalpiaz, and Eliana Leo. 2021. "Nasal biocompatible powder of Geraniol oil complexed with cyclodextrins for neurodegenerative diseases: physicochemical characterization and in vivo evidences of nose to brain delivery." *Journal of Controlled Release*. 335. 191–202. doi: 10.1016/J.JCONREL.2021.05.020

[110] Chavda, Vivek P., Lalitkumar K. Vora, Anjali K. Pandya, and Vandana B. Patravale. 2021. "Intranasal vaccines for SARS-CoV-2: From challenges to potential in COVID-19 management." *Drug Discovery Today*. 26. 2619–2636. doi: 10.1016/J.DRUDIS.2021.07.021

[111] Chavda, Vivek P., Aayushi B. Patel, Lalitkumar K. Vora, Rajeev K. Singla, Priyal Shah, Vladimir N. Uversky, and Vasso Apostolopoulos. 2022. "Nitric oxide and its derivatives containing nasal spray and inhalation therapy for the treatment of COVID-19." *Current Pharmaceutical Design*. 28. 3658–3670. doi: 10.2174/1381612829666221024124848.

[112] Chavda, Vivek P., Gargi Jogi, Nirav Shah, Mansi N. Athalye, Nirav Bamaniya, Lalitkumar K Vora, and Ana Cláudia Paiva-Santos. 2022. "Advanced particulate carrier-mediated technologies for nasal drug delivery." *Journal of Drug Delivery Science and Technology*. 74. 103569. doi: 10.1016/J.JDDST.2022.103569

[113] Wingrove, Jed, Magda Swedrowska, Regina Scherließ, Mark Parry, Mervin Ramjeeawon, David Taylor, Gregoire Gauthier, Louise Brown, Stephanie Amiel, Fernando Zelaya, and Ben Forbes. 2019. "Characterisation of nasal devices for delivery of insulin to the brain and evaluation in humans using functional magnetic resonance imaging." *Journal of Controlled Release*. 302. 140–147. doi: 10.1016/J.JCONREL.2019.03.032

[114] Parikh, Ankit, Utkarshini Anand, Malachy Ugwu, Tiam Feridooni, Emad Massoud, and Remigius Agu. 2014. "Drug-eluting nasal implants: Formulation, characterization, clinical applications and challenges." *Pharmaceutics*. 6. 249–267. doi: 10.3390/pharmaceutics6020249

[115] Stewart, Sarah, Juan Domínguez-Robles, Ryan Donnelly, and Eneko Larrañeta. 2018. "Implantable polymeric drug delivery devices: Classification, manufacture, materials, and clinical applications." *Polymers*. 10. 1379. doi: 10.3390/polym10121379

[116] Johnson, Ashley R., Seth P. Forster, David White, Graciela Terife, Michael Lowinger, Ryan S. Teller, and Stephanie E. Barrett. 2021. "Drug eluting implants in pharmaceutical development and clinical practice." *Expert Opinion on Drug Delivery*. 18. 577–593. doi: 10.1080/17425247.2021.1856072

[117] Quarterman, Juliana C., Sean M. Geary, and Aliasger K. Salem. 2021. "Evolution of drug-eluting biomedical implants for sustained drug delivery." *European Journal of Pharmaceutics and Biopharmaceutics*. 159. 21–35. doi: 10.1016/J.EJPB.2020.12.005

[118] Larrañeta, Eneko, Thakur Raghu Raj Singh, and Ryan F. Donnelly. 2022. "Overview of the clinical current needs and potential applications for long-acting and implantable

delivery systems." *Long-Acting Drug Delivery Systems: Pharmaceutical, Clinical, and Regulatory Aspects*. 1–16. doi: 10.1016/B978-0-12-821749-8.00005-7

[119] Higashi, Kyoko, Goran Medic, Kavi J. Littlewood, Teresa Diez, Ola Granström, and Marc De Hert. 2013. "Medication adherence in schizophrenia: factors influencing adherence and consequences of nonadherence, a systematic literature review." *Therapeutic Advances in Psychopharmacology*. 3. 200–218. doi: 10.1177/2045125312474019

[120] Padmakumar, Smrithi, Gregory Jones, Olga Khorkova, Jane Hsiao, Jonghan Kim, Benjamin S. Bleier, and Mansoor M. Amiji. 2021. "Osmotic core-shell polymeric implant for sustained BDNF AntagoNAT delivery in CNS using minimally invasive nasal depot (MIND) approach." *Biomaterials*. 276. 120989. doi: 10.1016/J.BIOMATERIALS.2021.120989

[121] Utomo, Emilia, Juan Domínguez-Robles, Natalia Moreno-Castellanos, Sarah A. Stewart, Camila J. Picco, Qonita Kurnia Anjani, Jon Ander Simón, Iván Peñuelas, Ryan F. Donnelly, and Eneko Larrañeta. 2022. "Development of intranasal implantable devices for schizophrenia treatment." *International Journal of Pharmaceutics*. 624. 122061. doi: 10.1016/J.IJPHARM.2022.122061

[122] Simón, Jon Ander, Emilia Utomo, Félix Pareja, María Collantes, Gemma Quincoces, Aarón Otero, Margarita Ecay, Juan Domínguez-Robles, Eneko Larrañeta, and Iván Peñuelas. 2023. "Radiolabeled risperidone microSPECT/CT imaging for intranasal implant studies development." *Pharmaceutics*. 15. 843. doi: 10.3390/pharmaceutics15030843

[123] Deruyver, Laura, Clément Rigaut, Pierre Lambert, Benoît Haut, and Jonathan Goole. 2021. "The importance of pre-formulation studies and of 3D-printed nasal casts in the success of a pharmaceutical product intended for nose-to-brain delivery." *Advanced Drug Delivery Reviews*. 175. 113826. doi: 10.1016/J.ADDR.2021.113826

[124] Beule, Achim G. 2010. "Physiology and pathophysiology of respiratory mucosa of the nose and the paranasal sinuses." *GMS Current Topics in Otorhinolaryngology, Head and Neck Surgery*. 9. Doc07. doi: 10.3205/CTO000071

[125] Corbo, Diane C., Jue-Chen -C Liu, and Yie W. Chienx. 1990. "Characterization of the barrier properties of mucosal membranes." *Journal of Pharmaceutical Sciences*. 79. 202–206. doi: 10.1002/JPS.2600790304

[126] Agrawal, Mukta, Swarnlata Saraf, Shailendra Saraf, Sophia G. Antimisiaris, Mahavir Bhupal Chougule, Sunday A. Shoyele, and Amit Alexander. 2018. "Nose-to-brain drug delivery: An update on clinical challenges and progress towards approval of anti-Alzheimer drugs." *Journal of Controlled Release*. 281. 139–177. doi: 10.1016/J.JCONREL.2018.05.011

[127] Mygind, Niels and Ronald Dahl. 1998. "Anatomy, physiology and function of the nasal cavities in health and disease." *Advanced Drug Delivery Reviews*. 29. 3–12. doi: 10.1016/S0169-409X(97)00058-6

[128] Schriever, Valentin A., Thomas Hummel, Johan N. Lundström, and Jessica Freiherr. 2013. "Size of nostril opening as a measure of intranasal volume." *Physiology & Behavior*. 110–111. 3–5. doi: 10.1016/J.PHYSBEH.2012.12.007

[129] Kim, Byung Guk, Jung Hyun Kim, Soo Whan Kim, Sung Won Kim, Kyung Suk Jin, Jin Hee Cho, Jun Myung Kang, and So Young Park. 2013. "Nasal pH in patients with chronic rhinosinusitis before and after endoscopic sinus surgery." *American Journal of Otolaryngology*. 34. 505–507. doi: 10.1016/J.AMJOTO.2013.04.015

[130] Ferreira, Natália N., Edilson de Oliveira Junior, Sara Granja, Fernanda I. Boni, Leonardo M. B. Ferreira, Beatriz S. F. Cury, Lilian C. R. Santos, Rui M. Reis, Eliana M. Lima, Fátima Baltazar, and Maria Palmira D. Gremião. 2021. "Nose-to-brain co-delivery

of drugs for glioblastoma treatment using nanostructured system." *International Journal of Pharmaceutics*. 603. 120714. doi: 10.1016/J.IJPHARM.2021.120714
[131] European Medicines Agency. *Guideline on the Pharmaceutical Quality of Inhalation and Nasal Products*. 2006. Accessed: Mar. 6, 2023. [Online]. Available: www.emea.eu.int
[132] le Guellec, S., S. Ehrmann, and L. Vecellio. 2021. "In vitro–in vivo correlation of intranasal drug deposition." *Advanced Drug Delivery Reviews*. 170. 340–352. doi: 10.1016/J.ADDR.2020.09.002
[133] Khan, Abdur Rauf, Mengrui Liu, Muhammad Wasim Khan, and Guangxi Zhai. 2017. "Progress in brain targeting drug delivery system by nasal route." *Journal of Controlled Release*. 268. 364–389. doi: 10.1016/J.JCONREL.2017.09.001
[134] Costa, Cláudia Pina, João Nuno Moreira, José Manuel Sousa Lobo, and Ana Catarina Silva. 2021. "Intranasal delivery of nanostructured lipid carriers, solid lipid nanoparticles and nanoemulsions: A current overview of in vivo studies." *Acta Pharmaceutica Sinica B*. 11. 925–940. doi: 10.1016/J.APSB.2021.02.012
[135] Sakane, Toshiyasu, Sachi Okabayashi, Shunsuke Kimura, Daisuke Inoue, Akiko Tanaka, and Tomoyuki Furubayashi. 2020. "Brain and nasal cavity anatomy of the cynomolgus monkey: Species differences from the viewpoint of direct delivery from the nose to the brain." *Pharmaceutics*. 12. 1227. doi: 10.3390/pharmaceutics12121227
[136] Jiao, Jian and Luo Zhang. 2019. "Influence of intranasal drugs on human nasal mucociliary clearance and ciliary beat frequency." *Allergy, Asthma & Immunology Research*. 11. 306–319. doi: 10.4168/AAIR.2019.11.3.306
[137] Meng, Huan, Wei Leong, Kam W. Leong, Chunying Chen, and Yuliang Zhao. 2018. "Walking the line: The fate of nanomaterials at biological barriers." *Biomaterials*. 174. 41–53. doi: 10.1016/J.BIOMATERIALS.2018.04.056
[138] Food and Drug Administration. *Guidance for Industry Changes to an Approved NDA or ANDA*. 2004. Accessed: Mar. 6, 2023. [Online]. Available: www.fda.gov/cder/guidance/index.htm
[139] Santos, Carlos, Gustavo Marco, Lee M. Nagao, Eva Castro, and Tim Chesworth. 2018. "European regulatory developments for orally inhaled and nasal drug products." *AAPS PharmSciTech*. 19. 3134–3140. doi: 10.1208/S12249-018-1154-5/TABLES/3
[140] Vitorino, Carla, Soraia Silva, Joana Bicker, Amílcar Falcão, and Ana Fortuna. 2019. "Antidepressants and nose-to-brain delivery: drivers, restraints, opportunities and challenges." *Drug Discovery Today*. 24. 1911–1923. doi: 10.1016/J.DRUDIS.2019.06.001

5 Mesoporous Silica Nanoparticles for Drug Delivery in Brain Disorders

Abhay Dev Tripathi, Aditi Bhatnagar, Soumya Katiyar, and Abha Mishra

5.1 INTRODUCTION

The World Health Organization forecasts that by the year 2040, neurological illnesses will overtake cancer cases as the second leading cause of mortality after cardiovascular illnesses in senior citizens due to increased life span across most people globally [1]. The gradual impairment of neuronal activity caused by neuron degeneration in the central nervous system (CNS) characterizes a variety of neurological disorders (NDs), such as Alzheimer's disease (AD), meningitis, Parkinson's disease, multiple sclerosis (MS), Huntington's disease, and many more [2]. Efficient options for therapy are still lacking, possibly due to the complexities of the CNS and the hypothesized multiple pathogenic pathways, despite significant advancements in the delivery of medicinal drugs and the knowledge of the etiology of neurological illnesses. As a consequence, the presently accessible therapeutic medicines, which primarily attempt to reduce neurological degeneration and decrease disease development, but have not been able to revert it and fully recover normal neuronal activity completely, have largely been shown to be unsuccessful [3, 4].

Furthermore, the medical treatment of CNS illnesses requires the passage of pharmaceutical drugs to the brain in substantial amounts to reach therapeutic dosages. However, amino acids, hormones, ions, and electrolytes in plasma routinely vary considerably, especially following physical activity, meals, or stressful situations. Since numerous of these compounds govern nerve sensitivity, even a minor change in the interstitial fluid content in the CNS might cause an uncontrollable increase in brain function. Consequently, the blood–brain barrier (BBB), which guards neural cells against toxins, infections, and environmental alterations, is present at the blood–CNS level to stabilize the neuronal region. Therefore, the BBB may make it more difficult for most medications with CNS activity, particularly pharmaceutical drugs, to be delivered. The BBB restricts the delivery of therapeutic medications and the transit of potentially dangerous substances into the brain [5]. Additionally, it was previously shown that during the development stage, more than 50% of innovative medications were water insoluble [6, 7]. Thus, one of the foremost difficult challenges

 DOI: 10.1201/9781032661964-5

in developing drugs is to increase the solubility of the medicinal product and, in turn, its level of bioavailability. Recently, there has been a greater focus on creating innovative ways to deliver medications that can increase medication bioavailability [8–10].

Using nanometric-sized particles (NPs) is one of the most important aspects of nanotechnology. Particles of this size, in particular, have the ability to imitate and influence biological activities in the field of nanomedicine [11]. Mesoporous silica nanoparticles (MSNs) are among the most intriguing types of NPs. MSNs have become attractive nanocarriers for the administration of drugs in recent years [12, 13]; refer to Figure 5.1. According to research by Baghirov et al., copolymer-coated or uncoated MSNs with the lowest dimensions in the region of 100 nm were capable of crossing the BBB [14]. MSNs provide a huge surface area and pore volume for conceivably huge drug loading, a distinctive 3D structure for drug-regulated release,

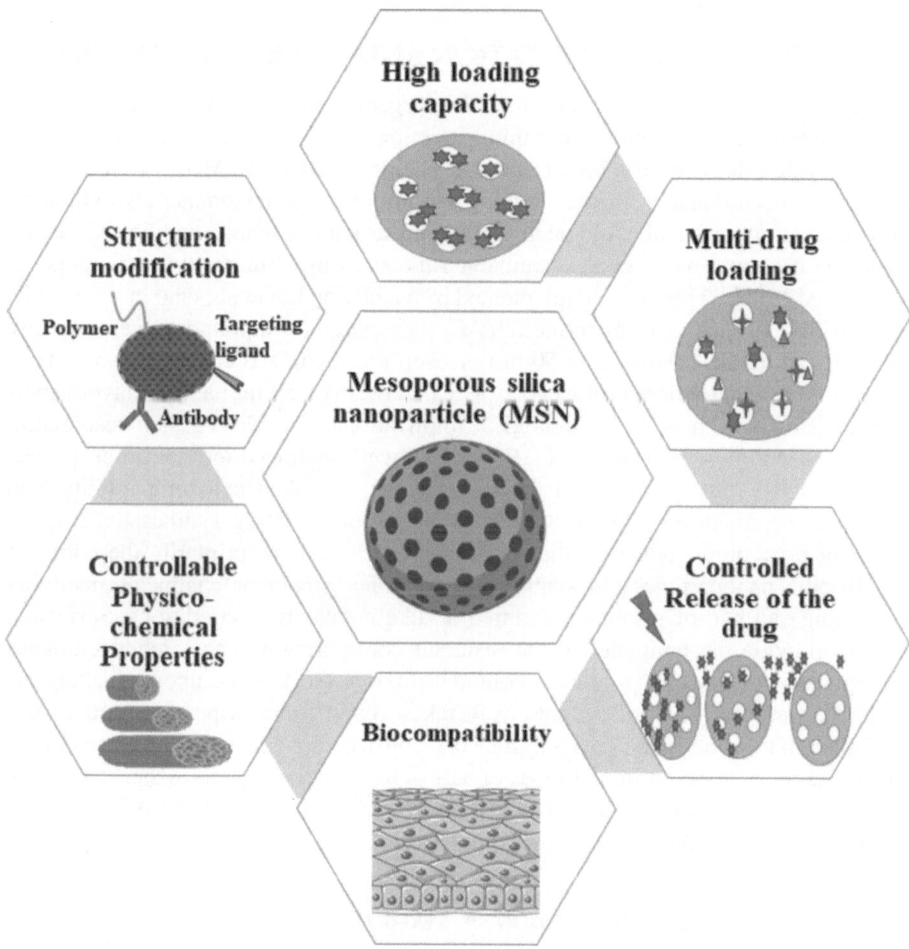

FIGURE 5.1 Advantages of using mMesoporous silica nanoparticle as a nano carrier for drug delivery applications.

and customizable surfaces that allow additional modification depending on diverse biological applications [15, 16]. Additionally, because the drug is trapped within the inner porosity, it is shielded from enzymes and metabolites that may alter it before reaching the intended target, resulting in unfavorable adverse reactions in unwanted organs and uncontrollable consequences [16].

Because of these attributes, MSNs are a great choice for the delivery of drugs and other bioactive agents to a specific site. Therefore, this chapter covers the production, biocompatibility, capacity, and processes by which MSNs traverse the BBB. In addition, we have emphasized the potential use of therapeutically drug-loaded MSNs in managing NDDs. We have also outlined the issues that must be resolved to advance the utilization of these prospective particles. We think that an extensive audience involved in the study of neurobiology and brain regeneration would benefit from the content of this article.

5.2 TYPES OF MSNS: FABRICATION AND CHARACTERIZATION

Numerous nanosized metallic, non-metallic, organic, and polymeric nanomaterials with surface functionalization are gaining traction in this context as top contenders for the targeted delivery of a broad range of chemotherapeutics. MSNs were initially designed in accordance with the growing requirement for nanomaterials exhibiting strong thermo-mechanical, biologically safer, and structure-tunable qualities. Cai et al., Nooney et al., and Fowler et al. documented the ever-initial impactful preparation of nano-scaled MSNs. This was complemented by a study by Lai et al., who introduced its name "MSN" [17]. According to the IUPAC, mesoporous compounds have a porosity that varies in diameter from 2 to 50 nm or even the organized configuration of pore spaces that gives an ordered framework. MSNs have evolved into a new class of inorganic constructs with potential biological implications, considering their resourceful dimensions, enormous surface area (~999 m^2/g), well-organized interior pores, porous capacity (0.5–1 cm^3/g), increased therapeutic load, excellent cytocompatibility, and affordable manufacturing cost [18]. MSNs are probably being synthesized using a variety of procedures; however, the sol-gel approach remains primarily the common one. Briefly, nanoparticles are synthesized by silica precursor chemicals involving condensing and hydrolysis under acidified or alkaline catalysis conditions. Surfactant micelles provide the template for the resultant configuration. Those latter templates subsequently condense to produce a colloidal mixture (sol), while upon adjusting the reaction's variables, the gel progressively takes shape from suspended particulates. A template-based technique uses a framework-constructing agent to synthesize hollow porous MSNs [19, 20]. Different types of MSNs have been reported to date, and some of these are the following: MCM41, MCM48, MCM50, SBA11, SBA12, SBA15, SBA16, FSM16, HMM33, FDU, TUD1, and COK12 [21–23].

5.2.1 MCM (Mobil Composition of Matter)

The Mobil Research & Development Corporation originally fabricated and termed MCM41. With the application of different surfactants, the microporosity diameter of nanomaterials was modified and controlled. With a pore width ranging from 2 to 6 nm, MCM41 is a hexagon and was created using positively charged surfactants as frameworks, whereas alternative MSNs were additionally constructed by altering the substrates used as well as the reaction parameters. Such MSNs differ in pore diameter or geometric configuration, just as MCM-50 and MCM-48 showcase a lamella-like and cubic-like layout respectively [17, 21]. The methodology for generating chemically synthesized MCMs depends on silica substrates' coalescence, usually sodium silicate $(Na_2O)_x \cdot SiO_2$ or tetraethylorthosilicate (TEOS), throughout the vicinity of cationic surfactants in an alkaline environment. The quintessential manufacturing combines a surfactant like a cetyltrimethylammonium bromide (CTAB) to TEOS at 80 °C and pH ≈ 11 adjusted by adding NaOH. The sol-gel technique creates nanomaterials [24–26].

5.2.2 SBA (Santa Barbara Amorphous)

Only a mere five to seven years after MCM synthesis in 1992, Stucky along with his team constructed a silica-based nanoparticle, a different form of nanoparticle, that is, the Santa Barbara Amorphous (SBA), with a different array-like arrangement of hexagonal pores. The SBA gained importance due to its arranged nanopores, significant pore diameter (4–32 nm), robust pore membrane, and high thermodynamic sustainability, resulting in an exquisite alternative for numerous possibilities in heterogeneous catalysts, entrapment, and controlled therapeutic release. Following the preliminary synthesis of SBA, there here have been various other reports of a broad range of SBA nanoparticles, including SBA-11 (cube), SBA-15 (hexagon shaped), and SBA-16 (cube shaped) [27]. Synthesis of basic SBA involves the following steps, described briefly. In order to synthesize SBA15, the framework scaffold must first dissolve in an acidified condition until a silica donor gets introduced. Later, the combination mixture should be first heated overnight at 40 °C, followed by 36 hours of aging at 85–90°C. Following this, a white precipitate is obtained. The resulting solid is then separated, carefully rinsed using deionized water, air-dried at 37 °C, and then oven-dried at 80°C for five to six hours. Later, it is calcined for 6 hours at 500°C to remove the scaffold [27–30]. For the materials, TEOS or tetra-methoxy silane (TMOS) are SiO_2 substrates throughout the coordinated self-building mechanism to generate a 2D array with a linear conduit. The SBA-15 synthesis (EO20PO70EO20) as a scaffold framework is a copolymer of non-ionic units of propylene oxide as a hydrophobic end, and ethylene oxide as a hydrophobic end and a hydrophilic end of the scaffold micelle [27, 31, 32].

5.2.3 Other Types of MSN

Other types of MSN include FSM-16, HMM-33, TUD-1, COK-12, and so on. To briefly describe their synthesis and structural characteristics one by one, FSM-16, a folded sheet of MSN nanomaterials, can be constructed by using layering of polysilicate (which is a silylation product of mono-, di-, and trichloro(alkyl)silanes) kanemite, in addition to a 4° cationic reagent to serve as a framework [33]. Besides

TABLE 5.1
MSN Types and Their Biomedical Applications

MSN class	MSN subtype	Pore size (nm)	Structure	Application	References
MCM (Mobil Composition of Matter)	MCM 41	a. 80–100 b. 1.5–8	Hexagonal 2D hexagonal P6mm	Drug delivery	[34, 35]
	MCM 48	a. 2–5	Cubic	Drug delivery	[36, 37]
	MCM 50	a. 2–5	Lamellar	Adsorbents; Catalysis	[38]
SBA (Santa Barbara amorphous)	SBA 11	a. 5.8	3D cubic	Drug delivery	[38–40]
	SBA 12	a. 3.1	3D hexagonal		
	SBA 15	a. 6–10	2D hexagonal		[41, 42]
	SBA 16	a. 5–15	Cubic		[43]
Other types of MSNs	FDU 11	a. 2.7	Tetragonal	Drug delivery	[45, 46, 47]
	FDU 12	a. 36	Cubic		
	FDU 13	a. 1.7	Orthorhombic		
	COK 12	a. 5.5–6	Hexagonal	Catalysis	[48, 49]
	TUD 1	a. 2.5–25	Disordered	Drug delivery; catalysis	[50, 51]
	FSM 16	a. 3.2–4	2D hexagonal	Sensing; Catalysis; Drug delivery	[52, 53]

this, for HMM-33 (Hiroshima Mesoporous Material 33), and COK-12 (Centrum Voor Oppervlaktechemie en Katalyse), on the basis of pores arrangement (randomly or arrayed), pore diameter, and structure, the above-mentioned MSN types are differentiated. The different types of MSN used in the various biological applications with their structural information are listed in Table 5.1.

5.3 OVERCOMING CHALLENGES IN DRUG DELIVERY OF MSN ACROSS THE BBB

An active regulatory juncture found amid the capillaries of the brain, nerve tissues, and the spine is the BBB. Only gas molecules and tiny lipid-soluble molecules can pass through the barrier under typical physiological circumstances. The BBB also has the power to pump particular hazardous or excessive chemicals out of the brain to keep the environment within the brain stable and allow the CNS to work correctly [52]. A laborious research topic for many years has been the safe and effective penetration of the BBB. Many neurodegenerative illnesses and gliomas can benefit from targeted medication delivery to the brain. Nano drug-targeted delivery systems have shown significant promise in solving this obstacle, thanks to recent microscale and nanotechnology breakthroughs. The potential of nanoparticles to cross the BBB and their transport to the brain is constantly being improved; biobased carriers, inorganic nanocarriers, liposomes, and organic polymer-carriers are manufactured in various sizes, shapes, and surface functional groups [53]. Kreuter et al. were the first to develop Poly(butyl cyanoacrylate) (PBCA) nanoparticles in 1995. They enabled the antinociceptive peptide dalargin to be distributed *in vivo*. PS80 is now accepted globally for increasing polymeric particle BBB crossing since it has been shown to increase apolipoprotein-nanoparticle engagement for a wide range of polymers without generating BBB toxicity [54].

Mesoporous silica nanoparticles (MSNs) are one type of inorganic nanoparticle that offers particular benefits in drug delivery. Recently, MSNs have received much interest due to their use in healthcare and as carriers of drugs. Their structural adaptability, large surface area, and ease of functionalization provide substantial advantages over traditional materials. These nanoparticles feature well-defined pore arrangements with controlled diameters of pores ranging from 2 to 50 nm [55]. The pockets in these nanostructures can constitute a significant proportion of the entire volume that can be designed to store medicinal dosages, imaging chemicals, or occasionally both. Besides providing a wide surface area for MSNs, porosity allows for the independent assimilation of intrinsic and extrinsic surfaces. The pores in MSNs can help with drug binding, while the external surface can aid in stabilizing the nanocarrier.

Several strategies for delivering MSN and other nanoparticles carrying remedial drugs, including peptides, and other small molecules, are being explored continuously. These approaches include temporarily breaching the BBB, changing the structure of the drug, and making alterations to the surface to enable it to traverse the BBB, circumventing the BBB, and transporting the medicine straight to the brain. Disrupting the BBB for targeted drug delivery via the intranasal route, Fonseca et al. created a mucoadhesive method for olanzapine delivery using a copolymer having amphiphilic methacrylic implemented poly(epsilon-caprolactone) nanocapsules. Another investigation looked into the mannitol-induced BBB opening process, in which vascular endothelial cell drying caused cell shrinkage and tight junction breach [56].

Ultrasound-based approaches rely on the vibrations of acoustically generated cavitation to create a brief and temporary perforation of the vascular endothelium, allowing targeted molecules to penetrate the BBB into the CNS. To interrupt the BBB in model rats having gliosarcoma, Atkins employed a 558 kHz transducer capable of producing pulsed ultrasound and microbubbles [57]. Aryal et al. discovered that utilizing the focused ultrasonic approach enhanced the delivery efficacy of liposomal doxorubicin, resulting in a boost in mean longevity of 100% and 72% relative to the non-treatment and DOX-alone control groups, respectively. The synergistic delivery approach might be used in healthy and sick brains, considerably improving drug-loaded magnetic nanoparticle brain accumulation [58].

Researchers have been performing many experiments to clarify drug permeability across the BBB. According to the findings of Nowak et al., the connection between nanoparticles and endothelial cells seems to depend majorly on particle size [59]. Silica nanoparticles act on specific targets and have a good drug release profile. They may aid in transporting various compounds across the BBB, such as phytochemicals, oligonucleotides, proteins, and peptides. Nevertheless, substantial challenges in employing these materials include their nonspecific aggregation and adhesion to various surfaces [60]. Turan and colleagues used a two-step reservoir-surging technique to construct a multicomponent nano vector made of a silica shell having an iron oxide core (Fe@MSN) to transport medications via the BBB for brain cancer therapy [61]. Kuang and colleagues used MSNs as a chemo-immuno therapeutic carrier for administering tumor microenvironment responsive release of the chemical medicine doxorubicin and the immunological checkpoint inhibitor 1-methyltryptophan (1-MT). Another study found that administering MSNPs and mesenchymal stem cells increased viability in U87MG xenograft rats with orthotopic glioblastomas [62].

The presence of a magnetic field and transferrin as the target ligand might increase the delivery and subsequent cellular absorption of doxorubicin-loaded paclitaxel nanoparticles modified with transferrin (DOX-PTX-NPs-Tf), resulting in the largest *in vitro* cytotoxicity [63]. In an experiment, SZI molecules were employed to penetrate the BBB. Despite having longer-conjugated bridges than ThT (commercial fluorescent probe-thioflavin T), SZIs cannot traverse the BBB to approach the brain for imaging. There was no fluorescence in the brain area, indicating that SZIs alone could not pass the BBB. Therefore, MSN-based nanocomposites were employed to deliver fluorescent dyes to the brain that helped in imaging for AD. In another study, MSN-based drug-delivery systems were produced and coupled with TAT peptide to improve brain tissue targeting and methotrexate permeability over the BBB and absorption by cancer cells [64]. The pH-responsive nano system used a cell-penetrating peptide (TAT) to breach the brain parenchyma. Yang et al. created H_2O_2-responsive controlled drug release of gold metal-capped mesoporous silica nanoparticles (MSN-CQ-AuNPs) for AD targeted clioquinol (CQ) delivery [63]. Mo et al. investigated nanoparticle absorption in glioma cells using MSNs of various sizes, employing the ability to change MSN size. MSNs were preloaded with doxorubicin, and their surfaces were coated with cRGD, a peptide widely used in nanomedicine due to its ability to bind to integrin receptors, which can be found upregulated in many cancerous cell lines. The findings demonstrated that MSNs (40nm) might cross the BBB and subsequently be quickly absorbed in glioma cells, avoiding damaging side effects in the healthy brain [53] [65]. Kim et al. discussed employing porous silica nanoparticles (Psi) decorated using the tripeptide RGD as a specific cancer photoluminescent two-photon NIR compound that produces enhanced spatial details of tumoral tissues in an animal model with deep localization ideal resolution. A PSi's surface can be modified with proteins to boost its selectivity toward tumor cells. Dox-loaded PSis adorned with transferrin could selectively kill glioma cells across the BBB [66].

Technologies like confocal microscopy and flow cytometry can be utilized for identifying fluorescein isothiocyanate (FITC)-labeled MSN uptake by cells. Surface plasmon resonance assessments can also be employed to track cell absorption of MSN in real time, having no labels [52]. Two types of copolymer-coated MSNs, that is, spherical and rod-shaped nanoparticle absorption, were found robust in both MDCK II and RBE4 cells, indicating that the copolymer coating was highly successful in enhancing intracellular delivery of spherical and rod-shaped MSNs. Uncoated particle delivery is substantially less pronounced. The existence of the BBB makes treatment of such disorders difficult since it is impenetrable by most

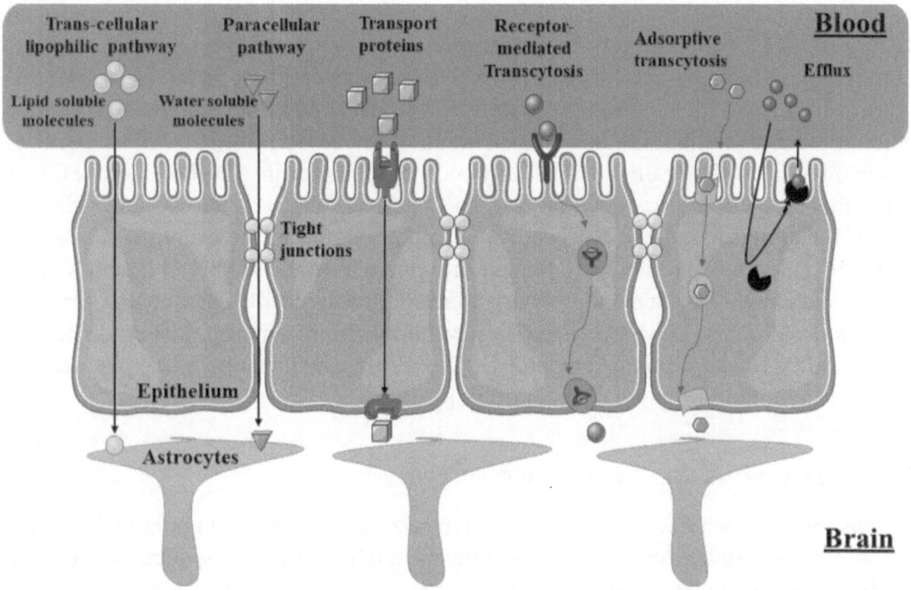

FIGURE 5.2 Transport mechanisms under the influence of the blood–brain barrier (BBB).

currently known and potentially beneficial medications. As a result, educational and pharmaceutical communities face significant challenges in discovering and developing innovative drug-delivery mechanisms for managing such disorders. Nanotechnology is an exciting and promising method. Nowadays, multiple varieties of NPs with various properties and applications are available for biomedical use, allowing the transport of neuroactive substances such as medicines, growth regulators and genes, and cells to the brain. NPs provide therapeutic benefits for medication delivery, including lower drug dosage, fewer adverse effects, extended drug half-life, and the potential to improve drug crossing over the BBB (See Figure 5.2).

5.4 APPLICATION OF MSN

5.4.1 Treatment of Alzheimer's Disease

AD is found to affect an estimated 15–20 million individuals globally. Among numerous therapeutic NP-based prototypes developed to suppress aggregation in AD, MSNs have the superiority of preferentially traversing the BBB and transporting considerably large quantities of target molecules into the brain if appropriately functionalized. Increased concentrations of trace metal ions, particularly iron, copper, and zinc, are a major metabolic characteristic of AD that leads to neurodegeneration. Various engineered MSNs using competitive binding, redox, pH, photon, and enzyme as activators have been demonstrated for drug delivery [67].

The curcumin (CCM)-loaded MSN-CCM and the thermos-responsive hydrogel (HG) (HG@MSN-CCM) successfully reversed the cognitive loss caused by streptozotocin-induced AD in mice. MSNs have been discovered to behave as nano scavengers and have been recommended as a possible therapy for various neurodegenerative illnesses because of their ability to bind and remove harmful compounds from the brain, such as amyloid beta plaques in AD [68]. For AD, it is found that the action of reactive oxygen species (ROS), such as H_2O_2, generation, is part of metabolic reactions that occur at a higher degree in the brain. In a research study, bioactive metabolites were loaded into phenylboronic acid-conjugated MSNs. The nanomaterial was then capped with adjacent diol molecules and human IgG and β-D-glucose-AuNPs. The ROS in the diseased brain micro-environment could help in the controlled release of metal chelator CQ, reducing the clustering of Aβ plaques and the Aβ accumulation-related neurotoxicity [69].

5.4.2 Diagnosis and Monitoring of Epilepsy

Epilepsy is an NDcharacterized by repetitive seizures which can hamper and damage the brain cells forever. Accompanying epilepsy, other dysfunctions, such as cognitive and behavioral changes, muscular tension, and autonomic and other systemic deficits, may occur. As a result, the intricacy of epilepsy is unquestionable, and authors concur that treating it remains a huge problem. Epileptic seizures are unexpected and can result in injury, hospitalization, and death, leading to a higher mortality rate than in the general population. The BBB is a crucial biological barrier that limits the delivery and transport of anti-seizure drugs (ASDs) to the brain. The BBB's restrictive permeability and active efflux of many therapeutic agents make the treatment of NDs difficult. In this connection, it has been claimed that epilepsy treatment issues may be caused by an inadequate concentration of ASDs in the CNS, which might be avoided with appropriate drug-delivery methods. Lopez et al. reported using a template approach to create mesoporous silica and titania nanotubes. They assembled MSNs (SBA-15) and titania nanotubes to include the antiepileptic medication phenytoin (PH) [70]. For monitoring drug delivery, very sensitive and selective K+ sensing could be adopted. In this regard, MSNs were coated with a one-of-a-kind ultrathin layer of a K^+ permeable membrane filter. This filter was created by controlled self-assembly of 3-D tripodal ligands, which could exclusively collect K^+, allowing the K^+ indicators implanted inside MSN to detect the dynamics of the K^+ level entirely without interference from other cations. The K^+ reactive nanosensors have shown tremendous promise in the early epilepsy diagnosis and to-the-point monitoring of epileptic convulsions, which can guide the sensible use of antiepileptic medicines for precise epilepsy therapy with minimal side effects [71].

5.4.3 Treatment of Brain Tumors

Gliomas are malignant tumors originating from brain and spinal cord glial cells. They are the second most significant cause of mortality in teenagers. It is the most common and aggressive primary intracranial neoplasm in the CNS.

MSNs with large surface area, tunable pore diameters, and greater pore volume have been widely used for controlled drug release and targeted cancer treatment. Researchers talk about paclitaxel lipid-coated MSNs, which have blended features of both MSNs and liposomes perfect for constructing a targeted drug-delivery system for therapeutics with various characteristics and action mechanisms [72]. MSN with tiny diameters could be preloaded with anticancer medicine, such as temozolomide

TABLE 5.2
Therapeutic-loaded MSNs for Brain-related Disorders

Drug	Carrier	Model	Disease targeted	Reference
Doxorubicin (DOX)	MSN-PEG-IP	C6-IL13Rα2 cell	Glioma	[74]
Leptin/pioglitazone	MSN-lep-pio	Tdp-43^{a315t} mice	Amyotrophic lateral sclerosis	[75]
L-dopa	MSN-*n*-oleyl-L-Dopa	Simulated body fluid system	Parkinson's	[76]
Doxorubicin (DOX)	Fe@MSN	CNS-1 glioma model in mice	Glioblastoma	[61]
Arctigenin	MSN-FC@ ARC-G	C57BL/6J mice	Brain and spinal cord injury	[77]
Thymoquinone	MSN	Male Wistar rats	Diagnostic purposes	[78]
Polydopamine and DOX	MSN-DOX-PDA-NGR	Brain capillary endothelial cells and c6 cells	Antitumor	[79]
Paclitaxel and DOX	Magnetic silica PLGA	U-87 MG-luc2 xenograft of BALB/c nude mice	Brain glioma	[80]
Metal chelators CQ	MSN-CQ-AuNP	Bend.3 cell	Alzheimer	[81]
Carbamazepine (CBZ), oxcarbazepine (OXC), and rufinamide (RFN)	SBA-16	3T3 endothelial cells	Anti-epileptic	[82]
Phenytoin (PH)	SBA 15) and nanostructured titania tubes tio_2	*In vitro* drug release	Anti-epileptic	[83]
Resveratrol	PLA-coated MSN	Rat brain microvascular endothelial cells	Oxidative stress therapy in CNS.	[84]

(TMZ). In an experiment, TMZ encapsulated with polydopamine (PDA) and coupled with Asn-Gly-Arg (NGR) was adopted to manage glioma treatment, the most common and invasive primary intracranial tumor in the CNS. NGR-MSN accumulation in rat glioma cell lines was greater than that of unaltered MSNPs. MSN-PEG-IP was successfully synthesized, an MSN-based vehicle coated with IL13Rα2-targeted peptide (IP) using polyethylene glycol (PEG). Its properties for delivering chemotherapeutic medicines were thoroughly examined. IP was shown to be a promising ligand for developing glioma-targeted drug-delivery systems. These nanocarriers were validated as the latest cargo for delivering the hydrophobic anticancer drug doxorubicin to glioma cells (Table 5.2) [73].

5.5 CONCLUSIONS

In light of the restrictions in the medical management of NDDs, nanotechnology provides a viable option for developing novel therapeutic solutions. MSNs, among the third generation of silica-based nanomaterials, offer a great deal of promise because of their special characteristics. This chapter serves as a status report on the benefits and possible uses of MSNs as a therapeutic drug-delivery system specifically suited to circumvent the BBB. Moreover, we have reviewed the appropriate transport and functionalization techniques required to pass through the crucial BBB in treating multiple NDDs, in light of the expanding scientific curiosity in the clinical application of these nanoparticles for diagnostics and imaging. Smart MSN nanocarriers may be modified quickly to target and deliver drugs at specific locations, hence increasing bioavailability and minimizing negative effects. However, owing to a shortage of comprehensive *in vivo* investigations and also clinical investigations, there is still a lot to be studied in terms of MSN-based nanoplatforms for NDs therapy. The designing and functioning of smart nanosystems must be understood in order to gain Food and Drug Administration or regulatory authority clearance and to go from laboratory to manufacturing facilities. Following on from the promise of MSNs, these nanosystems are intriguing tools for additional clinical investigation and, eventually, effective NDDs therapy.

ACKNOWLEDGMENTS

The authors are thankful to the School of Biochemical Engineering, IIT (BHU) Varanasi, for providing technical support. This work was financially supported by the Department of Biotechnology, India, under the DBT JRF PhD program, for providing a fellowship to author Abhay Dev Tripathi during the tenure of this study.

REFERENCES

1. Marques C, Fernandes I, Meireles M et al. (2018) Gut microbiota modulation accounts for the neuroprotective properties of anthocyanins. *Sci Rep* 8:1–9.
2. Xu X, Warrington AE, Bieber AJ, Rodriguez M (2011) Enhancing central nervous system repair-the challenges. *CNS Drugs* 25:555.

3. Mukherjee S, Madamsetty VS, Bhattacharya D et al. (2020) Recent advancements of nanomedicine in neurodegenerative disorders theranostics. *Adv Funct Mater* 30:2003054.
4. Savelieff MG, Nam G, Kang J et al. (2018) Development of multifunctional molecules as potential therapeutic candidates for Alzheimer's disease, Parkinson's disease, and amyotrophic lateral sclerosis in the last decade. *Chem Rev* 119:1221–1322.
5. Bourganis V, Kammona O, Alexopoulos A, Kiparissides C (2018) Recent advances in carrier mediated nose-to-brain delivery of pharmaceutics. *Eur J Pharm Biopharm* 128:337–362.
6. Čerpnjak K, Zvonar A, Gašperlin M, Vrečer F (2013) Lipid-based systems as promising approach for enhancing the bioavailability of poorly water-soluble drugs. *Acta pharmaceutica* 63:427–445.
7. Dizaj SM, Vazifehasl Z, Salatin S et al. (2015) Nanosizing of drugs: effect on dissolution rate. *Res Pharm Sci* 10:95.
8. Saraf S (2010) Applications of novel drug delivery system for herbal formulations. *Fitoterapia* 81:680–689.
9. Asil SM, Ahlawat J, Barroso GG, Narayan M (2020) Nanomaterial based drug delivery systems for the treatment of neurodegenerative diseases. *Biomater Sci* 8:4109–4128.
10. Akhtar A, Andleeb A, Waris TS et al. (2021) Neurodegenerative diseases and effective drug delivery: A review of challenges and novel therapeutics. *JCR* 330:1152–1167.
11. Hickey JW, Santos JL, Williford J-M, Mao H-Q (2015) Control of polymeric nanoparticle size to improve therapeutic delivery. *JCR* 219:536–547.
12. Vallet-Regí M, Schüth F, Lozano D et al. (2022) Engineering mesoporous silica nanoparticles for drug delivery: where are we after two decades? *Chem Soc Rev* 51 (13): 5365–5451.
13. Cauda V, Canavese G (2020) Mesoporous materials for drug delivery and theranostics. *Pharmaceutics* 12:1108.
14. Baghirov H, Karaman D, Viitala T et al. (2016) Feasibility study of the permeability and uptake of mesoporous silica nanoparticles across the blood brain barrier. *PLoS One* 11:e0160705.
15. Rizzi F, Castaldo R, Latronico T et al. (2021) High surface area mesoporous silica nanoparticles with tunable size in the sub-micrometer regime: Insights on the size and porosity control mechanisms. *Molecules* 26:4247.
16. Rajput S, Vadia N, Mahajan M (2022) Role of mesoporous silica nanoparticles as drug carriers: Evaluation of diverse mesoporous material nanoparticles as potential host for various applications. *Advanced Functional Porous Materials: From Macro to Nano Scale Lengths* 205–234.
17. Mendiratta S, Hussein M, Nasser HA, Ali AAA (2019) Multidisciplinary role of mesoporous silica nanoparticles in brain regeneration and cancers: From crossing the blood–brain barrier to treatment. *Part Part Syst Charact* 36:1900195.
18. Nigro A, Pellegrino M, Greco M et al. (2018) Dealing with skin and blood–brain barriers: The unconventional challenges of mesoporous silica nanoparticles. *Pharmaceutics* 10:250.
19. Jafari Z, Honarmand S, Rahimi F et al. (2021) Mesoporous Silica Nanoparticles as Versatile carrier platforms in therapeutic applications. *J Nanosci Technol* 20210:40–62.
20. Trewyn BG, Slowing II, Giri S et al. (2007) Synthesis and functionalization of a mesoporous silica nanoparticle based on the sol–gel process and applications in controlled release. *Acc Chem Res* 40:846–853.

21. Carvalho GC, Sábio RM, de Cássia Ribeiro T et al. (2020) Highlights in mesoporous silica nanoparticles as a multifunctional controlled drug delivery nanoplatform for infectious diseases treatment. *Pharm Res* 37:191.
22. Narayan R, Nayak UY, Raichur AM, Garg S (2018) Mesoporous silica nanoparticles: A comprehensive review on synthesis and recent advances. *Pharmaceutics* 10:118.
23. Øye G, Sjöblom J, Stöcker M (2001) Synthesis, characterization and potential applications of new materials in the mesoporous range. *Adv Colloid Interface Sci* 89:439–466.
24. Singh AK, Singh S Sen, Rathore AS et al. (2021) Lipid-coated MCM-41 mesoporous silica nanoparticles loaded with berberine improved inhibition of acetylcholine esterase and amyloid formation. *ACS Biomater Sci Eng* 7:3737–3753.
25. Sohrabnezhad S, Jafarzadeh A, Pourahmad A (2018) Synthesis and characterization of MCM-41 ropes. *Mater Lett* 212:16–19.
26. Martínez-Edo G, Balmori A, Pontón I et al. (2018) Functionalized ordered mesoporous silicas (MCM-41): Synthesis and applications in catalysis. *Catalysts* 8:617.
27. Chaudhary V, Sharma S (2017) An overview of ordered mesoporous material SBA-15: synthesis, functionalization and application in oxidation reactions. *Journal Porous Mater* 24:741–749.
28. Vernimmen J, Meynen V, Cool P (2011) Synthesis and catalytic applications of combined zeolitic/mesoporous materials. *Beilstein J Nanotechnol* 2:785–801.
29. Huirache-Acuña R, Nava R, Peza-Ledesma CL et al. (2013) SBA-15 mesoporous silica as catalytic support for hydrodesulfurization catalysts. *Materials* 6:4139–4167.
30. Yang C-M, Zibrowius B, Schmidt W, Schüth F (2004) Stepwise removal of the copolymer template from mesopores and micropores in SBA-15. *Chemistry of materials* 16:2918–2925.
31. Fulvio PF, Pikus S, Jaroniec M (2005) Short-time synthesis of SBA-15 using various silica sources. *J Colloid Interface Sci* 287:717–720.
32. Ulrich K, Galvosas P, Kärger J et al. (2010) Self-assembly and diffusion of block copolymer templates in SBA-15 nanochannels. *J Phys Chem B* 114:4223–4229.
33. Tozuka Y, Wongmekiat A, Kimura K et al. (2005) Effect of pore size of FSM-16 on the entrapment of flurbiprofen in mesoporous structures. *Chem Pharm Bull (Tokyo)* 53:974–977.
34. Karaman DŞ, Kettiger H (2018) Silica-based nanoparticles as drug delivery systems: Chances and challenges. In: *Inorganic frameworks as smart nanomedicines*. Elsevier, pp 1–40.
35. Narayan R, Nayak UY, Raichur AM, Garg S (2018) Mesoporous silica nanoparticles: A comprehensive review on synthesis and recent advances. *Pharmaceutics* 10:118.
36. Feng Y, Panwar N, Tng DJH et al. (2016) The application of mesoporous silica nanoparticle family in cancer theranostics. *Coord Chem Rev* 319:86–109.
37. Shah P V, Rajput SJ (2017) A comparative in vitro release study of raloxifene encapsulated ordered MCM-41 and MCM-48 nanoparticles: a dissolution kinetics study in simulated and biorelevant media. *J Drug Deliv Sci Technol* 41:31–44.
38. Ukmar T, Planinšek O (2010) Ordered mesoporous silicates as matrices for controlled release of drugs. *Acta Pharmaceutica* 60:373–385.
39. Kruk M, Jaroniec M, Sakamoto Y et al. (2000) Determination of pore size and pore wall structure of MCM-41 by using nitrogen adsorption, transmission electron microscopy, and X-ray diffraction. *J Phys Chem B* 104:292–301.
40. Aqeel T, Greer HF (2020) Quantum-sized zinc oxide nanoparticles synthesised within mesoporous silica (SBA-11) by humid thermal decomposition of zinc acetate. *Crystals (Basel)* 10:549.

41. Jangra S, Sharma B, Singh S (2021) Aloe-emodin-loaded SBA-15 and its in vitro release properties and cytotoxicity to cervical cancer cells. *Materials Research Innovations* 25:264–275.
42. Carmona D, Balas F, Santamaria J (2014) Pore ordering and surface properties of FDU-12 and SBA-15 mesoporous materials and their relation to drug loading and release in aqueous environments. *Mater Res Bull* 59:311–322.
43. Fekri MH, Soleymani S, Mehr MR, Akbari-adergani B (2022) Synthesis and characterization of mesoporous ZnO/SBA-16 nanocomposite: Its efficiency as drug delivery system. *J Non Cryst Solids* 591:121512.
44. Poyatos-Racionero E, González-Álvarez I, González-Álvarez M et al. (2020) Surfactant-triggered molecular gate tested on different mesoporous silica supports for gastrointestinal controlled delivery. *Nanomaterials* 10:1290.
45. Chircov C, Spoială A, Păun C et al. (2020) Mesoporous silica platforms with potential applications in release and adsorption of active agents. *Molecules* 25:3814.
46. Colmenares MG, Simon U, Cruz O et al. (2018) Batch and continuous synthesis upscaling of powder and monolithic ordered mesoporous silica COK-12. *Microporous Mesoporous Mater* 256:102–110.
47. Varkolu M, Velpula V, Ganji S et al. (2015) Ni nanoparticles supported on mesoporous silica (2D, 3D) architectures: highly efficient catalysts for the hydrocyclization of biomass-derived levulinic acid. *RSC Adv* 5:57201–57210.
48. Heikkilä T, Salonen J, Tuura J et al. (2007) Mesoporous silica material TUD-1 as a drug delivery system. *Int J Pharm* 331:133–138.
49. Keshri KS, Bhattacharjee S, Singha A et al. (2022) Synthesis of cyclic carbonates of different epoxides using CO2 as a C1 building block over Ag/TUD-1 mesoporous silica catalyst: A solvent free approach. *Molecular Catalysis* 522:112234.
50. Fukuoka A, Higashimoto N, Sakamoto Y et al. (2001) Preparation and catalysis of Pt and Rh nanowires and particles in FSM-16. *Microporous and Mesoporous Mater* 48:171–179.
51. Trewyn BG, Whitman CM, Lin VS-Y (2004) Morphological control of room-temperature ionic liquid templated mesoporous silica nanoparticles for controlled release of antibacterial agents. *Nano Lett* 4:2139–2143.
52. Baghirov H, Karaman D, Viitala T et al. (2016) Feasibility study of the permeability and uptake of mesoporous silica nanoparticles across the blood–brain barrier. *PLoS One* 11:1–22. https://doi.org/10.1371/journal.pone.0160705
53. Mendiratta S, Hussein M, Nasser HA et al. (2019) Multidisciplinary role of mesoporous silica nanoparticles in brain regeneration and cancers: from crossing the blood brain barrier to treatment. Part Part Syst Charact 36 (9), p. 1900195. https://doi.org/10.1002/ppsc.201900195
54. Petri B, Bootz A, Khalansky A et al. (2007) Chemotherapy of brain tumour using doxorubicin bound to surfactant-coated poly(butyl cyanoacrylate) nanoparticles: Revisiting the role of surfactants. *JCR* 117:51–58. https://doi.org/10.1016/j.jconrel.2006.10.015
55. Nagavarma BVN, Yadav HKS, Ayaz A et al. (2012) Different techniques for preparation of polymeric nanoparticles- A review. *Asian J Pharm and Clin Res* 5:16–23.
56. Fonseca FN, Betti AH, Carvalho FC et al. (2014) Mucoadhesive amphiphilic methacrylic copolymer-functionalized poly(ε-caprolactone) nanocapsules for nose-to-brain delivery of olanzapine. *J Biomed Nanotechnol* 11:1472–1481. https://doi.org/10.1166/jbn.2015.2078
57. Alkins RD, Brodersen PM, Sodhi RNS, Hynynen K (2013) Enhancing drug delivery for boron neutron capture therapy of brain tumors with focused ultrasound. *NeuroOncology* 15: 1225–1235. https://doi.org/10.1093/neuonc/not052

58. Wipt P, George KM (2008) 基因的改变NIH Public Access. *Bone* 23:1–7. https://doi.org/10.1016/j.jconrel.2013.04.007
59. Brown TD, Nowak M, Bayles AV et al. (2019) A microfluidic model of human brain (μHuB) for assessment of blood brain barrier. *Bioeng Transl Med* 4:1–13. https://doi.org/10.1002/btm2.10126
60. Yang Y, Yan X, Cui Y et al. (2008) Preparation of polymer-coated mesoporous silica nanoparticles used for cellular imaging by a "graft-from" method. *J Mater Chem* 18:5731–5737. https://doi.org/10.1039/b811573g
61. Turan O, Bielecki P, Perera V et al. (2019) Delivery of drugs into brain tumors using multicomponent silica nanoparticles. *Nanoscale* 11:11910–11921. https://doi.org/10.1039/c9nr02876e
62. Kuang J, Song W, Yin J et al. (2018) iRGD modified chemo-immunotherapeutic nanoparticles for enhanced immunotherapy against glioblastoma. *Adv Funct Mater* 28. https://doi.org/10.1002/adfm.201800025
63. Choudhury H, Pandey M, Chin PX et al. (2018) Transferrin receptors-targeting nanocarriers for efficient targeted delivery and transcytosis of drugs into the brain tumors: a review of recent advancements and emerging trends. Drug Deliv and Transl Res 8, 1545–1563. https://doi.org/10.1007/s13346-018-0552-2
64. Ma L, Yang S, Ma Y et al. (2021) Benzothiazolium derivative-capped silica nanocomposites for β-amyloid imaging in vivo. *Anal Chem* 93:12617–12627. https://doi.org/10.1021/acs.analchem.1c02289
65. Mo J, He L, Ma B, Chen T (2016) Tailoring particle size of mesoporous silica nanosystem to antagonize glioblastoma and overcome blood–brain barrier. *ACS Appl Mater Interfaces* 8:6811–6825. https://doi.org/10.1021/acsami.5b11730
66. Nigro A, Pellegrino M, Greco M et al. Dealing with skin and blood–brain barriers: The unconventional challenges of mesoporous silica nanoparticles. https://doi.org/10.3390/pharmaceutics10040250
67. Wang L, Yin YL, Liu XZ et al. (2020) Current understanding of metal ions in the pathogenesis of Alzheimer's disease. *Transl Neurodegener* 9:1–13. https://doi.org/10.1186/s40035-020-00189-z
68. Ribeiro T de C, Sábio RM, Luiz MT et al. (2022) Curcumin-loaded mesoporous silica nanoparticles dispersed in thermo-responsive hydrogel as potential Alzheimer disease therapy. *Pharmaceutics* 14. https://doi.org/10.3390/pharmaceutics14091976
69. Yang L, Yin T, Liu Y et al. (2016) Gold nanoparticle-capped mesoporous silica-based H2O2-responsive controlled release system for Alzheimer's disease treatment. *Acta Biomater* 46:177–190. https://doi.org/10.1016/j.actbio.2016.09.010
70. López T, Ortiz E, Meza D et al. (2011) Controlled release of phenytoin for epilepsy treatment from titania and silica based materials. *Mater Chem Phys* 126:922–929. https://doi.org/10.1016/j.matchemphys.2010.12.011
71. Octeau JC, Gangwani MR, Allam SL et al. (2019) Transient, Consequential Increases in Extracellular Potassium Ions Accompany Channelrhodopsin2 Excitation. *Cell Rep* 27:2249–2261.e7. https://doi.org/10.1016/j.celrep.2019.04.078
72. Zhu J, Zhang Y, Chen X et al. (2020) Biochemical and biophysical research communications angiopep-2 modi fi ed lipid-coated mesoporous silica nanoparticles for glioma targeting therapy overcoming BBB. *Biochem Biophys Res Commun* 2–7. https://doi.org/10.1016/j.bbrc.2020.10.076
73. Zhang P, Tang M, Huang Q et al. (2019) Combination of 3-methyladenine therapy and Asn-Gly-Arg (NGR)-modified mesoporous silica nanoparticles loaded with temozolomide for glioma therapy in vitro. *Biochem Biophys Res Commun* 509:549–556. https://doi.org/https://doi.org/10.1016/j.bbrc.2018.12.158

74. Shi J, Hou S, Huang J et al. (2017) An MSN-PEG-IP drug delivery system and IL13Rα2 as targeted therapy for glioma. Nanoscale, 9(26), pp. 8970–8981. https://doi.org/10.1039/c6nr08786h
75. Diana D, Ferrer-donato A, Jos MM et al. (2022) Design of mesoporous silica nanoparticles for the treatment of amyotrophic lateral sclerosis (ALS) with a therapeutic cocktail based on leptin and pioglitazone. https://doi.org/10.1021/acsbiomaterials.2c00865
76. Morales V, McConnell J, Pérez-Garnes M et al. (2021) L-Dopa release from mesoporous silica nanoparticles engineered through the concept of drug-structure-directing agents for Parkinson's disease. *J Mater Chem B* 9:4178–4189. https://doi.org/10.1039/d1tb00481f
77. Sun G, Zeng S, Liu X et al. (2019) Synthesis and characterization of a silica-based drug delivery system for spinal cord injury therapy. *Nanomicro Lett* 11:1–20. https://doi.org/10.1007/s40820-019-0252-6
78. Fahmy HM, Fathy MM, Abd-elbadia RA, Elshemey WM (2019) Targeting of thymoquinone-loaded mesoporous silica nanoparticles to different brain areas: In vivo study. *Life Sci* 222:94–102. https://doi.org/10.1016/j.lfs.2019.02.058
79. Hu J, Zhang X, Wen Z et al. (2016) Asn-Gly-Arg-modified polydopamine-coated nanoparticles for dual-targeting therapy of brain glioma in rats. *Oncotarget* 7:73681–73696. https://doi.org/10.18632/oncotarget.12047
80. Cui Y, Xu Q, Chow PKH et al. (2013) Transferrin-conjugated magnetic silica PLGA nanoparticles loaded with doxorubicin and paclitaxel for brain glioma treatment. *Biomaterials* 34:8511–8520. https://doi.org/10.1016/j.biomaterials.2013.07.075
81. Yang L, Yin T, Liu Y et al. (2016) Gold nanoparticle-capped mesoporous silica-based H2O2-responsive controlled release system for Alzheimer's disease treatment. *Acta Biomater* 46:177–190. https://doi.org/10.1016/j.actbio.2016.09.010
82. Thomas MJK, Slipper I, Walunj A et al. (2010) Inclusion of poorly soluble drugs in highly ordered mesoporous silica nanoparticles. *Int J Pharm* 387:272–277. https://doi.org/10.1016/j.ijpharm.2009.12.023
83. López T, Ortiz E, Meza D et al. (2011) Controlled release of phenytoin for epilepsy treatment from titania and silica based materials. *Mater Chem Phys* 126:922–929. https://doi.org/10.1016/j.matchemphys.2010.12.011
84. Shen Y, Cao B, Snyder NR et al. (2018) ROS responsive resveratrol delivery from LDLR peptide conjugated PLA-coated mesoporous silica nanoparticles across the blood–brain barrier. *J Nanobiotechnology* 16:1–17. https://doi.org/10.1186/s12951 018-0340-7

6 Polymeric Nanocarriers for Drug Delivery to the Central Nervous System

Aditya Kadam, Shradha Karande, Shreya Thakkar, Namdev More, and Dilip Sharma

6.1 INTRODUCTION

Over 600 different types of neurological diseases, such as Alzheimer's, Parkinson's, dementia, Huntington's, epilepsy, and stroke, affect the lives of millions of people and are a major cause of death [1, 2]. Often these diseases affect people resulting in chronic disability. Accurately diagnosing and treating these conditions is extremely difficult due to their underlying complex neural physiology and anatomy. Efforts have been directed by researchers toward developing therapeutic approaches for the treatment of these neurological diseases. As a result, numerous therapeutic approaches using drugs, proteins, and nucleic acids have been developed; however, treatments for neurological diseases are still limited because of the inability of therapeutic agents to cross barriers such as the blood–brain barrier (BBB) and the blood–cerebrospinal fluid barrier (BCFB) [1, 3]. For the most part, the BBB acts as a roadblock to macromolecules being transported from the bloodstream to the brain. The BBB, on the other hand, is able to transport molecules with a molecular weight of less than 400 Da that is lipid-soluble. Most therapeutic molecules cannot cross the BBB, which allows for the development of new drug-delivery methods for the brain. Therapeutic agents have been delivered across the BBB using a variety of invasive and noninvasive methods in recent years. BBB tight junctions are disrupted to facilitate drug delivery by invasive methods. Noninvasive methods utilize advanced drug-delivery systems/modified delivery systems (such as exosomes, liposomes, lipid carriers, and polymeric nanocarriers/nanoparticle-based approaches) [4, 5].

In the last few decades, nanocarrier-based delivery strategies have been developed to overcome the difficulties of therapeutic molecule transport over the BBB. There are numerous nanocarriers like liposomes, nano micelles, nanogels, polymeric nanocarriers, exosomes, and many more that can be used for the delivery of therapeutic agents in the treatment of neurological diseases [4]. Nanocarrier stragegies display improved drug delivery, improve solubility, improve targeting of a drug, improve drug kinetics, and enhance cellular internalization. Biocompatibility, biodegradability, and an abundance of surface groups are all advantages of polymeric nanocarriers. As a result, polymeric nanocarriers have drawn interest as a means of delivering drugs to the brain [5].

 DOI: 10.1201/9781032661964-6

In this chapter, we discuss the roadblocks in brain drug delivery and the new strategies to deliver drugs using polymeric nanocarriers, as well as examples of polymers used most frequently for drug-delivery purposes.

6.1.1 Blood–brain Barrier Physiology

The brain's microvascular endothelial cells (BMECs), pericytes, and astrocytes form the structural and functional BBB, which prevents and controls the flow of the majority of substances from the blood to the brain. It controls the movement of molecules in and out of the brain to retain the neural climate and concentration of L-dopa in the brain through metabolic activities such as L-dopa metabolism. The BBB is a vital structure that, like a computer firewall, preferentially permits substances into the brain while throwing out injurious materials [6].

The BBB function is indeed the product of a complex of these factors:

A physical barrier: Tight junctions among cells limit the flux through the paracellular or intercellular cavity.

B transport barrier: A specialized transmission system mediates solute flow and the specific targeting transport mechanism, as long as the intracellular component of the carriers and its intracellular ligands are not strongly affected by the technology. [7]

All components are blocked by the BBB, except those that use lipid solubility to cross cell membranes (such as oxygen, carbon dioxide, and ethanol). The brain consumes approximately 20% of the oxygen and glucose acquired by the body, despite its relatively low weight. This high metabolic demand is attributed to the extensive number of decisions and processes continually taking place within the brain, resulting in a rapid metabolism of the nervous system. The BBB and the BCFB are two types of barriers that protect the brain from various harmful substances [6, 8]. Because 98% of drugs weigh more than 500 molecular weight, many of them cannot pass the barrier. Except for the "circumventricular organs," Dalton hormones typically do not enter the brain from the blood. When brain infections do occur, they can be very serious and challenging to treat because antibodies cannot pass the BBB due to their size [9].

6.1.2 Obstacles of Drug Delivery to the Brain

The BBB acts as a permeability barrier, preventing the majority of substances from being transported from the blood to the brain while providing essential minerals for the brain. Physiological (tight junctions) and metabolic (enzymes) barriers restrict transport into the brain, with the exception of peripheral capillaries, where compounds can interact relatively freely across cells. Brain capillary endothelial cells (BCECs) are primarily responsible for BBB formation, although astrocytes, pericytes, and neuronal cells also play an important role in the functioning of the BBB. Tight junctions, one of the distinctive features of BMECs, inhibit the paracellular transport of small and large (aqueous) substances from the blood to the brain [7]. Furthermore, due to reduced vesicular transport, increased metabolic function, and insufficiency in fenestrate, transcellular transport from blood to the brain is constricted. The BBB's role is to protect the brain from detrimental extracellular substances while providing it with vital nutrients like ions, glucose, amino acids, purines, nucleosides, peptides, and proteins. There are various influx processes at the BBB, which are further classified as active or passive BBB transport mechanisms. Lipophilicity and molar mass influence passive diffusion. A compound's capacity to construct hydrogen bonds will also restrict its ability to diffuse through the BBB [10]. While the transcellular route allows lipophilic drugs with a molecular weight of 400–600 Dalton or less to enter the brain, the transport of hydrophilic substances is constrained via the paracellular route [11]. There are three types of active transport systems: receptor-mediated transcytosis (RMT), absorptive-mediated transcytosis (AMT), and carrier-mediated transcytosis (CMT). Nutrients like glucose, amino acids, and purine bases are transcytosis using CMT. For instance, the hexose transporter, which carries glucose and mannose, and the amino acid transporters, which can be roughly classified as neutral, cationic, or anionic amino acid carriers, are two examples. The transport rate for CMT is specific and is influenced by the carrier's invasion rate. Polycationic substances that bind to the negatively charged plasma membrane's surface begin the AMT process [12]. No particular plasma membrane receptors are involved in this process. Endocytosis and endosome formation eventuate after the cationic compound binds to the plasma membrane. RMT is capable of transporting both peptides and proteins to the brain. The insulin receptor, transferrin receptor, low-density lipoprotein transporters, and insulin-like growth factor transporters are a few examples of receptors involved in RMT [13]. The compound is exocytosed at the brain capillary vascular endothelium (brain) side through receptor-mediated endocytosis, mobility through the endothelial cytoplasm, and endocytosis at the luminal (blood) side. P-glycoprotein (Pgp) transmembrane protein is found at the BCEC's apical membrane (brain microvascular endothelial cells) [14].

6.1.3 Drug Targeting to the Brain

It is suggested that polymer-based nanotechnologies could replace the conventional formulations for drug delivery and targeting. The rate at which a drug can cross the BBB and enter the brain is commonly a significant constraint. This study evaluated the ability of surface-engineered long circular PLGA nanoparticles (NPs) to deliver to the brain [15]. The BBB blocks the delivery of many drugs to and from the brain. The tightly connected endothelial cells that make up the brain capillaries form the BBB. Therefore, paracellular solute transit across the BBB is blocked by tight junctions in the brain endothelial epithelium [7].

A number of efflux transport mechanisms, including p-glycoprotein and reactive organic acids, found in brain endothelial cells, work with tight junctions to remove unnecessary substances [16]. The use of polymeric nanoparticles as drug carriers has been widely used over the past decade, including in pharmaceutical and medical research. Owing to the principles of enhanced permeability and retention (EPR), drug carriers need to circulate in the bloodstream for an extended duration, allowing them to accumulate in specific pathological regions, such as tumors. This phenomenon enables drugs to reach and affect previously inaccessible areas within the body. [17].

Various methods of delivering the drug to the target can be divided into two groups:

- Passive targeting
- Active targeting (receptor-mediated targeting and physical targeting)

Passive targeting: When a delivery system targets the systemic circulation, it is said to be passive (i.e., targeting happens as a result of the body's physiological reaction to the physicochemical properties of the drug or drug-carrier system).

Active targeting: Active targeting uses drug carriers that have been altered or manipulated to revise their life. Chemical, biological, and physical methods are used to improve the drug carrier composites' natural pattern of distribution, which reaches out to and can be recognized by specific sites. Active transport processes are divided into three types: transporter-mediated transcytosis (TMT), uptake-mediated transcytosis (AMT), and receptor-mediated transcytosis (RMT). The main goal is the process of improving receptor-mediated drug localization and target-specific drug delivery by facilitating the binding of drug carriers to the target with the help of ligands or building blocks [18].

6.1.4 Approaches of Drug-targeting Delivery to the Brain

Multiple drug-delivery strategies have been implemented to bypass various obstacles preventing the delivery of potential therapeutic agents into the CNS. These methods typically come under the invasive, noninvasive, or other techniques categories [19]. The methods for delivering drugs to the brain are schematically shown in Figure 6.1. Only a small number of peptides, essential minerals, and low-molecular-weight, lipophilic molecules, either passively diffusing across the barrier or by using specialized transport processes, can penetrate this barrier to any significant extent using the invasive method. But with these procedures, medication must be infused directly into the brain. The tight junctions' opening is reduced by the endothelial cells [20]. Malignant glioma-disseminated CNS germ cell tumors, and cerebral lymphomas can all benefit from the effects, which last for 20 to 30 minutes [21]. Inadvertent anticancer agent delivery to healthy brain tissues, physiological stress, and brief increases in intracranial pressure are a few of the side effects [22].

Numerous noninvasive techniques for delivering drugs to the brain have been researched, and they all rely on the brain's extensive blood vessel network. Drug delivery to the brain via noninvasive systemic means is still difficult, which has led to the creation of new drug-targeting technologies as shown in Figure 6.1 [19]. Drug-targeting technologies are constantly being improved due to the difficulty of noninvasively delivering drugs to the brain [4]. Most noninvasive methods are based on the production of antibodies, lipophilic analogues, drug carriers, are drug receptor-mediated, and so on. It is based on the use of drugs that can lead to the formation of a drug delivery system. For this purpose, many strategies have been put forward to

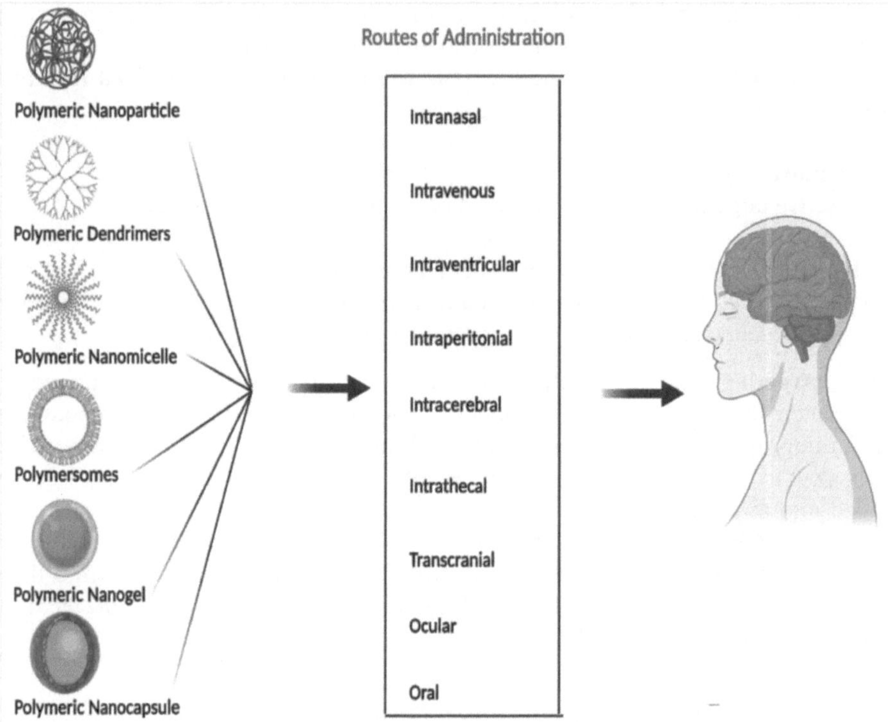

FIGURE 6.1 Schematic representation of approaches to brain drug delivery.

overcome this problem. One of the most exciting research questions is the study of polymeric nanocarriers as drug-delivery systems for effective local and therapeutic drug delivery to the CNS [20]. Processes of polymeric nanoparticles, including hybrid, natural-based, and synthetic nanoparticles, have been used for brain targeting as shown in Figure 6.2. Although nano-carriers have several benefits, including the capacity to transport medicines throughout the BBB and improved blood circulation retention times, their therapeutic applications are constrained by several issues [23]. The most important problem is the negative effects of long-term exposure to nanomaterials like polymers. Due to the higher structural proportion of nano-drugs, polymers may concentrate in the central CNS as a result of the prolonged administration of nano-carriers. Both immunogenic and harmful effects are possible. Therefore, strict experimental procedural regimens are necessary to deal with and control these problems before they become clinically significant. The long-term toxicity profile of NPs in the brain must be investigated in particular, as this could restrict the application of nano-drugs in clinical settings [24].

Second, it is necessary to assure that the encapsulation efficiency rate is maintained as the nano-drug formulation technique is scaled up for use in industrial manufacturing. Based on the dosage and the physicochemical characteristics of the pharmaceuticals conjugated or encapsulated, nano-drugs have varying therapeutic

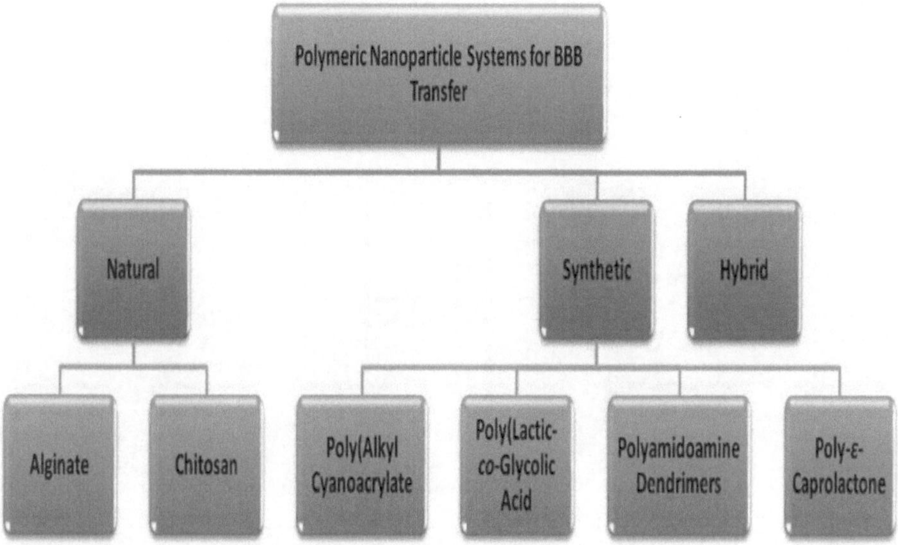

FIGURE 6.2 Polymeric nanoparticle system for BBB transfer.

effectiveness. Because of this, maintaining the encapsulation efficiency speed under the physiological environment depends on improving the formulation process for large-scale production [25]. Moreover, the procedure is constrained by the high expense of scaling up the synthesis of nano-drugs and the usage of organic solvents in that process. Finding alternatives is, therefore, essential to produce nanomaterials that are environmentally compatible [26, 27]. Another drawback is that the data may be difficult to interpret when exocytosed nanoparticles are detected using pH-dependent fluorescent tags, such as FITC. Utilizing naturally paramagnetic (ferrous oxide), luminous (gold), and fluorescent (quantum dots, nanodiamonds) materials can provide definite advantages to overcome this limitation [28].

6.2 CELLULAR TRANSPORT MECHANISMS INVOLVED IN NANOCARRIER ABSORPTION

The endocytosis process, which is strictly controlled, allows the BBB to connect with the outside environment and acquire nutrients. Adsorptive, receptor-mediated, and fluid-phase endocytosis are all examples of endocytotic processes. Various endocytic mechanisms effectively transfer components inside the brain vascular endothelium and are utilized in drug-delivery systems as shown in Figure 6.3, depending upon the nature of the substance and its physicochemical properties. Similar to this, the method by which NCs enter cells differs depending on their physicochemical characteristics, such as size, shape, surface tension, and surface chemistry. Only a small amount of fluid-phase endocytosis is involved in the BBB because the brain capillaries have lost their caveolae [4, 29].

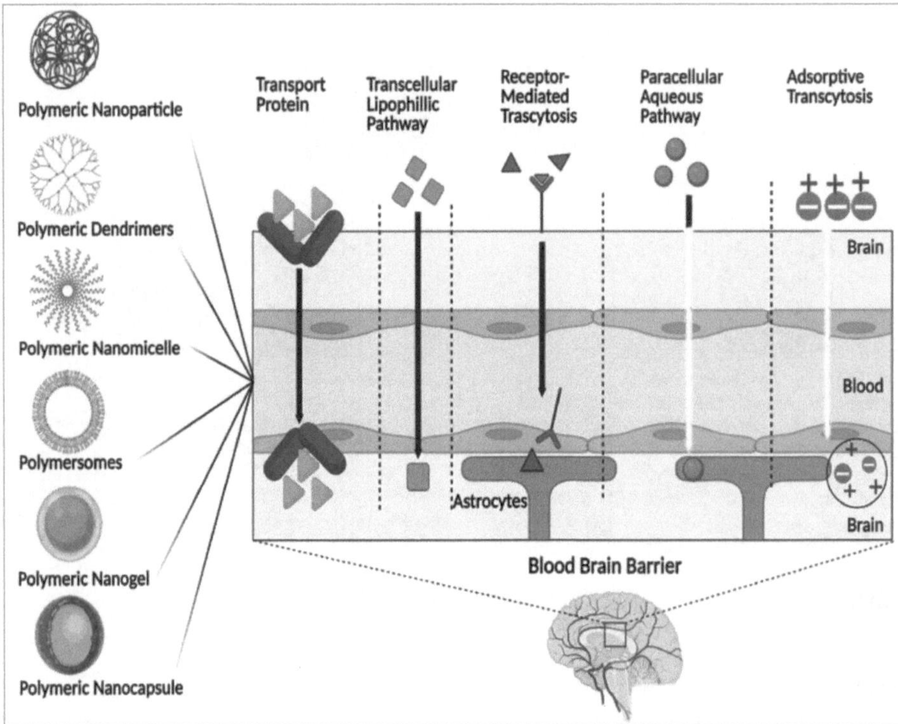

FIGURE 6.3 Transport mechanism of polymeric nanocarrier through blood brain barrier.

A detailed summary of the effects of the properties of polymeric NCs on brain conduction, advantages, and limitations is provided in Table 6.1. As a consequence, receptor-mediated and adsorptive-mediated endocytosis is the endocytosis process for the nanocarrier drug-delivery system. Additionally, conjugating nanocarrier to endothelial stimulation markers targeting ligands may be an effective strategy to enhance particle internalization in arterial flow as a potential substitute to clathrin and caveolae-dependent approaches. The mechanism of endocytosis facilitated by cell adhesion molecules (CAM) is independent of clathrin or caveolae [30].

6.2.1 Adsorptive Transcytosis

The BBB can be crossed using the process of adsorption-mediated transcytosis (AMT) to supply nanoparticles to the brain. The phospholipid-rich membrane of BBB endothelial cells is protected by a glycocalyx formed of the HSPGs glypican and syndecan [30]. Moreover, sialoglycolipids and sialoglycoproteins contain a variety of carboxyl groups on the side of the BBB [31]. Therefore, the lumen side of the BBB has a negative charge. AMT can be induced due to the electrostatic interaction between negative particles on the luminal surface of brain endothelial cells and cationic groups of ligands covalently attached to the nanoparticle surface [31]. Several studies have shown that clathrin-coated pits are the basis of AMT.

TABLE 6.1
Summary of the Effects of the Properties of Polymeric NCs on Brain Conduction, Advantages and Limitations in Use

Polymeric Nanocarrier Property	Effect on Delivery Brain	Advantages	Limitations
Size	Smaller sizes aid with transport across the BBB.	Different techniques can be used to control NC size.	For small-sized NPs, molecule loading may be minimal.
	Smaller NCs accumulate more brain tissue.	Size control may improve brain accumulation.	
Shape	Specific interactions might be promoted.	Particular NC shapes, like rods, may improve cell adhesion.	Synthesis methods are not quite simple or widely applicable.
Stiffness	NC brain deposition is dependent on stiffness.	A variety of methodologies are available to control stiffness.	Clear threshold for range of particles may not be possible due to the presence of other physicochemical properties.
	Effects are strongly influenced by the stiffness range (often Young's module).	Enhanced brain accumulation and avoid MPS by using softer particles.	The stiffness of NPs may not be uniform throughout the particle.
Charge	Positively charged particles interact more readily with the negatively charged endothelial cell surface.	Endothelial cell accumulation can be reduced and BBB transport can be improved by controlling the surface charge.	Positively charged particles may increase ROS, cause toxicity, and compromise the integrity of the BBB.
	Positively charged NPs show a higher rate of increase but less transport of cell material than negatively charged NPs.		Higher uptake does not always imply higher transcytosis, as positively charged particles may be trapped in endothelial cells to a greater extent.
Ligand	May increase targetability	Improves specifificity Variety of ligands. Use of multiple ligands for multi-targeting.	Non-specific site functionalization strategies can reduce receptor-ligand interactions; population heterogeneity is also required.

(Continued)

TABLE 6.1 (Continued)
Summary of the Effects of the Properties of Polymeric NCs on Brain Conduction, Advantages and Limitations in Use

Polymeric Nanocarrier Property	Effect on Delivery Brain	Advantages	Limitations
Avidity	It regulates the level and location of NP in the brain.	Improvement in the therapeutic index of drug and enhanced uptake by target cell.	Controlled ligand density is not trivial.
Corona	Specific proteins such as Apo E can improve NC transport across the BBB and accumulation in the brain.	May improve particle targetability.	Influences the predictability of NC-biological environment interactions.

Nanoparticles will then pass through endothelial cells due to the formation of membrane invagination vesicles and subsequent charge interactions [31, 32]. Clathrin-coated pits are particularly common in the brain capillary endothelium compared to peripheral endothelial cells. In addition, the fact that clathrin-coated pits are more abundant than normal pits indicates that clathrin-mediated processes play an important role in transcytosis [33]. Positive nanoparticles can be transferred to negative clathrin-coated pits on the luminal surface of endothelial cells. Therefore, the method relies on the electrostatic interaction between nanocarriers and the target, resulting in BBB adsorption of nanoparticles and their transport to the brain, where nanoparticles can work with good results. However, AMT alone does not provide specific targeting of the cell because positive electrons can be attracted rapidly and randomly to all cell membranes and thus invade many cells. However, many studies suggest using AMT as a brain transfer strategy. [34].

There are many brain capillary endothelial cells, and many of these cells have clathrin-coated vesicles or pits, which give the luminal surface of the cerebral endothelial membrane a negative charge to repel anionic molecules [35]. To form and synthesize essential NPs for adsorptive-induced transcytosis, cationic constituents like cationic bovine serum albumin (CBSA), RMP-7 peptides, TAT peptides, and MMP-2200 derivatives have been used. Cells can recognize and accumulate cationic substances with the aid of cationic substances that interact electrostatically with the anionic surface of the cerebral endothelium membrane at the luminal surface [36]. The engulfed NPs are then exocytosed in the direction of the luminal surface. The BBB could be crossed with the help of this technique for delivering therapeutic nanoparticles.

- Bovine serum albumin (BSA) functionalized nanoparticles
- TAT peptide functionalized nanoparticles
- MMP-2200 derivatives functionalized nanoparticles

6.2.2 Transporter-Mediated Transcytosis

An alternative approach for delivering medications to the brain is the use of carriers that are specific to the BBB for the efficient source of low-molecular nutrients from the systemic circulation to the CNS. In this regard, designing nanocarriers for brain delivery using transporter-mediated transcytosis (TMT) may be a useful method. It is possible to design nanoparticles with functionalized molecules on their surfaces that are readily recognized by carriers that are highly expressed in brain endothelial cells [37]. This strategy is still not prominent, because it can obstruct healthy nutrient absorption. However, the most frequently employed methods are amino acid, glucose, and glutathione transporters.

- Glucose Transporter
- Amino Acids Transporters
- Glutathione Transporter

6.2.3 Receptor-Mediated Transcytosis

Receptors highly expressed in the BBB can also be used to enter brain tissue, and this process is called receptor-mediated transcytosis (RMT) [38]. In the same concept as AMT, this process induces endocytosis from clathrin-coated pits. Nanoparticles are advantageous in terms of size, cost, composition, and ligand conjugation for different intracellular pathways [39]. The most common receptors that mediate RMT through the BBB are transferrin, lactoferrin, low-density lipoprotein, and nicotinic acetylcholine receptors. In addition, the potential strategy is to express insulin receptor and insulin-like growth factor receptor in the luminal membrane of brain capillary endothelial cells [31]. The results indicated that α-galactosidase is widely expressed in primate brains. However, the application of these receptors in nanotechnology has been constrained by the possibility of altering normal insulin regulation [31]. In consideration of this, brain endothelial cells can be stimulated to undertake nanoparticles that have been engineered with receptor ligands.

Active targeting can assist in helping nanoparticles locate the proper cell target after they have entered the brain. $\alpha v\beta 3$ integrins and CD13/APN receptors are well-known receptor elements regulated in the extracellular domain of tumor cells, while nicotinic acetylcholine receptors can be used to target specific cells and these receptors are used voluntarily to create specific treatments for cancer cells in the brain [40]. The most extensively researched receptors for receptor-mediated transcytosis on cerebral endothelial cells are insulin, integrin, iron-transferrin, low-density lipoprotein (LDL) cholesterol, nicotinic acetylcholine, metabolic nutrient transporters, and LDL cholesterol [41]. Particular ligands for such receptors have been extensively investigated as therapeutic logistics carriers across the BBB.

- Transferrin Receptor
- Lactoferrin Receptor
- Low-Density Lipoprotein Receptors
- Nicotinic Acetylcholine Receptors

6.2.4 Transcellular Transport

This is a potential method for delivering therapeutic agents to the brain. Using this method, drugs are delivered straight across the endothelial cells of the BBB. It is assumed that a large number of clinically accessible CNS medicines, including opioids and anticonvulsants, reach the brain by the transcellular lipophilic pathway, which can transport lipid-soluble substances smaller than 400 Da. The typical size of a CNS active medication is 357 Da. This strategy, however, has not been very effective because lipid solubility alterations typically cause chemicals' affinity for their target receptors to decrease or their molecular size to expand above 400 Da, although both are unfavorable to BBB permeability [11, 42]. Since all cell membranes are responsible for lipophilic transport, nonspecific absorption is another limitation of the lipophilic pathway for the BBB targets [43].

6.2.5 Paracellular Aqueous Pathway

The paracellular route includes the transfer of substances inside and outside of cells. Hormones, alcohol, and gases (CO_2, O_2) are examples of small, lipid-soluble substances with low molecular weights (400 Da) that can passively flow across the vascular endothelium. While paracellular channels are frequently used for distribution in peripheral capillaries, tight junctions in the BBB cause a large number of transports to occur through transcellular pathways [10].

6.3 TYPES OF POLYMERIC NANOCARRIERS

6.3.1 Polymeric Micelles

When introduced to an aqueous environment, amphiphilic block copolymers self-associate to generate nanoparticle molecules with a core-shell configuration known as polymeric micelles [44]. Polymeric micelles are employed in drug administration due to their intriguing properties, including biocompatibility, low cytotoxicity, a core-shell configuration, micellar association, shape, dimension, and considerably large stability. They are employed in the management of a variety of illnesses, including cancer, estrogen treatment, and anti-influenza antivirals [45]. The composition of the polymer micelles determines their function: The hydrophobic core delivers and protects the drug, while the hydrophilic shell controls and stabilizes the hydrophobic core in an aqueous environment, increasing the water solubility of the polymer, which facilitates drug delivery [46]. Polymeric micelles have a variety of potential therapeutic benefits, including the preservation of pharmaceuticals in capsules and the dissolution rate of medications with poor solubility. These carriers are typically generated using three methods: direct dissolution, solvent casting, or dialysis [46, 47]. The identification of polymeric micelles involves the use of three different polymer types. These are graft copolymers such as stearic acid and G-chitosan, triblock copolymers such as polyethylene oxide, and diblock copolymers such as polystyrene and polyethylene glycol (PEG). Depending on how the drug is used, polymeric micelles fall into two groups: polymeric micelles that physically encapsulate the drug, or those that chemically bond to the drug covalently [48].

The drug-binding copolymers featured in chemical form, which regulate the drug's delivery, make it more stable than the body attributes. Nevertheless, depending on the drug's polarity, the drug component can be confined in one of three sections of the polymer: the core if the drug is nonpolar, the shell if the drug is polar, or somewhere in between the core and the shell if the drug has moderate polarity [49]. Additionally, depending on the intermolecular tensions, polymeric micelles are classified into three types [44]:

- The conventional form, made from hydrophilic contacts, with poly(ethylene oxide) serving as an illustration of three types of micelles.
- The non-covalently linked polymeric micelles that are produced by self-assemblage of polymers; an instance of this kind is poly(4-vinyl pyridine).
- The polyion combination micelle form, which is created by electrostatic interactions between oppositely charged polymers, such as PEG.

6.3.2 Nanogels

Nanogels are made of a range of biological polymers, synthetic polymers, or a blend of both, and have a three-dimensional "nanoscopic" architecture [50]. The physio-chemical assembly of polymers carrying amphiphilic polymeric chains results in the formation of nanogels. Hydrogen bonds, electrostatic, van der Waals, and hydrophobic forces are used in the physical assembly, and covalent bonds are used in chemical cross-linking. OncoGel, a type of nanogel that contains paclitaxel, is one of the products of physical self-assembly [51]. Below the critical gelation temperature (CGT), PLGA-b-PEG-b-PLGA (ABA type) copolymers generate nanoscopic micelles in water by forming loops that share a hydrophobic PLGA center. The micelle's core contains paclitaxel (logP 3.0), which is physically confined there. Above the CGT, PLGA-b-PEG-b-PLGA gelates [52].

Temperature-dependent micelle formation decreases water mobility, and an apparent viscosity is the result of increased hydrophobic contacts between PLGA segments (gelation occurs). Pullulan serves as a carrier for hydrophobized cholesterol-based nanogels that are designed for the administration of insulin. When combined with insulin, these nanogels, typically ranging in size from 20 to 30 nanometers, undergo a self-assembly process. Another approach to creating nanogels involves the integration of nanoparticles into a hydrogel matrix, either suspending or immobilizing them within the structure. [53]. Due to the hydrogels' ability to limit the mobility of the nanoparticles and prevent their aggregation, nanogels containing silica and gold nanoparticles reduced the early drug release of loaded medicines. The ultimate stability of nanoparticles was increased by the addition of hydrogels [52].

6.3.3 Polymersomes

A polymersome is a remarkable method of delivery because it may carry a variety of medicines with different chemical characteristics [54]. These nanocarriers can hold amphiphilic substances because they have hydrophilic centers and hydrophobic walls. Polymersomes are one of the most potent delivery vehicles due to their versatility in drug loading, especially in combinational therapy where the ability to encapsulate numerous medicines with different chemical characteristics is extremely helpful [55]. They are made from artificial amphiphilic block copolymers that comprise both hydrophilic and hydrophobic key components, making them useful for entrapping both hydrophilic and hydrophobic therapeutics. The advantages of polymersomes over liposomes include higher colloidal stability, improved mechanical stability, high drug loading potential, prolonged blood circulation time, reduced drug leakage, and increased storage capacity [56].

Due to their capacity to reach the brain, polymersomes are regarded as effective carriers for combating glioma, and recent experiments have yielded positive results. [57]. In comparison to other innovative carriers, these nanocarriers have been discovered to be superior in terms of stability, storage space, release properties, and circulation duration. Block copolymers with different features can be used to create polymersomes [58]. By decreasing the adverse impacts on the healthy cells around them, their surface is changed with ligands targeting receptors found on the BBB, enabling precise delivery of the drug into the tumor sites. A variety of targeting techniques, including receptor-mediated, carrier-mediated, adsorption-mediated, and other physical mechanisms, are used to manage neurological conditions [59]. Among them, utilizing various specific receptors such as transferrin, lactoferrin, insulin, and endothelial growth factors found on the BBB, receptor-mediated endocytosis has been one of the principal strategies for targeting glioma [60].

6.3.4 Polymeric Nanoparticles

Polymeric nanoparticles comprise solid nanocrystals with a size between 10 and 1000 nm that are constructed of biocompatible and biodegradable polymers or copolymers [61, 62]. The substance can be physically adsorbed on the carrier's interface, chemically bound to the surface, or imprisoned or encapsulated inside the carrier. A compact size, biocompatibility, hydrophilicity, chemical inertness, biodegradability, and durability throughout preservation are just a few of these nanocarriers' appealing qualities [63]. For transporting medications, proteins, DNA, or genes to desired target tissues or organs, these properties make them significant. As a result, they are utilized in the treatment of cancer, in vaccination, and in genetic manipulation, for penetrating the BBB, in diagnostics, and in many other areas of medicine [64].

Polymeric nanoparticles are primarily used to deliver pharmacological drugs to a specific catalytic site, increasing drug concentration and enhancing the stability of volatile chemicals as well as the improved productivity of the treatment. Polymeric nanoparticles can be produced using one of three methods [65]:

1. Solvent evaporation, nanoprecipitation, emulsification, salting out, dialysis, and supercritical fluid are steps in the process of creating nanoparticles from a combination of produced polymers. [66]
2. Monomer-based polymerization, such as restricted radical polymerization, interfacial polymerization, and emulsion and microemulsion.
3. Coacervation of hydrophilic polymers or ionic gelatin.

Two distinct types of polymers are generally used to create polymeric nanoparticles: synthetic hydrophobic polymers, such as poly(methyl methacrylate) and poly(isobutyl cyanoacrylate), which are prepolymerized and polymerized-in-process materials; and naturally occurring hydrophilic polymers, which are made up of proteins like gelatin and albumin and polysaccharides like alginate and chitosan [47]. Polymeric nanoparticles are divided into groups according to how they are produced. These include nanospheres, which disperse the drug across a matrix system, and nanocapsules, which have a polymer membrane enclosing the drug [47].

6.3.5 Dendrimers

A novel category of polymeric nanomaterials is called dendrimers. They are 15 nm or smaller, 3D tree-shaped polymers that branch off of a central core [67]. Dendrimers are also known as cascade monomers and arborols. Size, shape, branching structure, and multivalency are desirable aspects that make dendrimers simple to functionalize, solubilize in water, and regulate their molecular weight [68]. Because of their ability to deliver a medicine to a specific tissue and inhibit its breakdown, nanoparticles are molecules of interest when trying to target cancer cells and damaged tissues. In addition, they demonstrate efficient functions such as boosting poorly soluble medications' solubility, lengthening the drug's half-life in circulation, and regulating the drug's release [69].

Three different synthetic strategies, divergent, convergent, and double-exponential and mixed growth, are used in the preparation of dendrimers.

1. The divergence strategy allows the dendrimers to grow from the central core and extend toward the surface. This strategy is used to prepare a large number of dendrimers. However, certain difficulties can be observed when cleaning the product.
2. In the convergent strategy, dendrimers grow from the tip or surface and extend inward until they coalesce to form a core. Unlike the divergent strategy, cleaning can be done easily.
3. The third strategy is a combination of the two previous strategies, in which two monomers, which are prepared by divergent and convergent methods, react together to form a protected trimer that can be used to repeat the growth process [70]. Many dendrimers have been successfully produced, and from their benefits, performance, and efficiency, it can be predicted that many more will be produced in the future, so the classification of dendrimers is very branched [71].

6.4 METHODS OF PREPARATION

6.4.1 Direct Dissolution

Direct dissolution, which involves dissolving both the drug and the amphiphilic copolymer in water, is the simplest technique for creating polymeric nanoparticles [47]. Limiting drug loading is a problem that can occur with this technique. To solve this challenge and increase the efficiency of drug delivery, this process increases the temperature or forms a thin layer before the copolymer is added [72]. The formation of polymeric micelles containing paclitaxel (PTX) is an example of this process. These micelles are formed by the self-assembly of amphiphilic copolymers in the aqueous phase, and PTX is physically embedded in the inner cores of the micelles due to the hydrophobic interaction between the drug and the copolymer. [46].

6.4.2 Dialysis

This approach involves incorporating a mixture of polymer and drug in an organic solvent using a dialysis bag. The dialysis bag is then immersed in water to recover the organic solvent and form the polymeric nanomaterial. For effective drug loading, the dialysis procedure required 36 hours. To overcome this restriction, we can employ a more economical method that involves dissolving the drug and the polymer, lyophilizing it, and then redispersing it in a compatible solvent to get the polymeric nanomaterial [73].

Dialysis is used, for instance, to prepare polymeric nanoparticles made of morin hydrate (MH). The process starts with the suspension of 15 mg of poly(butyl cyanoacrylate) block copolymer of hyaluronic acid in 3 ml of phosphate-buffered saline at pH 7.4. Next, a mixture of MH in 0.5 ml of dimethyl sulfoxide is introduced into the prepolymer suspension with constant stirring at a speed of 150 revolutions per minute at a temperature of 25°C. The resulting mixture is then sonicated for 30 minutes in an ice bath using an ultrasonic probe. The solution is further dialyzed for 12 hours against an excess of distilled water using a dialysis bag, followed by filtration and lyophilization. In this technique, a volatile solvent is used to combine the polymer with the drug to form an emulsion [74, 75]. Due to its non-toxic potential, ethyl acetate is the polymer most commonly used in this approach. The solvent further converts the emulsion into a suspension by evaporation. To remove contaminants and additives, solid molecules can be extracted by ultracentrifugation, rinsed and finally lyophilized. This technique is used to create poly(lactide, co-glycolide, co-PEG) (PLGA-PEG) nanoparticles [76].

6.4.3 Solvent Evaporation (Polymeric Nanoparticles)

In this technique, a volatile solvent is used to combine the polymer with the drug to make an emulsion. The non-cytotoxic nature of ethyl acetate makes it the most suitable polymer. The solvent transforms the emulsion into a suspension as it evaporates. The product is then lyophilized after the solid components have been recovered by ultracentrifugation and cleaned to eliminate additives and contaminants. This technique is used to create poly(lactide, co-glycolide, co-PEG) (PLGAePEG) nanoparticles [77]. To prepare particle dispersion, an acetone-soluble polymer is added to a poly(vinyl alcohol) aqueous phase that has already been agitated. After the acetone has completely evaporated, the mixture is maintained under agitation, and the resulting nanoparticle dispersion is compacted and purified. Before lyophilization, nanoparticles are separated by centrifugation for 25 min and twice rinsed with water.

6.4.4 Nanoprecipitation (Polymeric Nanoparticles)

The process of nanoprecipitation, which involves the polymer precipitating in an organic phase and the organic solvent diffusing into an aqueous environment, is known as solvent displacement and can occur with or without the use of a surfactant [78]. Some of the polymers that are used in this method of making polymeric nanomaterials are poly(lactic acid), PLGA, and poly(caprolactone). The water-miscible solvent is one of the limitations of the method, as it will cause some instability in the solution. Water miscible solvents must have sufficient diffusion rate to form spontaneous emulsification, if the coalescence rate is high spontaneous emulsification is not observed [79].

Since they improve the immobilization and particle density of the drug, acetone or dichloromethane are primarily utilized in this procedure when producing lipophilic drugs. Antifungal medications bifonazole and clotrimazole are formed using the nanoprecipitation process [80].

6.4.5 Interfacial Polymerization (Polymeric Nanoparticles)

This is one of the key processes for producing polymeric nanomaterials. There are two reactive agents that are disseminated in continuous and dispersed phases, where they polymerize. The reaction is initiated in-between two phases. The production of oil-containing nanocapsules with this technique involves polymerizing the substances found at the interface of the oil and water phases of o/w microemulsion. Acetonitrile, ethanol, and n-butanol are a few examples of aprotic solvents that are utilized in interfacial polymerization [81].

6.5 POLYMERIC CONSTRUCTS

There are a novel ways to cross the BBB by nanoparticles. These nanoparticles are known due to their small size, large surface area, ability to enhance bioavailability, and solubility. These nanoparticles are found in a less than 100 nm scale overall dimension [24]. In recent years, these nanoparticles have been shown to play an important role in modern medicine. The problem with treatment and diagnostic tools is crossing the BBB to achieve good results. There are two primary source of these polymers, which are natural and synthetic.

6.5.1 Natural Polymers

These polymers are naturally obtained and have abilities like biodegradation and are compatible with the body. This natural polymer comes from bacteria fungi plants and animals. There are two types of main polymers, which are polysaccharides and protein-based polymers. The similarity between them is they can form scaffolds and the extracellular matrix, which is viable. Because of these, nanoparticles can achieve high loading efficiency and targeted delivery [82].

6.5.1.1 Protein-based Polymer

These polymers are obtained from natural tissues. Polymers are formed with amino acids and these acids are stabilized by various bondings like hydrogen bonding and disulphide bonding with salt bridges. Protein-based polymers have good biodegradation capacity as well as good biocompatibility. Amino acids in protein-based polymers are linked with peptide bonds. But unlike polysaccharides, these compounds show low toxicity. Despite this, protein-based polymers show very minimum byproduct accumulation in the body. The most commonly used protein-based polymers are gelatin, collagen, and albumin [83].

6.5.1.1.1 Gelatin

Gelatin (GE), a byproduct of slightly dissolved and denatured collagen, is widely used in the administration of medicinal agents and tissue engineering. This product is formed after the hydrolysis of animal collagen. It is a natural, biodegradable, and bioavailable compound. Gelatin is mostly used in pharmaceutical products as well as in food products [84]. But for nanoparticles and drug delivery, gelatin needs to be modified and developed for better results. Gelatin has good water solubility, and this is required for long-term drug delivery. Additionally, GE has active molecules such as arginine-glycine-aspartic acid, which gives it a function that allows it to adhere to cells and adds to its value as a biomaterial [85]. GE and its mixtures are currently utilized in both the food sector and healthcare industries. GE is an appropriate drug-delivery mechanism due to its nontoxic, biodegradable, and bioactive qualities. It was observed that these nanoparticles (NPs) demonstrated a lethal effect on U87MG glioblastoma cancer cells. These NPs had a diameter in the range of 40–200 nm, a zeta potential of –40.1 mV, and entrapment effectiveness of 70% [86].

6.5.1.1.2 Collagen

Collagen is a widely presented extracellular matrix in animal tissues such as skin, small intestine, pericardium, tendon, bone, cartilage, and many others. Collagen is isolated from animal tissues using various chemical and physical techniques. There are 28 different types of collagen present in animal tissues. Collagen is biocompatible, biodegradable, mechanically stable, and can be crosslinked using chemical crosslinkers [87].

6.5.1.1.3 Albumin

The four main types of albumin present in the human and animal bodies are ovalbumin (OSA), rat serum albumin (RSA), bovine serum albumin (BSA), and human serum albumin (HSA) [88]. The BBB may be more easily penetrated with albumin due to its poor immunity and toxicity. Drugs can form conjugates with albumin due to the presence of numerous binding sites, enabling the formation of covalent connections.. The two most commonly used serum albumins for medication delivery are human and bovine. These kinds of organic polymers can be utilized to strengthen nanoparticles so they can pass across the BBB.

HSA is a protein with a molecular mass (66 kDa) that is hydrophilic [89]. This protein is very prevalent in the body and plays a variety of important roles, such as improving the bioavailability of long-chain fatty acids, transporting various ions and chemicals, including medications and hormones, and controlling osmolality in the bloodstream. It is a possible option for medication delivery due to these favorable traits and its lengthy half-life of about 20 days in the circulatory system. HSA-based nanoparticles have been researched and created for use in prophylactic and treatment medication delivery to the brain. Following BBB permeabilization, it was discovered that BSA enhanced medication retention in the glioma area [90].

6.5.1.2 Polysaccharide

This is the second major category of naturally occurring polymers. This is composed of a lengthy chain of polymeric carbohydrates and many monosaccharides, or sugars. Chitosan and chondroitin are two examples of polysaccharides derived from animal sources. Plants contain mannan, pectin, and guar gum as polymers. Algae and microorganisms, respectively, contain alginate, xanthan gum, and dextran. These polysaccharides have over 10 sugar monomer units in them. The main benefits are strong stability and biocompatibility, and another benefit is nontoxicity because it is derived from nature. In nanocarrier therapy, four polysaccharides with the names dextran, alginate, hyaluronic acid, and chitosan are frequently employed [82].

6.5.1.2.1 Dextran

This polymer is made up of a chain of branched glucan with a linkage between alpha 1,6 linkage of D glucose. This structure affects biological activities because of the molecular weight and branching. With medium water solubility and being easy to modify, dextran makes a good polymer for nanocarriers. Dextran has a lower toxicity rate and this can stabilize drug conjugates or DDS. Dextran shows good bioavailability, which is why it is suitable for modification in polymer nanocarriers [91].

6.5.1.2.2 Alginate

Alginate, which is produced from algae, is frequently utilized. The most used salt is sodium alginate because monovalent salts of alginic acid may be dissolved in water but alginic acid itself cannot. Alpha L glucuronic acid and beta D mannuronic acid, which have 1,4 glycosidic connections, combine to form the irregular structure of this alginate. The pH and temperature are just two of the many variables that affect this alginate. Alginate can form a gel under the right circumstances and at a constant pH temperature without the use of any harmful solvents. The gel's quality can be impacted by temperature, chemical makeup, and ions in solution [92]. Water can flow through the matrix when the gel forms. This alginate can perform exceptionally in hydrogel and developing nanocarriers, but the only problem with the alginate is that it is obtained from seaweed or algae, so it has more of a crude or impure form that includes heavy metal and protein inside the matrix of alginate. That is why it is hard to purify it.

6.5.1.2.3 Hyaluronic Acid

Glucuronic acid and N-acetylglucosamine are linked by beta 1,4 and beta 1,3 glycosidic bonds in this linear anionic glycosaminoglycan. This is mostly employed in the delivery of controlled-release medications. Hyaluronic acid has the unique ability to bind receptors like CD44. The development of tumors contains these kinds of receptors. Additionally, hyaluronic gel is beneficial when angiogenesis and tumor cell proliferation are occurring due to complex bioactivity [93].

6.5.1.2.4 Chitosan

Deacetylation of chitin results in the formation of chitosan. It is an amino polysaccharide that is linearly cationic. N-acetyl and beta-o-glucosamine molecules combine to create this chitosan. Chitosan is renowned for its mucoadhesive characteristics, biocompatibility, antibacterial and antifungal capabilities, and nontoxicity. When there is enzymatic activity, this can create monomers and oligomers. This compound can be changed to add more groups to the skeleton of its chemical structure. This adjustment will address the complex's issue of poor solubility. The technique can be applied to the treatment of microspheres, nanoparticles, and hydrogen [94].

CS is a positive-charged, water-soluble cationic polysaccharide that is both biocompatible and biodegradable. CS is a great alternative for drug carriers in pharmaceutical applications due to its benign and nonallergenic properties. Through its association with the tight junction, CS can render epithelial cells permeable, allowing them to pass through the epithelial barrier. Through the nasal epithelium, researchers have examined how various medications (such as proteins, peptides, hormones, etc.) are absorbed into the body [95].

6.5.2 Synthetic Polymers

These are frequently utilized to deliver medications and bioactive substances. Due to their biocompatibility and biodegradability, polyesters among them offer a lot of potential [96]. They are nontoxicologically hazardous, and the human body's metabolic processes remove both their monomers and byproducts. In medicine and pharmaceuticals, polylactic acid (PLA), polyglycolic acid (PGA), and PLGA are frequently utilized. The Food and Drug Administration has given PLA and PLGA the go ahead for clinical applications. These polymers break down in the human body without triggering any immunological or inflammatory responses. They have been used to create biodegradable medical devices such as scaffolds, drug-loaded nanoparticles, and implants [97].

6.5.2.1 PLA

In the human body, PLA biodegrades into its monomeric units and is a nontoxic polymer. Lactic acid's monomer is a stable and common intermediary in the metabolism of carbohydrates. PLA NPs are used for the delivery of neurotoxin-I (NT-I). After NT-I-PLA NPs were administered intranasally (IN) or intravenously (IV), it was discovered that the level of NT-I rose in the brain. Results showed that NT-I-PLA NPs administered IN were more efficient than those administered IV [98]. It has been suggested that cell-penetrating peptides (CPPs) with a low proportion of basic amino acids provide excellent candidates for PEG-PLA NP characterization and drug delivery to the brain. In the brain, polymeric NPs were shown to be accumulating more frequently. Studies conducted *in vitro* and *in vivo* were utilized to evaluate the hypothesis that the surface characteristics of NPs are related to their cellular distribution. Overall, it was determined that because of their low toxicity and rapid absorption by brain cells, PLA NPs are prospective options for the administration of drugs into the brain [99].

6.5.2.2 PLGA

An appropriate polymer for biomedical and pharmaceutical uses, poly(lactic-co-glycolic acid) PLGA has these common attributes: biodegradability, biocompatibility, and prolonged release [100]. Variations in molecular size and the molarity of lactic acid to glycolic acid can have an impact on the polymer breakdown and drug-releasing function [101]. During the regular metabolic activities of the cells, both monomers are digested and excreted. The detection, diagnosis, and therapy of diseases have all been performed using sustainable delivery methods based on the PLGA polymer [102]. PLGA NPs have been used to implicate a variety of medicines, including proteins, peptides, genes, and oncology medications. Acidic or elevated conditions can be harmful to medications made of proteins and peptides. The stability and bioavailability after polymer decomposition can be reduced when proteins and peptides are exposed over an extended period to the acidic by-products of PLGA [103]. Determining the physicochemical properties of proteins and peptides is essential. The potential for using PLGA NPs to treat brain disorders has been explored.

6.5.2.3 Poly(ε-caprolactone) (PCL)

A biodegradable polyester called Poly(-caprolactone) (PCL) is frequently used to increase the tensile strength and elasticity of several polymers, including PLA. Additionally, PCL has also been widely employed for cultured cell constructs as a typical polymer for electrospinning [104]. Because PCL degrades more slowly than PLA, it can be used to create structures and nanoparticles (NPs) for the sustained release of pharmacological drugs over an extended period [100]. Poly(N-isopropyl acrylamide)-b-poly(3-caprolactone) (PNPCL) block copolymers were employed as a thermosensitive nanosystem for clonazepam administration into the brain. Findings indicate that Poly(N-isopropyl acrylamide), when present in a copolymer, coats the interface of nanoparticles in a film and inhibits the drug's rapid onset of action. Clonazepam functions in the brain by enhancing the effects of GABA, which reduces or inhibits certain nerve signaling [105]. It has been demonstrated that these NPs are more bioavailable in the rat brain after IN injection and that this could help alleviate cerebral ischemia. For the management of glioblastoma tumors, the extended delivery of TMZ from electrospun PCL-Diol-b-PU/gold nanocomposite nanofibers is used [106, 107]. The outcome of the above-mentioned study showed that these NPs reduced the proliferation and mortality of glioblastoma cells.

6.6 CONCLUSION

This chapter has discussed the composition of the BBB, as understanding of the BBB is very important for brain drug delivery and understanding the BBB could widen thinking for the development of new drug-delivery systems. Various polymer-based nanocarrier strategies could be used for efficient drug delivery to the brain in various pathological conditions. Recent advances in polymeric nanocarrier-based research have yielded promising strategies for high drug loading and efficient delivery to the brain. Common nanocarriers such as polymeric nanoparticles, dendrimers, nanocapsule, nano gel, nano micelle, and polymersomes have been introduced for more efficient drug delivery. Moreover, polymers offer the advantage of fabrication of nanocarriers in a variety of sizes, and morphologies. Natural and synthetic polymers have their advantages in drug delivery.

REFERENCES

1. Mansoor, K., K. Sima, and K. Soheila, Advancement of polymer–based nanoparticles as smart drug delivery systems in neurodegenerative medicine. *Journal of Nanomedicine Reseasrch*, 2019. 8: p. 277–280.
2. Rabiee, N. et al., Polymeric nanoparticles for nasal drug delivery to the brain: relevance to Alzheimer's disease. *Advanced Therapeutics*, 2021. 4(3): p. 2000076.
3. Manek, E. and G.A. Petroianu, Brain delivery of antidotes by polymeric nanoparticles. *Journal of Applied Toxicology*, 2021. 41(1): p. 20–32.
4. Dong, X. Current Strategies for Brain Drug Delivery. *Theranostics*, 2018. 8(6): p. 1481–1493.
5. Gao, Y. et al., Natural polymeric nanocarriers in malignant glioma drug delivery and targeting. *Journal of Drug Targeting*, 2021. 29(9): p. 960–973.
6. Serlin, Y. et al., Anatomy and physiology of the blood–brain barrier. *Semin Cell Dev Biol*, 2015. 38: p. 2–6.
7. Daneman, R. and A. Prat, The blood–brain barrier. *Cold Spring Harb Perspect Biol*, 2015. 7(1): p. a020412.
8. Bernardo-Castro, S. et al., Pathophysiology of blood–brain barrier permeability throughout the different stages of ischemic stroke and its implication on hemorrhagic transformation and recovery. *Front Neurol*, 2020. 11: p. 594672.
9. Diamond, B. et al., Brain-reactive antibodies and disease. *Annu Rev Immunol*, 2013. 31: p. 345–85.

10. Upadhyay, R.K., Transendothelial transport and its role in therapeutics. *Int Sch Res Notices*, 2014. 2014: p. 309404.
11. Pardridge, W.M., Drug transport across the blood–brain barrier. *J Cereb Blood Flow Metab*, 2012. 32(11): p. 1959–72.
12. Tanaka, M. et al., Characterization of the AT2 receptor on rat ovarian granulosa cells. *Adv Exp Med Biol*, 1996. 396: p. 175–82.
13. Zhang, W. et al., Differential expression of receptors mediating receptor-mediated transcytosis (RMT) in brain microvessels, brain parenchyma and peripheral tissues of the mouse and the human. *Fluids Barriers CNS*, 2020. 17(1): p. 47.
14. Tsuji, A. et al., P-glycoprotein as the drug efflux pump in primary cultured bovine brain capillary endothelial cells. *Life Sci*, 1992. 51(18): p. 1427–37.
15. Cai, Q. et al., Systemic delivery to central nervous system by engineered PLGA nanoparticles. *Am J Transl Res*, 2016. 8(2): p. 749–64.
16. Davis, T.P., L. Sanchez-Covarubias, and M.E. Tome, P-glycoprotein trafficking as a therapeutic target to optimize CNS drug delivery. *Adv Pharmacol*, 2014. 71: p. 25–44.
17. Maeda, H., Vascular permeability in cancer and infection as related to macromolecular drug delivery, with emphasis on the EPR effect for tumor-selective drug targeting. *Proc Jpn Acad Ser B Phys Biol Sci*, 2012. 88(3): p. 53–71.
18. Yoo, J. et al., Active targeting strategies using biological ligands for nanoparticle drug delivery systems. *Cancers (Basel)*, 2019. 11(5).
19. Upadhyay, R.K., *Drug delivery systems, CNS protection, and the blood brain barrier*. Biomed Res Int, 2014. 2014: p. 869269.
20. Lu, C.T. et al., Current approaches to enhance CNS delivery of drugs across the brain barriers. *Int J Nanomedicine*, 2014. 9: p. 2241–57.
21. Wang, C.C., J. Carnevale, and J.L. Rubenstein, Progress in central nervous system lymphomas. *Br J Haematol*, 2014. 166(3): p. 311–25.
22. Thakkar, S. et al., Tumor microenvironment targeted nanotherapeutics for cancer therapy and diagnosis: A review. *Acta biomaterialia*, 2020. 101: p. 43–68.
23. Ahlawat, J. et al., Nanocarriers as potential drug delivery candidates for overcoming the blood–brain barrier: Challenges and possibilities. *ACS Omega*, 2020. 5(22): p. 12583–12595.
24. De Jong, W.H. and P.J. Borm, Drug delivery and nanoparticles:applications and hazards. *Int J Nanomedicine*, 2008. 3(2): p. 133–49.
25. Patra, J.K. et al., Nano based drug delivery systems: recent developments and future prospects. *J Nanobiotechnology*, 2018. 16(1): p. 71.
26. Gol, D., S. Thakkar, and M. Misra, Nanocrystal-based drug delivery system of risperidone: lyophilization and characterization. *Drug development and industrial pharmacy*, 2018. 44(9): p. 1458–1466.
27. Jeyaraj, M. et al., A comprehensive review on the synthesis, characterization, and biomedical application of platinum nanoparticles. *Nanomaterials (Basel)*, 2019. 9(12).
28. Nune, S.K. et al., Nanoparticles for biomedical imaging. *Expert Opin Drug Deliv*, 2009. 6(11): p. 1175–94.
29. Bareford, L.M. and P.W. Swaan, Endocytic mechanisms for targeted drug delivery. *Adv Drug Deliv Rev*, 2007. 59(8): p. 748–58.
30. Xu, S. et al., Targeting receptor-mediated endocytotic pathways with nanoparticles: rationale and advances. *Adv Drug Deliv Rev*, 2013. 65(1): p. 121–38.
31. Pinheiro, R.G.R. et al., Nanoparticles for targeted brain drug delivery: what do we know? *Int J Mol Sci*, 2021. 22(21).
32. Behzadi, S. et al., Cellular uptake of nanoparticles: journey inside the cell. *Chem Soc Rev*, 2017. 46(14): p. 4218–4244.

33. Villasenor, R. et al., Intracellular transport and regulation of transcytosis across the blood–brain barrier. *Cell Mol Life Sci*, 2019. 76(6): p. 1081–1092.
34. Stewart, M.P., R. Langer, and K.F. Jensen, Intracellular delivery by membrane disruption: mechanisms, strategies, and concepts. *Chem Rev*, 2018. 118(16): p. 7409–7531.
35. Herve, F., N. Ghinea, and J.M. Scherrmann, CNS delivery via adsorptive transcytosis. *AAPS J*, 2008. 10(3): p. 455–72.
36. Lu, W. et al., Cationic albumin conjugated pegylated nanoparticle with its transcytosis ability and little toxicity against blood–brain barrier. *Int J Pharm*, 2005. 295(1–2): p. 247–60.
37. Wiley, D.T. et al., Transcytosis and brain uptake of transferrin-containing nanoparticles by tuning avidity to transferrin receptor. *Proc Natl Acad Sci U S A*, 2013. 110(21): p. 8662–7.
38. Jones, A.R. and E.V. Shusta, Blood–brain barrier transport of therapeutics via receptor-mediation. *Pharm Res*, 2007. 24(9): p. 1759–71.
39. Hansen, C.G. and B.J. Nichols, Molecular mechanisms of clathrin-independent endocytosis. *J Cell Sci*, 2009. 122(Pt 11): p. 1713–21.
40. Desgrosellier, J.S. and D.A. Cheresh, Integrins in cancer: biological implications and therapeutic opportunities. *Nat Rev Cancer*, 2010. 10(1): p. 9–22.
41. Lajoie, J.M. and E.V. Shusta, Targeting receptor-mediated transport for delivery of biologics across the blood–brain barrier. *Annu Rev Pharmacol Toxicol*, 2015. 55: p. 613–31.
42. Pardridge, W.M., The blood–brain barrier: bottleneck in brain drug development. *NeuroRx*, 2005. 2(1): p. 3–14.
43. Bellettato, C.M. and M. Scarpa, Possible strategies to cross the blood–brain barrier. *Ital J Pediatr*, 2018. 44(Suppl 2): p. 131.
44. Hwang, D., J.D. Ramsey, and A.V. Kabanov, *P*olymeric micelles for the delivery of poorly soluble drugs: from nanoformulation to clinical approval. *Adv Drug Deliv Rev*, 2020. 156: p. 80–118.
45. Jhaveri, A.M. and V.P. Torchilin, Multifunctional polymeric micelles for delivery of drugs and siRNA. *Front Pharmacol*, 2014. 5: p. 77.
46. Xu, W., P. Ling, and T. Zhang, Polymeric micelles, a promising drug delivery system to enhance bioavailability of poorly water-soluble drugs. *J Drug Deliv*, 2013. 2013: p. 340315.
47. Zielinska, A. et al., Polymeric nanoparticles: production, characterization, toxicology and ecotoxicology. *Molecules*, 2020. 25(16).
48. Lu, Y. and K. Park, Polymeric micelles and alternative nanonized delivery vehicles for poorly soluble drugs. *Int J Pharm*, 2013. 453(1): p. 198–214.
49. Liechty, W.B. et al., Polymers for drug delivery systems. *Annu Rev Chem Biomol Eng*, 2010. 1: p. 149–73.
50. Stawicki, B., T. Schacher, and H. Cho, Nanogels as a versatile drug delivery system for brain cancer. *Gels*, 2021. 7(2).
51. Elstad, N.L. and K.D. Fowers, OncoGel (ReGel/paclitaxel) – clinical applications for a novel paclitaxel delivery system. *Adv Drug Deliv Rev*, 2009. 61(10): p. 785–94.
52. Tyler, B. et al., A thermal gel depot for local delivery of paclitaxel to treat experimental brain tumors in rats. *J Neurosurg*, 2010. 113(2): p. 210–7.
53. Torres, A.J. et al., Paclitaxel delivery to brain tumors from hydrogels: a computational study. *Biotechnol Prog*, 2011. 27(5): p. 1478–87.
54. Zheng, M. et al., Tuning the elasticity of polymersomes for brain tumor targeting. *Adv Sci (Weinh)*, 2021. 8(20): p. e2102001.

55. Ahmed, F. et al., Biodegradable polymersomes loaded with both paclitaxel and doxorubicin permeate and shrink tumors, inducing apoptosis in proportion to accumulated drug. *J Control Release*, 2006. 116(2): p. 150–8.
56. Anajafi, T. and S. Mallik, Polymersome-based drug-delivery strategies for cancer therapeutics. *Ther Deliv*, 2015. 6(4): p. 521–34.
57. Robbins, G.P. et al., Photoinitiated destruction of composite porphyrin-protein polymersomes. *J Am Chem Soc*, 2009. 131(11): p. 3872–4.
58. Ghoroghchian, P.P. et al., Bioresorbable vesicles formed through spontaneous self-assembly of amphiphilic poly(ethylene oxide)-block-polycaprolactone. *Macromolecules*, 2006. 39(5): p. 1673–1675.
59. Beduneau, A., P. Saulnier, and J.P. Benoit, Active targeting of brain tumors using nanocarriers. *Biomaterials*, 2007. 28(33): p. 4947–67.
60. Smith, M.W. and M. Gumbleton, Endocytosis at the blood–brain barrier: from basic understanding to drug delivery strategies. *J Drug Target*, 2006. 14(4): p. 191–214.
61. Ahire, E. et al., Parenteral nanosuspensions: a brief review from solubility enhancement to more novel and specific applications. *Acta pharmaceutica sinica B*, 2018. 8(5): p. 733–755.
62. Bolhassani, A. et al., Polymeric nanoparticles: potent vectors for vaccine delivery targeting cancer and infectious diseases. *Hum Vaccin Immunother*, 2014. 10(2): p. 321–32.
63. Thakkar, S. and M. Misra, Electrospray drying of docetaxel nanosuspension: A study on particle formation and evaluation of nanocrystals thereof. *Journal of Drug Delivery Science and Technology*, 2020. 60: p. 102009.
64. Akagi, T. et al., Preparation and characterization of biodegradable nanoparticles based on poly(gamma-glutamic acid) with l-phenylalanine as a protein carrier. *J Control Release*, 2005. 108(2–3): p. 226–36.
65. Begines, B. et al., Polymeric nanoparticles for drug delivery: recent developments and future prospects. *Nanomaterials (Basel)*, 2020. 10(7).
66. Pawar, A., S. Thakkar, and M. Misra, A bird's eye view of nanoparticles prepared by electrospraying: advancements in drug delivery field. *Journal of controlled release*, 2018. 286: p. 179–200.
67. Tambe, V. et al., Surface engineered dendrimers in siRNA delivery and gene silencing. *Current Pharmaceutical Design*, 2017. 23(20): p. 2952–2975.
68. Klajnert, B. and M. Bryszewska, Dendrimers: properties and applications. *Acta Biochim Pol*, 2001. 48(1): p. 199–208.
69. Bosman, A.W., H.M. Janssen, and E.W. Meijer, About dendrimers: structure, physical properties, and applications. *Chem Rev*, 1999. 99(7): p. 1665–1688.
70. Wolinsky, J.B. and M.W. Grinstaff, Therapeutic and diagnostic applications of dendrimers for cancer treatment. *Adv Drug Deliv Rev*, 2008. 60(9): p. 1037–55.
71. Svenson, S. and D.A. Tomalia, Dendrimers in biomedical applications – reflections on the field. *Adv Drug Deliv Rev*, 2005. 57(15): p. 2106–29.
72. Kamaly, N. et al., Degradable controlled-release polymers and polymeric nanoparticles: mechanisms of controlling drug release. *Chem Rev*, 2016. 116(4): p. 2602–63.
73. Krishnamoorthy, K. and M. Mahalingam, Selection of a suitable method for the preparation of polymeric nanoparticles: multi-criteria decision making approach. *Adv Pharm Bull*, 2015. 5(1): p. 57–67.
74. Anup, N., S. Thakkar, and M. Misra, Formulation of olanzapine nanosuspension based orally disintegrating tablets (ODT); comparative evaluation of lyophilization and electrospraying process as solidification techniques. *Advanced Powder Technology*, 2018. 29(8): p. 1913–1924.

75. Thakkar, S., D. Sharma, and M. Misra, Comparative evaluation of electrospraying and lyophilization techniques on solid state properties of erlotinib nanocrystals: assessment of In-vitro cytotoxicity. *Eur J Pharm Sci*, 2018. 111: p. 257–269.
76. Ryu, U. et al., Recent advances in process engineering and upcoming applications of metal-organic frameworks. *Coord Chem Rev*, 2021. 426: p. 213544.
77. Xue, J. et al., Electrospinning and Electrospun nanofibers: methods, materials, and applications. *Chem Rev*, 2019. 119(8): p. 5298–5415.
78. Salatin, S. et al., Development of a nanoprecipitation method for the entrapment of a very water soluble drug into eudragit RL nanoparticles. *Res Pharm Sci*, 2017. 12(1): p. 1–14.
79. Kumar, M. et al., Techniques for formulation of nanoemulsion drug delivery system: a review. *Prev Nutr Food Sci*, 2019. 24(3): p. 225–234.
80. Reis, C.P. et al., Nanoencapsulation I. Methods for preparation of drug-loaded polymeric nanoparticles. *Nanomedicine*, 2006. 2(1): p. 8–21.
81. Dallas, P. and V. Georgakilas, Interfacial polymerization of conductive polymers: generation of polymeric nanostructures in a 2-D space. *Adv Colloid Interface Sci*, 2015. 224: p. 46–61.
82. Torres, F.G. et al., Natural polysaccharide nanomaterials: an overview of their immunological properties. *Int J Mol Sci*, 2019. 20(20).
83. Varanko, A., S. Saha, and A. Chilkoti, Recent trends in protein and peptide-based biomaterials for advanced drug delivery. *Adv Drug Deliv Rev*, 2020. 156: p. 133–187.
84. Coppola, D. et al., Marine collagen from alternative and sustainable sources: extraction, processing and applications. *Mar Drugs*, 2020. 18(4).
85. Nitta, S.K. and K. Numata, Biopolymer-based nanoparticles for drug/gene delivery and tissue engineering. *Int J Mol Sci*, 2013. 14(1): p. 1629–54.
86. Caraway, C.A. et al., Polymeric nanoparticles in brain cancer therapy: a review of current approaches. *Polymers (Basel)*, 2022. 14(14).
87. Meyer, M., Processing of collagen based biomaterials and the resulting materials properties. *Biomed Eng Online*, 2019. 18(1): p. 24.
88. Raoufinia, R. et al., Overview of albumin and its purification methods. *Adv Pharm Bull*, 2016. 6(4): p. 495–507.
89. Hoogenboezem, E.N. and C.L. Duvall, Harnessing albumin as a carrier for cancer therapies. *Adv Drug Deliv Rev*, 2018. 130: p. 73–89.
90. Kiela, P.R. and F.K. Ghishan, Physiology of intestinal absorption and secretion. *Best Pract Res Clin Gastroenterol*, 2016. 30(2): p. 145–59.
91. Khalikova, E., P. Susi, and T. Korpela, Microbial dextran-hydrolyzing enzymes: fundamentals and applications. *Microbiol Mol Biol Rev*, 2005. 69(2): p. 306–25.
92. Lee, K.Y. and D.J. Mooney, Alginate: properties and biomedical applications. *Prog Polym Sci*, 2012. 37(1): p. 106–126.
93. Fallacara, A. et al., Hyaluronic acid in the third millennium. *Polymers (Basel)*, 2018. 10(7).
94. Cheung, R.C. et al., Chitosan: An update on potential biomedical and pharmaceutical applications. *Mar Drugs*, 2015. 13(8): p. 5156–86.
95. Wu, Q.X., D.Q. Lin, and S.J. Yao, Design of chitosan and its water soluble derivatives-based drug carriers with polyelectrolyte complexes. *Mar Drugs*, 2014. 12(12): p. 6236–53.
96. Thakkar, S. et al., Fast dissolving electrospun polymeric films of anti-diabetic drug repaglinide: formulation and evaluation. *Drug development and industrial pharmacy*, 2019. 45(12): p. 1921–1930.

97. Saghazadeh, S. et al., Drug delivery systems and materials for wound healing applications. *Adv Drug Deliv Rev*, 2018. 127: p. 138–166.
98. Shakeri, S. et al., Multifunctional polymeric nanoplatforms for brain diseases diagnosis, therapy and theranostics. *Biomedicines*, 2020. 8(1).
99. Xia, H. et al., Penetratin-functionalized PEG-PLA nanoparticles for brain drug delivery. *Int J Pharm*, 2012. 436(1–2): p. 840–50.
100. Makadia, H.K. and S.J. Siegel, Poly lactic-co-glycolic acid (PLGA) as biodegradable controlled drug delivery carrier. *Polymers (Basel)*, 2011. 3(3): p. 1377–1397.
101. Hines, D.J. and D.L. Kaplan, Poly(lactic-co-glycolic) acid-controlled-release systems: experimental and modeling insights. *Crit Rev Ther Drug Carrier Syst*, 2013. 30(3): p. 257–76.
102. Lu, J.M. et al., Current advances in research and clinical applications of PLGA-based nanotechnology. *Expert Rev Mol Diagn*, 2009. 9(4): p. 325–41.
103. Bruno, B.J., G.D. Miller, and C.S. Lim, Basics and recent advances in peptide and protein drug delivery. *Ther Deliv*, 2013. 4(11): p. 1443–67.
104. Sowmya, B., A.B. Hemavathi, and P.K. Panda, Poly (epsilon-caprolactone)-based electrospun nano-featured substrate for tissue engineering applications: a review. *Prog Biomater*, 2021. 10(2): p. 91–117.
105. Jeong, Y.I. et al., Clonazepam release from core-shell type nanoparticles in vitro. *J Control Release*, 1998. 51(2–3): p. 169–78.
106. Pena, E.S. et al., Design of biopolymer-based interstitial therapies for the treatment of glioblastoma. *Int J Mol Sci*, 2021. 22(23).
107. Thakkar, S. and M. Misra, Electrospun polymeric nanofibers: nNew horizons in drug delivery. *Eur J Pharm Sci*, 2017. 107: p. 148–167.

7 Lipid-Based Nanocarriers for Brain Delivery of Drugs in Neurodegenerative Disorders

Mukesh Kumar Yadav, Manish Singh, Pritee Chaudhary, and Shardendu Kumar Mishra

7.1 INTRODUCTION

Solid lipid nanoparticles (SLNs), nanostructured lipid carriers (NLCs), and liposomes are lipid-based nanocarriers that have shown promise as drug-delivery systems for the treatment of neurodegenerative diseases like Alzheimer's, Parkinson's, and Huntington's diseases. These nanocarriers offer several advantages, including the ability to encapsulate both hydrophilic and hydrophobic drugs, with the ability to cross the blood–brain barrier (BBB) for targeted drug delivery. One of the challenges in the treatment of neurodegenerative disorders is the limited ability of drugs to cross the BBB, which is a highly selective barrier that separates the brain from the circulating blood. Lipid-based nanocarriers have been shown to improve drug delivery across the BBB by taking advantage of the natural uptake mechanisms of brain cells, such as receptor-mediated endocytosis and transcytosis [1,2].

Additionally, lipid-based nanocarriers can be designed to target specific cells or regions within the brain, such as neurons or glial cells. This can be achieved by modifying the surface of the nanocarriers with ligands that bind to specific receptors on the target cells. Several studies have shown the potential of lipid-based nanocarriers for the delivery of drugs to treat neurodegenerative disorders, such as Alzheimer's disease (AD), Parkinson's disease (PD), and Huntington's disease (HD) [3,4]. For example, liposomes have been used to deliver anti-inflammatory drugs, such as curcumin, to reduce neuroinflammation in AD [5,6]. SLNs have been used to deliver the antioxidant resveratrol to protect neurons from oxidative stress in PD. NLCs have been used to deliver gene therapy to silence the mutant huntingtin gene in HD.

Lipid-based nanocarriers hold great promise for the treatment of neurodegenerative disorders by improving drug delivery across the BBB and enabling targeted drug

DOI: 10.1201/9781032661964-7

delivery to specific cells or regions within the brain [7–13]. However, further research is needed to optimize the design and formulation of lipid-based nanocarriers for effective and safe drug delivery in clinical settings.

7.2 NEURODEGENERATIVE DISEASES

Neurodegenerative diseases are a group of disorders characterized by the progressive loss of function and death of neurons in the brain and nervous system. These diseases are typically chronic and often incurable, and they can have a significant impact on a person's quality of life. There are many different types of neurodegenerative diseases, each with its own set of symptoms, causes, and treatments [14, 15]. Some of the most common neurodegenerative diseases include:

7.2.1 Alzheimer's Disease

The most common neurodegenerative condition and the main contributor to dementia is Alzheimer's disease (AD). Several additional cognitive domains, such as sensorimotor, visual-spatial, behavioral, or linguistic abilities are affected by AD, which is clinically defined by progressive memory loss and targets large-scale brain networks [16]. Depending on the severity of the disease and the individual, cognitive processes might be impacted to varying degrees [17]. Beta-amyloid (Aβ) plaques outside of cells and neurofibrillary tangles, which include tau inside of neurons, are both found in AD [18]. The pathogenesis of the illness appears to be triggered and amplified by oxidative stress and the buildup of free radicals, with an aggravated immunological response involving pro-inflammatory cytokines. As a result, the brain experiences excessive lipid peroxidation and neuronal degeneration, with the loss of cholinergic neurons being particularly noticeable [19,20]. The development of diseases may also include the glutamate pathway [21]. The accumulation of plaques and tangles, which results in the loss of synapses involved in cognition and memory functions, causes the classic behavioral symptoms of AD. It seems that many of the detrimental features of Aβ require tau, and that A and tau jointly cause healthy neurons to become unwell. Tau is present in AD pathogenesis before Aβ, but through a feedback loop, tau makes Aβ more toxic [22,23]. As seen in Figure 7.1, there are significant criteria for the assessment of neurodegenerative diseases. The disease typically begins with mild symptoms, such as difficulty remembering recent events, but gradually progresses to more severe symptoms, such as confusion, disorientation, and difficulty with language and communication. As the disease progresses, individuals with Alzheimer's may experience difficulty with basic activities of daily living, such as dressing, bathing, and eating.

Although the precise etiology of AD is unknown, it is thought to be a result of genetic, environmental, and lifestyle alterations. Although there is currently no cure for Alzheimer's, there are drugs and treatments that can help control the disease's symptoms and enhance the quality of life for patients.

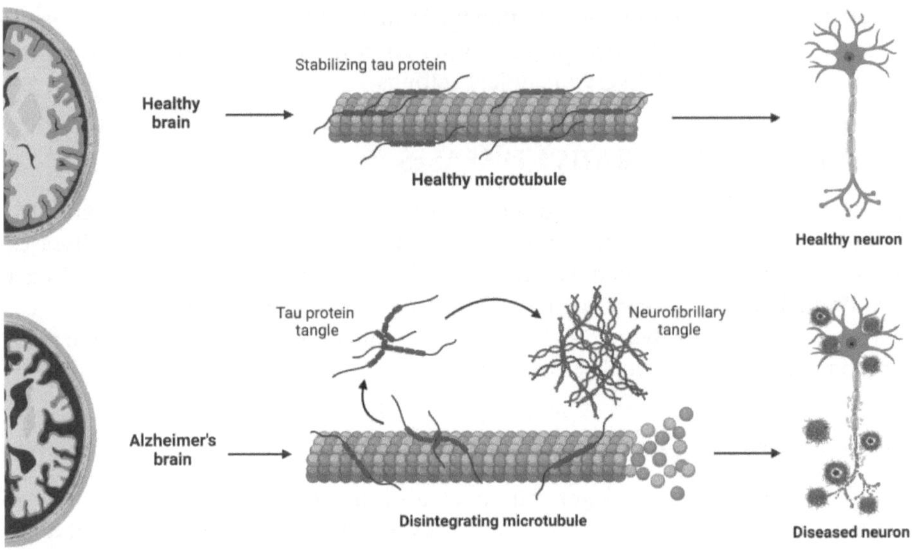

FIGURE 7.1 Scheme representation of pathogenesis for Alzheimer's disease.

7.2.2 Parkinson's Disease

The second-most prevalent adult-onset neurodegenerative disease is PD. The loss of dopaminergic neurons in the substantia nigra and intracellular inclusions containing synuclein aggregates are the PD neuropathological hallmarks that are linked to the disease's typical signs (Figure 7.2) [24]. The etiology of PD has been associated with several molecular pathways, although the exact reason is still uncertain [25,26]. These mechanisms include mitochondrial dysfunction, improper protein transport, inflammation, and oxidative stress.

PD is a chronic and progressive neurodegenerative disorder that affects the part of the brain that controls movement. It is characterized by a variety of motor symptoms, including tremors, rigidity, and difficulty with balance and coordination (Figure 7.3). The disease occurs when nerve cells in the brain that produce dopamine, a neurotransmitter that helps control movement, begin to die. As dopamine levels decrease, individuals with PD experience a range of movement problems and other symptoms. Other symptoms of PD may include a stooped posture, slowed movement, a shuffling gait, and difficulty with speech and writing. In addition, some individuals with PD may also experience non-motor symptoms, such as depression, anxiety, sleep disorders, and cognitive changes.

7.2.3 Huntington's Disease

A neurological condition with autosomal dominant inheritance is called HD. The condition is caused by an enlarged CAG trinucleotide repeat in the HTT gene on chromosome 4, which codes for the protein huntingtin [27,28]. As a result, mutant

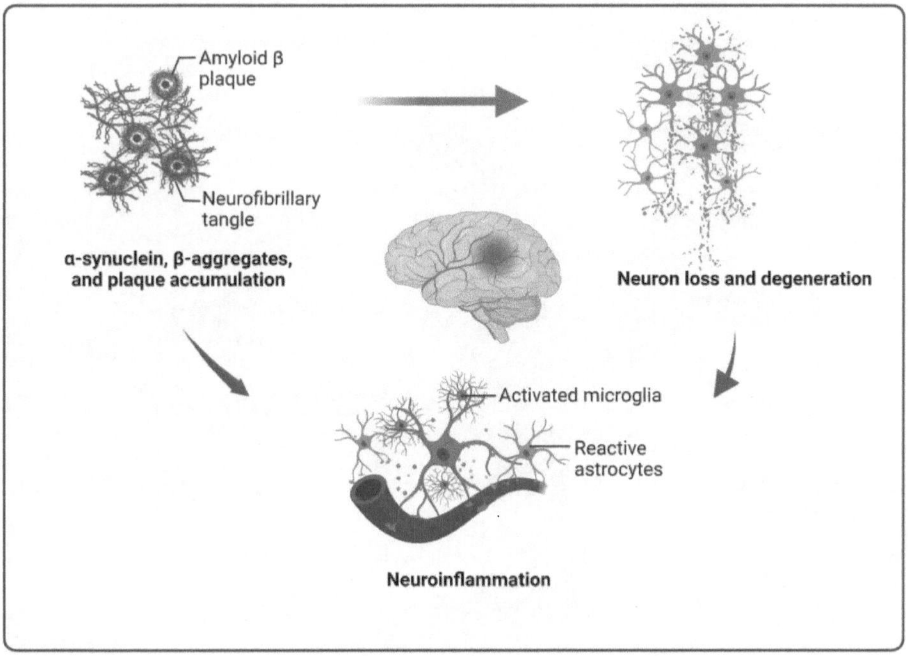

FIGURE 7.2 Scheme representation of pathogenesis for Parkinson's disease.

huntingtin (mHTT), a protein linked to protein aggregation and toxicity, develops. It has excessively long polyglutamine sequences. In addition to its inherent toxicity, mHTT also disrupts a wide range of cellular functions that can cause neuronal dysfunction and death [29–33], including protein homeostasis disruption, impaired protein degradation, transcriptional dysregulation of gene expression, disruption of synaptic signaling, mitochondrial dysfunction, impaired metabolism pathways, and aberrant activation of stress responses. The striatum's striatal atrophy and early macroscopic abnormalities can be seen before the disease manifests.

Cortical and subcortical brain regions are also affected [34,35]. A wide spectrum of symptoms, including motor, cognitive, and mental ones, are present in the disorder, which often manifests itself in mid-adulthood. Jerky, uncontrollable movements (chorea), as well as issues with balance and coordination, might be among the motor signs of HD. Planning and organizing challenges, as well as issues with memory and learning, are examples of cognitive symptoms. Depression, anxiety, impatience, and mood swings are a few examples of psychiatric symptoms.

7.2.4 Amyotrophic Lateral Sclerosis (ALS)

Lou Gehrig's disease, also known as amyotrophic lateral sclerosis (ALS), is a neurodegenerative condition that rapidly and steadily impairs lower and upper motor neurons that emerge from the brain and spinal cord [36,37]. The communication

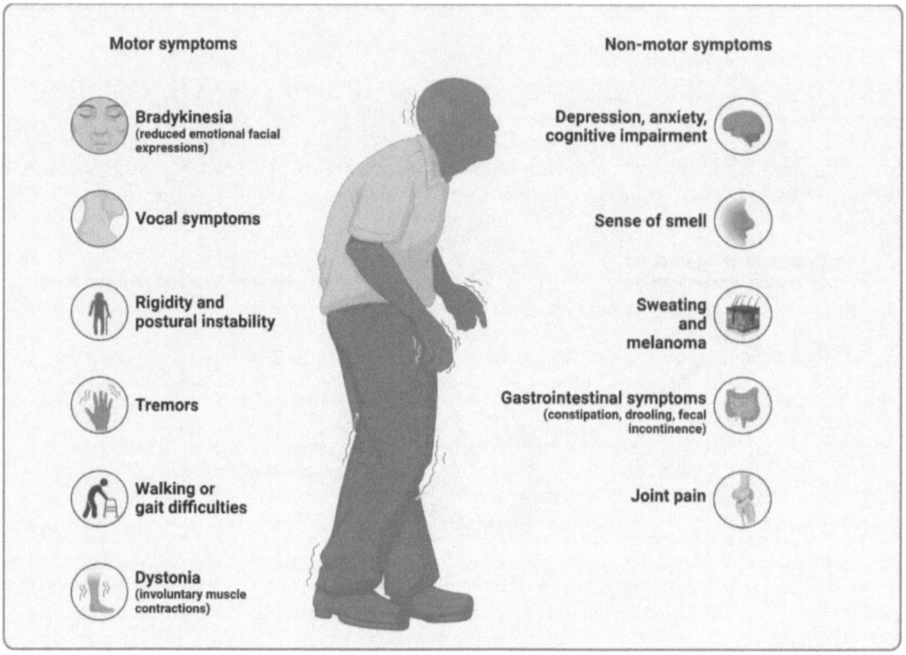

FIGURE 7.3 An overview of motor and non-motor symptoms in Parkinson's disease.

between a motor neuron and muscle is lost because of motor neuron degeneration, which causes muscle wasting and gradual weakness in the arms, legs, trunk, and bulbar region [38,39].

The two main types are (a) **the sporadic form** (**SALS**), which accounts for 90% of cases and develops spontaneously without a family history, and (b) **the familial form** (**FALS**), which accounts for the remaining 10% of cases and is caused by the genetic dominant inheritance component.

The middle to late 50s are the typical onset years for the first symptoms. Localized weakness is the initial symptom of ALS, which progresses to affect the majority of muscles [40]. Motor neurons, the nerve cells that control voluntary muscle movement, eventually degenerate and die in ALS, which is defined by the onset of more severe symptoms such difficulties speaking, eating, and breathing. ALS symptoms include muscle weakness, cramping, and twitching. Total paralysis and, in certain situations, respiratory failure are potential outcomes of ALS. Although the precise cause of ALS is unknown, it is thought to be the result of a mix of hereditary and environmental factors. In some instances, ALS may result from mutations in particular genes that have an impact on motor neuron function.

7.2.5 Multiple Sclerosis (MS)

The autoimmune disease known as multiple sclerosis (MS) primarily affects the central nervous system (CNS) and causes nerve demyelination and axonal destruction. The exact cause of MS has not yet been determined, along with many other neurodegenerative disorders. However, it is believed that both hereditary and environmental variables, such as bacterial and viral infections, smoking, toxins, and low vitamin D levels, might affect how this condition manifests [41–43].

In general, MS has three stages [44,45]:

(I) The preclinical stage, during which the disease is triggered.
(II) The relapsing-remitting stage, which is characterized by episodes of neurologic dysfunction that are partially or completely reversible and typically last days or weeks.
(III) The progressive clinical stage, during which, after typically 10–20 years, neurologic dysfunction worsens gradually and eventually impairs mobility and cognition [46].

The disease occurs when the immune system mistakenly attacks the myelin sheath, which is the protective coating around nerve fibers in the brain and spinal cord. The damage to the myelin sheath can cause a wide range of symptoms, including muscle weakness, difficulty with coordination and balance, sensory changes, and cognitive impairment. The symptoms of MS can vary widely from person to person and can range from mild to severe. The causes of neurodegenerative diseases are not yet fully understood, but they are believed to be the result of a combination of genetic, environmental, and lifestyle factors. Treatments for these diseases are currently limited and focus mainly on managing symptoms and slowing disease progression. Research into new treatments and potential cures for these diseases is ongoing.

7.3 EXISTING THERAPEUTIC INTERVENTIONS IN NEURODEGENERATIVE DISEASES

There are various therapeutic interventions currently available for neurodegenerative diseases, although most of them focus on managing symptoms rather than curing the underlying disease. Here are some of the existing therapeutic interventions for neurodegenerative diseases:

7.3.1 Medications

There are various medications available to manage the symptoms of neurodegenerative diseases such as Alzheimer's, Parkinson's, and Huntington's diseases. These medications include cholinesterase inhibitors, NMDA receptor antagonists, and dopamine agonists. Various medications can be used to manage the symptoms of neurodegenerative diseases, such as AD, PD, HD, and ALS. However, it is important to note that there is currently no cure for these diseases, and medications are aimed at managing symptoms and improving quality of life.

Some common medications for neurodegenerative diseases include:

7.3.1.1 Cholinesterase Inhibitors

These medications are used to treat symptoms of AD and improve memory and cognitive function. Examples include donepezil, rivastigmine, and galantamine [47,48].

7.3.1.2 NMDA Receptor Antagonists

These medications are used to treat moderate to severe symptoms of AD by blocking the activity of glutamate, a neurotransmitter that can cause damage to nerve cells. Memantine is an example of an NMDA receptor antagonist [49].

7.3.1.3 Dopamine Agonists

These medications are used to treat symptoms of PD by mimicking the effects of dopamine in the brain. Examples include pramipexole and ropinirole [41].

7.3.1.4 Levodopa

This medication is also used to treat symptoms of PD by increasing levels of dopamine in the brain. It is often combined with carbidopa, which helps prevent the breakdown of levodopa before it reaches the brain [50].

7.3.1.5 Antipsychotics

These medications are used to treat psychiatric symptoms of neurodegenerative diseases, such as hallucinations, delusions, and agitation. Examples include risperidone and quetiapine.

7.3.1.6 Muscle Relaxants

These medications are used to treat muscle stiffness and spasms in individuals with neurodegenerative diseases such as ALS. Examples include baclofen and tizanidine.

It is important to note that medication management for neurodegenerative diseases is complex and must be tailored to the individual's specific symptoms and needs. A healthcare provider with experience in managing neurodegenerative diseases is often needed to prescribe and manage medications.

7.3.2 Physical and Occupational Therapy

Physical and occupational therapy can help improve movement and reduce muscle stiffness and rigidity in PD. They can also help with mobility and balance in other neurodegenerative diseases. Physical and occupational therapy can be important components of care for individuals with neurodegenerative diseases. These therapies can help maintain or improve physical function, mobility, and independence, and can also help manage symptoms such as pain, stiffness, and muscle weakness.

Physical therapy may involve exercises and activities designed to improve strength, balance, coordination, and range of motion. For individuals with neurodegenerative diseases such as PD or ALS, physical therapy may focus on maintaining or improving mobility and reducing the risk of falls. Occupational therapy may involve activities and interventions designed to improve the ability to perform daily living tasks, such as dressing, grooming, and feeding oneself. This may involve strategies to adapt to the home environment, as well as the use of assistive devices such as wheelchairs or adaptive utensils. In addition to these traditional therapies, there are also newer approaches such as exercise programs specifically designed for individuals with neurodegenerative diseases. These programs may include activities such as dance, yoga, or tai chi, which can help improve physical function and quality of life.

7.3.3 Gene Therapy

Gene therapy is being researched as a potential treatment for neurodegenerative diseases such as HD. The aim is to silence the abnormal gene responsible for the disease, thus slowing or stopping disease progression. Gene therapy is a promising area of research for the treatment of neurodegenerative diseases. This approach involves using genetic engineering techniques to modify a patient's cells to produce or enhance a specific protein that is deficient or damaged in the disease. In some cases, gene therapy may involve using viral vectors to deliver the modified genes to the patient's cells. These viral vectors are designed to specifically target and infect the cells of interest and can be used to introduce new genes or modify existing ones.

Several clinical trials are currently underway to evaluate the safety and efficacy of gene therapy for neurodegenerative diseases such as HD, ALS, and PD. For example, one ongoing trial is testing a gene therapy approach for HD that involves using a virus to deliver a gene that produces a protein that can help protect nerve cells. While gene therapy holds great promise for the treatment of neurodegenerative diseases, there are still many challenges to overcome, such as developing safe and effective delivery methods, and ensuring that the modified genes are expressed in the appropriate cells at the right levels.

7.3.4 Deep Brain Stimulation (DBS)

Deep brain stimulation (DBS) is a type of therapy that involves the surgical implantation of electrodes in specific areas of the brain, followed by the delivery of electrical impulses to these areas. DBS is commonly used to treat symptoms of neurodegenerative diseases such as PD and essential tremor, but it may also be used for other conditions such as dystonia and epilepsy. The exact mechanism by which DBS works is not fully understood, but it is thought to involve the modulation of abnormal electrical activity in the brain. By delivering electrical impulses to specific regions of the brain, DBS can help improve symptoms such as tremors, rigidity, and bradykinesia (slowness of movement).

DBS is typically considered when medication management is no longer effective or is associated with significant side effects. The procedure involves the implantation of a small device, like a pacemaker, that delivers electrical impulses to the brain. The electrodes are placed in specific areas of the brain based on the patient's symptoms and the underlying neurodegenerative disease. While DBS can be effective in reducing symptoms, it is important to note that it is not a cure for neurodegenerative diseases. Additionally, the procedure carries some risks, such as infection, bleeding, and hardware malfunction. Therefore, it is important to carefully consider the potential risks and benefits of DBS in consultation with a healthcare provider who has experience with the procedure.

7.3.5 Stem Cell Therapy

Stem cell therapy is a promising area of research for the treatment of neurodegenerative diseases. Stem cells are unspecialized cells that have the potential to develop into different types of cells, and they can be used to replace or repair damaged tissues or cells in the body. In the context of neurodegenerative diseases, stem cells are being studied as a potential therapy to replace damaged or lost neurons. The goal of this approach is to use stem cells to replace the neurons that are lost in conditions such as PD, HD, and ALS. Different types of stem cells can be used for therapy, including embryonic stem cells, induced pluripotent stem cells, and adult stem cells. Each type of stem cell has its advantages and disadvantages, and the choice of cell type depends on the specific condition being treated and the goals of the therapy. While stem cell therapy is a promising area of research, there are still many challenges that need to be overcome before it can be widely used in clinical practice. These include developing safe and effective methods for delivering the stem cells to the brain, ensuring that the transplanted cells integrate properly into the existing neural circuitry, and preventing the immune system from attacking the transplanted cells.

Despite these challenges, there have been some encouraging results from early clinical trials of stem cell therapy for neurodegenerative diseases, particularly in the case of PD. However, further research is needed to fully understand the safety and efficacy of this approach before it can be used as a routine therapy for these conditions.

7.3.6 Lifestyle Interventions

Lifestyle interventions such as exercise, a healthy diet, and cognitive stimulation are beneficial in reducing the risk of neurodegenerative diseases and slowing disease progression in some cases. Lifestyle interventions are becoming increasingly recognized as an important part of the management of neurodegenerative diseases. These interventions involve making changes to an individual's daily habits and behaviors to improve their overall health and well-being.

Some examples of lifestyle interventions that may be beneficial for individuals with neurodegenerative diseases include:

7.3.6.1 Exercise: Regular physical activity has been shown to improve cognitive function and reduce the risk of dementia in older adults. Exercise may also help improve motor function in individuals with PD and other movement disorders.

7.3.6.2 **Healthy diet:** A diet that is high in fruits, vegetables, and whole grains, and low in processed foods and saturated fats, may help reduce the risk of cognitive decline and dementia.

7.3.6.3 **Sleep:** Getting adequate sleep is important for overall brain health. Sleep disturbances are common in neurodegenerative diseases, and treating sleep disorders may improve cognitive and motor function.

7.3.6.4 **Mental stimulation:** Engaging in activities that stimulate the brain, such as reading, doing puzzles, or learning a new skill, may help maintain cognitive function and reduce the risk of dementia.

7.3.6.5 **Social engagement:** Social isolation and loneliness are risk factors for cognitive decline and dementia. Maintaining social connections and engaging in meaningful activities with others may help protect against these conditions.

While lifestyle interventions are not a cure for neurodegenerative diseases, they may help improve quality of life and slow the progression of these conditions. It is important to work with a healthcare provider to develop a personalized plan that is tailored to the individual's needs and abilities.

In conclusion, while there are various therapeutic interventions available for neurodegenerative diseases, there is still a need for more effective treatments that can cure or slow the progression of these diseases. Research into new therapies and potential cures for neurodegenerative diseases is ongoing.

7.4 LIPID-BASED NANOCARRIERS

Lipid-based nanocarriers, also known as lipid nanoparticles, are a type of drug-delivery system that uses lipids as the main component. These nanocarriers are typically between 10 and 1,000 nanometers in size and can encapsulate both hydrophilic and hydrophobic drugs.

There are different types of lipid-based nanocarriers, including liposomes, SLNs, and NLCs (Figure 7.4). Liposomes are spherical structures made up of a lipid bilayer that can encapsulate drugs within their core or the lipid bilayer. SLNs are made up of solid lipids and surfactants, while NLCs contain a mixture of solid and liquid lipids.

7.4.1 Liposomes

Liposomes are a type of lipid-based nanocarrier that is composed of one or more lipid bilayers surrounding an aqueous core. These structures can be thought of as tiny spherical vesicles, ranging in size from 20 nanometers to several micrometers in diameter. Liposomes were first described in the 1960s, and since then, they have been widely studied for drug delivery and other biomedical applications. One of the key advantages of liposomes is their ability to encapsulate both hydrophilic and hydrophobic drugs, making them versatile carriers for a wide range of therapeutic agents. In addition, liposomes can be designed to target specific cells or tissues in the body by modifying their surface with ligands or other molecules that bind to receptors on the target cells. This allows for the selective delivery of drugs to the desired site, reducing the risk of side effects and improving therapeutic efficacy [51].

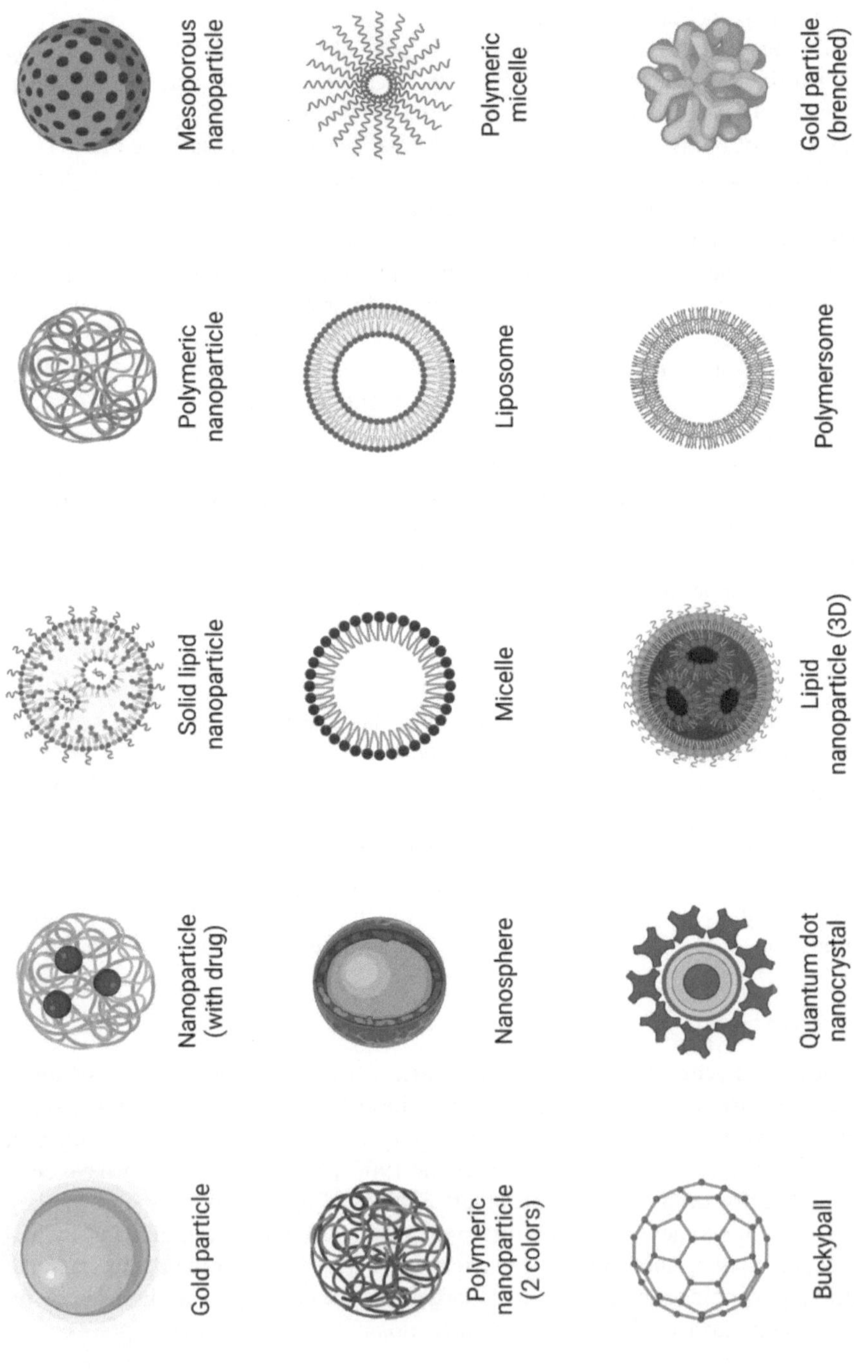

FIGURE 7.4 Different types of nanocarriers that can be designed to encapsulate drugs within their core, surface, or both.

Liposomes have been studied for the treatment of various diseases, including cancer, infectious diseases, and neurological disorders. For example, liposomal formulations of anticancer drugs have been shown to improve drug delivery to tumors and reduce side effects compared to traditional formulations. While liposomes have shown promise for drug delivery, there are still challenges that need to be addressed. These include optimizing the size, stability, and targeting capabilities of the nanoparticles, as well as ensuring their safety and biocompatibility (Figure 7.5). Nevertheless, liposomes remain a promising technology for drug delivery and other biomedical applications [52,53].

7.4.2 Solid Lipid Nanoparticles (SLNs)

Solid lipid nanoparticles are nanoparticles that can be used for drug delivery and associated biomedical applications. SLNs are made of a solid lipid core, typically made of natural or synthetic lipids, surrounded by a layer of surfactants and other stabilizing agents. One of the advantages of SLNs is their ability to encapsulate both hydrophilic and hydrophobic drugs, similar to liposomes [54]. However, unlike liposomes, SLNs have a solid core, which can provide increased stability and protection for the encapsulated drug. SLNs have several other advantages for drug delivery, including their ability to target specific cells or tissues in the body. This can be achieved by modifying the surface of the SLN with ligands or other molecules that bind to receptors on the target cells. In addition, SLNs can be designed to release their payload in a controlled manner, allowing for sustained drug release over a period of time. SLNs have been studied for the treatment of various diseases, including cancer, inflammatory disorders, and infectious diseases. For example, SLN formulations of antimicrobial drugs have been shown to improve drug delivery and reduce toxicity compared to traditional formulations [55].

7.4.3 Nanostructured Lipid Carriers (NLCs)

For drug delivery and other biomedical uses, one class of lipid-based nanoparticles is known as NLCs. NLCs are composed of a mixture of solid and liquid lipids, which form a structured matrix that can encapsulate drugs or other molecules. One of the benefits of NLCs is their ability to encapsulate both hydrophilic and hydrophobic drugs, like liposomes and SLNs. However, the structured matrix of NLCs provides increased stability and protection for the encapsulated drug compared to SLNs. NLCs can also be designed to target specific cells or tissues in the body by modifying the surface of the nanoparticle with ligands or other molecules that bind to receptors on the target cells. In addition, NLCs can be designed to release their payload in a controlled manner, allowing for sustained drug release over a period of time. NLCs have been investigated for therapy to treat several illnesses, including cancer, inflammatory conditions, and infectious infections. For example, NLC formulations of anticancer drugs have been shown to improve drug delivery to tumors and reduce side effects compared to traditional formulations [56].

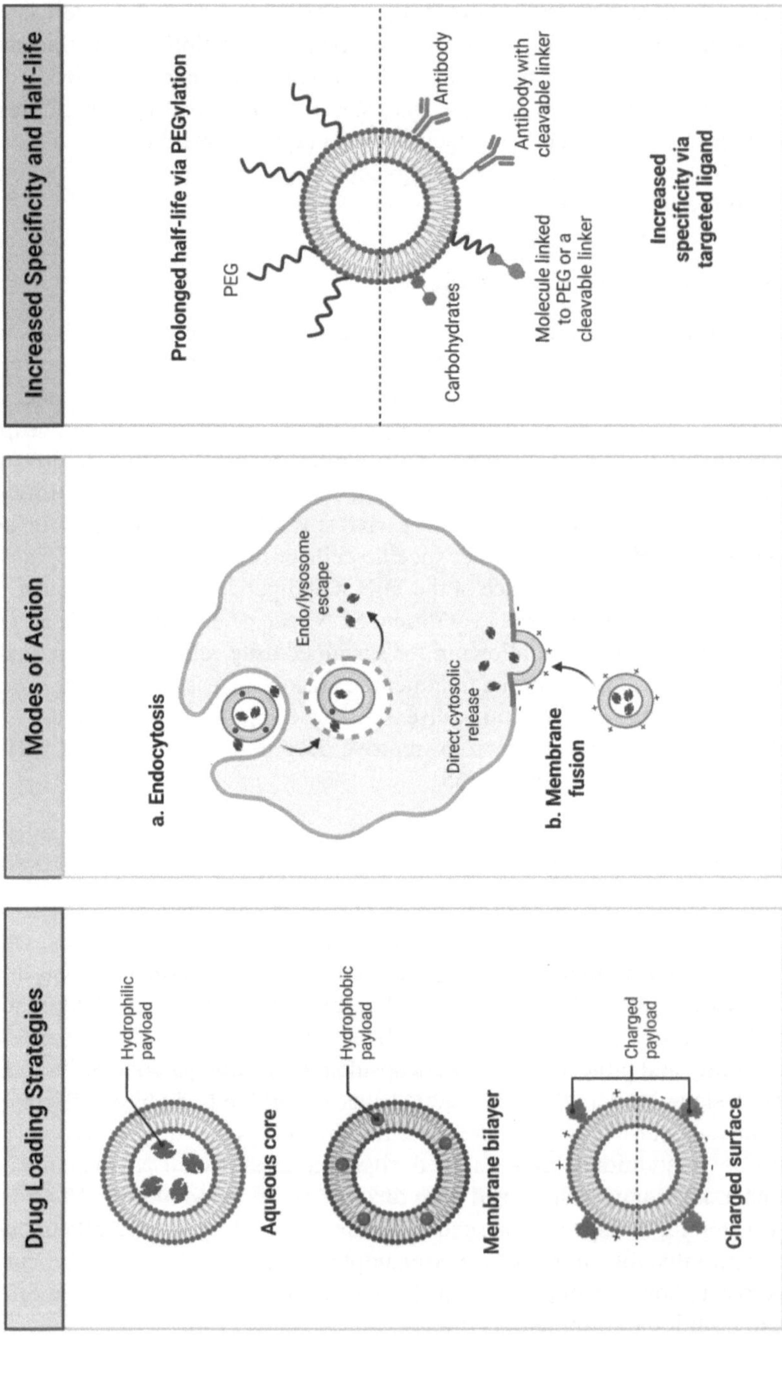

FIGURE 7.5 Schematic presentation of liposome based drug-delivery system.

7.4.4 Lipid-based Nanocarriers

Lipid-based nanocarriers have several advantages over other drug-delivery systems. They can protect the drug from degradation and increase its bioavailability. They can also improve drug targeting by delivering the drug directly to the site of action, such as the brain in the case of neurodegenerative diseases. In addition, they can reduce drug toxicity by allowing for the use of lower doses. In the case of neurodegenerative diseases, lipid-based nanocarriers are effective in delivering drugs to the brain. For example, liposomes have been used to deliver drugs such as tacrine and memantine to the brain in animal models of AD. SLNs have been used to deliver curcumin, a natural compound with neuroprotective properties, to the brain in a mouse model of PD.

Lipid-based nanocarriers have several advantages for drug delivery. For example, they can protect drugs from degradation and clearance in the body, and they can target specific cells or tissues by using surface modifications or ligands that bind to specific receptors. There are several types of lipid-based nanocarriers, including liposomes, SLNs, NLCs, and lipid-drug conjugates. Each type of nanocarrier has its advantages and disadvantages, and the choice of nanocarrier depends on the specific drug being delivered and the intended target.

Studies on lipid-based nanocarriers for the treatment of various illnesses, such as cancer, neurological conditions, and infectious diseases, have been conducted. For example, liposomal formulations of anticancer drugs have been shown to improve drug delivery to tumors and reduce side effects compared to traditional formulations. While lipid-based nanocarriers have shown promise for drug delivery, there are still challenges that need to be addressed. These include optimizing the size, stability, and targeting capabilities of the nanoparticles, as well as ensuring their safety and biocompatibility. Nevertheless, lipid-based nanocarriers have the potential to improve the efficacy and safety of drug delivery for a wide range of diseases [57].

7.5 NANOCARRIERS FOR BRAIN-TARGETED DRUG-DELIVERY SYSTEMS

Nanocarriers are being explored as promising drug-delivery systems for the treatment of neurodegenerative diseases. One of the main challenges in treating neurodegenerative diseases is getting drugs to cross the BBB, a protective barrier that prevents many substances from entering the brain. Nanocarriers can potentially overcome this challenge by delivering drugs across the BBB and directly to the brain. Various types of nanocarriers have been studied for brain-targeted drug delivery, including liposomes, polymeric nanoparticles, dendrimers, and carbon nanotubes. These nanocarriers can be designed to encapsulate drugs within their core, surface, or both (Table 7.1).

7.5.1 Liposomes

Liposomes are one of the most widely studied nanocarriers for brain-targeted drug delivery. They are spherical vesicles composed of a lipid bilayer that can encapsulate both hydrophilic and hydrophobic drugs. They are effective in delivering

TABLE 7.1
A Detailed List of Presently Available Nanocarrier-based Drugs for Neurodegenerative Diseases

Nanocarriers	Drug	*In vitro/in vivo* results
Liposomes	siRNA-4400	siRNA-dependent inhibition of neuronal nitric oxide synthases [58].
	Minocycline	When compared to a free medicine, ALS progression is effectively slowed [59].
	Riluzole and Verapamil	The biodistribution and uptake of riluzole in mouse brain endothelial bEND.3 and astrocyte C8D1A cells were improved by adding verapamil (a P-gp efflux pump inhibitor) to the liposomes [60].
	Bis-(pivaloyloxy)-dopamine (BPD)	Enhanced therapeutic effect in PD animal model, with no obvious systemic harm [61].
	Glial cell line-derived neurotrophic factor plasmid gene	Reducing the neurotoxicity caused by 6-OHDA and preventing the death of dopaminergic neurons [62].
	Polyethylene glycol/ Cholesterol	Preventing α-Syn fibrillation. decreased levels of ROS and α-Syn-induced neurotoxicity in PC12 and SHSY5Y dopaminergic cell lines [63].
	Maltodextrin and Levodopa	BBB permeability and cellular binding are improved [64].
	Levodopa Chlorotoxin	Greater drug dispersion in the brain, which significantly lessens behavioral defects [65].
SLN (Solid lipid nanoparticles)	Apomorphine	Rats with improved treatment effectiveness and behavioral outcomes [56].
	Methylprednisolone	Compared to PEGylated SLN, MS-induced mice's brain tissue was taken up more [66].
	Di-methyl fumarate	The effectiveness of SLN containing DMF in a once-daily dose regimen compared to thrice-daily administration of plain DMF on critical measures such locomotor activity, grip strength, mortality, and motor coordination in sick mice [67–71].
	Riluzole	When compared to rats treated with free Riluzole, those administered with SLN showed clinical indications of EAE later [72].
NLC (Nanostructured lipid carriers)	Ropirinole	When compared to the intranasal drug solution, the medication has a higher drug transport and penetration efficiency and an improved absolute bioavailability [56].
	Basic-FGF	Effectively exhibiting therapeutic benefits in hemi-parkinsonian rats by promoting dopaminergic activity in surviving synapses [73].

TABLE 7.1 (Continued)
A Detailed List of Presently Available Nanocarrier-based Drugs for Neurodegenerative Diseases

Nanocarriers	Drug	*In vitro/in vivo* results
	Teriflunomide	As compared to oral administration, intranasally delivered teriflunomide NLC improved neurological function in rats and more quickly reached the target region. It also reduced neuroinflammatory pathways more significantly [74].

drugs such as doxorubicin, paclitaxel, and curcumin to the brain in animal models of neurodegenerative diseases. Liposomes have been studied extensively as a brain-targeted drug-delivery system due to their ability to cross the BBB. The BBB is a highly selective membrane that separates the blood vessels in the brain from the surrounding tissue, and it can prevent many drugs from entering the brain. Liposomes can be modified to cross the BBB by attaching specific ligands or antibodies to their surface, which can bind to receptors on the BBB and facilitate transport across the membrane. In addition, liposomes can be engineered to release their cargo in response to specific stimuli, such as changes in pH or temperature, which can enhance their efficacy in the brain. Several studies have demonstrated the potential of liposomes for brain-targeted drug delivery. For example, liposomal formulations of anticancer drugs have been shown to improve drug delivery to brain tumors and reduce side effects compared to traditional formulations. Liposomes have also been studied for the delivery of drugs to treat neurological disorders such as AD, PD, and multiple sclerosis.

However, there are still challenges that need to be addressed in the advancement of liposomal drug-delivery systems for the brain. These include optimizing the size, stability, and targeting capabilities of the nanoparticles, as well as ensuring their safety and biocompatibility. Nevertheless, liposomes remain a promising technology for brain-targeted drug delivery and other biomedical applications.

7.5.2 Polymeric Nanoparticles

Polymeric nanoparticles are another type of nanocarrier that has been studied for brain-targeted drug delivery. They are composed of biocompatible and biodegradable polymers and designed to release drugs in a controlled manner. Polymeric nanoparticles are effective in delivering drugs such as curcumin, nerve growth factor, and glial cell line-derived neurotrophic factor to the brain in animal models of neurodegenerative diseases.

Polymeric nanoparticles have also been studied as a brain-targeted drug-delivery system due to their ability to cross the BBB. Like liposomes, polymeric nanoparticles can be engineered to carry drugs or other therapeutic agents and modified to target specific cells in the brain. Polymeric nanoparticles can be designed to overcome the limitations of liposomes, such as low stability and poor drug loading capacity. They can also be engineered to release their cargo in a controlled manner, allowing for sustained drug release over a period of time. Several studies have demonstrated the potential of polymeric nanoparticles for brain-targeted drug delivery. For example, polymeric nanoparticles have been used to deliver drugs for the treatment of neurodegenerative disorders such as AD and PD, as well as for brain tumors. Polymeric nanoparticles can also be modified with targeting ligands or antibodies to facilitate transport across the BBB. In addition, they can be devised to respond to specific stimuli, like changes in pH or temperature, which can enhance their efficacy in the brain.

7.5.3 Dendrimers

Dendrimers are highly branched, synthetic polymers that can be designed to encapsulate drugs within their core and surface. They are effective in delivering drugs such as methotrexate and acetylcholine esterase inhibitors to the brain in animal models of neurodegenerative diseases. Dendrimers are another class of nanoparticles that have been studied as a brain-targeted drug-delivery system. Dendrimers are highly branched, tree-like molecules that can be synthesized with precise control over their size, shape, and surface chemistry. These characteristics make them attractive for drug-delivery applications, including brain targeting.

Dendrimers can be modified with various functional groups, such as targeting ligands, which allow them to cross the BBB and selectively bind to specific cells in the brain. In addition, dendrimers can be designed to encapsulate drugs or other therapeutic agents and release them in a controlled manner. Several studies have demonstrated the potential of dendrimers for brain-targeted drug delivery. For example, dendrimers have been used to deliver drugs for the treatment of neurodegenerative disorders such as AD, PD, and multiple sclerosis. They have also been studied for the delivery of gene therapies to the brain. Dendrimers have several benefits over other nanoparticle-based drug-delivery systems, including their precise control over size and shape, their ability to carry large payloads, and their ability to target specific cells in the brain.

7.5.4 Carbon Nanotubes

Carbon nanotubes are another type of nanocarrier that has been investigated for brain-targeted drug delivery. They are composed of carbon atoms and have a unique structure that allows them to penetrate the BBB. Carbon nanotubes are effective in delivering drugs such as dopamine and nerve growth factor to the brain in animal models of neurodegenerative diseases. Carbon nanotubes are another type of nanomaterial that has been investigated as a potential brain-targeted drug-delivery system. Carbon nanotubes are cylinder-shaped structures comprised of carbon atoms organized in a tube-like pattern. They possess special qualities that make them appealing for drug-delivery applications, such as their high surface area, large aspect ratio, and capacity to cross the BBB. Carbon nanotubes can be functionalized with targeting moieties, such as antibodies or peptides, which allow them to selectively bind to specific cells in the brain. They can also be loaded with drugs or other therapeutic agents and designed to release them in a controlled manner. Several studies have demonstrated the potential of carbon nanotubes for brain-targeted drug delivery. For example, carbon nanotubes have been used to deliver drugs for the treatment of neurodegenerative disorders such as AD and brain tumors. They have also been studied for the delivery of gene therapies to the brain.

However, there are still concerns about the safety of carbon nanotubes as drug-delivery vehicles, particularly concerning their potential toxicity and biocompatibility. Some studies have shown that carbon nanotubes can induce oxidative stress, inflammation, and cell death *in vitro* and *in vivo*. Subsequently, more investigation is required to completely comprehend the safety and effectiveness of carbon nanotubes for the transport of drugs that are specifically intended for the brain as well as to create plans to reduce any potential negative effects. Overall, nanocarriers have great potential as drug-delivery systems for the treatment of neurodegenerative diseases. However, more research is needed to optimize their formulation, improve their effectiveness in delivering drugs to the brain, and ensure their safety.

7.6 FUTURE PERSPECTIVE

Nanocarriers hold great promise for the future of brain-targeted drug-delivery systems. Here are some potential prospects for nanocarriers:

a. **Personalized medicine:** With advances in nanotechnology, it may be possible to create personalized nanocarriers that are tailored to an individual's specific needs. This could help optimize drug delivery and minimize side effects.
b. **Combination therapies:** Nanocarriers could enable the delivery of multiple drugs simultaneously, which could lead to more effective treatment for neurodegenerative diseases. For example, combining a drug that targets inflammation with a drug that targets protein misfolding could potentially slow the progression of AD.
c. **Targeted gene therapy:** Nanocarriers could be used to deliver gene therapies directly to the brain. This could be particularly useful in the treatment of genetic forms of neurodegenerative diseases such as HD.
d. **Noninvasive drug delivery:** Nanocarriers could potentially enable noninvasive drug-delivery methods such as intranasal or oral administration, which would be more convenient for patients and could potentially improve compliance with treatment.
e. **Smart nanocarriers:** Researchers are exploring the use of "smart" nanocarriers that can respond to changes in the body or environment. For example, drugs may be released by nanocarriers in response to biomarkers linked to neurodegenerative disorders.

Overall, the prospects for nanocarriers in brain-targeted drug-delivery systems are exciting. As research in this field continues to advance, we may see significant improvements in the treatment of neurodegenerative diseases in the future.

REFERENCES

1. Gupta S, Bansal R, Gupta S, Jindal N, Jindal A. 2013. "Nanocarriers and nanoparticles for skin care and dermatological treatments." *Indian Dermatol Online J.* 4 (4): 267–72. doi: 10.4103/2229-5178.120635
2. Saleem S, Iqubal MK, Garg S, Ali J, Baboota S. 2020. "Trends in nanotechnology-based delivery systems for dermal targeting of drugs: an enticing approach to offset psoriasis." *Expert Opin Drug Deliv.* 17(6):817–38. doi: 10.1080/17425247.2020.1758665
3. Kakoty V, Sarathlal KC, Pandey M, Dubey SK, Kesharwani P, Taliyan R. 2022. "Biological toxicity of nanoparticles." *Nanoparticle Therapeutics, Academic Press.* 603–628, ISBN 9780128207574, doi:10.1016/B978-0-12-820757-4.00016-8
4. Taliyan R, Kakoty V, Sarathlal KC, Kharavtekar SS, Karennanavar CR, Choudhary YK, Singhvi G, Riadi Y, Dubey SK, Kesharwani P. 2022. "Nanocarrier mediated drug delivery as an impeccable therapeutic approach against Alzheimer's disease." *JCR,* 343, 528–550. doi.org/10.1016/j.jconrel.2022.01.044
5. Mishra G, Awasthi R, Singh AK, Singh S, Mishra SK, Singh SK, Nandi MK. 2022. "Intranasally co-administered berberine and curcumin loaded in transfersomal vesicles improved inhibition of amyloid formation and BACE-1." *ACS Omega.* 7(47):43290–43305. doi: 10.1021/acsomega.2c06215
6. Singh AK, Singh SS, Rathore AS, Singh SP, Mishra G, Awasthi R, Mishra SK, Singh SK. 2021. "Lipid-coated MCM-41 mesoporous silica nanoparticles loaded with Berberine improved inhibition of acetylcholine esterase and amyloid formation." *ACS Biomaterials Science & Engineering, ACS Publication.* 7 (8):3737–3753. doi: 10.1021/acsbiomaterials.1c00514
7. Singh AK, Mishra SK, Mishra G, Maurya A, Awasthi R, Yadav MK, Atri N, Pandey PK and Singh SK. 2019. "Inorganic clay nanocomposite system for improved cholinesterase inhibition and brain pharmacokinetics of donepezil." *Drug Development and Industrial Pharmacy, Taylor & Francis Online.* 46 (1):8–19. doi:10.1080/03639045.2019.1698594
8. Singh AK, Gothwal A, Rani S, Rana M, Sharma AK, Yadav AK and Gupta U. 2019. "Dendrimer donepezil conjugates for improved brain delivery and better *in vivo* pharmacokinetics." *ACS Omega, ACS Publication.* 4 (3):4519–4529. doi: 10.1021/acsomega.8b03445
9. Singh AK, Singh SK, Nandi MK, Mishra G, Maurya A, Rai A, Rai GK, Awasthi R, Sharma B, Kulkarni GT. 2019. "Berberine: A plant derived alkaloid with therapeutic potential to combat Alzheimer's disease." *Central Nervous System Agents in Medicinal Chemistry, Bentham Science.* 19 (3):154–170. doi: 10.2174/1871524919666190820160053
10. Maurya A, Singh AK, Mishra G, Kumari K, Rai A, Sharma B, Kulkarni GT, Awasthi R. 2018. "Strategic use of nanotechnology in drug targeting and its consequences on human health: A focused review." *Interventional Medicine and Applied Science,* AKjournals. 11 (1): 38–54. doi: 10.1556/1646.11.2019.04
11. Singh AK, Choudhary S, Rani S, Sharma AK, Gupta L and Gupta U. 2015. "Dendrimer-drug conjugates in drug delivery and targeting." *Pharmaceutical Nanotechnology, Bentham Science.* 3 (4): 239–260. doi: 10.2174/2211738504666160213000307
12. Singh AK, Sharma AK, Khan I, Gothwal A, Gupta L and Gupta U. 2016. "Oral drug delivery potential of dendrimers." In: *Alexandru Mihai Grumezescu Edited Nanostructures for Oral Medicine (Multi-Volume Set).* Elsevier. ISBN: 978-0-323-47720-8. doi: 10.1016/b978-0-323-47720-8.00010-9

13. Singh AK, Mishra G, Maurya A, Awasthi R, Kumari K, Thakur A, Rai A, Rai GK, Sharma B, Kulkarni GT, Singh SK. 2019. "Role of TREM2 in Alzheimer's disease and its consequences on β-amyloid, Tau and neurofibrillary tangles." *Current Alzheimer Research, Bentham Science.* 16 (13): 1216–1229. doi: 10.2174/1567205016666190903102822
14. Gitler AD, Dhillon P, Shorter J. 2017. "Neurodegenerative disease: models, mechanisms, and a new hope." *Dis Model Mech.* 10(5):499–502. doi: 10.1242/dmm.030205
15. Karande P, Trasatti JP, Chandra D. 2015. "Novel approaches for the delivery of biologics to the central nervous system." In: Singh M, Salnikova M (eds) *Novel Approaches and Strategies for Biologics, Vaccines and Cancer Therapies.* Academic Press, San Diego, CA, 59–88
16. Villemagne VL, Doré V, Burnham SC, Masters CL, Rowe CC. 2018. "Imaging tau and amyloid-β proteinopathies in Alzheimer disease and other conditions." *Nat Rev Neurol.* 14(4):225–36. doi: 10.1038/nrneurol.2018.9
17. Jones DT, Graff-Radford J, Lowe VJ, Wiste HJ, Gunter JL, Senjem ML, Botha H, Kantarci K, Boeve BF, Knopman DS, Petersen RC, Jack CR Jr. 2017. "Tau, amyloid, and cascading network failure across the Alzheimer's disease spectrum." *Cortex.* 97:143–159. doi: 10.1016/j.cortex.2017.09.018
18. Furcila D, DeFelipe J, Alonso-Nanclares L. 2018. "A Study of amyloid-β and phosphotau in plaques and neurons in the hippocampus of Alzheimer's disease patients." *J Alzheimers Dis.* 64(2):417–35. doi: 10.3233/JAD-180173
19. Peña-Bautista C, López-Cuevas R, Cuevas A, Baquero M, Cháfer-Pericás C. 2019. "Lipid peroxidation biomarkers correlation with medial temporal atrophy in early Alzheimer Disease." *Neurochem Int.* 129:104519. doi: 10.1016/j.neuint.2019.104519
20. Boza-Serrano A, Yang Y, Paulus A, Deierborg T. 2018. "Innate immune alterations are elicited in microglial cells before plaque deposition in the Alzheimer's disease mouse model 5xFAD." *Sci Rep.* 8(1):1550. doi: 10.1038/s41598-018-19699-y
21. Mi D.J., Dixit S., Warner T.A., Kennard J.A., Scharf D.A., Kessler E.S., Moore L.M., Consoli D.C., Bown C.W., Eugene A.J. 2018. "Altered glutamate clearance in ascorbate deficient mice increases seizure susceptibility and contributes to cognitive impairment in APP/PSEN1mice." *Neurobiol.Aging.* 71:241–254. doi: 10.1016/j.neurobiolaging.2018.08.002
22. Marciani DJ. 2015. "Alzheimer's disease vaccine development: A new strategy focusing on immune modulation." *J Neuroimmunol.* 15;287:54–63. doi:10.1016/j.jneuroim.2015.08.008
23. Bloom GS. 2014. "Amyloid-β and tau: the trigger and bullet in Alzheimer disease pathogenesis." *JAMA Neurol.* 71(4):505–8. doi: 10.1001/jamaneurol.2013.5847
24. Ryan BJ, Bengoa-Vergniory N, Williamson M, Kirkiz E, Roberts R, Corda G, Sloan M, Saqlain S, Cherubini M, Poppinga J, Bogtofte H, Cioroch M, Hester S, Wade-Martins R. 2021. "REST Protects Dopaminergic Neurons from Mitochondrial and α-Synuclein Oligomer Pathology in an Alpha Synuclein Overexpressing BAC-Transgenic Mouse Model." *J Neurosci.* 41(16):3731–46. doi: 10.1523/JNEUROSCI.1478-20.2021
25. Franco-Iborra S, Cuadros T, Parent A, Romero-Gimenez J, Vila M, Perier C. 2018. "Defective mitochondrial protein import contributes to complex I-induced mitochondrial dysfunction and neurodegeneration in Parkinson's disease." *Cell Death Dis.* 9(11):1122. doi: 10.1038/s41419-018-1154-0
26. Martínez JH, Fuentes F, Vanasco V, Alvarez S, Alaimo A, Cassina A, Coluccio Leskow F, Velazquez F. 2018. "Alpha-synuclein mitochondrial interaction leads to

irreversible translocation and complex I impairment." *Arch Biochem Biophys*. 651:1–12. doi: 10.1016/j.abb.2018.04.018

27. MacDonald ME, Ambrose CM, Duyao MP, Myers RH, Lin C, Srinidhi L, Barnes G, Taylor SA, James M, Groot N, MacFarlane H, Jenkins B, Anderson MA, Wexler NS, Gusella JF, Bates GP, Baxendale S, Hummerich H, Kirby S, North M, Youngman S, Mott R, Zehetner G, Sedlacek Z, Poustka A, Frischauf A, Lehrach H, Buckler AJ, Church D, Doucette-Stamm L, O'Donovan MC, Riba-Ramirez L, Shah M, Stanton VP, Strobel SA, Draths KM, Wales JL, Dervan P, Housman DE, Altherr M, Shiang R, Thompson L, Fielder T, Wasmuth JJ, Tagle D, Valdes J, Elmer L, Allard M, Castilla L, Swaroop M, Blanchard K, Collins FS, Snell R, Holloway T, Gillespie K, Datson N, Shaw D, Harper PS. 1993. "A novel gene containing a trinucleotide repeat that is expanded and unstable on Huntington's disease chromosomes." *Cell*. 72:971–983. doi: 10.1016/0092-8674(93)90585-E
28. Lieberman AP, Shakkottai VG, Albin RL. 2019. "Polyglutamine repeats in neurodegenerative diseases." *Annu Rev Pathol*. 14:1–27. doi: 10.1146/annurev pathmechdis-012418-012857
29. Ast A, Buntru A, Schindler F, Hasenkopf R, Schulz A, Brusendorf L, Klockmeier K, Grelle G, McMahon B, Niederlechner H, Jansen I, Diez L, Edel J, Boeddrich A, Franklin SA, Baldo B, Schnoegl S, Kunz S, Purfürst B, Gaertner A, Kampinga HH, Morton AJ, Petersén Å, Kirstein J, Bates GP, Wanker EE. 2018. "mHTT Seeding Activity: A Marker of Disease Progression and Neurotoxicity in Models of Huntington's Disease." *Mol Cell*. 71(5):675–688.e6. doi: 10.1016/j.molcel.2018.07.032
30. Lin L, Jin Z, Tan H, Xu Q, Peng T, Li H. 2016. "Atypical ubiquitination by E3 ligase WWP1 inhibits the proteasome-mediated degradation of mutant huntingtin." *Brain Res*. 1643:103–12. doi: 10.1016/j.brainres.2016.03.027
31. Taeger L, Bonin M, Stricker-Shaver J, Riess O, Nguyen HHP. 2017. "Dysregulation of gene expression in the striatum of BACHD rats expressing full-length mutant huntingtin and associated abnormalities on molecular and protein levels." *Neuropharmacology*. 117:260–272. doi: 10.1016/j.neuropharm.2017.01.029
32. Yu C, Li CH, Chen S, Yoo H, Qin X, Park H. 2018. "Decreased BDNF release in cortical neurons of a knock-in mouse model of Huntington's disease." *Sci Rep*. 8(1):16976. doi: 10.1038/s41598-018-34883-w
33. Askeland G, Dosoudilova Z, Rodinova M, Klempir J, Liskova I, Kuśnierczyk A, Bjørås M, Nesse G, Klungland A, Hansikova H, Eide L. 2018. "Increased nuclear DNA damage precedes mitochondrial dysfunction in peripheral blood mononuclear cells from Huntington's disease patients." *Sci Rep*. 8(1):9817. doi: 10.1038/s41598-018-27985-y
34. Patassini S, Begley P, Xu J, Church SJ, Kureishy N, Reid SJ, Waldvogel HJ, Faull RLM, Snell RG, Unwin RD, Cooper GJS. 2019. "Cerebral vitamin B5 (D-pantothenic acid) deficiency as a potential cause of metabolic perturbation and neurodegeneration in Huntington's disease." *Metabolites*. 9(6):113. doi: 10.3390/metabo9060113
35. Zhou X, Li G, Kaplan A, Gaschler MM, Zhang X, Hou Z, Jiang M, Zott R, Cremers S, Stockwell BR, Duan W. 2018. "Small molecule modulator of protein disulfide isomerase attenuates mutant huntingtin toxicity and inhibits endoplasmic reticulum stress in a mouse model of Huntington's disease." *Hum Mol Genet*. 27(9):1545–1555. doi: 10.1093/hmg/ddy061
36. Coppen EM, van der Grond J, Roos RAC. 2018. "Atrophy of the putamen at time of clinical motor onset in Huntington's disease: a 6-year follow-up study." *J Clin Mov Disord*. 5:2. doi: 10.1186/s40734-018-0069-3

37. Brown RH, Al-Chalabi A. 2017. "Amyotrophic lateral sclerosis." *N Engl J Med.* 377(2):162–172. doi: 10.1056/NEJMra1603471
38. Hardiman O, Al-Chalabi A, Chio A, Corr EM, Logroscino G, Robberecht W, Shaw PJ, Simmons Z, van den Berg LH. 2017. "Amyotrophic lateral sclerosis." *Nat Rev Dis Primers.* 3:17071. doi: 10.1038/nrdp.2017.71
39. Calvo AC, Manzano R, Mendonça DM, Muñoz MJ, Zaragoza P, Osta R. 2014. "Amyotrophic lateral sclerosis: a focus on disease progression." *Biomed Res Int.* 2014:925101. doi: 10.1155/2014/925101
40. Morgan S, Orrell RW. 2016. "Pathogenesis of amyotrophic lateral sclerosis." *Br Med Bull.* 119(1):87–98. doi: 10.1093/bmb/ldw026
41. Zarei S, Carr K, Reiley L, Diaz K, Guerra O, Altamirano PF, Pagani W, Lodin D, Orozco G, Chinea A. 2015. "A comprehensive review of amyotrophic lateral sclerosis." *Surg Neurol Int.* 6:171. doi: 10.4103/2152-7806.169561
42. Gironi, M., Arnò, C., Comi, G., Penton-Rol, G., & Furlan, R. 2016. "Multiple sclerosis and neurodegenerative diseases." *In Immune Rebalancing: The Future of Immunosuppression.*63–84. doi:10.1016/B978-0-12-803302-9.00004-X
43. Gadhave DG, Kokare CR. 2019. "Nanostructured lipid carriers engineered for intranasal delivery of teriflunomide in multiple sclerosis: optimization and in vivo studies." *Drug Dev Ind Pharm.* 45(5):839–851. doi: 10.1080/03639045.2019.1576724
44. Leray E, Moreau T, Fromont A, Edan G. 2016. "Epidemiology of multiple sclerosis." *Rev Neurol.* 172(1):3–13. doi: 10.1016/j.neurol.2015.10.006
45. Baecher-Allan C, Kaskow BJ, Weiner HL. 2018. "Multiple sclerosis: mechanisms and immunotherapy." *Neuron.* 97(4):742–768. doi: 10.1016/j.neuron.2018.01.021
46. Reich DS, Lucchinetti CF, Calabresi PA. 2018. "Multiple sclerosis." *N Engl J Med.* 378(2):169–180. doi: 10.1056/NEJMra1401483
47. Dargahi N, Katsara M, Tselios T, Androutsou ME, de Courten M, Matsoukas J, Apostolopoulos V. 2017. "Multiple sclerosis: immunopathology and treatment update." *Brain Sci.* 7(7):78. doi: 10.3390/brainsci7070078
48. Dou KX, Tan MS, Tan CC, Cao XP, Hou XH, Guo QH, Tan L, Mok V, Yu JT. 2018. "Comparative safety and effectiveness of cholinesterase inhibitors and memantine for Alzheimer's disease: a network meta-analysis of 41 randomized controlled trials." *Alzheimers Res Ther.* 10(1):126. doi: 10.1186/s13195-018-0457-9
49. Di Stefano A, Iannitelli A, Laserra S, Sozio P. 2011. "Drug delivery strategies for Alzheimer's disease treatment." *Expert Opin Drug Deliv.* 8(5):581–603. doi: 10.1517/17425247.2011.561311
50. Dash RP, Babu RJ, Srinivas NR. 2018. "Two decades-long journey from riluzole to edaravone: revisiting the clinical pharmacokinetics of the only two amyotrophic lateral sclerosis therapeutics." *Clin Pharmacokinet.* 57(11):1385–1398. doi: 10.1007/s40262-018-0655-4
51. Connolly BS, Lang AE. 2014. "Pharmacological treatment of Parkinson disease: a review." *JAMA.* 311(16):1670–83. doi: 10.1001/jama.2014.3654
52. Walunj M, Doppalapudi S, Bulbake U, Khan W. 2020. "Preparation, characterization, and *in vivo* evaluation of cyclosporine cationic liposomes for the treatment of psoriasis." *J Liposome Res.* 30(1):68–79. doi: 10.1080/08982104.2019.1593449
53. Wang AZ, Langer R, Farokhzad OC. 2012. "Nanoparticle delivery of cancer drugs." *Annu Rev Med.* 63:185–98. doi: 10.1146/annurev-med-040210-162544
54. Sercombe L, Veerati T, Moheimani F, Wu SY, Sood AK, Hua S. 2015. "Advances and challenges of liposome assisted drug delivery." *Front Pharmacol.* 6:286. doi: 10.3389/fphar.2015.00286

55. Raza K, Singh B, Lohan S, Sharma G, Negi P, Yachha Y, Katare OP. 2013. "Nano-lipoidal carriers of tretinoin with enhanced percutaneous absorption, photostability, biocompatibility and anti-psoriatic activity." *Int J Pharm.* 456(1):65–72. doi: 10.1016/j.ijpharm.2013.08.019
56. Tsai MJ, Huang YB, Wu PC, Fu YS, Kao YR, Fang JY, Tsai YH. 2011. "Oral apomorphine delivery from solid lipid nanoparticles with different monostearate emulsifiers: pharmacokinetic and behavioral evaluations." *J Pharm Sci.* 100(2):547–57. doi: 10.1002/jps.22285
57. Gabal YM, Kamel AO, Sammour OA, Elshafeey AH. 2014. "Effect of surface charge on the brain delivery of nanostructured lipid carriers in situ gels via the nasal route." *Int J Pharm.* 473(1–2):442–57. doi: 10.1016/j.ijpharm.2014.07.025
58. Lebwohl M, Menter A, Koo J, Feldman SR. Combination therapy to treat moderate to severe psoriasis. *J Am Acad Dermatol.* 2004 Mar;50(3):416–30. doi: 10.1016/j.jaad.2002.12.002
59. Titze-de-Almeida R, Titze-de-Almeida SS, Ferreira NR, Fontanari C, Faccioli LH, Del Bel E. 2019. "Suppressing nNOS enzyme by small-interfering RNAs protects SH-sy5y cells and nigral dopaminergic neurons from 6-OHDA injury." *Neurotox Res.* 36(1):117–131. doi: 10.1007/s12640-019-00043-9
60. Wiley N.J., Madhankumar A.B., Mitchell R.M., Neely E.B., Rizk E., Douds G.L., Simmons Z., Connor J.R. 2012. "Lipopolysaccharide modified liposomes for amyotropic lateral sclerosis therapy: Efficacy in SOD1 mouse model." *Adv. Nanoparticles.*1:44–53. doi: 10.4236/anp.2012.13007
61. Yang T, Ferrill L, Gallant L, McGillicuddy S, Fernandes T, Schields N, Bai S. 2018. "Verapamil and riluzole cocktail liposomes overcome pharmacoresistance by inhibiting P-glycoprotein in brain endothelial and astrocyte cells: A potent approach to treat amyotrophic lateral sclerosis." *Eur J Pharm Sci.* 120:30–39. doi: 10.1016/j.ejps.2018.04.026
62. Qu M, Lin Q, He S, Wang L, Fu Y, Zhang Z, Zhang L. 2018. "A brain targeting functionalized liposomes of the dopamine derivative N-3,4-bis(pivaloyloxy)-dopamine for treatment of Parkinson's disease." *J Control Release.* 277:173–182. doi: 10.1016/j.jconrel.2018.03.019
63. Yue P, Miao W, Gao L, Zhao X, Teng J. 2018. "Ultrasound-triggered effects of the microbubbles coupled to GDNF plasmid-loaded pegylated liposomes in a rat model of Parkinson's disease." *Front Neurosci.* 12:222. doi: 10.3389/fnins.2018.00222
64. Schlichtmann BW, Hepker M, Palanisamy BN, John M, Anantharam V, Kanthasamy AG, Narasimhan B, Mallapragada SK. 2021. "Nanotechnology-mediated therapeutic strategies against synucleinopathies in neurodegenerative disease." *Curr Opin Chem Eng.* 31:*100673.* doi: 10.1016/j.coche.2021.100673
65. Gurturk Z, Tezcaner A, Dalgic AD, Korkmaz S, Keskin D. 2017. "Maltodextrin modified liposomes for drug delivery through the blood–brain barrier." *Med Chem Comm.* 8(6):1337–1345. doi: 10.1039/c7md00045f
66. Xiang Y, Wu Q, Liang L, Wang X, Wang J, Zhang X, Pu X, Zhang Q. 2012. "Chlorotoxin-modified stealth liposomes encapsulating levodopa for the targeting delivery against Parkinson's disease in the MPTP-induced mice model." *J Drug Target.* 20(1):67–75. doi: 10.3109/1061186X.2011.595490
67. Ghahremani MH, Sharifzadeh M, Amini M, Dinarvand R. 2017. "Solid lipid nanoparticles surface modified with anti-Contactin-2 or anti-Neurofascin for brain-targeted delivery of medicines." *Pharm Dev Technol.* 22(3):426–435. doi: 10.1080/10837450.2016.1226901

68. Kumar P, Sharma G, Gupta V, Kaur R, Thakur K, Malik R, Kumar A, Kaushal N, Raza K. 2018. "Preclinical explorative assessment of dimethyl fumarate-based biocompatible nanolipoidal carriers for the management of multiple sclerosis." *ACS Chem Neurosci.* 9(5):1152–1158. doi: 10.1021/acschemneuro.7b00519
69. Esposito E, Cortesi R, Drechsler M, Fan J, Fu BM, Calderan L, Mannucci S, Boschi F, Nastruzzi C. 2017. "Nanoformulations for dimethyl fumarate: Physicochemical characterization and in vitro/in vivo behavior." *Eur J Pharm Biopharm.* 115:285–296. doi: 10.1016/j.ejpb.2017.04.011
70. Ojha S, Kumar B. 2018. "Preparation and statistical modeling of solid lipid nanoparticles of dimethyl fumarate for better management of multiple sclerosis." *Adv Pharm Bull.* 8(2):225–233. doi: 10.15171/apb.2018.027
71. Kumar P, Sharma G, Kumar R, Malik R, Singh B, Katare OP, Raza K. 2017. "Vitamin-derived nanolipoidal carriers for brain delivery of dimethyl fumarate: A novel approach with preclinical evidence." *ACS Chem Neurosci.* 8(6):1390–1396. doi: 10.1021/acschemneuro.7b00041
72. Kumar P, Sharma G, Kumar R, Malik R, Singh B, Katare OP, Raza K. 2017. "Stearic acid based, systematically designed oral lipid nanoparticles for enhanced brain delivery of dimethyl fumarate." *Nanomedicine.* 12(23):2607–2621. doi: 10.2217/nnm-2017-0082
73. Bondì ML, Craparo EF, Giammona G, Drago F. 2010. "Brain-targeted solid lipid nanoparticles containing riluzole: preparation, characterization and biodistribution." *Nanomedicine.* 5(1):25–32. doi: 10.2217/nnm.09.67
74. Zhao YZ, Li X, Lu CT, Lin M, Chen LJ, Xiang Q, Zhang M, Jin RR, Jiang X, Shen XT, Li XK, Cai J. 2014. "Gelatin nanostructured lipid carriers-mediated intranasal delivery of basic fibroblast growth factor enhances functional recovery in hemiparkinsonian rats." *Nanomedicine.* 10(4):755–64. doi: 10.1016/j.nano.2013.10.009

8 Combination of Drug Delivery through Nanocarriers for Brain Diseases

Hagera Dilnashin, Shekhar Singh, Richa Singh, and Surya Pratap Singh

8.1 COMBINATIONAL DRUG DELIVERY THROUGH NANOCARRIERS FOR BRAIN DISEASES

The blood–brain barrier (BBB) is a barrier that prevents the majority of available therapies for neurodegenerative diseases from entering the brain and relieving symptoms [1]. Hence, owing to the devastating impacts of neurodegenerative diseases, researchers from across the world are concentrating on creating new carrier systems that will carry neuroprotective drugs to the target areas without having an adverse influence on healthy tissues [2]. By inciting, reacting to, and interacting with target sites to stimulate physiological responses while significantly reducing side effects, nanotechnology uses designed materials and devices that interact with biomolecules at the molecular level [3]. This could vastly improve the management of neurodegenerative diseases (NDs). Nanotechnology is the design, characterisation, formulation, and use of materials by controlling their size and shape in the nanoscale range (1 to 100 nm) [4]. Due to their large surface-to-volume ratio, nanocarriers exhibit a variety of optical, magnetic, and biological characteristics when incorporated into living things like human tissue [5]. To create a unique, highly drug-loaded nanocarrier, the existing problems and potential difficulties in nanocarrier-mediated drug delivery are also taken into consideration [6]. The continuous drug release from these nanocarriers will outpace the endosome–lysosome process, resulting in a long-term circulation period [7]. Nanocarriers have several distinctive qualities like the following: improvements in biodistribution and pharmacokinetics, increased stability, improved solubility, toxicity reduction, and medication delivery that is focused and sustained [8].

8.2 TYPES OF NANOCARRIERS

On the basis of surface-to-volume ratio, nanocarriers are divided into three types, such as: inorganic, organic, and hybrid nanocarriers.

DOI: 10.1201/9781032661964-8

8.2.1 Inorganic Nanocarriers

Inorganic nanocarriers include mesoporous silica nanoparticles (MSNs), carbon nanotubes, magnetic, copper oxide, noble metal, silver, and gold-based nanocarriers [9] [10] [11].

8.2.1.1 Gold Nanocarriers

Gold nanocarriers (NCs) are among the most researched metal nanoparticles because of their comparatively low cytotoxicity, optical characteristics that make them ideal for imaging and detection, and well-established production techniques [12]. They have the potential to cross the BBB by changing their size or coupling different modified ligands.

Gold NCs are advantageous in imaging as well [13]. Insulin-targeted gold nanoparticles can be used as contrast agents in computed tomography (CT) scans to draw attention to certain brain areas where they concentrate [14]. The size of gold NCs makes a difference in biodistribution and circulation time [15]. In a study, 20 nm gold NCs exhibited the highest levels of migration and accumulation in the brain, highlighting the significance of nanoparticle size in the development of gold NCs for neurodegenerative disorders [16].

8.2.1.2 Silver Nanocarriers

Another common metallic nanoparticle with several biological uses is silver nanocarriers (AgNCs), which has unique physical and chemical characteristics [15]. Several scientists examined the neurological and inflammatory effects of Ag NCs on microglia [17]. According to previous findings, when silver nanoparticles are taken up, they become covered with non-reactive silver sulphide (Ag_2S), which has an anti-inflammatory impact by lowering reactive oxygen species (ROS), nitric oxide, and tumour necrosis factor (TNF). Ag ion toxicity was discovered to be caused by the production of Ag_2S [18]. The formulation proved successful in protecting the medicine, enhancing its stability and bioavailability.

8.2.1.3 Silica Nanocarriers

The use of silica nanoparticles (SiO_2-NCs) in the diagnosis, imaging, and therapeutic administration of central nervous system illnesses is widespread [19]. To improve the absorption by BBB, silica nanoparticles were additionally coupled with various ligands. Lactoferrin (Lf), a cationic iron-binding glycoprotein, was produced by Song et al. as PEGsilica nanoparticles [20]. This functionalisation enabled more nanoparticle transport across the BBB in the *in vitro* model, indicating that this sort of conjugation may be advantageous for nanocarriers for diseases of the brain [21]. However, according to certain studies, silica nanoparticles have negative effects on brain cells, induce neurotoxicity, and cause neurodegeneration [22]. It was discovered that there was cognitive impairment and an increase in anxiety after intranasal application of SiO_2-NCs into mice models [23]. Karimzadeh et al. created MSNs that were modified with succinic anhydride and 3-aminopropyltriethoxysilane and loaded with rivastigmine hydrogen tartrate [24]. Nevertheless, additional improvement is required to lessen the viability loss linked to these nanocarriers.

8.2.1.4 Iron Nanocarriers

Fe_3O_4 magnetic nanoparticles (MNPs), which are superparamagnetic, non-toxic, and biocompatible, are among the iron nanoparticles that have undergone substantial research [25]. Moreover, iron nanoparticles naturally have advantages in imaging [26]. For the purpose of performing magnetic resonance imaging of various NDs, several superparamagnetic iron oxide nanoparticles have been coupled with therapeutic substances or modified components (PEG and 1,1-dicyano-2-[6-(dimethylamino) naphthalene-2-yl]propene car-boxyl derivative) [27].

8.2.1.5 Cerium Oxide Nanocarriers

Nanoceria, or cerium oxide nanocarriers (CeONCs), exhibit antioxidant and radical-scavenging properties that may be useful in the treatment of neurological disorders [28]. Nevertheless, biodistribution studies unequivocally showed that the liver, kidney, and spleen are the principal organs of accumulation, which may provide a safety issue in further research [28]. CeO_2NCs might therefore use the targeting method to improve effectiveness and reduce potential toxicity [29].

8.2.2 Organic Nanocarriers

8.2.2.1 Liposomes

Liposomes are nanocarriers made up of an aqueous core and a phospholipid bilayer, having low toxicity [30]. Therapeutic substances can be encapsulated in them in both hydrophilic and hydrophobic forms [31]. They can be either multilamellar vesicles, little unilamellar vesicles, or big unilamellar vesicles (MLV) [32]. They are able to pass across the BBB by transcytosis or active transport after attaching to a particular receptor [33]. Another advantageous delivery of liposome is the intranasal route, which easily reaches the brain via olfactory and trigeminal nerves [34]. Rivastigmine liposomes were administered to the brain orally and intranasally by Arumugam et al. The findings that the intranasal route of administration produced larger levels of the medication in the brain suggest that this route has a better bioavailability [35]. The liposomal surface has undergone several changes recently in order to enhance its capacity for brain targeting [36]. A liposome can effectively cross the BBB and carry the medication to the desired place with the aid of some specialised ligands (glucose, lactoferrin, transferrin, and specific peptides) [37].

8.2.2.2 Transferin-mediated Liposomes

One of the receptors, the transferrin receptor (TfR), is of particular relevance for the distribution of medicinal drugs across the BBB in order to improve the targeting effectiveness [38]. Both *in vivo* and *in vitro* Tf liposome administration in the brain have been shown to pass through the BBB and enhance brain function. A transmembrane glycoprotein, comprising two 90 kDa subunits of TfR, can bind to one molecule of transferrin [39]. A disulfide bridge connects these subunits. There are various issues with TfR that must be highlighted as a target delivery system [39]. 1) Together with the BBB, TfR is expressed on neurons, hepatocytes, RBC, intestinal cells, monocytes, and choroid plexus epithelial cells [40]. As a result, TfR-targeted liposomes are widely distributed in the liver and kidneys as well [41]. 2) An elevated level of Tf in blood serum (2 mol/l) creates a serious problem because in healthy conditions, endogenous Tf generally saturates the TfR expressed on endothelial cells. Thus, the ability to target is insufficiently effective [42].

8.2.2.3 Cationic Liposome

The most widely used modified liposomes are cationic liposomal drug carriers because they may interact electrostatically to take advantage of the BBB's negative charge and so start the cell internalisation processes [43]. By injecting anionic, cationic, and charge-neutral liposomes into the internal carotid arteries of Sprague-Dawley rats, it was possible to determine how a liposome surface charge affected brain tissue uptake [43]. According to a previous study, a liposome surface charge influences cellular connections. Both positively and negatively charged liposomes interacted with cells more intensely than uncharged liposomes; cationic liposomes were most prevalent in the brain [44].

8.2.2.4 PEG-modified Liposome

Polyethylene glycol (PEG)-coated liposomes has been often used and extensively documented to boost their chemical stability in serum and further provide an extended circulation period in plasma, enabling longer dose intervals [45]. Importantly, the effectiveness of brain targeting is affected by the chain length of PEG [46]. In order to examine their differences and identify the ideal length of PEG for drug administration, the properties of glucose-modified liposomes utilizing PEGs with various chain lengths (PEG200, PEG400, PEG1000, and PEG2000) as the linkers were compared and analysed both *in vitro* and *in vivo* [47]. The results showed that longer chain length PEGs connected to glucose-modified liposomes were more effective at promoting drug transport through the BBB. At every stage of the *in vivo* trial, liposomes connected by PEG1000 showed the best brain-targeted property [48]. Due to steric hindrance, PEG with greater chain length may reduce the brain-targeted effectiveness of the liposome, whereas PEG with shorter chain length may prevent the ligand from being exposed [49].

8.2.2.5 Multifunctional Liposome

Using successive targeting, multifunctional liposomes were also employed to treat AD [50]. The BBB was targeted using a peptide generated from the apolipoprotein-E receptor-binding domain of liposomes, and the BBB and peripheral clearance of the peptide were both improved by phosphatidic acid for Aβ-binding, which also destabilised brain Aβ-aggregates [50]. To achieve a dual targeting impact and precise distribution in the brain, multifunctional liposomes were also employed in the treatment of gliomas [51]. Doxorubincin (Dox) liposomes with dual targeting were created by combining liposomes with both folate and transferrin [52]. These liposomes have been effectively employed to traverse the BBB and target tumours [53].

8.3 SELECTIVE NANOCARRIERS AND BRAIN DISEASE

8.3.1 Epilepsy

Epilepsy is a chronic neurological disorder that affects over 50 million people worldwide. Despite the availability of many anti-epileptic drugs, up to 30% of epilepsy patients remain unresponsive to current treatments [53]. Combination drug therapy has emerged as a promising approach to treat epilepsy patients who are resistant to monotherapy. However, the challenge of combining multiple drugs is the increased risk of drug-to-drug interactions and toxicity. Nanocarriers have recently gained attention as a potential solution for combination drug delivery, offering targeted and controlled release of multiple drugs with reduced toxicity [54].

Several studies have investigated the use of nanocarriers for combination drug delivery in epilepsy. In one study, researchers developed a liposome-based nanocarrier that contained two anti-epileptic drugs, valproic acid and levetiracetam. The nanocarrier exhibited sustained release of both drugs over 48 hours and showed enhanced anticonvulsant activity in a mouse model of epilepsy compared to monotherapy with either drug alone [55].

Another study investigated the use of a dendrimer-based nanocarrier for combination drug delivery in epilepsy. The nanocarrier was loaded with two antiepileptic drugs, phenytoin and phenobarbital, and was functionalised with a peptide ligand that targeted the BBB-exhibited targeted delivery to the brain and prolonged release of both drugs, resulting in improved seizure control in a rat model of epilepsy [60].

In addition to liposomes and dendrimers, other nanocarriers have been explored for combination drug delivery in epilepsy, including polymer-based nanoparticles and mesoporous silica nanoparticles [57]. Polymer-based nanoparticles can be designed to release drugs in response to specific stimuli, such as changes in pH or temperature. Mesoporous silica nanoparticles can be loaded with multiple drugs and functionalised with targeting ligands for selective delivery to specific cells or tissues.

8.3.2 Alzheimer's Disease

Alzheimer's disease is a progressive and irreversible neurological disorder affecting millions of people worldwide. The disease is characterised by the accumulation of abnormal proteins in the brain, leading to brain cell death and a decline in cognitive function. Currently, there is no cure for Alzheimer's disease, and the available treatments only provide temporary relief from the symptoms. Therefore, there is a critical need to develop new therapies that can slow down or halt the progression of the disease.

One promising approach for the treatment of Alzheimer's disease is the use of combination drug delivery through nanocarriers. Nanocarriers are tiny particles that can encapsulate drugs and deliver them to specific cells or tissues in the body. They can also protect the drugs from degradation and improve their bioavailability, which can enhance their therapeutic efficacy.

Combination drug delivery through nanocarriers involves the simultaneous delivery of two or more drugs to target multiple pathways involved in the pathogenesis of Alzheimer's disease. The use of combination therapy can enhance the therapeutic efficacy of the drugs and reduce the risk of drug resistance, which is a common problem with single-drug therapies.

One example of combination drug delivery through nanocarriers for Alzheimer's disease is the use of cholinesterase inhibitors and N-methyl-D-aspartate (NMDA) receptor antagonists. Cholinesterase inhibitors are currently used to treat the cognitive symptoms of Alzheimer's disease, while NMDA receptor antagonists can protect the brain cells from excitotoxicity, which is a common problem in Alzheimer's disease [58].

The combination of cholinesterase inhibitors and NMDA receptor antagonists has shown promise in preclinical studies, but the clinical application of this combination therapy has been limited by the low bioavailability of the drugs and their poor ability to cross the BBB. However, the use of nanocarriers can overcome these limitations and enhance the therapeutic efficacy of the drugs.

Several types of nanocarriers have been investigated for the delivery of drugs to the brain, including liposomes, polymeric nanoparticles, and dendrimers. These nanocarriers can be functionalised with specific ligands that can target the drugs to the brain and enhance their BBB-crossing ability.

One example of nanocarrier-based combination therapy for Alzheimer's disease is the use of curcumin and resveratrol. Curcumin and resveratrol are two natural compounds that have been shown to have neuroprotective effects in preclinical studies. However, their therapeutic efficacy is limited by their poor solubility and bioavailability. Therefore, researchers have encapsulated curcumin and resveratrol in liposomes and tested their efficacy in a mouse model of Alzheimer's disease [59].

The results of the study showed that the liposomal formulation of curcumin and resveratrol significantly reduced the accumulation of amyloid-beta (Aβ) plaques in the brain and improved cognitive function in the mice. The study also showed that the combination therapy was more effective than the individual drugs alone, indicating the potential of nanocarrier-based combination therapy for the treatment of Alzheimer's disease [53].

8.3.3 Parkinson's Disease (PD)

Parkinson's disease (PD) is a progressive neurodegenerative disorder characterised by the loss of dopaminergic neurons in the substantia nigra region of the brain. Currently, the primary treatment for PD involves dopamine replacement therapy with L-dopa, but this treatment has limitations and can lead to long-term side effects such as dyskinesia. Combination drug delivery through nanocarriers has emerged as a promising strategy for improving the effectiveness of PD treatment while reducing side effects. In the case of PD, nanocarriers can be used to simultaneously deliver multiple drugs to different regions of the brain to address the multiple pathological processes associated with the disease.

For example, nanocarriers can be used to deliver L-dopa along with other drugs that target different aspects of PD, such as neuroinflammation, oxidative stress, and mitochondrial dysfunction [60]. This approach has been shown to improve the therapeutic efficacy of L-dopa and reduce the risk of side effects. Additionally, nanocarriers can be designed to cross the BBB, which is a major challenge for traditional drug-delivery methods.

8.3.4 Traumatic Brain Injury (TBI)

Nanocarriers can be used to deliver neuroprotective agents, anti-inflammatory agents, and growth factors to promote neuroregeneration and reduce neuronal damage. Additionally, nanocarriers can be engineered to cross the BBB, which is a major challenge for traditional drug-delivery methods.

Recent studies have demonstrated the potential of nanocarriers in TBI treatment. For instance, a study on rats showed that a combination of two drugs (a neuroprotective agent and an anti-inflammatory agent) delivered through nanocarriers improved cognitive function and reduced brain damage after TBI [61]. Another study showed that nanocarriers loaded with a growth factor and an anti-inflammatory agent improved motor function and reduced brain damage in mice after TBI.

8.3.5 Stroke

Nanocarriers can be used to deliver neuroprotective agents, anti-inflammatory agents, and growth factors to reduce the extent of brain damage and promote recovery.

Recent studies have shown the potential of nanocarriers in stroke treatment. For example, a study on rats showed that a combination of two drugs (a neuroprotective agent and an anti-inflammatory agent) delivered through nanocarriers improved functional outcomes and reduced brain damage after stroke [62]. Another study showed that nanocarriers loaded with a growth factor and an anti-inflammatory agent improved functional recovery and reduced brain damage in mice after stroke.

8.3.6 Huntington's Disease

Huntington's disease (HD) is a rare genetic disorder that affects the central nervous system and leads to the progressive loss of cognitive and motor function. Currently, there is no cure for HD, and treatment is limited to symptomatic relief. Combination drug delivery through nanocarriers is an emerging approach for HD treatment that has the potential to improve outcomes by delivering multiple drugs to the site of injury.

Recent studies have shown the potential of nanocarriers in HD treatment. For example, a study on mice showed that nanocarriers loaded with two drugs (a neuroprotective agent and a drug that targets the abnormal protein accumulation) improved motor function and reduced brain damage in HD mice [63]. Another study showed that nanocarriers loaded with an anti-inflammatory agent and a drug that promotes neuroregeneration improved motor function and reduced brain damage in HD mice.

8.3.7 Other Brain Disorders

Rare brain diseases, such as Niemann-Pick disease, Tay-Sachs disease, and Batten disease, are a group of devastating and often fatal genetic disorders that affect the central nervous system. Current treatments for these diseases are limited, and there is an urgent need for new and effective therapies [63]. Combination drug delivery through nanocarriers is an emerging approach that shows promise for the treatment of rare brain diseases.

8.4 CONCLUSION

In conclusion, combination drug delivery through nanocarriers holds great promise for the treatment of brain diseases. The use of nanocarriers can enhance the bioavailability of the drugs and target them to specific cells or tissues in the body. The combination of multiple drugs can enhance the therapeutic efficacy of the drugs and reduce the risk of drug resistance. While there are still challenges to overcome, such as optimizing the nanocarrier design and ensuring their safety, the use of nanocarrier-based combination therapy has the potential to revolutionise the treatment of brain diseases and improve the lives of millions of people affected by this devastating condition. However, further research is needed to optimise the design of nanocarriers and evaluate their safety and efficacy in clinical trials.

REFERENCES

1. Wu Ying-Chieh, Tuuli-Maria Sonninen, Sanni Peltonen, Jari Koistinaho, and Šárka Lehtonen. 2021. "Blood–brain barrier and neurodegenerative diseases – modeling with iPSC-derived brain cells". *International Journal of Molecular Sciences*, *22*(14), 7710.
2. Ajay Kumar, Ravi K. Chaudhary, Rachita Singh, Satya P. Singh, Shao-Yu Wang, Zheng-Yu Hoe, Cheng-Tang Pan, Yow-Ling Shiue, Dong-Qing Wei, Aman C. Kaushik, and Xiaofeng Dai. 2020. "Nanotheranostic applications for detection and targeting neurodegenerative diseases". *Frontiers in Neuroscience,* 14, 305.
3. Ian Y. Wong, Sangeeta N. Bhatia, and Mehmet Toner. 2013. "Nanotechnology: Emerging tools for biology and medicine". *Genes & Development*, *27*(22), 2397–2408.
4. Deepak K. Dash, Rajni K. Panik, Anil K. Sahu, and Vaibhav Tripathi. 2020. "Role of nanobiotechnology in drug discovery, development and molecular diagnostic". In *Applications of Nanobiotechnology*. IntechOpen.
5. V. Chandrakala, Valmiki Aruna, and Gangadhara Angajala. 2022. "Review on metal nanoparticles as nanocarriers: Current challenges and perspectives in drug delivery systems". *Emergent Materials*, 1–23.
6. Fakhar ud Din, Waqar Aman, Izhar Ullah, Omer S. Qureshi, Omer Mustapha, Shumaila Shafique, and Alam Zeb. 2017. "Effective use of nanocarriers as drug delivery systems for the treatment of selected tumors". *International Journal of Nanomedicine*, 7291–7309.
7. Jinhyun H. Lee, and Yoon Yeo. 2015. "Controlled drug release from pharmaceutical nanocarriers". *Chemical Engineering Science, 125*, 75–84.
8. Shi Su, and Peter M. Kang. 2020. "Recent advances in nanocarrier-assisted therapeutics delivery systems". *Pharmaceutics*, *12*(9), 837.

9. Miguel Gisbert-Garzarán, Miguel Manzano, and Maria Vallet-Regí. 2020. "Mesoporous silica nanoparticles for the treatment of complex bone diseases: Bone cancer, bone infection and osteoporosis". *Pharmaceutics*, *12*(1), 83.
10. P. N. Navya, Anubhav Kaphle, S. P. Srinivas, Suresh K. Bhargava, Vincent M. Rotello, and Hemant K. Daima. 2019. "Current trends and challenges in cancer management and therapy using designer nanomaterials". *Nano Convergence, 6*, 1–30.
11. Panoraia I. Siafaka, Neslihan U. Okur, Ioannis D. Karantas, Mehmet E. Okur, and Evren A. Gündoğdu. 2021. "Current update on nanoplatforms as therapeutic and diagnostic tools: A review for the materials used as nanotheranostics and imaging modalities". *Asian Journal of Pharmaceutical Sciences*, *16*(1), 24–46.
12. Alexandre P. Muller, Gabriela K. Ferreira, Allison J. Pires, Gustavo de Bem Silveira, Debora L. de Souza, Joice de Abreu Brandolfi, Claudio T. de Souza, Marcos M. S. Paula, and Paulo C. L. Silveira. 2017. "Gold nanoparticles prevent cognitive deficits, oxidative stress and inflammation in a rat model of sporadic dementia of Alzheimer's type". *Materials Science and Engineering: C, 77*, 476–483.
13. Julie Ruff, Sabine Hüwel, Marcelo J. Kogan, Ulrich Simon, and Hans-Joachim Galla. 2017. "The effects of gold nanoparticles functionalized with ß-amyloid specific peptides on an in vitro model of blood–brain barrier". *Nanomedicine: Nanotechnology, Biology and Medicine*, *13*(5), 1645–1652.
14. Malka Shilo, Menachem Motiei, Panet Hana, and Rachela Popovtzer. 2014. "Transport of nanoparticles through the blood–brain barrier for imaging and therapeutic applications". *Nanoscale*, *6*(4), 2146–2152.
15. Saurabh Bhatia. 2016. "Nanoparticles types, classification, characterization, fabrication methods and drug delivery applications". *Natural Polymer Drug Delivery Systems: Nanoparticles, Plants, and Algae*, 33–93.
16. Oshra Betzer, Malka Shilo, Renana Opochinsky, Eran Barnoy, Menachem Motiei, Eitan Okun, Gal Yadid and Rachela Popovtzer. 2017. "The effect of nanoparticle size on the ability to cross the blood–brain barrier: an in vivo study". *Nanomedicine*, *12*(13), 1533–1546.
17. Daniel A. Gonzalez-Carter, Bey F. Leo, Pakatip Ruenraroengsak, Shu Chen, Angela E. Goode, Ioannis G. Theodorou, Kian F. Chung, Raffaella Carzaniga, Milo S. P. Shaffer, David T. Dexter, Mary P. Ryan and Alexandra E. Porter. 2017. "Silver nanoparticles reduce brain inflammation and related neurotoxicity through induction of H2S-synthesizing enzymes". *Scientific Reports*, *7*(1), 42871.
18. Li Xu, Yi-Yi Wang, Jie Huang, Chen Chun-Yuan, Zhen-Xing Wang, and Hui Xie. 2020. "Silver nanoparticles: Synthesis, medical applications and biosafety". *Theranostics*, *10*(20), 8996.
19. Ran You, Yuen-Shan Ho, Clara H. Hung, Yan Liu, Chun-Xia Huang, Hei-Nga Chan, See-Lok Ho, Sheung-Yeung Lui, Hung-Wing Li, and Raymond C. Chang. 2018. "Silica nanoparticles induce neurodegeneration-like changes in behavior, neuropathology, and affect synapse through MAPK activation". *Particle and Fibre Toxicology*, *15*(1), 28. https://doi.org/10.1186/s12989-018-0263-3
20. Yang Song, Dan Du, Lei Li, Jun Xu, Prashanta Dutta, and Yuehe Lin. 2017. "In vitro study of receptor-mediated silica nanoparticles delivery across blood–brain barrier". *ACS Applied Materials & Interfaces*, *9*(24), 20410–20416. https://doi.org/10.1021/acsami.7b03504
21. Maria Vallet-Regí, Montserrat Colilla, Isabel Izquierdo-Barba, and Miguel Manzano. 2017. "Mesoporous silica nanoparticles for drug delivery: Current insights". *Molecules*, *23*(1), 47.

22. Vanitha Selvarajan, Sybil Obuobi, and Pui L. R. Ee. 2020. "Silica nanoparticles – a versatile tool for the treatment of bacterial infections". *Frontiers in Chemistry, 8*, 602.
23. Diana Díaz-García, Agueda Ferrer-Donato, Jose M. Méndez-Arriaga, Marta Cabrera-Pinto, Miguel Díaz-Sánchez, Sanjiv Prashar, Carmen M. Fernandez-Martos, and Santiago Gómez-Ruiz. 2022. "Design of mesoporous silica nanoparticles for the treatment of amyotrophic lateral sclerosis (ALS) with a therapeutic cocktail based on leptin and pioglitazone". *ACS Biomaterials Science & Engineering*, *8*(11), 4838–4849.
24. Mahmonir Karimzadeh, Ladan Rashidi, and Fariba Ganji. 2017. "Mesoporous silica nanoparticles for efficient rivastigmine hydrogen tartrate delivery into SY5Y cells". *Drug Development and Industrial Pharmacy*, *43*(4), 628–636. https://doi.org/10.1080/03639045.2016.1275668
25. Minh D. Nguyen, Hung-Vu Tran, Shoujun Xu, and T. R. Lee. 2021. "Fe3O4 nanoparticles: structures, synthesis, magnetic properties, surface functionalization, and emerging applications". *Applied Sciences*, *11*(23), 11301.
26. S. A. Shah, G. H. Yoon, S. S. Chung, M. N. Abid, T. H. Kim, H. Y. Lee, and M. O. Kim. 2017. "Novel osmotin inhibits SREBP2 via the AdipoR1/AMPK/SIRT1 pathway to improve Alzheimer's disease neuropathological deficits". *Molecular Psychiatry*, *22*(3), 407–416.
27. Jingting Zhou, Huanbao Fa, Wei Yin, Jin Zhang, Changjun Hou, Danqun Huo, Dong Zhang and Haifeng Zhang. 2014. "Synthesis of superparamagnetic iron oxide nanoparticles coated with a DDNP-carboxyl derivative for in vitro magnetic resonance imaging of Alzheimer's disease". *Materials Science and Engineering: C, 37*, 348–355.
28. Beverly A. Rzigalinski, Charles S. Carfagna, and Marion Ehrich. 2017. "Cerium oxide nanoparticles in neuroprotection and considerations for efficacy and safety". *Wiley Interdisciplinary Reviews: Nanomedicine and Nanobiotechnology*, *9*(4), e1444.
29. William DeCoteau, Karin L. Heckman, Ana Y. Estevez, Kenneth J. Reed, K, Wendi Costanzo, David Sandford, Paige Studlack, Jennifer Clauss, Elizabeth Nichols, Jennifer Lipps, Matthew Parker, Bonnie Hays-Erlichman, J. C. Leiter, and Joseph S. Erlichman. 2016. "Cerium oxide nanoparticles with antioxidant properties ameliorate strength and prolong life in mouse model of amyotrophic lateral sclerosis". *Nanomedicine: Nanotechnology, Biology and Medicine*, *12*(8), 2311–2320.
30. Nikolay Dimov, Elisabeth Kastner, Maryam Hussain, Yvonne Perrie, and Nicolas Szita. 2017. "Formation and purification of tailored liposomes for drug delivery using a module-based micro continuous-flow system". *Scientific reports*, *7*(1), 12045.
31. Jiawei Sun, Lei Jiang, Yi Lin, Ethan M. Gerhard, Xuehua Jiang, Li Li, Jian Yang, and Zhongwei Gu. 2017. "Enhanced anticancer efficacy of paclitaxel through multistage tumor-targeting liposomes modified with RGD and KLA peptides". *International Journal of Nanomedicine, 12*, 1517–1537. https://doi.org/10.2147/IJN.S122859
32. Hamdi Nsairat, Dima Khater, Usama Sayed, Fadwa Odeh, Abeer Al Bawab, Walhan Alshaer. 2022. "Liposomes: structure, composition, types, and clinical applications". *Heliyon*, *8*(5), e09394.
33. Domenico Lombardo, and Mikhail A. Kiselev. 2022. "Methods of liposomes preparation: Formation and control factors of versatile nanocarriers for biomedical and nanomedicine application". *Pharmaceutics*, *14*(3), 543.
34. Abdur R. Khan, Mengrui Liu, Muhammad W. Khan, and Guangxi Zhai. 2017. "Progress in brain targeting drug delivery system by nasal route". *Journal of Controlled Release, 268*, 364–389.
35. Soon-Seok Hong, Kyung T. Oh, Han-Gon Choi, and Soo-Jeong Lim. 2019. "Liposomal formulations for nose-to-brain delivery: Recent advances and future perspectives". *Pharmaceutics*, *11*(10), 540. https://doi.org/10.3390/pharmaceutics11100540

36. Amjad A. Khan, Khaled S. Allemailem, Saleh A. Almatroodi, Ahmed Almatroudi, and Arshad H. Rahmani. 2020. "Recent strategies towards the surface modification of liposomes: An innovative approach for different clinical applications". *3 Biotech, 10*, 1–15.
37. Debora B Vieira, and Lionel F. Gamarra. 2016. "Getting into the brain: Liposome-based strategies for effective drug delivery across the blood–brain barrier". *International Journal of Nanomedicine, 11*, 5381.
38. Jason M. Lajoie, and Eric V. Shusta. 2015. "Targeting receptor-mediated transport for delivery of biologics across the blood–brain barrier". *Annual Review of Pharmacology and Toxicology, 55*, 613–631.
39. Zhi-Lan Chen, Man Huang, Xia-Rong Wang, Jun Fu, Min Han, You-Qing Shen, Zheng Xia, and Jia-Qing Gao. 2016. "Transferrin-modified liposome promotes α-mangostin to penetrate the blood–brain barrier". *Nanomedicine: Nanotechnology, Biology and Medicine, 12*(2), 421–430.
40. Xiaoqian Niu, Jeijian Chen, Jianqing Gao. 2019. "Nanocarriers as a powerful vehicle to overcome blood–brain barrier in treating neurodegenerative diseases: Focus on recent advances". *Asian Journal of Pharmaceutical Sciences, 14*(5), 480–496.
41. Gitanjali Sharma, Sushant Lakkadwala, Amit Modgil, and Jagdish Singh. 2016. "The role of cell-penetrating peptide and transferrin on enhanced delivery of drug to brain". *International Journal of Molecular Sciences, 17*(6), 806.
42. Keith E. Maier, Rohit K. Jangra, Kevin R Shieh, David K. Cureton, Hui Xiao, Erik L. Snapp, Sean P. Whelan, Kartik Chandran, and Matthew Levy. 2016. "A new transferrin receptor aptamer inhibits new world hemorrhagic fever mammarenavirus entry". *Molecular Therapy-Nucleic Acids, 5*, e321.
43. Shailendra Joshi, Rajinder P. Singh-Moon, Mei Wang, Durba B. Chaudhuri, Mark Holcomb, Ninfa L. Straubinger, Jeffrey N. Bruce, Irving J. Bigio, and Robert M. Straubinger. 2014. "Transient cerebral hypoperfusion assisted intraarterial cationic liposome delivery to brain tissue". *Journal of Neuro-Oncology, 118*(1), 73–82. https://doi.org/10.1007/s11060-014-1421-6
44. Shailendra Joshi, Rajinder P. Singh-Moon, Mei Wang, Durba B. Chaudhuri, Jason A. Ellis, Jeffrey N. Bruce, Irving J. Bigio, and Robert M. Straubinger. 2014. "Cationic surface charge enhances early regional deposition of liposomes after intracarotid injection". *Journal of Neuro-Oncology, 120*, 489–497.
45. Kai K. Ewert, Venkata R. Kotamraju, Ramsey N. Majzoub, Victoria M. Steffes, Emily A. Wonder, Tambet Teesalu, Erkki Ruoslahti, and Cyrus R. Safinya. 2016. "Synthesis of linear and cyclic peptide–PEG–lipids for stabilization and targeting of cationic liposome–DNA complexes". *Bioorganic & Medicinal Chemistry Letters, 26*(6), 1618–1623.
46. Marwa Mohamed, Amr S. Abu Lila, Taro Shimizu, Eman Alaaeldin, Amal Hussein, Hatem A. Sarhan, Janos Szebeni, and Tatsuhiro Ishida. 2019. "PEGylated liposomes: immunological responses". *Science and Technology of Advanced Materials, 20*(1), 710–724.
47. Magdalena Kowalska, Marcin Broniatowski, Marzena Mach, Lukasz Płachta, and Pawel Wydro. 2021. "The effect of the polyethylene glycol chain length of a lipopolymer (DSPE-PEGn) on the properties of DPPC monolayers and bilayers". *Journal of Molecular Liquids, 335*, 116529.
48. Koki Ogawa, Naoya Kato, and Shigeru Kawakami. 2020. "Recent strategies for targeted brain drug delivery". *Chemical and Pharmaceutical Bulletin, 68*(7), 567–582.

49. Jung Soo Suk, Qingguo Xu, Namho Kim, Justin Hanes, and Laura M. Ensign. 2016. "PEGylation as a strategy for improving nanoparticle-based drug and gene delivery". *Advanced Drug Delivery Reviews*, *99*, 28–51.
50. Claudia Balducci, Simona Mancini, Stefania Minniti, Pietro La Vitola, Margherita Zotti, Giulio Sancini, Mario Mauri, Alfredo Cagnotto, Laura Colombo, Fabio Fiordaliso, Emanuele Grigoli, Mario Salmona, Anniina Snellman, Marja Haaparanta-Solin, Gianluigi Forloni, Massimo Masserini, and Francesca Re. 2014. "Multifunctional liposomes reduce brain β-amyloid burden and ameliorate memory impairment in Alzheimer's disease mouse models". *Journal of Neuroscience: The Official Journal of the Society for Neuroscience*, *34*(42), 14022–14031. https://doi.org/10.1523/JNEUROSCI.0284-14.2014
51. Bahare Salehi, Daniela Calina, Anca O. Docea, Niranjan Koirala, Sushant Aryal, Domenico Lombardo, Luigi Pasqua, Yasaman Taheri, Carla M. S. Castillo, Miquel Martorell, Natalia Martins, Marcello Iriti, Hafiz A. R. Suleria, and Javad Sharifi-Rad. 2020. "Curcumin's nanomedicine formulations for therapeutic application in neurological diseases". *Journal of Clinical Medicine*, *9*(2), 430.
52. Jian-Qing Gao, Qing Lv, Li-Ming Li, Xing-Jiang Tang, Fan-Zhu Li, Yu-Lan Hu, and Min Han. 2013. "Glioma targeting and blood–brain barrier penetration by dual-targeting doxorubincin liposomes". *Biomaterials*, *34*(22), 5628–5639.
53. Pranali P. Deshpande, Swati Biswas, and Vladimir P. Torchilin. 2013. "Current trends in the use of liposomes for tumor targeting". *Nanomedicine*, *8*(9), 1509–1528.
54. Abdul Wahab. 2010. "Difficulties in treatment and management of epilepsy and challenges in new drug development". In *Pharmaceuticals* (Vol. 3, Issue 7, pp. 2090–2110). MDPI AG. https://doi.org/10.3390/ph3072090
55. Lorena Bonilla, Gerard Esteruelas, Miren Ettcheto, Marta Espina, María L. García, Antoni Camins, Eliana B. Souto, Amanda Cano, Elena Sánchez-López. 2022. "Biodegradable nanoparticles for the treatment of epilepsy: From current advances to future challenges". *Epilepsia Open*, *7 Suppl 1*(Suppl 1), S121–S132. https://doi.org/10.1002/epi4.12567
56. Yuefei Zhu, Chunying Liu, and Zhiqing Pang. 2019. "Dendrimer-based drug delivery systems for brain targeting". *Biomolecules*, *9*(12), 790. https://doi.org/10.3390/biom9120790
57. Mosa Alsehli. 2020. "Polymeric nanocarriers as stimuli-responsive systems for targeted tumor (cancer) therapy: Recent advances in drug delivery". *Saudi Pharmaceutical Journal: SPJ: The Official Publication of the Saudi Pharmaceutical Society*, *28*(3), 255–265. https://doi.org/10.1016/j.jsps.2020.01.004
58. Marissa E. Wechsler, Julia E. V. Ramirez, and Nicholas A. Peppas. 2019. "110(th) anniversary: Nanoparticle mediated drug delivery for the treatment of Alzheimer's disease: Crossing the blood–brain barrier". *Industrial & Engineering Chemistry Research*, *58*(33), 15079–15087. https://doi.org/10.1021/acs.iecr.9b02196
59. Gabriela Mazzanti, and Silvia Di Giacomo. 2016. "Curcumin and resveratrol in the management of cognitive disorders: What is the clinical evidence?" *Molecules (Basel, Switzerland)*, *21*(9), 1243. https://doi.org/10.3390/molecules21091243
60. Obaydah A. A. Alabrahim, and Hassan M. E. S. Azzazy. 2022. "Polymeric nanoparticles for dopamine and levodopa replacement in Parkinson's disease". *Nanoscale Advances*, *4*(24), 5233–5244. https://doi.org/10.1039/d2na00524g
61. Badrul A. Bony, and Forrest M. Kievit. 2019. "A role for nanoparticles in treating traumatic brain injury". *Pharmaceutics*, *11*(9), 473. https://doi.org/10.3390/pharmaceutics11090473

62. Alkaff, S. A., Radhakrishnan, K., Nedumaran, A. M., Liao, P., & Czarny, B. (2020). "Nanocarriers for stroke therapy: Advances and obstacles in translating animal studies". *International Journal of Nanomedicine, 15*, 445–464. https://doi.org/10.2147/IJN.S231853
63. Kabanov, A. V, & Gendelman, H. E. (2007). "Nanomedicine in the diagnosis and therapy of neurodegenerative disorders". *Progress in Polymer Science, 32*(8–9), 1054–1082. https://doi.org/10.1016/j.progpolymsci.2007.05.014

9 Targeting Brain Cancer Using Advanced Nanoparticulate Drug-Delivery Systems

Vikash Kumar

9.1 INTRODUCTION

Cancer is the second leading cause of human mortality [1, 2]. Brain cancer (central nervous system (CNS)-related cancers) is one of the most difficult cancers to treat. Brain tumors are responsible for more than 200,000 deaths worldwide each year [2, 3]. Clinicians treating patients with brain cancer face a number of challenges that can have an impact on the treatment's outcome. Some of the major issues in brain cancer treatment include [4]: 1) Location of the tumor: The location of the brain tumor can make treatment difficult, particularly if it is in a sensitive area of the brain. In such cases, surgical removal of the tumor is highly risky and dangerous. 2) Tumor heterogeneity: Brain tumors are highly heterogeneous in nature, which means that different areas of the tumor may exhibit different characteristics with diverse cell population and microenvironment. This make targeting the tumor with a single treatment modality highly difficult. 3) Blood–brain barrier (BBB): The BBB can block drugs from entering the brain and reaching the tumor. This can reduce the effectiveness of therapy. The BBB is a specialized structure that protects the brain from toxins and pathogens. However, it also limits drug delivery to the brain. 4) Treatment resistance: Brain tumors are known to develop resistance to chemotherapy and radiation therapy, making tumors difficult to treat. 5) Lack of effective therapies: Despite advances in treatment modalities, some types of brain cancer remain difficult to treat, and patients with recurrent or metastatic disease have fewer to no treatment options. Therefore, the successful treatment of brain cancer necessitates a multidisciplinary approach to tackle these issues.

The development of multifunctional nanoparticles that can deliver drugs and imaging agents at the same time could revolutionize brain cancer management. Furthermore, combining nanoparticle-based therapies with immunotherapy and gene therapy may improve their efficacy and patient outcomes. Overall, nanoparticle-based drug delivery and imaging hold great promise for treating difficult cancers like brain cancer. Different types of brain tumors exist based on their cellular origin [5, 6, 7]. Below are examples of cell-origin-specific major brain cancer types Figure 9.1.

DOI: 10.1201/9781032661964-9

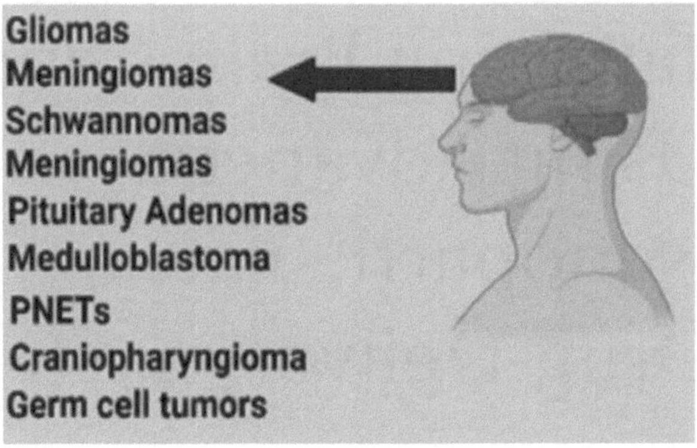

FIGURE 9.1 Figure illustrating major types of human brain tumors. Image was created using Biorender app.

9.1.1 Gliomas

This tumor is developed in glial cells and is characterized by brain or spinal cord based cellular origin. Gliomas include the following tumor subtypes: astrocytoma, glioblastoma, oligoastrocytoma, ependymoma, and oligodendroma. Astrocytoma: Astrocytomas arise from astrocytes, cells involved in the support and nourishment of the brain's nerve cells. Astrocytoma tumors are highly common in adult individuals, with higher incidences in men than women. In the US alone, about 15,000 new astrocytoma cases are reported every year. Astrocytomas are classified into different grades based on the level of tumor size and invasion. Generally, grade IV astrocytomas are referred to as glioblastoma, and have a very high potential to invade distant organs. Astrocytomas cause a wide range of symptoms, including seizures, memory loss, and vision problems, depending on their size and location in the brain. An oligoastrocytoma is rare type of brain cancer that appears to be of mixed glial cell origin, similar to astrocytomas and oligodendrogliomas. An ependymoma is a tumor that develops from the ependyma, a CNS tissue. In most cases, the location is intracranial in children and spinal in adults. The fourth ventricle is a common location for intracranial ependymomas. It is usually observed in people over 40 years of age and is more common in men than women. Tumor reoccurrence in ependymomas is associated with a poor prognosis. Oligodendromas are a subtype of gliomas, which originate from oligodendrocytes or from a glial precursor cell in the brain. Oligodendromas are common in adults and the outcome of therapy depends on the tumor's location, grade, and age (Figure 9.2).

9.1.2 Meningiomas

These tumors develop in the meninges, which are membranes that cover the brain and spinal cord. Meningiomas are usually slow growing and often benign in nature. Some meningiomas can be malignant, aggressive, and difficult to treat. They can develop at

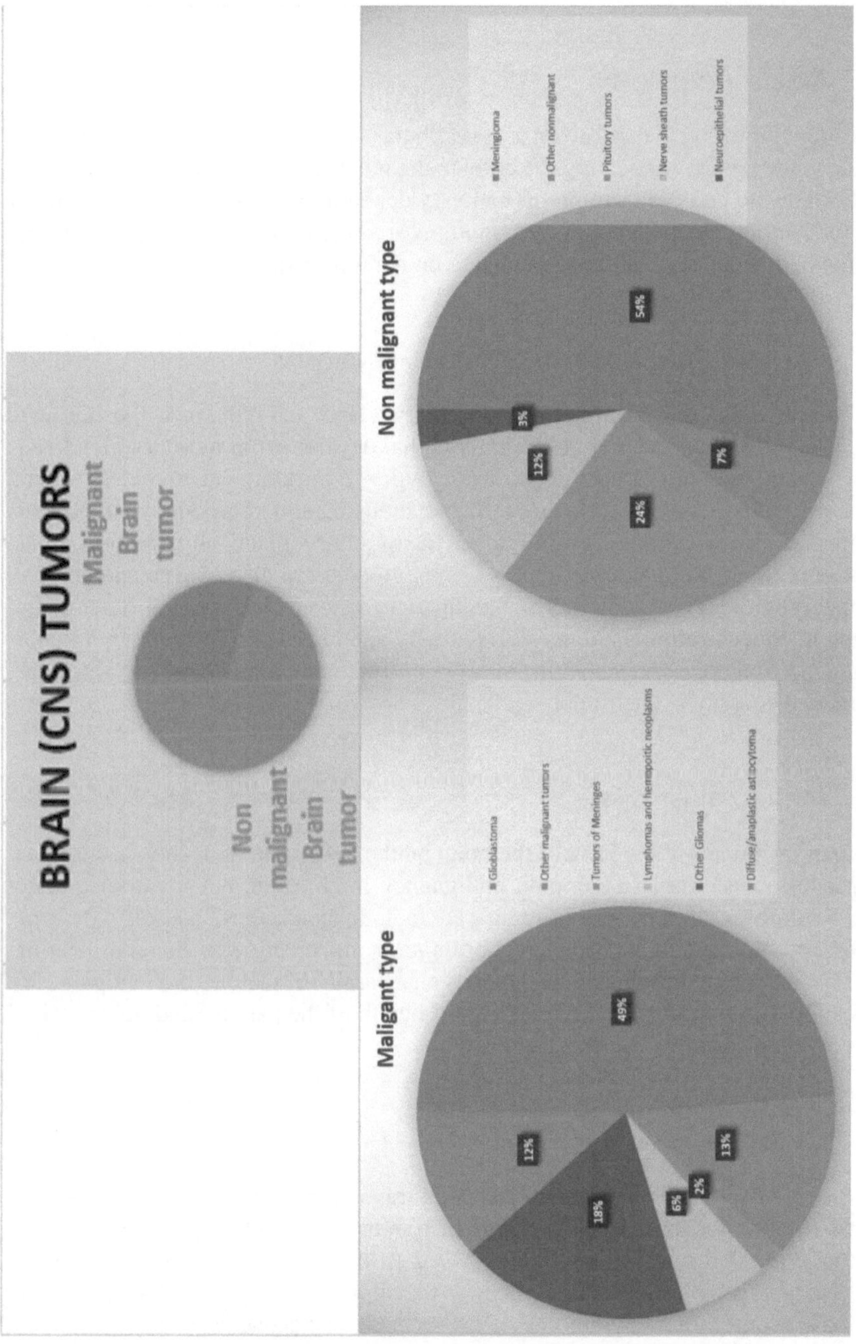

FIGURE 9.2 Classification chart of malignant and non-malignant brain tumor type.

Source: This image was adapted from [8].

any age and are common in older adults, especially women. Treatment for meningiomas is determined by the tumor's size, location, and type.

9.1.3 Acoustic Neuromas

This is a rare tumor type also known as a vestibular schwannoma. Acoustic neuromas originate in the nerves connecting the brain to the inner ear and are usually benign and curable. Acoustic neuroma symptoms can vary depending on the size and location of the tumor. Among the most common symptoms are hearing loss, dizziness or vertigo, problems with balance, and facial weakness on the tumor side.

9.1.4 Pituitary Adenomas and Craniopharyngiomas

These tumors arise in and around the pituitary gland and influence the hormone secreted by it. Pituitary adenomas are tumors that develop from pituitary gland cells and are usually benign. Depending on the type of pituitary adenoma, hormonal imbalances can occur, affecting growth, metabolism, and reproductive functions. Craniopharyngioma tumors develop from the pituitary gland and hypothalamus. Similar to pituitary tumors, craniopharyngioma tumors are also benign and curable. Craniopharyngiomas can cause hormonal imbalance, headache, vision problems, and difficulty in concentrating. Patients with pituitary adenomas and craniopharyngiomas show a good prognosis; however, the success of treatment depends on the type, size, location, and severity of the tumor.

9.1.5 Medulloblastomas

This tumor originates in the back of the brain on the lower part and reaches the spinal cord. Medulloblastoma is a common malignancy in children, but it can also affect adults. Symptoms of medulloblastoma can include headaches, nausea, vomiting, dizziness, problems with balance and coordination, and changes in vision or hearing. The prognosis for medulloblastoma depends on a variety of factors, including the size and location of the tumor, the age and overall health of the patient, and how much of the tumor can be removed surgically.

9.1.6 Germ Cell Tumors (GCTs)

This type of tumor arises from germ cells that travel to the brain from the testes and ovaries during tumor spread. GCTs can be benign or malignant. Malignant GCTs can be further classified into different types based on their cellular origin. In the brain, GCTs typically arise in the pineal gland or the suprasellar region, which is located at the base of the brain. Symptoms of GCTs include headache, visual disruption, nausea, and hormonal imbalance.

9.2 RISK FACTORS

9.2.1 Genetic Factors

Genetically, brain tumors are highly diverse and heterogeneous [9]. There are many genes that have been associated with the progression of brain cancer. Some of them are very well studied and have been implicated in the development of brain cancer, which includes TP53, EGFR, PTEN, and CDKN2A.

TP53: *TP53* is one of the most studied tumor suppressor genes in the human genome and has been implicated in a variety of cancers. *TP53* is involved in regulating cell cycle checkpoints, DNA damage and repair, and cell death. Mutations in this gene have been linked to increased incidences of different types of cancers in many organisms including humans. Germline *TP53* mutations have been associated with many childhood brain cancers [10, 11] and this mutation has been linked to poor disease outcome [12].

EGFR: This gene codes for a receptor involved in epidermal growth factor (EGF) signaling. Dysregulated EGFR signaling is a common phenomenon in cancer and has been associated with poor patient survival [13, 14]. Amplification of EGFR has been associated with more than 40% of glioblastoma cases [15].

IDH1 and IDH2: Isocitrate dehydrogenase (IDH) genes encode enzymes involved in Kreb's cycle and are important for the maintenance of cellular homeostasis. Mutations in these genes are found in various types of cancers, including brain cancer [16]. IDH1 and IDH2 mutations in lower-grade glioblastoma have been associated with better patient outcomes and longer survival [17].

PTEN: Phosphatase and tensin homolog (PTEN) is a PIP3 phosphatase that is involved in oncogenic PI3-kinase signaling regulation [18]. It is involved in the regulation of various cell processes like growth and division, metastasis, and chemoresistance. Mutations in PTEN have been found in a variety of cancers, including glioblastoma. Frequent PTEN mutation has been observed in glioblastoma and is associated with drug resistance [19].

CDKN2A: CDKN2A gene is involved in regulating the cell cycle and preventing the formation of tumors. Mutations in CDKN2A can disrupt the normal function of this gene and lead to uncontrolled cell growth and increased rate of tumor formation [20]. CDKN2A is a commonly mutated gene found in certain types of brain tumors, such as glioblastomas and meningiomas. Patients with glioblastomas who have mutations in CDKN2A tend to have a poorer prognosis and shorter survival times than those without these mutations [21].

9.2.2 Non-genetic/Environmental Factors

Some of the major risk factors associated with brain cancer include radiation exposure, N-nitroso compound-rich food items, viral infection, pesticides, socioeconomic status, age, sex, allergies, and anthropometric factors like body mass index and height. Structural birth defects and familial history of genetics and epigenetics also play an important role in brain cancer incidences [22, 23]. Diet has also been linked to increased and decreased incidences of many cancers. One meta-analysis showed that increased vitamin A, C, D, E, and β-carotene uptake has been linked to lower incidences of brain tumors [24]. Among all brain tumors, glioblastoma is the most prevalent and lethal subtype, having the lowest survival rate and contributing to the majority of brain tumor cases. The five-year survival rate of brain cancer varies from 5% to 20%, making it one of the deadliest cancer types [25]. Conventional treatment modalities for treating brain tumors include surgical tumor removal, radiotherapy, and chemotherapy [26, 27]. However, conventional treatment options are associated with various side effects like increased neurotoxicity, cognitive decline, and dysfunction in neurosensory and neuroendocrine functions. One of the difficulties clinicians face in treating brain cancer patients effectively is delivering the therapeutic payload to the tumor site because of the BBB. The BBB comprises plasma and different types of brain cells, which create a selective environment for the exchange of molecules between blood and brain tissue. This selectivity is important for protecting the brain from pathogens and toxic substances. However, this also blocks the entry of therapeutic molecules like chemotherapeutics, nucleotides, peptides, and other drugs from reaching the brain tumor, thus reducing the efficacy of the anti-cancer treatment and simultaneously increasing the systemic toxicity in the body [28, 29, 30]. Therefore, there is an urgent need to develop improved treatment regimes for addressing these issues. In recent years, NDDS have shown promising results in treating different types of cancers, including brain cancer in preclinical models. The following types of NDDS are being explored by researchers and clinicians for better brain cancer management. A list of Food and Drug Administration (FDA)-approved nanoparticle-based drugs for cancer treatment is shown in Table 9.1.

TABLE 9.1
FDA-approved Nanoparticle Based Drug for Cancer Treatment

Name	Description	Disease	Approved year
DaunoXome	Lipososmal Daunorubicin	HIVassociated Kaposi sarcoma	FDA 96
DepoCyt	Liposomal cytarabin	Lymphomatous meningitis	FDA 96
Oncaspar	PEG asparaginase	Acute lymphoblastic leukemia	FDA 94
Abraxane	Albumin bound paclitaxel nanospheres	Various cancers	FDA 05, EMEA 13, FDA 13
Myocet	Liposomal doxorubicin	Breast cancer	Europe, Canada
Marqibo	Liposomal vincristin	Acute lymphoblastic leukemia	FDA 12
Genexol	Paclitaxel loaded polymeric micelle	Breast cancer, small cell lung cancer	Europe, Korea
Onivyde	Liposomal irinotecan	Pancreatic cancer	FDA 15

TABLE 9.2
Important Physiological Properties of Nanoparticles

Physiological properties of nanoparticles
Low toxic
Biocompatible/Biodegradable
Enhanced stability
Increased retention in circulation
Low immunogenicity
Easily conjugated with drugs, peptides, proteins and oligonucleotides
Less expensive

9.3 IMPORTANT PHYSIOLOGICAL PROPERTIES OF NANOPARTICLES

Nanoparticles possess a number of physiologically important properties that make them an ideal target for drug-delivery applications. Some of these ideal properties are: **Size:** Nanoparticles typically have a diameter of 1–100 nanometers, allowing them to easily pass through biological barriers such as cell membranes and the BBB. Because nanoparticles have a large surface area, they have a higher drug-loading capacity, which means that more drug molecules can be loaded onto a single nanoparticle. **Surface charge:** Nanoparticles' surface charge can be manipulated to improve their cellular uptake and targeting. Positively charged nanoparticles can interact with negatively charged cell membranes, while negatively charged nanoparticles can interact with positively charged proteins. **Surface modification:** The surface of nanoparticles can be modified with targeting ligands, such as antibodies or peptides, which allow for specific recognition and binding to cancer cells or other diseased tissues. **Stability:** Nanoparticles can be designed to have long circulation times in the body, allowing for sustained drug release and increased efficacy. Overall, these physiologically important properties of nanoparticles allow for targeted and effective drug delivery, with the potential to overcome biological barriers and reduce toxicity associated with traditional chemotherapy agents (Table 9.2).

9.4 NANOPARTICLES AS A THERANOSTICS IN BRAIN CANCER MANAGEMENT

Nanoparticles are being investigated as potential theranostic agents in the management of brain cancer. Theranostics is the integration of diagnostic and therapeutic functions into a single entity, and labeled nanoparticles can fulfill both functions [31]. Labeled nanoparticles can be used to directly target and deliver drugs to brain tumor cells, as well as provide real-time imaging of the tumor and surrounding tissues. This can help clinicians diagnose and treat brain cancer more precisely, as well as track the effectiveness of treatment over time. Iron oxide nanoparticles, Gold nanoparticles, and carbon nanotubes are among the labeled nanoparticles that have been studied for use as theranostics for brain cancer [32]. These particles can be engineered to target specific cancer cells and deliver drugs directly to them while remaining detectable by imaging techniques such as magnetic resonance imaging (MRI) and computed tomography (CT) [33, 34, 35]. Overall, labeled nanoparticles have great potential to be exploited as a theranostic tool for brain cancer management, and ongoing research is likely to uncover and throw more light on how to use them more efficiently in brain cancer management.

9.5 NANOPARTICLE-BASED THERAPEUTICS IN BRAIN CANCER TREATMENT

9.5.1 Gold Nanoparticles

Gold nanoparticles (NPs) are usually < 10 nm in size and are used for delivering chemotherapeutic drugs, oligos/nucleotides, and siRNAs in different disease settings. [36]. Gold NPs are FDA approved and have been used in the clinic as a photothermal, contrast, and radiosensitizing agent [37, 38, 39]. The benefits of employing Gold NPs include their controlled release to a specific location, their ability to be altered to increase drug-delivery efficacy, their ability to be passively given, and their potential to be conjugated with receptors like transferrin that are highly expressed in brain tissue [40]. In a recent study, Ruan et al. showed increased efficacy of doxorubicin delivery *in vivo* in glioma mice model using Gold NPs coated with angiopep-2, which can bind to highly expressing low-density lipoprotein related-receptor-1(LRP-1) in brain tumors [41]. Temozolomide (TMZ) has been used in the clinic to treat glioblastoma; however, the tumor eventually develops resistance against TMZ. To increase its efficacy, Yu et al. tethered Gold NPs-TMZ with anti-ephrin and integrated it for chemical and auxiliary plasma photothermal treatment (GNPs-PPTT), which showed increased uptake by glioma cells and induced cell death via apoptosis [42]. Another study used short interfering RNA (siRNA) packed with Gold NPs delivered in the glioblastoma mice model to target Bcl2Like12 (Bcl2L12) oncoprotein. Interestingly, they observed rapid accumulation of Gold NPs-siRNA complex in the glioblastoma tumor, which activated p53 and caspase activity and led to decreased tumor load and increased survival of mice [43]. When combined with other well-known treatments like radiotherapy, Gold NPs have also shown their anti-cancer potential as an adjuvant. A study by Chen et al. indicated that when Gold NPs were combined with radiotherapy, it led to a significant decrease in the tumor burden and improved overall survival of glioma mice [44]. Additionally, Gold NPs can increase the effectiveness of radiation therapy on cancer cells and can significantly lower the radiation doses given to patients, thus reducing adverse effects [45]. Furthermore, Gold NPs can be combined with various biomolecules, drugs and therapeutics like nucleic acid, different drug formulations, photothermal therapy, and X-ray-based computed tomography for better cancer management. Apart from the use of Gold NPs in cancer treatment, it also has the potential to be used in the diagnosis of malignant tumors. [46]. Overall, using Gold NPs in brain cancer management holds promise for enhancing the efficiency of current medicines and lowering their side effects. To completely comprehend the possible advantages and restrictions of utilizing Gold NPs in managing brain cancer, more research is nonetheless required (Figure 9.3).

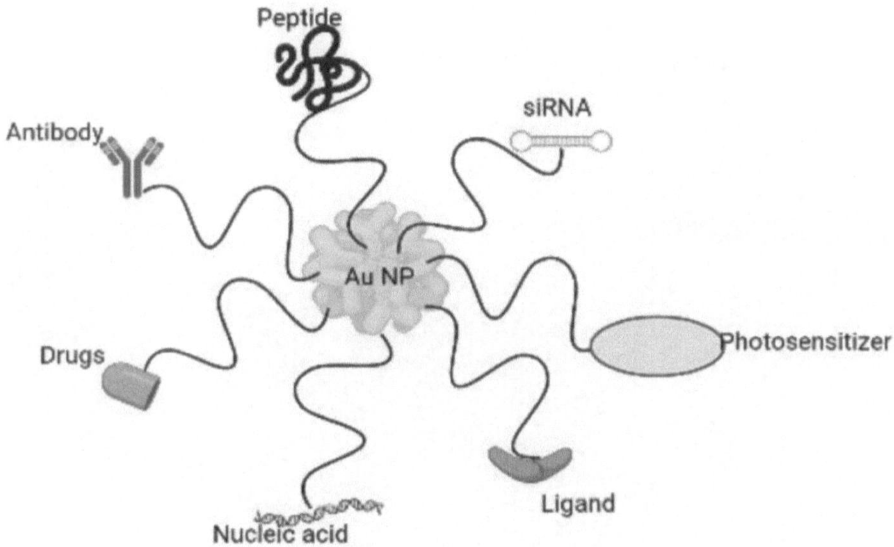

FIGURE 9.3 Gold NPs conjugated with drugs, peptides, antibody, siRNA, nucleic acid, ligand and photosensitizer. Image was created using Biorender app.

9.5.2 Silver Nanoparticles

Silver nanoparticles (NPs) have been extensively studied for their therapeutic potential to manage cancer in preclinical models. Silver NPs have a size ranging from 1 nm to 100 nm [47]. A major part of Silver NPs is silver oxide due to the high surface-to-bulk silver atom ratio. Functionally, Silver NPs induce cell death mostly by generating free radicals. Owing to their smaller size, they can cross nuclear and mitochondrial pores, disrupting the membrane potential and subsequently leading to an unbalanced respiratory chain and the generation of free radicals [48]. In a study conducted by AshaRani et al., it was shown that Silver NP treatment leads to chromosomal abnormalities, increased DNA damage, and changes in the overall morphology of glioblastoma cells [49]. In addition, Silver NPs also showed a potent killing effect on nonhuman glioma cells [50]. In a unique approach, Ubranska et al. grew glioma cells on a chicken embryo chorioallantoic membrane and after 8 days treated it with Silver NPs and found that compared to vehicle control, Silver NP treatment led to significant cell death by caspase induction [51]. Abass et al. investigated the potential of magnetic hyperthermia in combination with silver-doped lanthanum manganite nanoparticles to improve radiation therapy and target radio-resistant brain cancer cells. Real-time imaging after the combined application of radiation and undoped lanthanum manganite nanoparticles showed that 9LGS (glioma cells) growth was inhibited, while MDCK (normal cells) was unaffected. This was the first study to show the biological, in-depth potential of silver-doped lanthanum manganite as a brain cancer selective chemotherapeutic and radiation dose enhancer [52]. Moreover, Ag NPs have also been investigated to build a better cancer diagnostic and detection

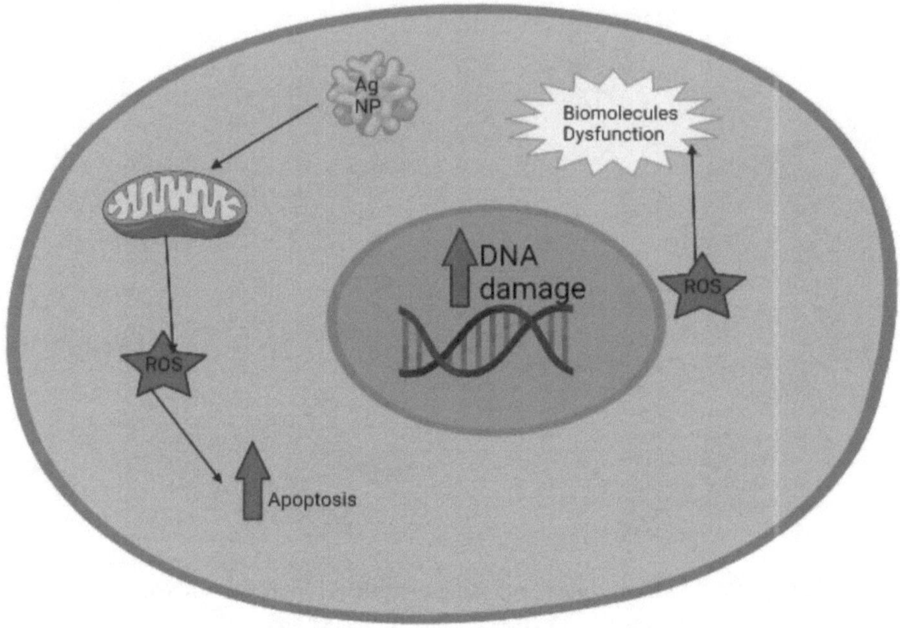

FIGURE 9.4 Treatment of cancer cells with Silver NPs. Silver NPs induce cell death mostly by generating free radicals, which damages DNA and various biomolecules. Image was created using Biorender app.

system [53]. However, it is important to validate optimal dose, route of administration, and potential side effects of Silver NPs, before it can be used in clinical settings for human cancer management (Figure 9.4).

9.5.3 Iron Oxide Nanoparticles in Brain Cancer Management

Iron oxide nanoparticles (IONPs) have been investigated as a potential tool to manage brain tumors due to their modifiable nature, ability to cross the BBB, low toxicity, and effective drug delivery. IONPs are biodegradable and after decomposition, they can get integrated into the physiological iron cycle of the body. Additionally, the surface of IONPs can also be modified and altered to increase their biocompatibility, enhance retention time in blood circulation, and increase surface area for conjugating it with different drugs. This can be achieved by loading it with various polymers like polyethylene glycol (PEG), polyethylene imine (PEI), dextran, and chitosan [54, 55, 56, 57]. In one study, Noorouzi et al. developed a carrier for doxorubicin delivery by using IONPs conjugated and stabilized with trimethoxysilylpropyl-ethylenediamine tri acetic acid (EDT). This combination showed greater efficacy in killing neuroblastoma cells [58]. Yoshida et al. used anti-sense oligonucleotide (ASO) against the MXD3 gene and delivered it after conjugating it with superparamagnetic Fe3O4 NPs (SPIONs), which led to increased apoptosis of neuroblastoma cells. Grillone et al.

encapsulated nutlin-3 and IONPs to target and degrade the MDM2 gene using glioblastoma as a model. MDM2 is an antagonist of p53 and is known to downregulate its expression and function in many cancer types, and has been linked to chemo resistance and poor prognosis. Importantly, it can elicit a strong immune response in mice, when given in combination with immunogenic biomolecules like toll-like receptors (TLR) receptors and CpG DNA [59, 60, 61]. Another approach for using IONPs in brain cancer therapy is through magnetic hyperthermia, a technique that involves applying an alternating magnetic field to IONPs in the tumor region, causing them to generate heat and kill tumor cells. Furthermore, iron oxide-related NPs have shown the potential to be used as a diagnostic tool when employed in combination with known imaging techniques to diagnose and detect brain tumors with increased accuracy [62, 63]. While the use of IONPs in managing brain cancer is still in the early stages of research, it shows promise as a potentially effective and targeted therapy. However, more studies are warranted to fully understand the safety and efficacy of this approach before it can be used to treat human patients.

9.5.4 Zinc Oxide Nanoparticles in Brain Cancer Management

Besides Gold and Silver NPs, zinc oxide nanoparticles (ZnO NPs) have also been studied for their potential use in managing brain cancer. ZnO NPs have unique properties that make them attractive for cancer therapy, including their small size, high surface area to volume ratio, and ability to cross the BBB [64, 65]. Previous research has shown that ZnO NPs can induce cell death in cancer cells through various mechanisms, including the generation of reactive oxygen species, loss of mitochondrial membrane potential, and inhibition of cell division [66, 67]. Also, ZnO NPs have shown tremendous potential in killing circulating tumor cells, which is responsible for metastasis and tumor relapse. Importantly, these nanoparticles have been shown to have low toxicity to healthy cells [68]. Ostrovsky et al. examined the effect of ZnO NPs on human cancer and normal cells. The results showed that the ZnO NPs were cytotoxic to human glioma cancer cells and breast and prostate cancer cell lines, but had no effect on normal cells. The study also found that the ZnO NPs caused an increase in the generation of free radicals in the cancer cells. Based on these results, the study suggests that ZnO NPs could be used as a selective agent for killing different types of cancer cells [69, 70]. Wahab et al. investigated the potential mechanisms of apoptosis induced by self-designed zinc oxide nanostructures (ZnO-NSts) on human T98G glioma cells. Their study included four types of ZnO-NSts: nanoplates (NPls), nanorods (NRs), nanosheets (NSs), and nanoflowers (NFs). They found that NRs induced oxidative stress and caspase activation, which led to cytotoxicity and inhibitory effects on cancer cells in a dose-dependent manner. These findings could provide new insights into the research of targeted cancer nanotechnology and may have the potential to improve therapeutic outcomes [71]. Another study investigated the therapeutic potential of ZnO NPs conjugated with folic acid (FA) on glioblastoma multiform (GBM) U87MG cell line *in vitro*. The MTT assay showed that after 12 hours, the viability of GBM U87MG cells significantly decreased at concentrations of 1.25 and 2.5 mg/ml, while no such effect was observed in normal astrocytes. These findings suggest that dose-dependent conjugated ZnO NPs could play a therapeutic role in cancer therapy [72]. However, it is important to note that the use of nanoparticles in cancer therapy is still in its early stages, and further research is needed to fully understand their potential benefits and risks.

9.6 ORGANIC NANOPARTICLE-BASED BRAIN CANCER MANAGEMENT

9.6.1 Lipid-based Nanoparticles in Brain Tumor Treatment

Micelles and liposomes are organic NPs made up of different types of physiological lipid formulations. Based on biophysical properties, micelles are single lipid bilayer NPs that are smaller than liposomes and can encapsulate or bind hydrophobic medicines, whereas liposomes are made up of one or multiple lipid bilayers that form an internal aqueous compartment and an exterior lipophilic layer. Recently, liposomes have been used to deliver drugs to treat brain tumors in preclinical models, because of their higher biocompatibility and biodegradability, low toxicity, and ability to load both hydrophilic and hydrophobic drugs [73, 74]. There is evidence showing that lipid nanoparticles (NPs) can build up specifically in the tumor tissue as a result of increased permeability and retention. [75]. Liposomes conjugated with a specific ligand, such as transferrin, glucose transporter, or endothelial growth factor, can target the CNS through receptor-mediated endocytosis, allowing the positively charged lipid-derived NPs to cross the BBB efficiently [76]. Aberrant hedgehog (Hh) signaling is known to be involved in medulloblastoma carcinogenesis and progression. To target this, Infante et al. developed amphiphilic self-assembling micelles to deliver Glabrescione B (Gla B), an Hh inhibitor, to deliver it to the tumor tissue. This led to significant inhibition of tumor growth in both allograft and orthotopic models of Hh-dependent medulloblastoma in mice [77]. In another study, Bell et al. [78] developed high-density lipoprotein (HDL) NPs to target the scavenger receptor class B type 1 (SCARB1). Interestingly, HDL-NPs-SCARB1 showed antineoplastic effects against the sonic hedgehog subtype of medulloblastoma (SHH-MB) and potent inhibitory effects on cancer stem cells. Targeting cancer stem cells is clinically important as it can prevent tumor recurrence and drug resistance. To increase bioavailability and reduce off-targets, Kim et al. created high-density lipoprotein-mimetic nanoparticles that could cross the BBB and deliver a sonic hedgehog (SHH) inhibitor *in vivo*. These NPs were created by combining anti-CD15 and apolipoprotein A1 to achieve dual-targeted delivery by binding to SCARB1 and CD15, both of which have SHH-expressing medulloblastoma cells. This formulation showed the potential of lipid NPs in the successful *in vivo* delivery of therapeutics with minimal off-target effects [79]. Lipid-based NPs have various advantages, including easy formulation, biocompatibility, and the ability to conjugate both lipophilic and hydrophilic drugs. However, despite these advantages, lipid NPs can cause systemic toxicity as they have shown high accumulation in various regions of the body, which persisted for a very long period of time [80, 81]. Several modifications of lipid NPs have been reported to decrease systemic toxicity and increase retention time in the body. One of the modifications wherein lipid NPs are coated by polyethylene glycol (PEGylation)

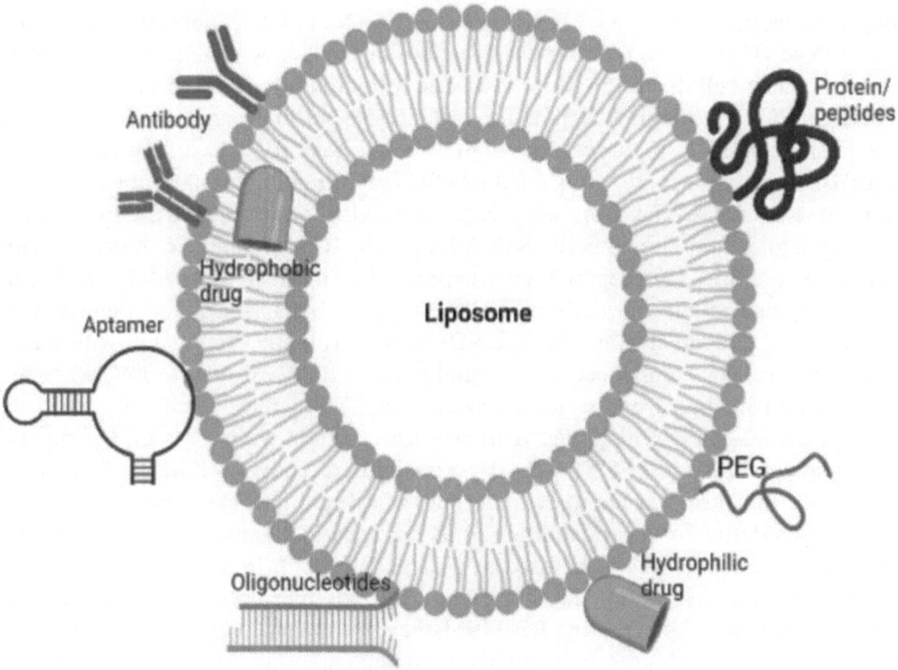

FIGURE 9.5 Liposome conjugated with drugs, protein/peptides, PEG, antibody, and oligonucleotides. Image was created using Biorender app.

showed significantly reduced microglia activation and neuro-inflammation, and increased biocompatibility. Another study showed successful delivery of antisense oligonucleotide using receptor-coated pegylated immunoliposome, which showed indicated inhibition in glioma cell growth [82, 83]. In one recent study, Li et al. screened more than 700 physilogical lipids and successfully delivered gene-editing therapies (CRISPR RNA-LNPs) to the lungs via inhalation. This breakthrough not only enables therapeutic CRISPR applications for gene editing but also for gene therapy to treat cancer and other complicated diseases [84]. Additionally, lipid NPs have the potential to be used in cancer diagnosis. Overall, lipid NPs show significant potential as a drug-delivery system in preclinical models; however, more studies are needed to validate their safety and efficacy before they can be used in human brain cancer management (Figure 9.5).

9.6.2 Carbon Nitride Dots in Brain Cancer Treatment and Diagnosis

Carbon dots are small, biocompatible, low toxic, and have the potential to be used in diagnosis and therapy. Carbon nitride dots (CNDs) are a novel subclass of carbon dots, which has recently gained attention in cancer treatment and diagnosis, including brain cancer [85]. CNDs have interesting physiochemical and optical properties, which make it an ideal candidate for fluorescene-based cancer diagnosis [86]. CNDs, along with gadolinium or Fe3+, have been used as a tool to detect breast tumors [87]. Gemcitabine (GM), a commonly used nucleoside analog with anti-cancer properties, can induce cell death in cancer cells due to its inhibitory effect on DNA polymerase activity. Although GM is highly effective in killing cancer cells, however, it has a short half-life in circulation, high systemic toxicity, and difficulty crossing the BBB, which has severely impacted its efficacy in treating brain tumors. To overcome these issues, CNDs were conjugated with GM, which increased its potency in killing high-grade glioma cells [88]. Additionally, CNDs can be conjugated with transferrin receptors (a receptor highly expressed in brain tumor cells), which can increase their specificity for delivery and crossing the BBB. In a study conducted by Li et al. using Zebrafish as a model, CNDs were covalently conjugated with transferrin receptor, which enhanced its potential to cross the BBB and reach CNS tissue via a receptor-mediated endocytosis process [89]. To increase specificity for drug delivery, Liyanage et al. conjugated transferrin receptor with CND-GM complex. This triple combination of CND-GM-Tf was highly effective in killing tumor cells. Importantly, this dose was not toxic to normal cells, highlighting its specific nature in targeted drug delivery [90]. In addition to its therapeutic potential, carbon dot-based NPs also possess potential to be used as a diagnostic tool. In a study conducted by Liu et al., to examine the potential of carbonized polymer dots (CPDs) in marking tumor boundaries and penetrating BBB [91], they found that CPDs possess long excitation/emission wavelengths, low toxicity, high photostability, and excellent biocompatibility. In time- and dose-dependent processes, CPDs showed high internalization in glioma cells. Both *in vitro* and *in vivo* studies confirmed the BBB permeability of CPDs, which visualized tumors in the brain without compromising the BBB. Moreover, under *ex vivo* conditions, the high tumor-to-normal tissue ratio of CPDs provides potential for guiding brain-tumor resection through real-time fluorescence imaging during surgery. While various carbon dot-based NPs have shown promise as a potential theranostic target for brain cancer management, more research is needed to fully understand their efficacy and safety in humans.

9.6.3 Dendrimers in the Treatment of Brain Cancer

Dendrimers range from 1 to 100 nm in size and are highly organized, radially symmetric, and branched organic polymers. The molecular structure, physicochemical stability, and water solubility of dendrimers make them an ideal target for drug delivery. In recent years, dendrimers have become increasingly popular as a drug-delivery system due to their ability to be highly modifiable nature [92, 93]. Dendrimers have also been used in the delivery of various molecules like short oligonucleotides, siRNAs, and antibodies [94, 95]. The dual-targeting drug carrier PEGylated Poly(amidoamine) combined with wheat germ agglutinin and transferrin (PAMAM)-PEG-WGA-Tf) offers an improved way to deliver therapeutic compounds to tumor tissue such as doxorubicin, enabling greater efficiency for effective delivery in the tumor tissue and less toxicity to the surrounding tissue [96]. He et al., using TEM microscopy, showed that PAMAM-PEG-WGA-Tf was very small in size, which made it cross the BBB, allowing it to effectively deliver a drug payload to the tumor tissue. Moreover, it reduced toxicity to normal cells and showed significantly higher doxorubicin delivery, and inhibited growth of glioma cells compared to conventional methods. In another approach to enhance penetration and retention, Zhao et al. created a nanoparticle that targets extracellular fibrin in brain tumors by conjugating PAMAM dendrimers with the fibrin-binding peptide CREKA. CREKA-modified PAMAM achieved higher accumulation and deeper penetration in glioblastoma multiforme (GBM) tissue than unmodified PAMAM, showing that this strategy might be very helpful in increasing drug permeability and retention for brain tumor therapy [97]. While dendrimers have shown promise for treating brain cancer, more research is needed to fully understand their efficacy and safety in humans.

9.7 RNA-BASED NANOPARTICLES FOR BRAIN CANCER MANAGEMENT

In the past decade, RNA as a therapeutic target has been studied extensively in different disease settings [98]. The unique property of RNA to target a specific gene makes it an attractive candidate for targeted cancer therapy. RNA species that have the potential to be used in cancer management are **siRNA**: These are double-stranded artificially synthesized RNA species that mimic cellular miRNA and are used to target and degrade messenger RNA (mRNA) transcripts to silence specific genes. In brain cancer, siRNAs can be programmed to target oncogenes or other genes involved in tumor growth and survival. Aberrant miRNA expression in cancer can contribute to tumor growth and progression. Therapeutic siRNAs can be used to restore normal levels of mRNA expression or to block the expression of specific oncogenic mRNAs. **ASOs:** ASOs are single-stranded DNA/RNA molecules that bind to specific mRNA transcripts and prevent them from being translated into proteins. ASOs can be designed to target overexpressed genes in brain cancer, such as the epidermal growth factor receptor (EGFR), or to target mRNAs that are upregulated in cancer. Few studies have also been conducted in treating brain tumors using RNA as a target. In one of the studies, Sayour et al. created a clinically translatable nanoparticle (NP) formulation, wherein they coupled tumor-derived total RNA with NPs to induce systemic anti-tumor t-cell immunity against medulloblastoma. This led to increased expression of co-stimulatory signaling molecules and subsequent induction of anti-tumor t-cell immunity. This outcome is crucial as brain tumors are known to dampen t-cell-mediated anti-tumor response during tumor progression. Now, Sayour et al. are trying to test this formulation for its safety, stability, effectiveness, and immunologic effects in a malignant canine brain tumor model, before it can be tested in human brain cancer patients [99]. One of the most recent approaches for treating human cancers, including GBM, is RNA interference (RNAi). Small RNA oligonucleotides are used in RNAi-based therapeutics to control protein expression at the post-transcriptional stage [100]. Despite the therapeutic potential of RNAi molecules, their progress into the clinic has been hindered by various issues such as decreased stability in circulation and poor release into the tumor tissue [101]. Another difficulty is getting RNAi molecules to cross the BBB effectively. Recently, Grafal-Ruiz et al. showed that small

RNA oligonucleotides targeting miRNA 92-b (an aberrantly expressed miRNA in glioblastoma cell lines and tumors) encapsulated in Gold NPs can successfully reduce its expression and overall tumor load. This shows the potential of nanoparticle-based drug delivery to target and ablate genes specific to brain tumors [102, 103]. In another interesting study, Hector Mendez-Gomez et al. modified an mRNA backbone transcript epigenetically to induce rapid anti-tumor activity against gliomas. This approach was successful in delivering positive immunomodulators like GM-CSF along with siRNA-targeting negative regulators like PD-L1. This formulation induced glioma-specific immune cell activation. Interestingly, this led to a human trial for treating children with lower-grade gliomas [104]. Another issue that has been observed in using messenger RNA (mRNA) vaccines in the clinic is that it can cause liver-related side effects such as reversible liver damage and t-cell-mediated hepatitis, which can lead to unintended antigen expression in the liver. To address this issue, Chen et al. used a lymphoid-organ-specific mRNA vaccine that should be investigated as a potential strategy for developing a next-generation mRNA vaccine, 113-O12B, a lymph-node-targeting mRNA based on lipid nanoparticles. This mRNA vaccine's targeted delivery effectively induced strong CD8+ T cell responses, resulting in impressive protective and therapeutic effects against B16F10 melanoma. Furthermore, 113-O12B is capable of delivering both full-length protein and short-peptide-based antigen-encoded mRNA, making it a versatile antigen delivery system [105]. In preclinical studies and early-phase clinical trials for the treatment of brain cancer, RNA-based therapeutics have shown promising results. However, more research is needed to fully understand their efficacy, safety, and physiological/immunological consequences before they can be used in brain cancer management.

9.8 IMMUNOTHERAPY-BASED BRAIN CANCER MANAGEMENT

Brain cancer is immunologically "cold," making it unsuitable for conventional immunotherapeutic approaches. [106]. In an approach to make such tumors immune responsive, Turco et al. used an NP-based formulation in a glioma mice model to target immune suppressive cells. Briefly, they used toll-like receptors 7 and 8 (TLR7/8) agonist R848, encapsulated in a formulation of cyclodextrin nanoparticles (CDNP-R848) that is intended to rewire myeloid cell signaling in the glioma microenvironment. They demonstrated that intravenous monotherapy with CDNP-R848 caused regression of a syngeneic experimental glioma tumor, leading to higher survival rates of mice when compared to CDNP controls that are not loaded. This anti-tumor effect was independent of t-cells and NK cells. Instead, CDNP-R848 therapy alters the immunosuppressive tumor microenvironment and orchestrates tumor clearance by pro-inflammatory tumor-associated myeloid cells. Mechanistically, a radiomic signature was detected in response after CDNP-R848 treatment using serial magnetic resonance imaging, and ultra-small superparamagnetic iron oxide (USPIO) imaging, which showed a reduction in the recruitment of immunosuppressive macrophages in the tumor microenvironment [107]. In another approach to activate cytotoxic t-cells and inhibit PD-L1, Tian et al. engineered extracellular vesicles (EVs) by coating them with the peptide RGDyK, targeting brain tumor cells, and encapsulated siRNA against PD-L1. They co-treated glioma tumor cells with modified EVs with bursts of radiation and found increased targeting efficiency of RGD-EV to murine GBM, reversed radiation-induced PD-L1 expression, and increased activity of cytotoxic t-cells, which led to reduced tumor load and increased survival of mice [108]. Immunotherapy-based approaches hold great potential and have been used in the clinic for treating different types of cancers; however, further studies and thorough investigations are needed before they can be used in brain cancer management.

9.9 CONCLUSION

Despite significant achievements in understanding cancer as a disease, however, the treatment modalities have not been improved significantly, especially for lethal cancers like brain cancer, which still relies heavily on conventional therapy. This approach leads to substantial adverse effects like nephrotoxicity, cardiotoxicity, and infertility, which is linked to the poor quality of life of patients' undergoing anti-cancer therapy. Effective and targeted drug delivery in brain tumors can minimize this problem. The field of NDDS has been growing rapidly in terms of its uses in various disease settings and has the potential to be exploited as a drug-delivery system to transport various prophylactics and therapeutic formulations in different parts of the body including the brain. During the Covid-19 outbreak, several vaccine formulations based on nanoparticle technology were developed and approved for use in emergency situations around the world. The Pfizer-BioNTech Covid-19 vaccine, for example, uses lipid nanoparticles to deliver a small piece of genetic material called messenger RNA (mRNA), which encodes for the SARS-CoV-2 virus's spike protein. An NDDS has shown promising results in treating different types of cancer, including brain cancer in various preclinical models. Also, NDDS have shown potential to be programmed to release drugs in response to specific signals within the body, allowing for personalized and precise brain cancer diagnosis and treatment. While more research is needed, limited studies have shown that NDDS may provide several advantages for better management of brain tumors, which includes its ability to cross the BBB and effectively deliver a therapeutic payload in the tumor, thus causing less systemic toxicity and increasing drug bioavailability. However, despite a few encouraging preclinical results, NDDS is still at its early stages of development. Although limited formulations have been made to clinical trials, none of them have reached the clinic for treating brain cancer patients. Some of the disadvantages that might render its slow progress to the clinic include differences in physiology between humans and the models used in a study, reduced therapeutic delivery, recognition by the immune system, and inconsistency in results reported in different studies. These issues should be addressed to make NDDS a better delivery model. In conclusion, a NDDS holds great potential in brain cancer management; however, further studies are warranted to address the remaining challenges and optimize the use of nanoparticles in clinical settings.

REFERENCES

1. "The global burden of cancer attributable to risk factors, 2010–19: a systematic analysis for the Global Burden of Disease Study 2019," VOLUME 400, ISSUE 10352, P563–591, AUGUST 20, 2022. GBD 2019 Cancer Risk Factors Collaborators: Lancet. 2022 Aug 20;400(10352):563–591. doi: 10.1016/S0140-6736(22)01438-6
2. Miller KD, Ostrom QT, Kruchko C, Patil N, Tihan T, Cioffi G, Fuchs HE, Waite KA, Jemal A, Siegel RL, Barnholtz-Sloan JS. "Brain and other central nervous system tumor statistics," 2021. *CA Cancer J Clin.* 2021 Sep;71(5):381–406. doi: 10.3322/caac.21693. Epub 2021 Aug 24. PMID: 34427324.
3. "Global, regional, and national burden of brain and other CNS cancer, 1990–2016: a systematic analysis for the Global Burden of Disease Study 2016," VOLUME 18, ISSUE 4, P376–393, APRIL 2019 GBD 2016 Brain and Other CNS Cancer Collaborators. Lancet Neurol 2019; 18: 376–93 DOI:https://doi.org/10.1016/S1474-4422(18)30468-X
4. Mellinghoff, Ingo K, and Richard J. Gilbertson. "Brain tumors: challenges and opportunities to cure." *J Clin Oncol* 35, no. 21 (2017): 2343–2345.
5. Louis D, Ohgaki H, Wiestler O et al. "The 2007 WHO Classification of Tumours of the Central Nervous System." *Acta Neuropathol.* 2007;114(2):97–109.
6. Louis D, Perry A, Reifenberger G et al. "The 2016 World Health Organization Classification of Tumors of the Central Nervous System: A Summary." *Acta Neuropathol.* 2016;131(6):803–20.
7. Louis D, Perry A, Wesseling P et al. "The 2021 WHO Classification of Tumors of the Central Nervous System: A Summary." *Neuro-Oncology.* 2021;23(8):1231–51.
8. Miller, Kimberly D, Quinn T Ostrom, Carol Kruchko, Nirav Patil, Tarik Tihan, Gino Cioffi, Hannah E Fuchs et al. "Brain and other central nervous system tumor statistics, 2021." *CA: A Cancer Journal for Clinicians* 71, no. 5 (2021): 381–406.
9. Sottoriva, Andrea, Inmaculada Spiteri, Sara GM Piccirillo, Anestis Touloumis, V Peter Collins, John C Marioni, Christina Curtis, Colin Watts, and Simon Tavaré. "Intratumor heterogeneity in human glioblastoma reflects cancer evolutionary dynamics." *Proceedings of the National Academy of Sciences* 110, no. 10 (2013): 4009–4014.
10. Stark, AM, P Witzel, RJ Strege, HH Hugo, and HM Mehdorn. "p53, mdm2, EGFR, and msh2 expression in paired initial and recurrent glioblastoma multiforme." *Journal of Neurology, Neurosurgery & Psychiatry* 74, no. 6 (2003): 779–783.
11. Fulci, Giulia, Nobuaki Ishii, and Erwin G Van Meir. "p53 and brain tumors: from gene mutations to gene therapy." *Brain Pathology* 8, no. 4 (1998): 599–613.
12. York, D, RJ Higgins, RA LeCouteur, AN Wolfe, R Grahn, N Olby, M Campbell, and PJ Dickinson. "TP53 mutations in canine brain tumors." *Veterinary Pathology* 49, no. 5 (2012): 796–801.
13. Ruano, Yolanda, Teresa Ribalta, Ángel Rodríguez de Lope, Yolanda Campos-Martín, Concepción Fiaño, Elisa Pérez-Magán, José-Luis Hernández-Moneo, Manuela Mollejo, and Bárbara Meléndez. "Worse outcome in primary glioblastoma multiforme with concurrent epidermal growth factor receptor and p53 alteration." *American Journal of Clinical Pathology* 131, no. 2 (2009): 257–263.
14. Hatanpaa, Kimmo J, Sandeep Burma, Dawen Zhao, and Amyn A Habib. "Epidermal growth factor receptor in glioma: signal transduction, neuropathology, imaging, and radioresistance." *Neoplasia* 12, no. 9 (2010): 675–684.
15. Liu, Haijing, Bo Zhang, and Zhifu Sun. "Spectrum of EGFR aberrations and potential clinical implications: insights from integrative pan-cancer analysis." *Cancer communications* 40, no. 1 (2020): 43–59.

16. Yan, Hai, D. Williams Parsons, Genglin Jin, Roger McLendon, B. Ahmed Rasheed, Weishi Yuan, Ivan Kos et al. "IDH1 and IDH2 mutations in gliomas." *New England Journal of Medicine* 360, no. 8 (2009): 765–773.
17. Han, Sue, Yang Liu, Sabrina J Cai, Mingyu Qian, Jianyi Ding, Mioara Larion, Mark R Gilbert, and Chunzhang Yang. "IDH mutation in glioma: molecular mechanisms and potential therapeutic targets." *British Journal of Cancer* 122, no. 11 (2020): 1580–1589.
18. Yang, JR-M, Paula Schiapparelli, Hoai-Nghia Nguyen, Atsushi Igarashi, Qiang Zhang, Sara Abbadi, L Mario Amzel, Hiromi Sesaki, Alfredo Quinones-Hinojosa, and Miho Iijima. "Characterization of PTEN mutations in brain cancer reveals that pten mono-ubiquitination promotes protein stability and nuclear localization." *Oncogene* 36, no. 26 (2017): 3673–3685.
19. Koul, Dimpy. "PTEN signaling pathways in glioblastoma." *Cancer Biology & Therapy* 7, no. 9 (2008): 1321–1325.
20. Funakoshi, Yusuke, Nobuhiro Hata, Kosuke Takigawa, Hideyuki Arita, Daisuke Kuga, Ryusuke Hatae, Yuhei Sangatsuda et al. "Clinical significance of CDKN2A homozygous deletion in combination with methylated MGMT status for IDH-wildtype glioblastoma." *Cancer Medicine* 10, no. 10 (2021): 3177–3187.
21. Fortin Ensign, Shannon P, Robert B Jenkins, Caterina Giannini, Jann N Sarkaria, Evanthia Galanis, and Sani H Kizilbash. "Translational significance of CDKN2A/B homozygous deletion in isocitrate dehydrogenase-mutant astrocytoma." *Neuro-Oncology* 25, no. 1 (2023): 28–36.
22. Rasheed S, Rehman K, Akash MSH. "An insight into the risk factors of brain tumors and their therapeutic interventions." *Biomed Pharmacother. 2021* Nov;143:112119. doi: 10.1016/j.biopha.2021.112119. Epub 2021 Aug 30. PMID: 34474351.
23. Ostrom QT, Adel Fahmideh M, Cote DJ, Muskens IS, Schraw JM, Scheurer ME, Bondy ML. "Risk factors for childhood and adult primary brain tumors." *Neuro Oncol.* 2019 Nov 4;21(11):1357–1375. doi: 10.1093/neuonc/noz123. PMID: 31301133; PMCID: PMC6827837.
24. Zhang W, Jiang J, He Y, Li X, Yin S, Chen F, Li W. Association between vitamins and risk of brain tumors: A systematic review and dose-response meta-analysis of observational studies. *Front Nutr.* 2022 Jul 29;9:935706. doi: 10.3389/fnut.2022.935706. PMID: 35967781; PMCID: PMC9372437.
25. Davis ME. "Glioblastoma: overview of disease and treatment." *Clin J Oncol Nurs.* 2016 Oct 1;20(5 Suppl):S2–8. doi: 10.1188/16.CJON.S1.2-8. PMID: 27668386; PMCID: PMC5123811.
26. Naser, R, Dilabazian, H, Bahr, H, Barakat, A, El-Sibai, M. "A guide through conventional and modern cancer treatment modalities: A specific focus on glioblastoma cancer therapy (Review)." *Oncology Reports* 48, no. 5 (2022): 190. Doi:10.3892/or.2022.8405
27. Mo F, Pellerino A, Soffietti R, Rudà R. "Blood–brain barrier in brain tumors: biology and clinical relevance." *Int J Mol Sci.* 2021 Nov 23;22(23):12654. Doi:10.3390/ijms222312654
28. Hajal, C., Offeddu, G.S., Shin, Y. et al. "Engineered human blood–brain barrier microfluidic model for vascular permeability analyses." *Nat Protoc* 17, 95–128 (2022).
29. Aldape, Kenneth, Kevin M Brindle, Louis Chesler, Rajesh Chopra, Amar Gajjar, Mark R Gilbert, Nicholas Gottardo et al. "Challenges to curing primary brain tumours." *Nature Reviews Clinical Oncology* 16, no. 8 (2019): 509–520.
30. Cerna, Tereza, Marie Stiborova, Vojtech Adam, Rene Kizek, and Tomas Eckschlager. "Nanocarrier drugs in the treatment of brain tumors." *Journal of Cancer Metastasis and Treatment* 2 (2016): 407–416.

31. Biddlestone-Thorpe, Laura, Nicola Marchi, Kathy Guo, Chaitali Ghosh, Damir Janigro, Kristoffer Valerie, and Hu Yang. "Nanomaterial-mediated CNS delivery of diagnostic and therapeutic agents." *Advanced Drug Delivery Reviews* 64, no. 7 (2012): 605–613.
32. Kelkar, Sneha S, and Theresa M Reineke. "Theranostics: combining imaging and therapy." *Bioconjugate Chemistry* 22, no. 10 (2011): 1879–1903.
33. Kelkar, Sneha S, and Theresa M Reineke. "Theranostics: combining imaging and therapy." *Bioconjugate Chemistry* 22, no. 10 (2011): 1879–1903.
34. Bernd, Hamm, Eric De Kerviler, Sophie Gaillard, and Bruno Bonnemain. "Safety and tolerability of ultrasmall superparamagnetic iron oxide contrast agent: comprehensive analysis of a clinical development program." *Investigative Radiology* 44, no. 6 (2009): 336–342.
35. Meyers, Joseph D, Tennyson Doane, Clemens Burda, and James P Basilion. "Nanoparticles for imaging and treating brain cancer." *Nanomedicine* 8, no. 1 (2013): 123–143.
36. Singh, Priyanka, Santosh Pandit, VRSS Mokkapati, Abhroop Garg, Vaishnavi Ravikumar, and Ivan Mijakovic. "Gold nanoparticles in diagnostics and therapeutics for human cancer." *International Journal of Molecular Sciences* 19, no. 7 (2018): 1979.
37. Meola, Antonio, Jianghong Rao, Navjot Chaudhary, Mayur Sharma, and Steven D Chang. "Gold nanoparticles for brain tumor imaging: a systematic review." *Frontiers in Neurology* 9 (2018): 328.
38. Bloise, Nora, Silvia Strada, Giacomo Dacarro, and Livia Visai. "Gold nanoparticles contact with cancer cell: a brief update." *International Journal of Molecular Sciences* 23, no. 14 (2022): 7683.
39. Sibuyi, NRS, Moabelo, KL, Fadaka, AO et al. "Multifunctional gold nanoparticles for improved diagnostic and therapeutic applications: a review." *Nanoscale Res Lett* 16, 174 (2021). https://doi.org/10.1186/s11671-021-03632-w
40. Ruan, Shaobo, Mingqing Yuan, Li Zhang, Guanlian Hu, Jiantao Chen, Xingli Cun, Qianyu Zhang, Yuting Yang, Qin He, and Huile Gao. "Tumor microenvironment sensitive doxorubicin delivery and release to glioma using angiopep-2 decorated gold nanoparticles." *Biomaterials* 37 (2015): 425–435.
41. Yu, Yawen, Aiping Wang, Siqi Wang, Yuchen Sun, Liuxiang Chu, Lin Zhou, Xiaoyue Yang et al. "Efficacy of temozolomide-conjugated gold nanoparticle photothermal therapy of drug-resistant glioblastoma and its mechanism study." *Molecular Pharmaceutics* 19, no. 4 (2022): 1219–1229.
42. Jensen, Samuel A, Emily S Day, Caroline H Ko, Lisa A Hurley, Janina P Luciano, Fotini M Kouri, Timothy J Merkel et al. "Spherical nucleic acid nanoparticle conjugates as an RNAi-based therapy for glioblastoma." *Science Translational Medicine* 5, no. 209 (2013): 209ra152–209ra152.
43. Chen, Yao, Juan Yang, Shaozhi Fu, and Jingbo Wu. "Gold nanoparticles as radiosensitizers in cancer radiotherapy." *International Journal of Nanomedicine* (2020): 9407–9430.
44. Antosh, Michael P, Dayanjali D Wijesinghe, Samana Shrestha, Robert Lanou, Yun Hu Huang, Thomas Hasselbacher, David Fox et al. "Enhancement of radiation effect on cancer cells by gold-pHLIP." *Proceedings of the National Academy of Sciences* 112, no. 17 (2015): 5372–5376.
45. New. Yang, Yan, Xi Zheng, Lu Chen, Xuefeng Gong, Hao Yang, Xingmei Duan, and Yuxuan Zhu. "Multifunctional gold nanoparticles in cancer diagnosis and treatment." *International Journal of Nanomedicine* (2022): 2041–2067.

46. Nguyen, Ngan NT, Colleen McCarthy, Darlin Lantigua, and Gulden Camci-Unal. "Development of diagnostic tests for detection of SARS-CoV-2." *Diagnostics* 10, no. 11 (2020): 905.
47. Graf C, Vossen DL, Imhof A, van Blaaderen A (July 11, 2003). "A general method to coat colloidal particles with silica." *Langmuir*. 19 (17): 6693–6700. doi:10.1021/la0347859
48. Verano-Braga, Thiago, Rona Miethling-Graff, Katarzyna Wojdyla, Adelina Rogowska-Wrzesinska, Jonathan R Brewer, Helmut Erdmann, and Frank Kjeldsen. "Insights into the cellular response triggered by silver nanoparticles using quantitative proteomics." *ACS Nano* 8, no. 3 (2014): 2161–2175.
49. Asharani, PV, M Prakash Hande, and Suresh Valiyaveettil. "Anti-proliferative activity of silver nanoparticles." *BMC Cell Biology* 10 (2009): 1–14.
50. Salazar-García, Samuel, Jose Fernando García-Rodrigo, Gabriel A Martínez-Castañón, Victor Manuel Ruiz-Rodríguez, Diana Patricia Portales-Pérez, and Carmen Gonzalez. "Silver nanoparticles (AgNPs) and zinc chloride (ZnCl 2) exposure order determines the toxicity in C6 rat glioma cells." *Journal of Nanoparticle Research* 22 (2020): 1–13.
51. Urbańska K, Pająk B, Orzechowski A, Sokołowska J, Grodzik M, Sawosz E, Szmidt M, Sysa P. "The effect of silver nanoparticles (AgNPs) on proliferation and apoptosis of in ovo cultured glioblastoma multiforme (GBM) cells." *Nanoscale Res Lett*. 2015 Mar 1;10:98. doi: 10.1186/s11671-015-0823-5
52. Khochaiche, Abass, Matt Westlake, Alice O'Keefe, Elette Engels, Sarah Vogel, Michael Valceski, Nan Li et al. "First extensive study of silver-doped lanthanum manganite nanoparticles for inducing selective chemotherapy and radio-toxicity enhancement." *Materials Science and Engineering*: C 123 (2021): 111970.
53. Huy, Tran Q, Pham Huyen, Anh-Tuan Le, and Matteo Tonezzer. "Recent advances of silver nanoparticles in cancer diagnosis and treatment." *Anti-Cancer Agents in Medicinal Chemistry (Formerly Current Medicinal Chemistry-Anti-Cancer Agents)* 20, no. 11 (2020): 1276–1287.
54. Israel, Liron L., Anna Galstyan, Eggehard Holler, and Julia Y. Ljubimova. "Magnetic iron oxide nanoparticles for imaging, targeting and treatment of primary and metastatic tumors of the brain." *Journal of Controlled Release* 320 (2020): 45–62.
55. Sheervalilou, Roghayeh, Milad Shirvaliloo, Saman Sargazi, and Habib Ghaznavi. "Recent advances in iron oxide nanoparticles for brain cancer theranostics: From in vitro to clinical applications." *Expert Opinion on Drug Delivery* 18, no. 7 (2021): 949–977.
56. Marekova, Dana, Karolina Turnovcova, Tolga H Sursal, Chirag D Gandhi, Pavla Jendelova, and Meena Jhanwar-Uniyal. "Potential for treatment of glioblastoma: new aspects of superparamagnetic iron oxide nanoparticles." *Anticancer Research* 40, no. 11 (2020): 5989–5994.
57. Shevtsov, Maxim, Boris Nikolaev, Yaroslav Marchenko, Ludmila Yakovleva, Nikita Skvortsov, Anton Mazur, Peter Tolstoy, Vyacheslav Ryzhov, and Gabriele Multhoff. "Targeting experimental orthotopic glioblastoma with chitosan-based superparamagnetic iron oxide nanoparticles (CS-DX-SPIONs)." *International Journal of Nanomedicine* 13 (2018): 1471.
58. Zhang, Yun, Hwa Jeong Lee, Ruben J. Boado, and William M Pardridge. "Receptor-mediated delivery of an antisense gene to human brain cancer cells." *Journal of Gene Medicine: A Cross-Disciplinary Journal for Research on the Science of Gene Transfer and Its Clinical Applications* 4, no. 2 (2002): 183–194.
59. Norouzi, Mohammad, Vinith Yathindranath, James A Thliveris, Brian M Kopec, Teruna J Siahaan, and Donald W Miller. "Doxorubicin-loaded iron oxide nanoparticles

for glioblastoma therapy: A combinational approach for enhanced delivery of nanoparticles." *Scientific Reports* 10, no. 1 (2020): 11292.
60. Yoshida, Sakiko, Connie Duong, Michael Oestergaard, Michael Fazio, Cathy Chen, Rachael Peralta, Shuling Guo et al. "MXD3 antisense oligonucleotide with superparamagnetic iron oxide nanoparticles: A new targeted approach for neuroblastoma." *Nanomedicine: Nanotechnology, Biology and Medicine* 24 (2020): 102127.
61. Grillone, Agostina, Matteo Battaglini, Stefania Moscato, Letizia Mattii, César de Julián Fernández, Alice Scarpellini, Mario Giorgi, Edoardo Sinibaldi, and Gianni Ciofani. "Nutlin-loaded magnetic solid lipid nanoparticles for targeted glioblastoma treatment." *Nanomedicine* 8, no. 3 (2019): 727–752.
62. Gu, L, Zhu, N, Findley, H. et al. "MDM2 antagonist nutlin-3 is a potent inducer of apoptosis in pediatric acute lymphoblastic leukemia cells with wild-type p53 and overexpression of MDM2." *Leukemia* 22, 730–739 (2008). https://doi.org/10.1038/leu.2008.11
63. Zhang, Jinsong, Tianyuan Zhang, and Jianqing Gao. "Biocompatible iron oxide nanoparticles for targeted cancer gene therapy: A review." *Nanomaterials* 12, no. 19 (2022): 3323.
64. Crespo, Ines, Ana Louisa Vital, María Gonzalez-Tablas, María del Carmen Patino, Alvaro Otero, María Celeste Lopes, Catarina de Oliveira, Patricia Domingues, Alberto Orfao, and Maria Dolores Tabernero. "Molecular and genomic alterations in glioblastoma multiforme." *American Journal of Pathology* 185, no. 7 (2015): 1820–1833.
65. Rasmussen, John W, Ezequiel Martinez, Panagiota Louka, and Denise G Wingett. "Zinc oxide nanoparticles for selective destruction of tumor cells and potential for drug delivery applications." *Expert Opinion on Drug Delivery* 7, no. 9 (2010): 1063–1077.
66. Bisht, Gunjan, and Sagar Rayamajhi. "ZnO nanoparticles: a promising anticancer agent." *Nanobiomedicine* 3, no. Godište 2016 (2016): 3–9.
67. Dang, Zechun, Jizheng Sun, Jiaqi Fan, Jinqi Li, Xinlei Li, and Tongsheng Chen. "Zinc oxide spiky nanoparticles: A promising nanomaterial for killing tumor cells." *Materials Science and Engineering*: C 124 (2021): 112071.
68. Xie, Shichen, Jingyao Zhu, Dicheng Yang, Yan Xu, Jun Zhu, and Dannong He. "Low concentrations of zinc oxide nanoparticles cause severe cytotoxicity through increased intracellular reactive oxygen species." *Journal of Biomedical Nanotechnology* 17, no. 12 (2021): 2420–2432.
69. Li, Jinqi, Xinlei Li, Yangfeng Zhang, Kun Jin, Ye Yuan, Ruiqi Ming, Yuhua Yang, and Tongsheng Chen. "An intravascular needle coated by ZnO nanoflowers for in vivo elimination of circulating tumor cells." *Nano Research* 16, no. 1 (2023): 873–881.
70. Ostrovsky, Stella, Gila Kazimirsky, Aharon Gedanken, and Chaya Brodie. "Selective cytotoxic effect of ZnO nanoparticles on glioma cells." *Nano Research* 2 (2009): 882–890.
71. Wahab, Rizwan, Neha Kaushik, Farheen Khan, Nagendra Kumar Kaushik, Eun Ha Choi, Javed Musarrat, and Abdulaziz A Al-Khedhairy. "Self-styled ZnO nanostructures promotes the cancer cell damage and supresses the epithelial phenotype of glioblastoma." *Scientific Reports* 6, no. 1 (2016): 1–13.
72. Marfavi, Zahra Hamod, Mona Farhadi, Seyed Behnamedin Jameie, Masoomeh Zahmatkeshan, Vahid Pirhajati, and Manasadat Jameie. "Glioblastoma U-87MG tumour cells suppressed by ZnO folic acid-conjugated nanoparticles: an in vitro study." *Artificial Cells, Nanomedicine, and Biotechnology* 47, no. 1 (2019): 2783–2790.
73. Nsairat, Hamdi, Dima Khater, Fadwa Odeh, Fedaa Al-Adaileh, Suma Al-Taher, Areej M Jaber, Walhan Alshaer, Abeer Al Bawab, and Mohammad S Mubarak. "Lipid nanostructures for targeting brain cancer." *Heliyon* 7, no. 9 (2021): e07994.

74. Iturrioz-Rodríguez, Nerea, Rosalia Bertorelli, and Gianni Ciofani. "Lipid-based nanocarriers for the treatment of glioblastoma." *Advanced Nanobiomed Research* 1, no. 2 (2021): 2000054.
75. Juillerat-Jeanneret, Lucienne. "The targeted delivery of cancer drugs across the blood–brain barrier: chemical modifications of drugs or drug-nanoparticles?" *Drug Discovery Today* 13, no. 23–24 (2008): 1099–1106.
76. Bhaskar, Sonu, Furong Tian, Tobias Stoeger, Wolfgang Kreyling, Jesús M de la Fuente, Valeria Grazú, Paul Borm, Giovani Estrada, Vasilis Ntziachristos, and Daniel Razansky. "Multifunctional nanocarriers for diagnostics, drug delivery and targeted treatment across blood–brain barrier: perspectives on tracking and neuroimaging." *Particle and Fibre Toxicology* 7, no. 1 (2010): 1–25.
77. Infante, Paola, Alessio Malfanti, Deborah Quaglio, Silvia Balducci, Sara De Martin, Francesca Bufalieri, Francesca Mastrotto et al. "Glabrescione B delivery by self-assembling micelles efficiently inhibits tumor growth in preclinical models of Hedgehog-dependent medulloblastoma." *Cancer Letters* 499 (2021): 220–231.
78. Bell JB, Rink JS, Eckerdt F, Clymer J, Goldman S, Thaxton CS, Platanias LC. "HDL nanoparticles targeting sonic hedgehog subtype medulloblastoma." *Sci. Rep.* 2018;8:1211. Doi: 10.1038/s41598-017-18100-8
79. Kim J, Dey A, Malhotra A, Liu J, Ahn SI, Sei YJ, Kenney AM, MacDonald TJ, Kim Y. "Engineered biomimetic nanoparticle for dual targeting of the cancer stem-like cell population in sonic hedgehog medulloblastoma." *Proc. Natl. Acad. Sci. USA.* 2020;117:24205–24212. Doi: 10.1073/pnas.1911229117
80. Hegde, MM, Prabhu, S, Mutalik, S et al. "Multifunctional lipidic nanocarriers for effective therapy of glioblastoma: recent advances in stimuli-responsive, receptor and subcellular targeted approaches." *J. Pharm. Investig*. 52, 49–74 (2022). https://doi.org/10.1007/s40005-021-00548-6
81. Bibhash, CM, Narahari, NP, Vijayaraj, S, Subas, CD, Jayaraman, R, Jyotirmoy, D, and Biswa, MS (2019) "Lipid based nanoparticles: current strategies for brain tumor targeting." *Current Nanomaterials*, 4(2), 84–100
82. Zhu, Feng-Dan, Yu-Jiao Hu, Lu Yu, Xiao-Gang Zhou, Jian-Ming Wu, Yong Tang, Da-Lian Qin, Qing-Ze Fan, and An-Guo Wu. "Nanoparticles: a hope for the treatment of inflammation in CNS." *Frontiers in Pharmacology* 12 (2021): 683935.
83. Huang, Ji-yun, Ying-mei Lu, Huan Wang, Jun Liu, Mei-hua Liao, Ling-juan Hong, Rong-rong Tao et al. "The effect of lipid nanoparticle PEGylation on neuroinflammatory response in mouse brain." *Biomaterials* 34, no. 32 (2013): 7960–7970.
84. Li, B, Manan, RS, Liang, SQ et al. "Combinatorial design of nanoparticles for pulmonary mRNA delivery and genome editing." *Nat Biotechnol* (2023). https://doi.org/10.1038/s41587-023-01679-x
85. Singh, Gurpal, Harinder Kaur, Akanksha Sharma, Joga Singh, Hema Kumari Alajangi, Santosh Kumar, Neha Singla, Indu Pal Kaur, and Ravi Pratap Barnwal. "Carbon based nanodots in early diagnosis of cancer." *Frontiers in Chemistry* 9 (2021): 669169.
86. Wang, Weiping, Ya-Chun Lu, Hong Huang, Jiu-Ju Feng, Jian-Rong Chen, and Ai-Jun Wang. "Facile synthesis of water-soluble and biocompatible fluorescent nitrogen-doped carbon dots for cell imaging." *Analyst* 139, no. 7 (2014): 1692–1696.
87. Jiang, Qunjiao, Li Liu, Qiuying Li, Yi Cao, Dong Chen, Qishi Du, Xiaobo Yang et al. "NIR-laser-triggered gadolinium-doped carbon dots for magnetic resonance imaging, drug delivery and combined photothermal chemotherapy for triple negative breast cancer." *Journal of Nanobiotechnology* 19, no. 1 (2021): 1–15.

88. Bastiancich, C, Bastiat, G, Lagarce, F. "Gemcitabine and glioblastoma: Challenges and current perspectives." *Drug Discov. Today* 2018, 23, 416–423. Doi.org/10.1016/j.drudis.2017.10.010
89. Li, Shanghao, Zhili Peng, Julia Dallman, James Baker, Abdelhameed M Othman, Patrica L Blackwelder, and Roger M Leblanc. "Crossing the blood–brain barrier with transferrin conjugated carbon dots: a zebrafish model study." *Colloids and Surfaces B: Biointerfaces* 145 (2016): 251–256.
90. Liyanage, PY, Zhou, Y, Al-Youbi, AO, Bashammakh, AS, El-Shahawi, MS, Vanni, S, Graham, RM, Leblanc, RM. "Pediatric glioblastoma target-specific efficient delivery of gemcitabine across the blood–brain barrier via carbon nitride dots." *Nanoscale* 2020, 12, 7927–7938. Doi:10.1039/D0NR01647K
91. Liu, Yang, Junjun Liu, Jiayi Zhang, Xiucun Li, Fangsiyu Lin, Nan Zhou, Bai Yang, and Laijin Lu. "Noninvasive brain tumor imaging using red emissive carbonized polymer dots across the blood–brain barrier." *ACS Omega* 3, no. 7 (2018): 7888–7896.
92. Tetteh-Quarshie, Samuel, Eric R Blough, and Cynthia B Jones. "Exploring dendrimer nanoparticles for chronic wound healing." *Frontiers in Medical Technology* 3 (2021): 661421.
93. Abbasi, Elham, Sedigheh Fekri Aval, Abolfazl Akbarzadeh, Morteza Milani, Hamid Tayefi Nasrabadi, Sang Woo Joo, Younes Hanifehpour, Kazem Nejati-Koshki, and Roghiyeh Pashaei-Asl. "Dendrimers: synthesis, applications, and properties." *Nanoscale Research Letters* 9, no. 1 (2014): 1–10.
94. Biswas, Swati, and Vladimir P Torchilin. "Dendrimers for siRNA delivery." *Pharmaceuticals* 6, no. 2 (2013): 161–183.
95. Wu, Jiangyu, Weizhe Huang, and Ziying He. "Dendrimers as carriers for siRNA delivery and gene silencing: a review." *Scientific World Journal* 2013 (2013).
96. He, Hai, Yan Li, Xin-Ru Jia, Ju Du, Xue Ying, Wan-Liang Lu, Jin-Ning Lou, and Yan Wei. "PEGylated Poly (amidoamine) dendrimer-based dual-targeting carrier for treating brain tumors." *Biomaterials* 32, no. 2 (2011): 478–487.
97. Zhao, Jingjing, Bo Zhang, Shun Shen, Jun Chen, Qizhi Zhang, Xinguo Jiang, and Zhiqing Pang. "CREKA peptide-conjugated dendrimer nanoparticles for glioblastoma multiforme delivery." *Journal of Colloid and Interface Science* 450 (2015): 396–403.
98. Zhu, Yiran, Liyuan Zhu, Xian Wang, and Hongchuan Jin. "RNA-based therapeutics: An overview and prospectus." *Cell Death & Disease* 13, no. 7 (2022): 644.
99. Sayour EJ, De Leon G, Pham C, Grippin A, Kemeny H, Chua J, Huang J, Sampson JH, Sanchez-Perez L, Flores C et al. "Systemic activation of antigen-presenting cells via RNA loaded nanoparticles." *Oncoimmunology*. 2016;6:e1256527. Doi: 10.1080/2162402X.2016.1256527
100. Feng, Rundong, Suryaji Patil, Xin Zhao, Zhiping Miao, and Airong Qian. "RNA therapeutics-research and clinical advancements." *Frontiers in Molecular Biosciences* 8 (2021): 710738.
101. Lozada-Delgado, Eunice L, Nilmary Grafals-Ruiz, and Pablo E Vivas-Mejía. "RNA interference for glioblastoma therapy: Innovation ladder from the bench to clinical trials." *Life Sciences* 188 (2017): 26–36.
102. Wang, Kun, Xuan Wang, Jian Zou, Anling Zhang, Yingfeng Wan, Peiyu Pu, Zhengfei Song et al. "miR-92b controls glioma proliferation and invasion through regulating Wnt/beta-catenin signaling via Nemo-like kinase." *Neuro-oncology* 15, no. 5 (2013): 578–588.
103. Grafals-Ruiz, Nilmary, Christian I Rios-Vicil, Eunice L Lozada-Delgado, Blanca I Quiñones-Díaz, Ricardo A Noriega-Rivera, Gabriel Martínez-Zayas, Yasmarie Santana-Rivera, Ginette S Santiago-Sánchez, Fatma Valiyeva, and Pablo E

Vivas-Mejía. "Brain targeted gold liposomes improve RNAi delivery for glioblastoma." *International Journal of Nanomedicine* (2020): 2809–2828.

104. Mendez-Gomez, Hector, James McGuiness, Frances Weidert, Sheila Carrera-Justiz, Duane Mitchell, and Elias Sayour. "IMMU-13. Customizable multi-lamellar RNA-nanoparticles for pediatric glioma." *Neuro-Oncology* 23, no. Suppl 1 (2021): i29.
105. Chen, Jinjin, Zhongfeng Ye, Changfeng Huang, Min Qiu, Donghui Song, Yamin Li, and Qiaobing Xu. "Lipid nanoparticle-mediated lymph node-targeting delivery of mRNA cancer vaccine elicits robust CD8+ T cell response." *Proceedings of the National Academy of Sciences* 119, no. 34 (2022): e2207841119.
106. Mitchell, Duane A, and John H Sampson. "Toward effective immunotherapy for the treatment of malignant brain tumors." *Neurotherapeutics* 6, no. 3 (2009): 527–538.
107. Nguyen, David N, Kerry P Mahon, Ghania Chikh, Phillip Kim, Hattie Chung, Alain P Vicari, Kevin T Love et al. "Lipid-derived nanoparticles for immunostimulatory RNA adjuvant delivery." *Proceedings of the National Academy of Sciences* 109, no. 14 (2012): E797–E803.
108. Tian, Tian, Ruyu Liang, Gulsah Erel-Akbaba, Lorenzo Saad, Pierre J Obeid, Jun Gao, E Antonio Chiocca, Ralph Weissleder, and Bakhos A Tannous. "Immune checkpoint inhibition in GBM primed with radiation by engineered extracellular vesicles." *ACS nano* 16, no. 2 (2022): 1940–1953.

10 Herbal Medicines
A Boon for a Healthy Brain

Fajar Sofyantoro, Andri Frediansyah, Wahyu Aristyaning Putri, Winda Adipuri Ramadaningrum, Firzan Nainu, and Rohit Sharma

10.1 INTRODUCTION

Traditional herbal medicine refers to practices derived from Indigenous knowledge and used to treat both physical and mental disorders. Traditional medicine is predicated on the notion that prevention is preferable to treatment. Utilization of medicinal plants is a vital aspect of traditional medicine found throughout the world [1–3]. Large-scale production of chemically synthesized pharmaceuticals has revolutionized the medical industry [4, 5]. In developing nations, nonetheless, considerable segments of the population continue to obtain primary care via traditional medicinal plants [6, 7]. However, there has been a considerable increase in public interest in natural medicines in affluent countries during the past two decades [7, 8]. The most common justifications for choosing traditional herbal therapy are that it is readily accessible, less expensive, consistent with people's Indigenous culture, and less likely to cause adverse side effects [7, 9].

Numerous methods exist for preparing and employing plants and herbs. Therefore, due to the absence of standardization, the constituents of a plant extract or product may vary significantly [7, 10]. In addition, evaluation and regulation of herbal medicines are highly challenging due to the variety of regional processing techniques. The absence of research data, safety monitoring, and established production processes are obstacles to incorporating herbal medicines into the healthcare system [7, 10, 11].

Herbal therapies can currently be used to treat acute and chronic conditions, including neurological disorders. Parkinson's disease (PD), multiple sclerosis (MS), and Alzheimer's disease (AD) are examples of neurodegenerative disorders that cause neuronal death and cognitive or sensory decline [12, 13]. Antioxidant and anti-inflammatory plant extracts have been utilized as complementary and alternative treatments for a variety of nervous system disorders [14–16]. However, plant extracts from herbs contain a variety of active chemicals, including isoprenoids, alkaloids, and flavonoids. Consequently, it is usually challenging to determine which plant components have the most biological activity [16–18].

In this chapter, herbal remedies and treatments for brain diseases and neurodegenerative disorders are examined in depth. The history of traditional medicine in many cultures will also be examined in order to offer a suitable context for the

 DOI: 10.1201/9781032661964-10

recent increase in herbal intake. Finally, limitations and obstacles associated with the use of herbal medicine to improve brain function will be discussed.

10.2 BRAIN DISEASE AND NEURODEGENERATIVE DISORDERS

The brain, a mass of nerve cells, is the command centre of the central nervous system (CNS), which includes the cerebrum, brainstem, and cerebellum [19, 20]. It coordinates numerous types of stimuli acquired by the sensory organs and regulates the cerebral functions of organisms [21, 22]. In general, two types of cells, neurons and glial cells, compose the brain's structure. Neurons in the brain transmit and receive electrical and metabolic impulses [23]. Oligodendrocytes, microglia, and astrocytes comprise the glial cells, which are essential to the proper functioning of neurons [24, 25]. The blood–brain barrier (BBB), which is composed of the brain capillary endothelium in the CNS, regulates the particle movement between the blood and the brain [26, 27]. The BBB enables the supply of vital nutrients to the brain while protecting it from circulating pathogens and toxins [27, 28]. Nevertheless, the BBB makes it difficult for many diagnostic and therapeutic chemicals to enter the brain [26, 28].

Neurons, which branch throughout the body, are necessary for communication and regulation of numerous biological functions [23, 29, 30]. Early in life, neural stem cells actively proliferate into neurons and then diminish with age [31, 32]. Neurodegeneration disorders, a severe health concern, are caused by disruptions in synapses, abnormalities in the brain's functioning proteins, or diminishing neuronal activities [33–36]. The risk for neurodegenerative illnesses may be influenced by a combination of environmental exposures and genetic features, according to a growing body of studies [37–39].

10.2.1 Alzheimer's Disease (AD)

The formation of amyloid-beta (Aβ) plaques and the build-up of aberrant tau proteins have been hypothesized to initiate AD [40–43]. Memory loss and damage to other brain processes are the most common characteristic of the early stages of AD [44]. Other factors, such as extended exposure to oxidative stress and elevated levels of inflammatory cytokines, may also aggravate the formation of plaques [45–47]. Emerging evidence suggests that multiple signalling pathways, including nerve growth factor (NGF), the Janus kinase/signal transducer and activator of transcription (JAK/STAT), and Fibroblast Growth Factors/Fibroblast Growth Factor Receptors (FGF/FGFR), are involved in the pathophysiology of AD, which is shown in Figure 10.1 [48].

Adult NGF acts by maintaining the peripheral nervous system's (PNS) homeostasis [49–51]. ProNGF, the precursor of NGF, is secreted from cells and cleaved to produce the mature form (mNGF) [52]. The release of acetylcholine is caused by the binding of mNGF to its receptors. AD patients have been shown to have mutations in the proNGF to mNGF conversion, downregulation of the mNGF receptor, reduced mNGF transport, and accelerated mNGF degradation. Numerous therapeutic initiatives are being developed to supply NGF to the brain, in order to

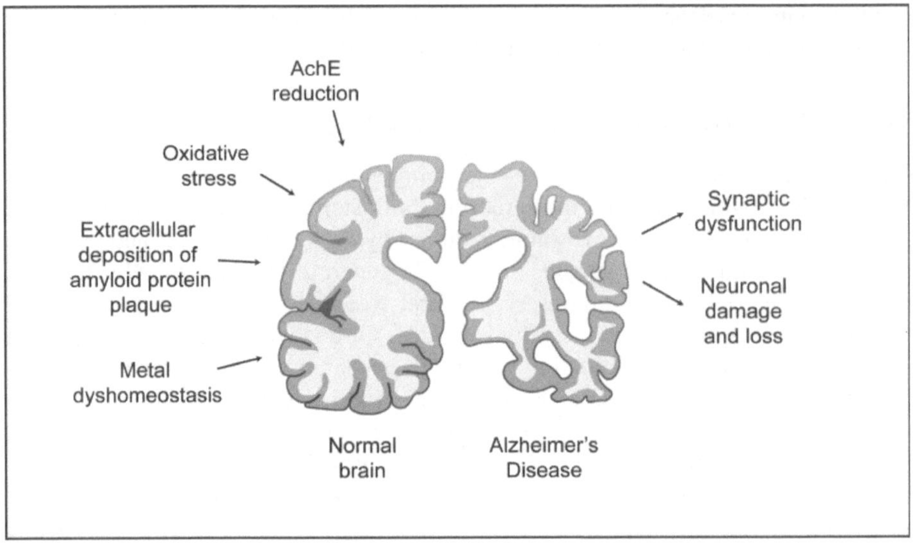

FIGURE 10.1 Schematic diagram of Alzheimer's diseases pathophysiology.

alleviate the pathologic symptoms of AD [53–56]. JAK/STAT signalling, which primarily regulates cytokine-responsive genes, is another AD-related pathway. JAK/STAT signalling is known to regulate cell proliferation and death. It has been proven that pharmacological medicines that suppress the JAK/STAT pathway have a protective effect against AD through Nrf2 signalling [57, 58]. In animal models of AD, colivelin and humanin peptides have been shown to protect neuronal function by activating the JAK2/STAT3 signalling pathway. AD has also been linked to fibroblast growth factors (FGFs), which regulate proliferation by interacting with high-affinity tyrosine kinase receptors (FGFRs). The growth of the brain is governed by FGF/FGFR signalling, and its dysregulation is associated with a variety of disorders, including AD. FGF7, a member of the FGF family, shows elevated mRNA levels in AD patients [59].

Targeting several molecular pathways is a crucial strategy for developing anti-AD treatments. Currently, the US Food and Drug Administration has approved three types of drugs that target specific pathways associated with AD, including glutamate receptor antagonists, cholinesterase inhibitors, and antibodies that target Aβ plaques. Combining memantine, a non-competitive glutamate receptor antagonist, with acetylcholinesterase inhibitors improved the treatment of AD symptoms [60–62]. Similarly, cholinesterase inhibitors, such as rivastigmine, donepezil, and galantamine, has been used to treat AD patients. These drugs reduce the breakdown of acetylcholine in the brain [63, 64]. Intravenous aducanumab, a monoclonal antibody designed to eliminate extracellular plaques in the brain, has been administered to AD patients as well. Recent clinical trials have shown that aducanumab reduces plaques without impairing the cognitive function of AD patients [65–68].

10.2.2 Parkinson's Disease (PD)

PD is typically diagnosed in older people with tremors and unstable movements [69, 70]. Even though the exact mechanisms remain unknown, genetic inheritance is widely regarded as the primary cause of PD, which is compounded by unhealthy lifestyle choices, such as smoking and excessive coffee intake [71–74]. Enlargement of the ventricles and loss of pigmentation in the locus coeruleus are pathophysiologic features of the PD. Furthermore, frontal cortex atrophy has been identified as an early sign of PD onset [75].

PD is caused by a combination of genetic and non-genetic factors [76, 77]. The accumulation of misfolded proteins, oxidative stress, inactivation of protein degradation pathways, mitochondrial abnormalities, and genetic mutations are among the primary causes that contribute to the emergence of PD symptoms [78–80]. The aggregation of alpha-synuclein (SNCA), as shown in Figure 10.2, and the accumulation of hyperphosphorylated tau proteins are two examples of how misfolded proteins contribute to PD. The intracellular accumulation of misfolded SNCA, which induces hole

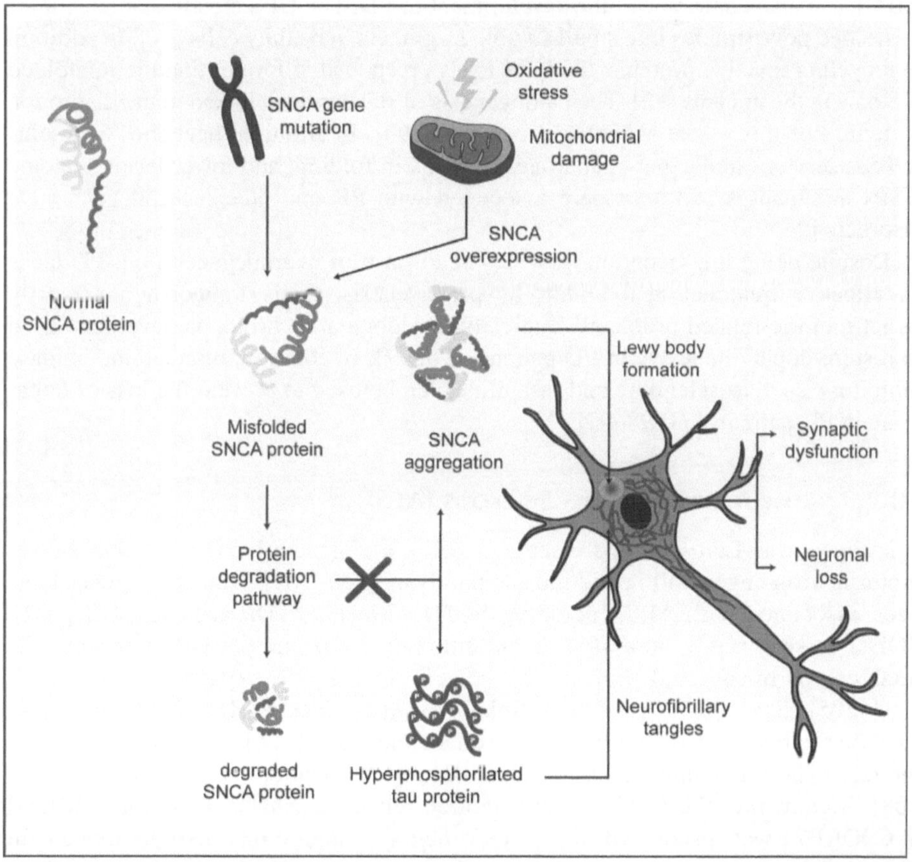

FIGURE 10.2 Schematic pathogenesis of Parkinson's disease.

formation and neuronal death, is one of the defining characteristics of PD [79, 81]. It has been suggested that mutations in the SNCA gene, which are also associated with the onset of dementia, are the primary cause of PD [79]. Overexpression of SNCA results in altered mitochondrial structure and membrane potential [82]. Similarly, tau hyperphosphorylation results in the formation of neurofibrillary tangles (NFT), a well-documented feature of PD [83]. Recent studies indicate that hereditary factors impact around 10% of late-onset PD [76, 84]. Parkin, DJ-1, and PINK1 are some of the most prevalent PD-related genes [76]. Parkin is an important protein associated with the ubiquitin-proteasome system, which aids in the destruction of misfolded proteins within the cell [85]. As a result, misfolded amyloid proteins accumulate due to parkin mutations [86]. DJ-1, which is associated with the early start of PD, is localized in multiple intracellular compartments, such as the nucleus and cytoplasm [87]. DJ-1 is considered essential for the control of transcriptional regulation and protease activity [88]. The PTEN-induced putative kinase-1 (PINK1) protects neurons from mitochondrial damage caused by stress [89]. Numerous PD patients have a mutation in the PINK1 gene, which enhances cell vulnerability [89, 90].

Inhibition of protein breakdown pathways, such as the ubiquitin-proteasome system (UPS), can also contribute to the development of PD. The UPS mostly degrades short misfolded polypeptides into small soluble fragments in healthy cells [91]. In addition to recycling inactive proteins, the UPS is also responsible for eliminating misfolded proteins in the nucleus [92]. The pathogenesis of PD has been linked to the disruption or failure of this essential biological process [93]. In addition, heat-shock proteins (HPSs) serve as molecular chaperones for protein folding, and lower levels of some HSPs in synapses and axons are associated with PD and other neurodegenerative disorders [94, 95].

Despite being the second most widespread form of neurodegeneration, PD lacks an effective treatment that affects its pathogenesis. Current medications mostly target motoric-related problems. Typically, levodopa and carbidopa have been used to restore dopamine levels in PD patients [96, 97]. In addition, monoamine oxidase inhibitors, such as selegiline and rasagiline, can be used to prevent the loss of dopamine in PD patients [71, 98, 99].

10.2.3 Amyotrophic Lateral Sclerosis (ALS)

Also known as Lou Gehrig's disease, ALS is a degenerative disease that causes motor neuron degeneration and muscle paralysis [100, 101]. Numerous genes have been associated with ALS, including SOD1, C9orf72, TDP-43, and FUS [102]. SOD1, as shown in Figure 10.3, is an antioxidant enzyme present in several cellular compartments and protects the cells from reactive oxygen species (ROS) [103–105]. The SOD1 gene was linked to ALS since SOD1 mutations cause oxidative stress and deregulation in iron metabolism [106]. In addition, animal models expressing mutant SOD1 also showed mitochondrial dysfunction [107, 108]. Meanwhile, the G4C2 hexanucleotide repeat expansion mutation (HREM) at C9ORF72 was discovered to be a detrimental mutation that disrupts movement of molecules between nucleus and cytoplasm, and thus it might contribute in the

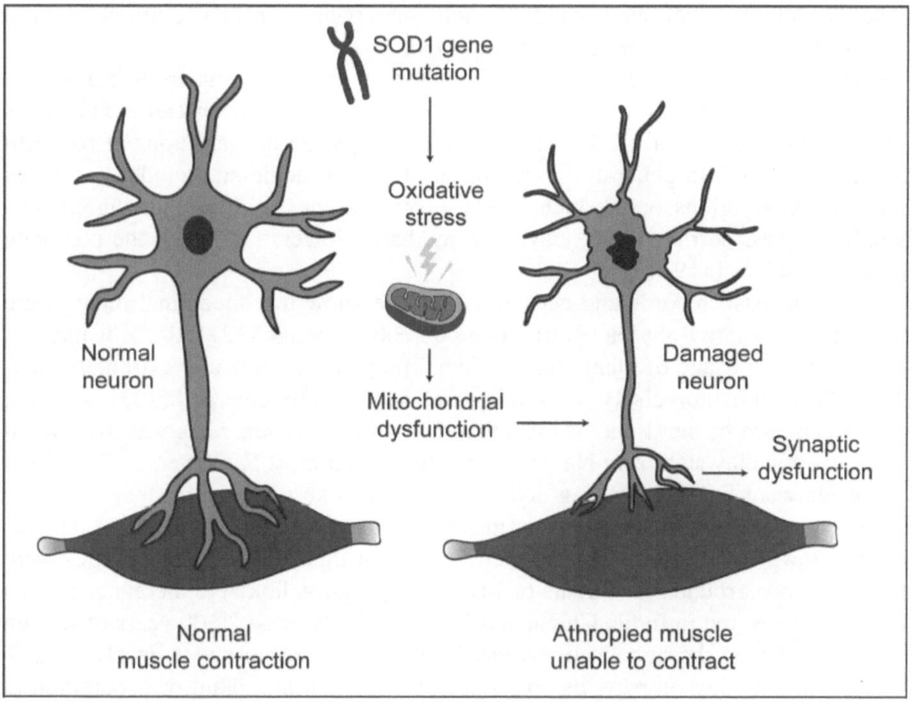

FIGURE 10.3 Schematic amyotrophic lateral sclerosis pathophysiology.

impairment of RNA processing machinery in ALS patients [109–111]. The nuclear ribonucleoprotein TDP-43, in which its mutations are found in ALS patients, is involved in exon splicing and mRNA transcription [112]. The clinical symptoms of ALS caused by FUS mutations were different between patients [113, 114]. ALS-related mutations result in mislocalization of FUS from the nucleus to the cytoplasm, thus drastically reducing FUS chromatin binding and leading to a loss of nuclear FUS function [115, 116]. Riluzole, a glutamate-receptor antagonist, is one of the therapy alternatives for ALS and has been proved to increase patients' lifespans. Similarly, edaravone, a substance with a high free-radical scavenger activity, helps suppress the disease progression [117].

10.3 THE HISTORY OF TRADITIONAL MEDICINAL USE OF HERBAL PLANTS

When it comes to the production of medicinal compounds, nature is, without a doubt, the best potential source. The treatment of illness by humans frequently involves the utilization of natural medicines such as plants, animals, minerals, microbes, and marine species. The use of medicinal plants for the treatment of illnesses dates all the way back to the beginning of human history. This means that ever since humans have looked for a tool in their environment to help them recover from a condition, the use of plants has been their preferable choice [118].

Plants, which make up the bulk of traditional medicine materials across the globe, are one of the primary forms of life that can be found on earth. The terms phytomedicine, botanical medicine, and phytotherapy are all variations of the term "herbal medicine." In general, the definition of herbal medicine includes any types of herbal preparations or products that use plant organs as the main ingredients, including seeds, berries, roots, leaves, fruits, bark, flowers, and even the complete plants themselves [119–121].

Based on fossil records and carbon dating, we know that medicinal plants were cultivated in ancient Babylon (Iraq) around 60,000 years ago [122]. Records like this demonstrate the usage of plants for medicinal purposes even if it is extremely challenging to establish precisely when this practice originally emerged [123]. The first written evidence of the usage of medicinal herbs to create remedies was discovered on a Sumerian clay slab from Nagpur that dates back almost 5,000 years [124]. Over 250 plants were listed, including alkaloid-rich ones like poppy, henbane, and mandrake, with step-by-step directions for making 12 distinct medicines [124]. Plants like laurel, caraway, and thyme that are well known for their medicinal properties were also discussed. Around 5,000 years of written information linked to therapeutic herbs has been discovered in India, China, and Egypt [125]. At least 2,500 years of written documentation on therapeutic herbs can be found in Greece and Asia [125, 126]. Writing and painting on papyrus, the fibrous stem of a water plant, was common in ancient times. The Berlin (1200 BC), Ebers (1500 BC), Edwin Smith (1600 BC), and Kahun (1900 BC) papyruses are all examples of papyrus utilized by the Egyptians [127, 128]. The "Ebers papyrus" is the most well-known Egyptian medicinal record, with over 800 different recipes, including gargles, snuff, and other remedies. Natural remedies were first recorded in cuneiform on clay tablets in Mesopotamia around 2600 BCE [129, 130]. Oils extracted from cypress trees (*Cupressus sempervirens*) and myrrh trees (*Commiphora* species) were used to make these tablets.

Explorers, preachers, and merchants have played a significant role in the spread of modern medicine during the past few centuries. They explored events in transcontinental history and human migration, as well as more modern developments like the Industrial Revolution and the globalization of the pharmaceutical industry. However, most of the world's population still depends on traditional medicine. Traditional treatments of ancient civilizations like Egypt, Mesopotamia, Greece, India, and China laid the groundwork for modern medicine, which relies on empirical evidence from laboratories and hospitals [131].

Traditional, complementary, and alternative medicine has been also commonly referred to as traditional knowledge-based medicine (TKBM) [131]. Traditional Chinese medicine, Kampo, and Ayurvedic practices all have deep roots in the societies and cultures of China, Japan, and India, respectively, making TKBM a hot commodity in these regions [131, 132]. There are various ways in which TKBM diverges from standard Western medicine (WM). WM focuses on relieving symptoms; TKBM practitioners put their patients' health first, using procedures like chiropractic manipulation and herbal supplements [131, 133]. Although TKBM was founded on scientific evidence in terms of diagnosis and therapy, it was severely confined by the rudimentary techniques available for medical observation and evaluation, which led to less precise understanding of the human health and illness state. However, clinical trials, the discovery of active substances, receptors, and associated pathways are currently being used to address these problems [134–136]. In the context of Western cultures, modern medicine developed in response to ancient TKBM [131].

After the introduction of "experimental medicine" as a prototypical contemporary medical system in 1900, traditional medicine flourished in several parts of the world, each with its own distinctive qualities. It is generally agreed that both traditional medicine (TM) and herbal medicine (HM) play an important part in maintaining people's health, with HM having its roots in the Middle Ages and TM in the Renaissance [137]. Traditional medical systems from around the world are listed and their key characteristics are summarized in Table 10.1 and Figure 10.4.

10.3.1 Herbal Treatments for Brain Ischemia

Ischemia of the brain is one of the most common causes of dementia [145], which occurs in over 50% of individuals following an ischemic event [146]. It is believed that degenerative changes in the hippocampus, particularly in the CA1 region, are responsible for the poor episodic memory which is the initial and most important clinical hallmark of post-ischemic dementia [147–149]. Cerebral ischemia caused by a substantial decrease in cerebral blood flow is a common and well-understood cause of permanent brain injury [150, 151]. Based on clinical experience, the brain cells are more resistant to ischemic disease than was previously hypothesized [152, 153]. Cellular acidosis and metabolic abnormalities caused by aberrant intracellular ion homeostasis may play a significant role in deciding the survival of neurons [150, 152].

Systematically, cerebral ischemia reduces immunological function, resulting in infectious complications [154–156]. Cerebral ischemia involves several pathways, such as the formation of free radicals, oxidative stress, membrane dysfunction disruption, neurotransmitter release, and death [157]. There is uncertainty over whether different immunological changes happen in the brain and periphery after a stroke and whether the same mechanisms are operating in both compartments [158, 159]. Natural killer (NK) cells exhibit significant changes in transcriptional activities in patients with ischemic stroke and in mice with middle cerebral artery blockage [155, 160]. NK cell responses in the brain are suppressed by cholinergic mediators involved in RUNX3, whereas catecholaminergic and hypothalamic-pituitary-adrenal axis activation results in splenic atrophy and restriction of peripheral NK cell populations through modifying SOCS3 expression [161]. It is important to note that genetic or pharmaceutical modification of NK cells reduces post-stroke infection [162]. As a result, cerebral ischemia impairs neurodevelopment and raises the likelihood of post-stroke infection in the brain, where it has a different impact than in the periphery, on NK cell-mediated immune defence [163].

Due to cerebral vascular blockage, a cerebral infarction causes ischemic tissue death, and current research indicates that post-stroke inflammation greatly contributes to the development of ischemic illness [156, 164]. Since secondary damages may require

TABLE 10.1
Characteristics of Several Important Traditional Medicine Systems

Name	Nation of Origin & Development	Information and Features	Examples
Traditional Chinese medicine (TCM)	• China • Thousands of years ago	• TCM is built on the Yin Yang Wu Xing concepts [138]. • For optimal efficacy, a TCM formula would typically combine multiple medications that work well together [139]. • According to their respective functions, a conventional formula contains four components: monarch (king), minister, assistant, and servant [140]	*Rheum rhabarbarum* is used as a laxative for acute constipation and in smaller dosages for digestive issues; *Panax ginseng* is particularly useful for the immune system, neurological system, and cardiovascular system; *Cinnamomum ceylanicum* is effective in treating persistent *Helicobacter pylori* infections due to its antifungal, antibacterial, and antiplasmodial properties; *Ephedra sinica* (Ma Huang) is used to treat asthma, bronchitis, and feverish conditions; *Wolfiporia cocos* is a diuretic, antimicrobial, blood sugar regulator, and enhancer of cardiac contractility; Chinese caterpillar mushroom *Cordyceps sinensis* is utilized to strengthen the lungs and kidneys, as well as tonify yin and yang and to alleviate emotional distress, eliminate mucus, and stop bleeding.
Ayurveda	• India • dating back to pre-Vedic eras (4000 BCE–1500 BCE)	• Ayurveda restores health by focusing on the body's innate ability to heal itself by natural remedies [141]. • Ayurveda promotes a healthy lifestyle as a means of warding off disease and discomfort [141, 142]. • Many Ayurvedic remedies involve the combination of multiple plants in a unique proportion to maximize therapeutic efficacy and minimize side effects [141].	*Asparagus racemosus* (Shavatari) for urinary tract health, immune system support, and blood purification; *Commiphora mukul* (Guggul) to prevent the common cold; reduce cholesterol and triglycerides while maintaining the HDL-to-LDL ratio; *Cyperus scariosus* (Nagarmusta) has hepatoprotective effects and promotes a healthy genitourinary system. *Garcinia cambogia* lowers hunger by stimulating glycogen production; *Glycyrrhiza glabra* (Yashtimadhu) protects genetic material from damage that might lead to cancer. *Gymnema sylvestre* (Gurmarar) helps subdue and negate sugar cravings; *Momordica charantia* inhibits the brain reactions to stimuli with a sweet taste; *Zingiber officinale* promotes bowel movements and relaxes the muscles that regulate digestion.

Unani medicine	• Greece • originated from Greco-Arabic medicine some 2,500 years ago and gained prominence during the emergence of the Arab civilization.	• All aspects of a person's being (physical, mental, and spiritual) are given equal consideration [143, 144]. • According to Unani medical theory, the human body is considered a unified whole made up of four constituent parts with distinct personalities [144]. • In the same way that a person's appearance and disposition are reflected in their temperament, so too is the body's susceptibility to illness in the event of a mismatch between the two [144].	*Aloe vera* (L.) to treat constipation; *Crocus sativus* for immune-modulating and health-protective benefits; *Juglans regia* for throat infection prevention.
Kampo (Japanese traditional medicine)	• Japan • In the fifth or sixth century, Kampo was brought to Europe from China via the Korean peninsula.	• Over the past 1,400 years, kampo has evolved and merged with traditional Japanese treatments. • Kampo treats every human being as a complete and self-controlled whole in which body and mind impact mutually. • Herbal remedies are believed to have an equal impact on the soul and the body, since diseases are believed to develop from mental and physical issues. • Kampo therapy places emphasis on the sufferer instead of on the illness.	*Luffa cylindrica* (Hechima) for sunburn relief; *Artemisia indica* (Yomogi) for dry skin and acne; *Eriobotrya japonica* (biwa) for heat rash reduction; *Perilla frutescens* (shiso) for eczema and acne; *Houttuynia cordata* (dokudami) for laxative and diuretic; *Cnidium officinale* (senkyu) for anemia and menstrual irregularity; *Citrus junos* (Yuzu) for circulation improvement, cold prevention, backache, neuralgia; *Acorus calamus* (Syobu) for neuralgia; and *Matricaria recutita* (kamitsure) for inflammation reduction.

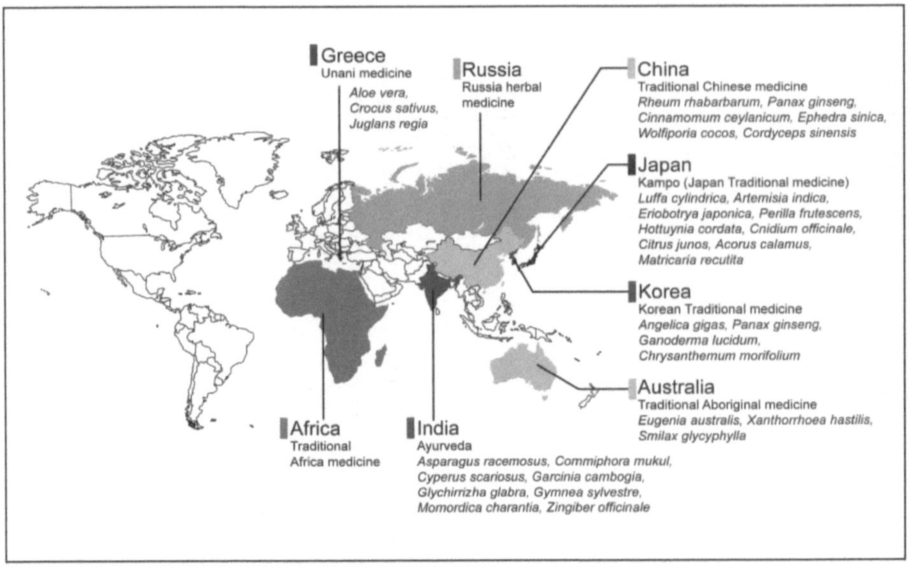

FIGURE 10.4 Traditional use of medicinal plants around the world.

lengthier therapy than original damage following artery blockage, inflammation control would be an apparent therapeutic objective [164]. Acute neuritis develops rapidly after several days of cerebral ischemia [165]. Neutrophils and macrophages are recruited to the site of inflammation in the brain by cytokines and chemokines [165, 166]. Subacute neuritis lasts between 2 and 6 weeks, whereas chronic post-ischemic inflammation persists for months or years [167]. In chronic neuroinflammation, macrophages, lymphocytes, and plasma cells predominate, whereas neutrophils predominate in acute neuroinflammation [148, 168]. In addition to their detrimental effects on the ischemic brain, inflammatory mediators may potentially promote stroke recovery [168, 169].

The most common treatment for cerebral ischemia is thrombolytic therapy [170–172]. The use of natural ingredients from conventional herbal remedies for neuroprotection seems to be a promising therapy alternative for cerebral ischemia with little risk of systemic side effects, which might restrict their long-term use [173]. This scenario needs additional study that may one day lead to the development of molecules with enhanced neuroprotective properties. It has been demonstrated that antioxidant, anti-inflammatory, calcium antagonist, and anti-apoptotic capabilities of natural compounds alter brain function [174]. Curcumin, resveratrol, EGb761, and epigallocatechin-3-gallate have all demonstrated notable medicinal benefits for cerebral ischemia [175]. However, as prospective treatments for cerebral ischemia, only ligustilide, tanshinone, scutellarin, and shikonin have been extensively studied in recent years [175].

The neuroprotective properties of herbal compounds are being given more attention in the realm of drug discovery. The cornerstone for developing neuroprotectants from conventional herbal remedies is a promising intervention for cerebral ischemia, a complex disease process that involves several pathways.

On experimental ischemia traumatic brain injury, natural substances with antioxidant, anti-inflammatory, calcium antagonist, anti-apoptotic, and neuromodulator properties have preventative or therapeutic effects [176]. Evaluation of traditional herbal remedies with neuroprotective properties against ischemic brain injury are summarized in Table 10.2.

TABLE 10.2
Pharmacological Action of Commonly Used Herbs for Ischemia

No	Herbal	Compound	Function	References
1	The root of *Salvia miltiorrhiza*	Salvianolic acid A and B; tanshinone IIA	enlarge coronary arteries, upregulate blood flow, and scavenges free radicals	[177]
2	Root of *Panax ginseng*	fquercetin 3-O-β-Dxylopyranosyl-β-D-galactopyranoside; saponins; ginsenosides Rg1 and Rb1	regulate production of cytokines, apoptotic pathways, and proteins associated to oxidative stress	[178]
3	*Pueraria lobata*	Puerarin	regulating the build-up of free fatty acids	[179]
4	Japanese Kampo (traditional herbal)	baicalein	minimizing inflammation and damage of neurons	[180]
5	Green tea	catechins	prevents cell deterioration and neurological impairments in the brain	[181]
6	*Nigella sativa* seeds	Thymoquinone	protective effects on hippocampus	[182]
7	*Astragalus membranaceus*	Astragaloside IV	reduce inflammation, control cytokine production, and increase regulatory T cell expression	[183]
8	*Ligusticum wallichii* Franchat (Chung Xiong)	Tetramethylpyrazine	increase antioxidant capacity and boost immune profile	[184]
9	*Angelica sinensis* (Oliv.) Diels (AS) and *Ligusticum chuanxiong* Hort. (LC)	Ferulic acid	protection of blood vessels, reduction of oxidative stress and inflammation	[185]

10.3.2 Herbal Remedies for Memory and Cognitive Impairment

Memory is the capacity of an individual to retain sensory stimuli for a predetermined period of time and recall them [186]. Memory function is vulnerable to a number of pathologic processes, including ageing, depression, pharmacological side effects, as well as neurodegenerative diseases [186]. Memory loss can range in intensity from mild to severe, and may happen suddenly (caused by a brain injury) or gradually (due to a neurodegenerative disease). Almost all are associated with partial or total impairment to neuroanatomical structures, which affects memory acquisition, formation, and retrieval [43]. Numerous studies have shown that the cholinergic system is essential for memory and learning. Additionally, studies have shown that AD is related to the degeneration of cholinergic neurons and impaired choline-acetyltransferase activity in the brain [187]. Acetylcholinesterase (AChE) inhibitors were synthesized as a treatment for patients with dementia caused by AD, which was triggered by decreased levels of cholinergic activity. Based on these findings, the routinely prescribed AChE inhibitors Donepezil®, Rivastigmine, and Galantamine were developed [187]. As memory involves numerous interconnected brain functions, there are various types of memories, and practically every sort of brain impairment can lead to one or more types of memory loss.

Cognitive enhancers are prescription medications and herbal supplements that work to improve the cognitive abilities of thought, memory, creativity, motivation, attentiveness, and focus. The cognitive enhancers, sometimes referred to as nootropics, or smart drugs, can be used to treat medical conditions that impair motor coordination, learning, and the ability to maintain a stable emotional state. Pharmacological properties of several plants as cognitive enhancers have reportedly been discovered [188]. Ayurveda, the Indian medical system which addresses the maintenance of health by considering the whole body, mind, and spirit, is gaining popularity in the field of cognitive enhancer supplements [189].

To treat cognitive problems, including neurodegenerative diseases like AD and other memory-related disorders, various herbs have been used in traditional medicine. Many studies have been carried out to find potential new plant-based drugs, including those for memory problems. Alkaloids from plant sources, for example, which have been researched for their possibilities in AD therapy and are already in clinical use, are just a few of the drugs that are currently available on the market. Although they could have negative consequences, such as drug interactions, herbal medicines are typically well tolerated [190]. Memory-boosting herbal medicines like *Ginkgo biloba* and *Bacopa moniera* (Bramhi) have been consumed regularly around the world [191, 192]. Evaluation of traditional herbal remedies for memory and cognitive impairment summaries are shown in Table 10.3.

10.3.3 Medicinal Plants as an Alternative Therapy for Alzheimer's, Dementia, and Parkinson's

Dementia is a slowly progressive disease that impairs memory and cognitive function [207]. Dementia is characterized as an acquired cognitive decline in many domains that is severe enough to limit daily functioning, such as the ability to engage in social

TABLE 10.3
Pharmacological Action of Commonly Used Herbs for Memory and Cognitive Impairment

No	Herbal	Compound	Function	Sources
1	*Glycyrrhiza glabra*	Glycyrrhizin	anti-inflammatory and antioxidant effects	[193]
2	*Caesalpinia crista*	furanoditerpenes- ά-, ß-, γ-, δ-, ε-, and F-caesalpins	learning and memory enhancer (nootropic drug)	[194]
3	*Ginkgo biloba*	Quercetin, kaemprofol, ginkgolides B and C, bilobalide	free radical-scavenging activities	[195]
4	*Centella asiatica*	triterpenes and caffeoylquinic acids	reduce oxidative stress, improved the health of neurons	[196]
5	*Tinospora cordifolia*	Phenolics, alkaloids, glycosides, steroids, diterpenoid lactones, sesquiterpenoid, polysaccharides, aliphatic compounds	nootropic activity	[197]
6	*Zingiber officinale*	gingerin, gingerol, shogaol and zingerone	antioxidant activity	[198]
7	*Bacopa monniera*	Bacosides: bacoside A and B, brahmine, nicotine, herpestine	enhance memory, attention, and cognitive processing in part by inhibiting AChE activity	[199]
8	*Ilex paraguariensis*	Purine alkaloids, flavonoids, and vitamins.	influences memory and learning by acting as an adenosine receptor antagonist.	[200]
9	*Evolvulus alsinoides*	Alkaloids betaine, sankhapushpine and evolvine, scopoletis, copoline, umbelliferone, 6-methory-7-0-β-glucophyranoside coumarin queretine-3-o-β glucophyrenoside	suppression of AChE activity and enhancement of spatial memory formation	[201]
10	*Acorus calamus*	α-and β-asarone	modulating inflammation and oxidative stress	[202]
11	*Commiphora wightii*	steroid guggulsterone	neuroprotective against oxidative damage	[203]
12	*Emblica officinalis*	major active constituents of vit-C, phyllemblin	enhancing cognition, reducing cholesterol, and anticholinesterase effects.	[204]

(Continued)

TABLE 10.3 (Continued)
Pharmacological Action of Commonly Used Herbs for Memory and Cognitive Impairment

No	Herbal	Compound	Function	Sources
13	*Salvia lavandulaefolia*	1, 8- cineole, linalool, α- and β-pinene, carvacrol, luteolin	antioxidant, oestrogenic, anti-inflammatory properties	[205]
14	*Magnolia officinalis*	Magnolol, honokiol, and obovatol	inhibition of acetylcholinesterase activity	[206]

or professional activities [208, 209]. People with dementia suffer cognitive abnormalities and impairments in executive functions such as abstract thought, planning, concentration, limb movements, and language [210]. Dementia may also appear together with age-related comorbidities such as stroke, arthritis, and heart disease [211].

According to the World Health Organization (WHO), the majority of persons with dementia reside in East Asia [212]. A high number of dementia patients have also been reported in England and Scotland [213]. Currently, in total, more than 50 million individuals worldwide suffer from dementia [214]. According to recent estimates, the frequency of dementia will triple by 2050, with a projected 131.5 million cases [214–216].

Unfortunately, diagnosing dementia is challenging and necessitates more comprehensive evaluations due to the wide variety of dementia symptoms. Cognitive function and neuroimaging studies are necessary for a correct diagnosis of dementia [217]. In Western countries, AD is the most prevalent form of dementia, followed by vascular dementia (VaD). Due to the same etiology, symptoms, and risk factors, VaD and AD are difficult to distinguish. VaD is a complex set of clinical disorders characterized by dementia caused by haemorrhagic, ischemic, hypoxic, or anoxic brain injury [218]. AD is characterized by the presence of excessive amyloid plaques and neurofibrillary tangles in the brain, which impair the activity of brain cells. In addition, the neurotransmitter acetylcholine, which is essential for memory and learning, is diminished [213]. VaD and AD can occur together; this is known as mixed dementia (MD). Typically, multiple medical factors contribute to the development of MD. AD and vascular diseases such as multiple infarcts are the most prevalent. Moreover, vascular disease is present in Parkinson's dementia (PD) [215].

AD is a progressive dementia characterized by memory, speech, and behavioural problems [219]. AD is currently the third largest cause of death in the United States and one of the major health issues in the world [220–222]. The WHO predicts that by 2050, the rated prevalence in the global population will have quadrupled, reaching 114 million patients [219, 223]. While the exact cause of AD is unknown, hereditary factors account for 5%–10% of family instances, with the remaining 90%–95% being random [223]. Homozygous or heterozygous for the ApoE 4 allele raises the risk of getting AD considerably [223]. To date, efforts to find a cure for AD have been unsuccessful, and the currently available medications to treat the condition have limited efficacy, particularly if the disease is in its moderate to severe stages [223]. The goal of AD treatments is to stop or delay the disease's progression. Cholinesterase inhibitors have a moderate effect on dementia symptoms, whereas memantine – the currently available N-methyl-d-aspartate receptor antagonist – does not prevent dementia deterioration [224, 225].

PD is another disease that attacks the CNS. It is characterized by rest tremor, myotonia, rigidity, bradykinesia (particularly difficulty initiating movement), hypokinesia (loss of facial expression), postural autonomic instability, and

TABLE 10.4
Pharmacological Action of Commonly Used Herbs for Alzheimer's, Dementia, and Parkinson's

No	Herbal	Compound	Function	Sources
1	*Lavandula angustifolia*	linalool, linalyl acetate, caffeic acid and luteolin	inhibition of A polymerization, inhibition of AChE	[229, 230]
2	*Ginkgo biloba*	ginkgolide, flavonoids, terpenic lactone	prevents ROS production, mitochondrial malfunction, and apoptosis; safeguarding brain cells from the toxicity caused by Aβ plaques.	[231–233]
3	*Melissa officinalis*	triterpenes, phenolic acids, and flavonoids	decrease Aβ-induced neurotoxicity and matrix metalloproteinase-2 activity	[234, 235]
4	*Salvia miltiorrhiza*	tanshinone IIA, caffeic acid, salvianolic acid B, rosmarinic acid, and salvianic acid A	inhibit glutamate-induced oxytosis, ROS, and mitogen-activated protein kinases	[236]
5	*Paeonia alba*	paeoniflorin, albiflorin, oxypaeoniflorin, benzoylpaeoniflorin	improve dopaminergic neurons cell growth	[237]
6	*Crocus sativus*	crocin	inhibit formation of Aβ	[238, 239]
7	*Panax Ginseng*	triterpene glycosides	reduce Aβ levels, rescue the activity of choline acetyltransferase	[240, 241]
8	*Magnolia officinalis*	magnolol, 4-O-methylhonokiol, honokiol, obovatol	prevent of Aβ induced cell death, rescue from ROS stress	[242, 243]

non-motor features such as depression, psychosis, and autonomic [226]. PD is a neurodegenerative condition of the substantia nigra in the midbrain that is associated with ageing dopaminergic neurons that deteriorate progressively, resulting in a decline in striatal dopaminergic levels. A comprehensive review of 25 prevalence studies revealed that the mean age of symptom onset was 60–65 years in eight studies and > 65 years in five [227]. In most Western nations, PD is often treated symptomatically with medications such as levodopa (LD), dopamine agonists, MAO-B inhibitors, COMT inhibitors, antimuscarinics, and amantadine [228]. Evaluation of traditional herbal remedies for Alzheimer's, dementia, and PD is summarized in Table 10.4, and the example of an herbal remedy that is important as an AChE inhibitor in Alzheimer's and memory dysfunction is shown in Figure 10.5.

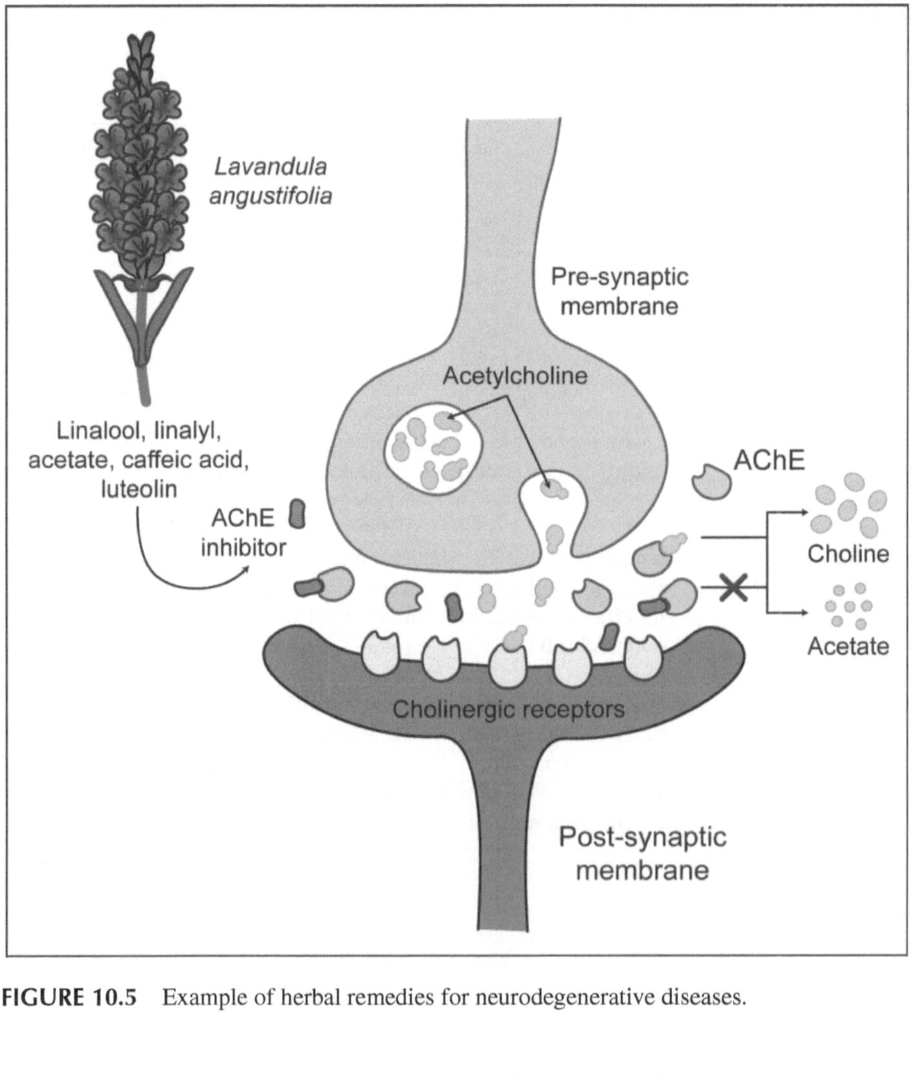

FIGURE 10.5 Example of herbal remedies for neurodegenerative diseases.

10.3.4 Limitations on the Consumption of Herbal Medicine for Enhancement of Brain Function or Disease Recovery

In recent decades, the consumption of therapeutic plants has increased significantly on a global basis [244, 245]. The assumption that "herbal" means "safe" promotes the global proliferation of herbal medications [7, 246, 247]. Unfortunately, this assumption is erroneous, as the pharmacologically active components of medicinal herbs may generate undesirable side effects [248, 249]. A rising number of studies have shown apparent harmful neurological and psychiatric effects as a result of herbal medication consumption, ranging from mild to severe in intensity, as shown in Table 10.5.

In addition to the above-mentioned negative effects of typical herbal supplements, incidences of poisoning due to the brain-enhancing benefits of herbal medications have also been documented. One example is the use of *Piper methysticum*, also known as kava, a crop native to the Pacific Islands. *P. methysticum*'s ability to relax the CNS makes it a popular anxiolytic medication. However, excessive consumption of *P. methysticum* may produce diplopia and photophobia [265]. Additionally, the combination of *P. methysticum* with other CNS-related medications may result in coma [266, 267]. Similarly, the unfavourable effect of *Hypericum perforatum*, a member of the family *Hypericaceae* and popularly referred to as St. John's wort, has been observed in the past. In recent years, the number of patients treated with *H. perforatum* for depression has increased significantly [268, 269]. However, comprehensive analysis of its adverse effects revealed that some patients had headache, nausea, and tremors [269]. In addition to the detrimental effects of undiscovered pharmacological substances in medicinal plants, it should be emphasized that contamination and herb-drug interactions may also have consequences [270, 271]. Concerns regarding the safety of medical plants are becoming more generally acknowledged as the global market for herbal therapeutic products grows.

TABLE 10.5
Lists of Reported Mild, Moderate, and Severe Adverse Effects from Herbal Medicine

No	Category	Symptoms
1	Mild or moderate	Dizziness and drowsiness [250–254]
		Drowsiness and headache [250, 255, 256]
		Nausea [257, 258]
		Sleep disorders [255]
2	Severe	Acute psychosis [256]
		Cerebral haemorrhage [259–261]
		Coma [262, 263]
		Loss of consciousness [264]
		Hallucinations [256]
		Seizures and epilepsy [251, 253, 254]

Even though they are extensively consumed, many herbal-based products have not yet been scientifically confirmed to be effective. Herbal products' safety is further compromised by the absence of standards, inadequate labelling, and lack of information [272]. Prior to introducing therapeutic herbs to the market, most countries do not require safety or toxicological testing. Moreover, many countries also lack government agencies capable of regulating industrial operations and enforcing quality standards. Furthermore, herbal medications are frequently marketed as prescription-free remedies, which increases the risk of taking substandard items [273].

Standardization, contamination or adulteration, and unlawful marketing are among the obstacles that have created worries over the future regulation of medicinal herbs. Since the quality of herbal ingredients varies based on a variety of factors, standardization is essential to ensure that the same product can be consistently manufactured. Variable amounts and concentrations of alkaloids, saponins, flavonoids, and bioactive are obtained during the manufacturing of herbal medicines. Most of the time, herb producers name their products based on a presumed active ingredient, as opposed to checking and identifying the precise active ingredient. In addition, product labelling regulations are rarely observed [274, 275]. Multiple routes are responsible for contamination and adulteration to occur. The application of pesticides to herb plants is one of the primary contamination problems. In several countries, herb plants are gathered from the wild and extracted using a variety of methods, hence increasing the likelihood of contamination during the production process. Previous accounts of the contamination of herbal items with pesticides, heavy metals, and other poisons are well documented [276–279]. In addition, there have been several reports that unlisted compounds, such as chlormethiazole, indomethacin, and sildenafil citrate have been introduced to herbal products [280, 281]. In poor nations, deceptive advertising has a significant impact on the use of herbal medicine. Even though common standards in food and medicine prohibit making claims that herbal remedies may heal diseases, some of them have been caught putting misleading labels on their products and selling them online [282, 283].

10.4 CONCLUSIONS AND PROSPECTS

More than three-quarters of all herbal medications currently in use were first identified using clues from traditional medicine. A combination of factors, including rising public costs associated with the day-to-day maintenance of personal health and the widespread acceptance of plant-derived products, has contributed to the growth in popularity of herbal medicines. The demand for herbals for treating neurodegenerative disorders and brain diseases is rising, even though establishing the effectiveness of herbs calls for the development of a quality consciousness with respect to evaluation-related evidence. Medical systems that include the use of herbal medications and therapies have been adopted in recent years by even the most economically developed nations. Herbal remedies and supplements for the healthy brain are becoming increasingly popular, which is expected to increase demand in the coming years. For the sake

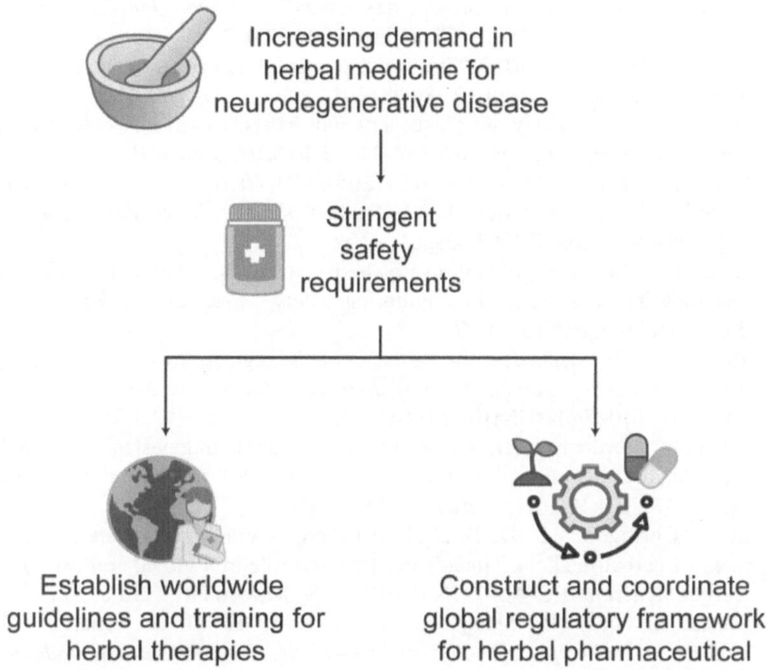

FIGURE 10.6 Future perspectives in the application of herbal medicine for a healthy brain.

of avoiding an uptick in complaints of negative side effects, it is crucial to establish guidelines and training for herbal therapies that are approved worldwide [284, 285], as illustrated in Figure 10.6. To reiterate, strict regulatory frameworks must be constructed and coordinated globally to ensure that stringent safety requirements for herbal pharmaceuticals are met (Figure 10.6). It is up to the proper regulatory bodies in various nations to make the required efforts to ensure the safety of commercially available products, especially herbal medications intended for enhancement of brain function and disease recovery.

REFERENCES

[1] Conboy L, Kaptchuk TJ, Eisenberg DM, Gottlieb B, Acevedo-Garcia D. 2017. "The relationship between social factors and attitudes toward conventional and CAM practitioners." *Complementary Therapies in Clinical Practice*. 13(3):146–157. doi:10.1016/j.ctcp.2006.12.003

[2] Engebretson J. 2002. "Culture and complementary therapies." *Complementary Therapies in Nursing and Midwifery*. 8(4):177–184. doi:10.1054/ctnm.2002.0638

[3] Rishton GM. 2008. "Natural products as a robust source of new drugs and drug leads: Past successes and present day issues." *American Journal of Cardiology*. 101(10):S43–S49. doi:10.1016/j.amjcard.2008.02.007

[4] Mathur S, Hoskins C. 2017. "Drug development: Lessons from nature." *Biomedical Reports*. 6(6):612–614. doi:10.3892/br.2017.909

[5] Jones AW. 2011. "Early drug discovery and the rise of pharmaceutical chemistry." *Drug Testing and Analysis*. 3(6):337–344. doi:10.1002/dta.301

[6] Oyebode O, Kandala N-B, Chilton PJ, Lilford RJ. 2016. "Use of traditional medicine in middle-income countries: A WHO–SAGE study." *Health Policy and Planning*. 31(8):984–991. doi:10.1093/heapol/czw022

[7] Ekor M. 2014. "The growing use of herbal medicines: Issues relating to adverse reactions and challenges in monitoring safety." *Frontiers in Pharmacology*. 4. doi:10.3389/fphar.2013.00177

[8] Tang TY, Li F, Afseth J. 2014. "Review of the regulations for clinical research in herbal medicines in USA." *Chinese Journal of Integrative Medicine*. 20(12):883–893. doi:10.1007/s11655-014-2024-y

[9] Elfahmi, Woerdenbag HJ, Kayser O. 2014. "Jamu: Indonesian traditional herbal medicine towards rational phytopharmacological use." *Journal of Herbal Medicine*. 4(2):51–73. doi:10.1016/j.hermed.2014.01.002

[10] Sen S, Chakraborty R, De B. 2011. "Challenges and opportunities in the advancement of herbal medicine: India's position and role in a global context." *Journal of Herbal Medicine*. 1(3–4):67–75. doi:10.1016/j.hermed.2011.11.001

[11] Zhang J, Wider B, Shang H, Li X, Ernst E. 2012. "Quality of herbal medicines: Challenges and solutions." *Complementary Therapies in Medicine*. 20(1–2):100–106. doi:10.1016/j.ctim.2011.09.004

[12] Dugger BN, Dickson DW. 2017. "Pathology of neurodegenerative diseases." *Cold Spring Harbor Perspectives in Biology*. 9(7):a028035. doi:10.1101/cshperspect.a028035

[13] Lamptey RNL, Chaulagain B, Trivedi R, Gothwal A, Layek B, Singh J. 2022. "A review of the common neurodegenerative disorders: Current therapeutic approaches and the potential role of nanotherapeutics." *International Journal of Molecular Sciences*. 23(3):1851. doi:10.3390/ijms23031851

[14] Virmani A, Pinto L, Binienda Z, Ali S. 2013. "Food, nutrigenomics, and neurodegeneration – Neuroprotection by what you eat!" *Molecular Neurobiology*. 48(2):353–362. doi:10.1007/s12035-013-8498-3

[15] Ratheesh G, Tian L, Venugopal JR, Ezhilarasu H, Sadiq A, Fan T-P, Ramakrishna S. 2017. "Role of medicinal plants in neurodegenerative diseases." *Biomanufacturing Reviews*. 2(1):2. doi:10.1007/s40898-017-0004-7

[16] Sharifi-Rad M, Lankatillake C, Dias DA, Docea AO, Mahomoodally MF, Lobine D, Chazot PL, Kurt B, Boyunegmez Tumer T, Catarina Moreira A et al. 2020. "Impact of natural compounds on neurodegenerative disorders: From preclinical to pharmacotherapeutics." *Journal of Clinical Medicine*. 9(4):1061. doi:10.3390/jcm9041061

[17] Khazdair MR, Anaeigoudari A, Hashemzehi M, Mohebbati R. 2019. "Neuroprotective potency of some spice herbs, a literature review." *Journal of Traditional and Complementary Medicine*. 9(2):98–105. doi:10.1016/j.jtcme.2018.01.002

[18] Adams M, Gmünder F, Hamburger M. 2007. "Plants traditionally used in age related brain disorders – A survey of ethnobotanical literature." *Journal of Ethnopharmacology*. 113(3):363–381. doi:10.1016/j.jep.2007.07.016

[19] Raichle ME. 2010. "Two views of brain function." *Trends in Cognitive Sciences*. 14(4):180–190. doi:10.1016/j.tics.2010.01.008

[20] Batista-García-Ramó K, Fernández-Verdecia C. 2018. "What we know about the brain structure–function relationship." *Behavioral Sciences*. 8(4):39. doi:10.3390/bs8040039

[21] Roth G, Dicke U. 2005. "Evolution of the brain and intelligence." *Trends in Cognitive Sciences*. 9(5):250–257. doi:10.1016/j.tics.2005.03.005

[22] Jones EG, Mendell LM. 1999. "Assessing the decade of the brain." *Science*. 284(5415):739–739. doi:10.1126/science.284.5415.739

[23] Sidiropoulou K, Pissadaki EK, Poirazi P. 2006. "Inside the brain of a neuron." *EMBO Reports*. 7(9):886–92. doi:10.1038/sj.embor.7400789

[24] Jäkel S, Dimou L. 2017. "Glial cells and their function in the adult brain: A journey through the history of their ablation." *Frontiers in Cellular Neuroscience*. 11. doi:10.3389/fncel.2017.00024

[25] Barres BA. 2008. "The mystery and magic of glia: A perspective on their roles in health and disease." *Neuron*. 60(3):430–440. doi:10.1016/j.neuron.2008.10.013

[26] Kadry H, Noorani B, Cucullo L. 2020. "A blood–brain barrier overview on structure, function, impairment, and biomarkers of integrity." *Fluids and Barriers of the CNS*. 17(1):69. doi:10.1186/s12987-020-00230-3

[27] Daneman R, Prat A. 2015. "The blood–brain barrier." *Cold Spring Harbor Perspectives in Biology*. 7(1):a020412. doi:10.1101/cshperspect.a020412

[28] Ballabh P, Braun A, Nedergaard M. 2004. "The blood–brain barrier: An overview." *Neurobiology of Disease*. 16(1):1–13. doi:10.1016/j.nbd.2003.12.016

[29] Pino A, Fumagalli G, Bifari F, Decimo I. 2017. "New neurons in adult brain: distribution, molecular mechanisms and therapies." *Biochemical Pharmacology*. 141:4–22. doi:10.1016/j.bcp.2017.07.003

[30] van den Heuvel MP, Sporns O. 2013."Network hubs in the human brain." *Trends in Cognitive Sciences*. 17(12):683–696. doi:10.1016/j.tics.2013.09.012

[31] Ganat YM, Silbereis J, Cave C, Ngu H, Anderson GM, Ohkubo Y, Ment LR, Vaccarino FM. 2006. "Early postnatal astroglial cells produce multilineage precursors and neural stem cells in vivo." *Journal of Neuroscience*. 26(33):8609–21. doi:10.1523/JNEUROSCI.2532-06.2006

[32] Houston SM, Herting MM, Sowell ER. 2014. "The neurobiology of childhood structural brain development: Conception through adulthood." *Current Topics in Behavioral Neurosciences*. 2014;16:3–17. doi:10.1007/7854_2013_265.

[33] Hoover BR, Reed MN, Su J, Penrod RD, Kotilinek LA, Grant MK, Pitstick R, Carlson GA, Lanier LM, Yuan L-L et al. 2010. "Tau mislocalization to dendritic spines mediates synaptic dysfunction independently of neurodegeneration." *Neuron*. 68(6):1067–1081. doi:10.1016/j.neuron.2010.11.030

[34] Milnerwood AJ, Raymond LA. 2010. "Early synaptic pathophysiology in neurodegeneration: Insights from Huntington's disease." *Trends in Neurosciences*. 33(11):513–523. doi:10.1016/j.tins.2010.08.002

[35] Przedborski S, Vila M, Jackson-Lewis V. 2003. "Series introduction: Neurodegeneration: What is it and where are we?" *Journal of Clinical Investigation*. 111(1):3–10. doi:10.1172/JCI200317522

[36] Würfel M, Breitfeld J, Gebhard C, Scholz M, Baber R, Riedel-Heller SG, Blüher M, Stumvoll M, Kovacs P, Tönjes A. 2022. "Interplay between adipose tissue secreted proteins, eating behavior and obesity." *European Journal of Nutrition*. 61(2):885–899. doi:10.1007/s00394-021-02687-w

[37] Jain N, Chen-Plotkin AS. 2018. "Genetic modifiers in neurodegeneration." *Current Genetic Medicine Reports*. 6(1):11–19. doi:10.1007/s40142-018-0133-1

[38] Jain V, Baitharu I, Barhwal K, Prasad D, Singh SB, Ilavazhagan G. 2012. "Enriched environment prevents hypobaric hypoxia induced neurodegeneration and is independent of antioxidant signaling." *Cellular and Molecular Neurobiology*. 32(4):599–611. doi:10.1007/s10571-012-9807-5

[39] Markello RD, Hansen JY, Liu Z-Q, Bazinet V, Shafiei G, Suárez LE, Blostein N, Seidlitz J, Baillet S, Satterthwaite TD et al. 2022. "Neuromaps: structural and functional interpretation of brain maps." *Nature Methods*. 19(11):1472–1479. doi:10.1038/s41592-022-01625-w

[40] Mondragón-Rodríguez S, Perry G, Zhu X, Boehm J. 2012. "Amyloid beta and tau proteins as therapeutic targets for Alzheimer's disease treatment: Rethinking the current strategy." *International Journal of Alzheimer's Disease*. 2012:1–7. doi:10.1155/2012/630182

[41] Chen G, Xu T, Yan Y, Zhou Y, Jiang Y, Melcher K, Xu HE. 2017. "Amyloid beta: Structure, biology and structure-based therapeutic development." *Acta Pharmacologica Sinica*. 38(9):1205–1235. doi:10.1038/aps.2017.28

[42] Rhein V, Eckert A. 2007. "Effects of Alzheimer's amyloid-beta and tau protein on mitochondrial function – Role of glucose metabolism and insulin signalling." *Archives of Physiology and Biochemistry*. 113(3):131–141. doi:10.1080/13813450701572288

[43] Kumar S, Walter J. 2011. "Phosphorylation of amyloid beta (Aβ) peptides – A trigger for formation of toxic aggregates in Alzheimer's disease." *Aging*. 3(8):803–812. doi:10.18632/aging.100362

[44] Spires-Jones TL, Hyman BT. 2014. "The intersection of amyloid beta and tau at synapses in Alzheimer's disease." *Neuron*. 82(4):756–771. doi:10.1016/j.neuron.2014.05.004

[45] Hollingworth P, Harold D, Jones L, Owen MJ, Williams J. 2011. "Alzheimer's disease genetics: Current knowledge and future challenges." *International Journal of Geriatric Psychiatry*. 26(8):793–802. doi:10.1002/gps.2628

[46] López González I, Garcia-Esparcia P, Llorens F, Ferrer I. 2016. "Genetic and transcriptomic profiles of inflammation in neurodegenerative diseases: Alzheimer, Parkinson, Creutzfeldt-Jakob and Tauopathies." *International Journal of Molecular Sciences*. 17(2):206. doi:10.3390/ijms17020206

[47] Megha K, Deshmukh PS, Banerjee BD, Tripathi AK, Ahmed R, Abegaonkar MP. 2015. "Low intensity microwave radiation induced oxidative stress, inflammatory response and DNA damage in rat brain." *NeuroToxicology*. 51:158–165. doi:10.1016/j.neuro.2015.10.009

[48] Abubakar MB, Sanusi KO, Ugusman A, Mohamed W, Kamal H, Ibrahim NH, Khoo CS, Kumar J. 2022. "Alzheimer's disease: An update and insights into pathophysiology." *Frontiers in Aging Neuroscience*. 14:742408. doi:10.3389/fnagi.2022.742408

[49] Aloe L, Rocco ML, Bianchi P, Manni L. 2012. "Nerve growth factor: From the early discoveries to the potential clinical use." *Journal of Translational Medicine*. 10(1):239. doi:10.1186/1479-5876-10-239

[50] Rocco ML, Soligo M, Manni L, Aloe L. 2018. "Nerve growth factor: Early studies and recent clinical trials." *Current Neuropharmacology*. 16(10):1455–1465. doi:10.2174/1570159X16666180412092859

[51] Tiberi A, Capsoni S, Cattaneo A. 2022. "A microglial function for the nerve growth factor: Predictions of the unpredictable." *Cells*. 11(11):1835. doi:10.3390/cells11111835

[52] Bruno MA, Cuello AC. 2006. "Activity-dependent release of precursor nerve growth factor, conversion to mature nerve growth factor, and its degradation by a protease cascade." *Proceedings of the National Academy of Sciences*. 103(17):6735–6740. doi:10.1073/pnas.0510645103

[53] Xu C-J, Wang J-L, Jin W-L. 2016. "The emerging therapeutic role of NGF in Alzheimer's disease." *Neurochemical Research*. 41(6):1211–1218. doi:10.1007/s11064-016-1829-9

[54] Giacobini E, Becker RE. 2007. "One hundred years after the discovery of Alzheimer's disease. A turning point for therapy?" *Journal of Alzheimer's Disease*. 12(1):37–52. doi:10.3233/JAD-2007-12105

[55] J. Allen S, J. Watson J, Dawbarn D. 2011. "The neurotrophins and their role in Alzheimers disease." *Current Neuropharmacology*. 9(4):559–573. doi:10.2174/157015911798376190

[56] Cuello AC, Pentz R, Hall H. 2019. "The brain NGF metabolic pathway in health and in Alzheimer's pathology." *Frontiers in Neuroscience*. 13:62. doi:10.3389/fnins.2019.00062

[57] Sharma V, Kaur A, Singh TG. 2020. "Counteracting role of nuclear factor erythroid 2-related factor 2 pathway in Alzheimer's disease." *Biomedicine & Pharmacotherapy*. 129:110373. doi:10.1016/j.biopha.2020.110373

[58] Nevado-Holgado AJ, Ribe E, Thei L, Furlong L, Mayer M-A, Quan J, Richardson JC, Cavanagh J, NIMA Consortium, Lovestone S. 2019. "Genetic and real-world clinical data, combined with empirical validation, nominate Jak-Stat signaling as a target for Alzheimer's disease therapeutic development." *Cells*. 8(5):425. doi:10.3390/cells8050425

[59] Chen W, Wu L, Hu Y, Jiang L, Liang N, Chen J, Qin H, Tang N. 2020. "MicroRNA-107 ameliorates damage in a cell model of Alzheimer's disease by mediating the FGF7/FGFR2/PI3K/Akt pathway." *Journal of Molecular Neuroscience*. 70(10):1589–1597. doi:10.1007/s12031-020-01600-0

[60] Johnson JW, Kotermanski SE. 2006. "Mechanism of action of memantine." *Current Opinion in Pharmacology*. 6(1):61–7. doi:10.1016/j.coph.2005.09.007

[61] Folch J, Busquets O, Ettcheto M, Sánchez-López E, Castro-Torres RD, Verdaguer E, Garcia ML, Olloquequi J, Casadesús G, Beas-Zarate C et al. 2018. "Memantine for the treatment of dementia: A review on its current and future applications." *Journal of Alzheimer's Disease*. 62(3):1223–1240. doi:10.3233/JAD-170672

[62] Reisberg B, Doody R, Stöffler A, Schmitt F, Ferris S, Möbius H. 2003. "Memantine in moderate-to-severe Alzheimer's disease." *New England Journal of Medicine*. 348(14):1333–41. doi:10.1056/NEJMoa013128

[63] Deardorff W, Feen E, Grossberg G. 2015. "The use of cholinesterase inhibitors across all stages of Alzheimer's disease." *Drugs & Aging*. 32(7):537–47. doi:10.1007/s40266-015-0273-x

[64] Hampel H, Mesulam M, Cuello A, Khachaturian A, Vergallo A, Farlow M, Snyder P, Giacobini E, Khachaturian ZS. 2019. "Revisiting the cholinergic hypothesis in Alzheimer's disease: Emerging evidence from translational and clinical research." *Journal of Prevention of Alzheimer's Disease*. 6(1):2–15. doi:10.14283/jpad.2018.43

[65] Dunn B, Stein P, Cavazzoni P. 2021. "Approval of aducanumab for Alzheimer disease – the FDA's perspective." *JAMA Internal Medicine*. 181(10):1276–1278. doi:10.1001/jamainternmed.2021.4607

[66] Walsh S, Merrick R, Milne R, Brayne C. 2021. "Aducanumab for Alzheimer's disease?" *BMJ*. 5:n1682. doi:10.1136/bmj.n1682

[67] Dunn B, Stein P, Temple R, Cavazzoni P. 2021. "An appropriate use of accelerated approval – Aducanumab for Alzheimer's disease." *New England Journal of Medicine.* 385(9):856–857. doi:10.1056/NEJMc2111960

[68] Parthasarathy G, Pattison MB, Midkiff CC. 2023. "The FGF/FGFR system in the microglial neuroinflammation with Borrelia burgdorferi: Likely intersectionality with other neurological conditions." *Journal of Neuroinflammation.* 20(1):10. doi:10.1186/s12974-022-02681-x

[69] Spires-Jones TL, Attems J, Thal D.2017. "Interactions of pathological proteins in neurodegenerative diseases." *Acta Neuropathol.* 134(2):187–205. doi:10.1007/s00401-017-1709-7

[70] Kouli A, Torsney KM, Kuan W-L. 2018. "Parkinson's disease: Etiology, neuropathology, and pathogenesis." In: *Parkinson's Disease: Pathogenesis and Clinical Aspects.* Brisbane, Australia: Codon Publications; 2018. p. 24.

[71] Emamzadeh FN, Surguchov A. 2018. "Parkinson's disease: Biomarkers, treatment, and risk factors." *Frontiers in Neuroscience.* 12:612. doi:10.3389/fnins.2018.00612

[72] Gorell JM, Peterson EL, Rybicki BA, Johnson CC. 2004. "Multiple risk factors for Parkinson's disease." *Journal of the Neurological Sciences.* 217(2):169–74. doi:10.1016/j.jns.2003.09.014

[73] Priyadarshi A, Khuder S, Schaub E, Priyadarshi S. 2001. "Environmental risk factors and Parkinson's disease: A metaanalysis." *Environmental Research.* 86(2):122–127. doi:10.1006/enrs.2001.4264

[74] Kuopio A-M, Marttila RJ, Helenius H, Rinne UK. 1999. "Environmental risk factors in Parkinson's disease." *Movement Disorders.* 14(6):12. doi:https://doi.org/10.1002/1531-8257(199911)14:6<928::AID-MDS1004>3.0.CO;2-Z

[75] Bartels AL, Leenders KL. 2009. "Parkinson's disease: The syndrome, the pathogenesis and pathophysiology." *Cortex.* 45(8):915–921. doi:10.1016/j.cortex.2008.11.010

[76] Klein C, Westenberger A. 2012. "Genetics of Parkinson's disease." *Cold Spring Harbor Perspectives in Medicine.* 2(1):a008888–a008888. doi:10.1101/cshperspect.a008888

[77] Cannon JR, Greenamyre JT. 2011. "The role of environmental exposures in neurodegeneration and neurodegenerative diseases." *Toxicological Sciences.* 124(2):225–250. doi:10.1093/toxsci/kfr239

[78] Abou-Sleiman PM, Muqit MMK, Wood NW. 2006. "Expanding insights of mitochondrial dysfunction in Parkinson's disease." *Nature Reviews Neuroscience.* 7(3):207–219. doi:10.1038/nrn1868

[79] Kim WS, Kågedal K, Halliday GM. 2014. "Alpha-synuclein biology in Lewy body diseases." *Alzheimer's Research & Therapy.* 6(5–8):73. doi:10.1186/s13195-014-0073-2

[80] Malkus KA, Tsika E, Ischiropoulos H. 2009. "Oxidative modifications, mitochondrial dysfunction, and impaired protein degradation in Parkinson's disease: How neurons are lost in the Bermuda triangle." *Molecular Neurodegeneration.* 4(1):24. doi:10.1186/1750-1326-4-24

[81] Marques O, Outeiro TF. 2012. "Alpha-synuclein: From secretion to dysfunction and death." *Cell Death & Disease.* 3(7):e350–e350. doi:10.1038/cddis.2012.94

[82] Parihar MS, Parihar A, Fujita M, Hashimoto M, Ghafourifar P. 2009. "Alpha-synuclein overexpression and aggregation exacerbates impairment of mitochondrial functions by augmenting oxidative stress in human neuroblastoma cells." *International Journal of Biochemistry & Cell Biology.* 41(10):2015–2024. doi:10.1016/j.biocel.2009.05.008

[83] Schraen-Maschke S, Sergeant N, Dhaenens C-M, Bombois S, Deramecourt V, Caillet-Boudin M-L, Pasquier F, Maurage C-A, Sablonnière B, Vanmechelen E et al. 2008. "Tau as a biomarker of neurodegenerative diseases." *Biomarkers in Medicine*. 2(4):363–384. doi:10.2217/17520363.2.4.363

[84] Coune PG, Schneider BL, Aebischer P. 2012. "Parkinson's disease: Gene therapies." *Cold Spring Harbor Perspectives in Medicine*. 2(4):a009431–a009431. doi:10.1101/cshperspect.a009431

[85] Chan NC, Salazar AM, Pham AH, Sweredoski MJ, Kolawa NJ, Graham RLJ, Hess S, Chan DC. 2011. "Broad activation of the ubiquitin–proteasome system by Parkin is critical for mitophagy." *Human Molecular Genetics*. 20(9):1726–1737. doi:10.1093/hmg/ddr048

[86] Schlossmacher MG, Frosch MP, Gai WP, Medina M, Sharma N, Forno L, Ochiishi T, Shimura H, Sharon R, Hattori N et al. 2002. "Parkin localizes to the Lewy bodies of Parkinson disease and dementia with Lewy bodies." *American Journal of Pathology*. 160(5):1655–1667. doi:10.1016/S0002-9440(10)61113-3

[87] Ariga H, Takahashi-Niki K, Kato I, Maita H, Niki T, Iguchi-Ariga SMM. 2013. "Neuroprotective function of DJ-1 in Parkinson's disease." *Oxidative Medicine and Cellular Longevity*. 2013:1–9. doi:10.1155/2013/683920

[88] Canet-Avilés RM, Wilson MA, Miller DW, Ahmad R, McLendon C, Bandyopadhyay S, Baptista MJ, Ringe D, Petsko GA, Cookson MR. 2004. "The Parkinson's disease protein DJ-1 is neuroprotective due to cysteine-sulfinic acid-driven mitochondrial localization." *Proceedings of the National Academy of Sciences*. 101(24):9103–9108. doi:10.1073/pnas.0402959101

[89] Wu W, Xu H, Wang Z, Mao Y, Yuan L, Luo W, Cui Z, Cui T, Wang XL, Shen YH. 2015. "PINK1-parkin-mediated mitophagy protects mitochondrial integrity and prevents metabolic stress-induced endothelial injury." *PLOS One*. 10(7):e0132499. doi:10.1371/journal.pone.0132499

[90] Dias V, Junn E, Mouradian MM. 2013. "The role of oxidative stress in Parkinson's disease." *Journal of Parkinson's Disease*. 3(4):461–491. doi:10.3233/JPD-130230

[91] McNaught KSP, Olanow CW, Halliwell B, Isacson O, Jenner P. 2001. "Failure of the ubiquitin–proteasome system in Parkinson's disease." *Nature Reviews Neuroscience*. 2(8):589–594. doi:10.1038/35086067

[92] Ciechanover A, Kwon YT. 2015. "Degradation of misfolded proteins in neurodegenerative diseases: Therapeutic targets and strategies." *Experimental & Molecular Medicine*. 47(3):e147–e147. doi:10.1038/emm.2014.117

[93] Rubinsztein DC. 2006. "The roles of intracellular protein-degradation pathways in neurodegeneration." *Nature*. 443(7113):780–786. doi:10.1038/nature05291

[94] Dokladny K, Myers OB, Moseley PL. 2015. "Heat shock response and autophagy – cooperation and control." *Autophagy*. 11(2):200–213. doi:10.1080/15548627.2015.1009776

[95] Karunanithi S, Brown IR. 2015. "Heat shock response and homeostatic plasticity." *Frontiers in Cellular Neuroscience*. 9. doi:10.3389/fncel.2015.00068

[96] Dhall R, Kreitzman DL. 2016. "Advances in levodopa therapy for Parkinson disease: Review of RYTARY (carbidopa and levodopa) clinical efficacy and safety." *Neurology*. 86((14 Suppl 1)):S13–S24.

[97] Rinne UK, Molsa P. 1979. "Levodopa with benserazide or carbidopa in Parkinson disease." *Neurology*. 29(12):1584–1589. doi:10.1212/WNL.29.12.1584

[98] Szökö É, Tábi T, Riederer P, Vécsei L, Magyar K. 2018. "Pharmacological aspects of the neuroprotective effects of irreversible MAO-B inhibitors, selegiline and rasagiline, in Parkinson's disease." *Journal of Neural Transmission*. 125(11):1735–1749. doi:10.1007/s00702-018-1853-9

[99] Naoi M, Maruyama W, Inaba-Hasegawa K. 2013. "Revelation in the neuroprotective functions of rasagiline and selegiline: the induction of distinct genes by different mechanisms." *Expert Review of Neurotherapeutics*. 13(6):671–684. doi:10.1586/ern.13.60

[100] Abel EL. 2007. "Football increases the risk for Lou Gehrig's disease, amyotrophic lateral sclerosis." *Perceptual and Motor Skills*. 104(3):1251–1254. doi:10.2466/pms.104.4.1251-1254

[101] Barinaga M. 1994. "Neurotrophic factors enter the clinic." *Science*. 264(5160):772–774. doi:10.1126/science.8171331

[102] Hardiman O, Al-Chalabi A, Chio A, Corr EM, Logroscino G, Robberecht W, Shaw PJ, Simmons Z. 2017. "Amyotrophic lateral sclerosis." *Nature Reviews Disease Primers*. 3:17071. doi:10.1038/nrdp.2017.71

[103] Azadmanesh J, Borgstahl G. 2018. "A review of the catalytic mechanism of human manganese superoxide dismutase." *Antioxidants*. 7(2):25. doi:10.3390/antiox7020025

[104] Saccon RA, Bunton-Stasyshyn RKA, Fisher EMC, Fratta P. 2013. "Is SOD1 loss of function involved in amyotrophic lateral sclerosis?" *Brain*. 136(8):2342–2358. doi:10.1093/brain/awt097

[105] Zelko IN, Mariani TJ, Folz RJ. 2002. "Superoxide dismutase multigene family: A comparison of the CuZn-SOD (SOD1), Mn-SOD (SOD2), and EC-SOD (SOD3) gene structures, evolution, and expression." *Free Radical Biology and Medicine*. 33(3):337–349. doi:10.1016/S0891-5849(02)00905-X

[106] Hayashi Y, Homma K, Ichijo H. 2016. "SOD1 in neurotoxicity and its controversial roles in SOD1 mutation-negative ALS." *Advances in Biological Regulation*. 60:95–104. doi:10.1016/j.jbior.2015.10.006

[107] Miquel E, Cassina A, Martínez-Palma L, Bolatto C, Trías E, Gandelman M, Radi R, Barbeito L, Cassina P. 2012. "Modulation of astrocytic mitochondrial function by dichloroacetate improves survival and motor performance in inherited amyotrophic lateral sclerosis." *PLoS ONE*. 7(4):e34776. doi:10.1371/journal.pone.0034776

[108] Szelechowski M, Amoedo N, Obre E, Léger C, Allard L, Bonneu M, Claverol S, Lacombe D, Oliet S, Chevallier S et al. 2018. "Metabolic reprogramming in amyotrophic lateral sclerosis." *Scientific Reports*. 8(1):3953. doi:10.1038/s41598-018-22318-5

[109] DeJesus-Hernandez M, Mackenzie IR, Boeve BF, Boxer AL, Baker M, Rutherford NJ, Nicholson AM, Finch NA, Flynn H, Adamson J et al. 2011. "Expanded GGGGCC hexanucleotide repeat in noncoding region of C9ORF72 causes chromosome 9p-linked FTD and ALS." *Neuron*. 72(2):245–256. doi:10.1016/j.neuron.2011.09.011

[110] Prpar Mihevc S, Darovic S, Kovanda A, Bajc Česnik A, Župunski V, Rogelj B. 2017. "Nuclear trafficking in amyotrophic lateral sclerosis and frontotemporal lobar degeneration." *Brain*. 140(1):13–26. doi:10.1093/brain/aww197

[111] Renton AE, Majounie E, Waite A, Simón-Sánchez J, Rollinson S, Gibbs JR, Schymick JC, Laaksovirta H, van Swieten JC, Myllykangas L et al. 2011. "A hexanucleotide repeat expansion in C9ORF72 is the cause of chromosome 9p21-linked ALS-FTD." *Neuron*. 72(2):257–268. doi:10.1016/j.neuron.2011.09.010

[112] Kametani F, Obi T, Shishido T, Akatsu H, Murayama S, Saito Y, Yoshida M, Hasegawa M. 2016. "Mass spectrometric analysis of accumulated TDP-43 in amyotrophic lateral sclerosis brains." *Scientific Reports*. 6(1):23281. doi:10.1038/srep23281

[113] Kwiatkowski TJ, Bosco DA, LeClerc AL, Tamrazian E, Vanderburg CR, Russ C, Davis A, Gilchrist J, Kasarskis EJ, Munsat T et al. 2009. "Mutations in the *FUS/TLS* gene on chromosome 16 cause familial amyotrophic lateral sclerosis." *Science*. 323(5918):1205–1208. doi:10.1126/science.1166066

[114] Vance C, Rogelj B, Hortobágyi T, De Vos KJ, Nishimura AL, Sreedharan J, Hu X, Smith B, Ruddy D, Wright P et al. 2009. "Mutations in FUS, an RNA processing protein, cause familial amyotrophic lateral sclerosis Type 6." *Science*. 323(5918):1208–1211. doi:10.1126/science.1165942

[115] Yang L, Gal J, Chen J, Zhu H. 2014. "Self-assembled FUS binds active chromatin and regulates gene transcription." *Proceedings of the National Academy of Sciences*. 111(50):17809–17814. doi:10.1073/pnas.1414004111

[116] Gal J, Zhang J, Kwinter DM, Zhai J, Jia H, Jia J, Zhu H. 2011. "Nuclear localization sequence of FUS and induction of stress granules by ALS mutants." *Neurobiology of Aging*. 32(12):2323.e27-2323.e40. doi:10.1016/j.neurobiolaging.2010.06.010

[117] Jaiswal MK. 2019. "Riluzole and edaravone: A tale of two amyotrophic lateral sclerosis drugs." *Medicinal Research Reviews*. 39(2):733–748. doi:10.1002/med.21528

[118] Halberstein RA. 2005. "Medicinal plants: Historical and cross-cultural usage patterns." *Annals of Epidemiology*. 15(9):686–699. doi:10.1016/j.annepidem.2005.02.004

[119] Jiofack T, Ayissi I, Fokunang C, Guedje N, Kemeuze V. 2009. "Ethnobotany and phytomedicine of the upper Nyong valley forest in Cameroon." *African Journal of Pharmacy and pharmacology*. 3(4):144–150.

[120] Kamboj VP. 2000. "Herbal medicine." *Current Science*. 78(1):35–39.

[121] Schulz V, Hänsel R, Blumenthal M, Tyler VE. 2004. "Rational phytotherapy: A reference guide for physicians and pharmacists." *Springer Science & Business Media*.

[122] Al-Ameri TK, Jasim SY, Al-Khafaji AJS. 2011. "Middle Paleolithic to Neolithic cultural history of North Iraq." *Arabian Journal of Geosciences*. 4(5):945–972.

[123] Fabricant DS, Farnsworth NR. 2001. "The value of plants used in traditional medicine for drug discovery." *Environmental Health Perspectives*. 109.

[124] Petrovska B. 2012. "Historical review of medicinal plants' usage." *Pharmacognosy Reviews*. 6(11):1. doi:10.4103/0973-7847.95849

[125] Pan S-Y, Litscher G, Gao S-H, Zhou S-F, Yu Z-L, Chen H-Q, Zhang S-F, Tang M-K, Sun J-N, Ko K-M. 2014. "Historical perspective of traditional indigenous medical practices: The current renaissance and conservation of herbal resources." *Evidence-Based Complementary and Alternative Medicine*. 2014:1–20. doi:10.1155/2014/525340

[126] Msomi NZ, Simelane BC. 2019. "Herbal medicine." *IntechOpen*.

[127] Alamgir ANM, Alamgir ANM. 2017. "Origin, definition, scope and area, subject matter, importance, and history of development of pharmacognosy." *Therapeutic Use of Medicinal Plants and Their Extracts*. 19–60.

[128] Weckowicz TE. 1990. *A history of great ideas in abnormal psychology. Elsevier*.

[129] Aboelsoud NH. 2010. "Herbal medicine in ancient Egypt." *Journal of Medicinal Plants Research*. 42(2):82–86.

[130] Shoeb M. 2006. "Anticancer agents from medicinal plants." *Bangladesh Journal of Pharmacology*. 1(2):35–41. doi:10.3329/bjp.v1i2.486

[131] Lemonnier N, Zhou G-B, Prasher B, Mukerji M, Chen Z, Brahmachari SK, Noble D, Auffray C, Sagner M. 2017. "Traditional knowledge-based medicine: a review of history, principles, and relevance in the present context of P4 systems medicine." *Progress in Preventive Medicine*. 2(7):e0011. doi:10.1097/pp9.0000000000000011

[132] Kloos S, Blaikie C. 2022. *Asian medical industries: contemporary perspectives on traditional pharmaceuticals. Routledge*.

[133] Chaudhuri B. 2015. "Science in society: Challenges and opportunities for indigenous knowledge in the present-day context." *Global Bioethics*. 26(2):78–85. doi:10.1080/11287462.2015.1037140

[134] Corson TW, Crews CM. 2007. "Molecular understanding and modern application of traditional medicines: Triumphs and trials." *Cell*. 130(5):769–774. doi:10.1016/j.cell.2007.08.021

[135] Challand S, Willcox M. 2009. "A clinical trial of the traditional medicine *Vernonia amygdalina* in the treatment of uncomplicated malaria." *Journal of Alternative and Complementary Medicine*. 15(11):1231–1237. doi:10.1089/acm.2009.0098

[136] Mirzaie A, Halaji M, Dehkordi FS, Ranjbar R, Noorbazargan H. 2020. "A narrative literature review on traditional medicine options for treatment of corona virus disease 2019 (COVID-19)." *Complementary Therapies in Clinical Practice*. 40:101214. doi:10.1016/j.ctcp.2020.101214

[137] Liu C. 2021. "Overview on development of ASEAN traditional and herbal medicines." *Chinese Herbal Medicines*. 13(4):441–450. doi:10.1016/j.chmed.2021.09.002

[138] Zhang Y. 2011. "Mathematical reasoning of treatment principle based on 'Yin Yang Wu Xing' theory in traditional Chinese medicine (II)." *Chinese Medicine*. 2(4):158–170. doi:10.4236/cm.2011.24026

[139] Wang X, Xu X, Tao W, Li Y, Wang Y, Yang L. 2012. "A systems biology approach to uncovering pharmacological synergy in herbal medicines with applications to cardiovascular disease." *Evidence-Based Complementary and Alternative Medicine*. 2012:1–15. doi:10.1155/2012/519031

[140] Zhang A, Sun H, Wang X. 2014. "Potentiating therapeutic effects by enhancing synergism based on active constituents from traditional medicine." *Phytotherapy Research*. 28(4):526–533. doi:10.1002/ptr.5032

[141] Yuan H, Ma Q, Ye L, Piao G. 2016. "The traditional medicine and modern medicine from natural products." *Molecules*. 21(5):559. doi:10.3390/molecules21050559

[142] Chattopadhyay K. 2017. "Ayurveda and lifestyle modification: Research to practice." *International Journal of Medicine and Public Health*. 7(3):132–133. doi:10.5530/ijmedph.2017.3.27

[143] Alam MdA, Quamri MA, Sofi G, Tarique BMd. 2019. "Understanding hypothyroidism in Unani medicine." *Journal of Integrative Medicine*. 17(6):387–391. doi:10.1016/j.joim.2019.05.006

[144] Husain A, Sofi GD, Tajuddin, Dang R, Kumar N. 2010. "Unani system of medicine – Introduction and challenges." *Medical Journal of Islamic World Academy of Sciences*. 18(1):27–30.

[145] Román GC. 2002. "Vascular dementia may be the most common form of dementia in the elderly." *Journal of the Neurological Sciences*. 203–204:7–10. doi:10.1016/S0022-510X(02)00252-6

[146] Sattin RW, Lambert Huber DA, Devito CA, Rodriguez JG, Ros A, Bacchelli S, Stevens JA, Waxweiler RJ. 1990. "The incidence of fall injury events among the elderly in a defined population." *American Journal of Epidemiology*. 131(6):1028–1037. doi:10.1093/oxfordjournals.aje.a115594

[147] Escobar I, Xu J, Jackson CW, Perez-Pinzon MA. 2019. "Altered neural networks in the Papez circuit: Implications for cognitive dysfunction after cerebral ischemia." *Journal of Alzheimer's Disease*. 67(2):425–446. doi:10.3233/JAD-180875

[148] Pluta R, Bogucka-Kocka A, Ułamek-Kozioł M, Bogucki J, Januszewski S, Kocki J, Czucwar SJ. 2018. "Ischemic tau protein gene induction as an additional key factor driving development of Alzheimer's phenotype changes in CA1 area of hippocampus in an ischemic model of Alzheimer's disease." *Pharmacological Reports*. 70(5):881–884. doi:10.1016/j.pharep.2018.03.004

[149] Radenovic L, Nenadic M, Ułamek-Kozioł M, Januszewski S, Czuczwar SJ, Andjus PR, Pluta R. 2020. "Heterogeneity in brain distribution of activated microglia and astrocytes in a rat ischemic model of Alzheimer's disease after 2 years of survival." *Aging*. 12(12):12251–12267. doi:10.18632/aging.103411

[150] Tobin MK, Bonds JA, Minshall RD, Pelligrino DA, Testai FD, Lazarov O. 2014. "Neurogenesis and inflammation after ischemic stroke: What is known and where we go from here." *Journal of Cerebral Blood Flow & Metabolism*. 34(10):1573–1584. doi:10.1038/jcbfm.2014.130

[151] Plesnila N. 2013. "Pathophysiological role of global cerebral ischemia following subarachnoid hemorrhage: The current experimental evidence." *Stroke Research and Treatment*. 2013:1–7. doi:10.1155/2013/651958

[152] Raichle ME. 1983. "The pathophysiology of brain ischemia." *Annals of Neurology*. 13(1):2–10. doi:10.1002/ana.410130103

[153] Gürer G, Gursoy-Ozdemir Y, Erdemli E, Can A, Dalkara T. 2009. "Astrocytes are more resistant to focal cerebral ischemia than neurons and die by a delayed necrosis." *Brain Pathology*. 19(4):630–641. doi:10.1111/j.1750-3639.2008.00226.x

[154] Haeusler KG, Schmidt WUH, Föhring F, Meisel C, Helms T, Jungehulsing GJ, Nolte CH, Schmolke K, Wegner B, Meisel A et al. 2008. "Cellular immunodepression preceding infectious complications after acute ischemic stroke in humans." *Cerebrovascular Diseases*. 25(1–2):50–58. doi:10.1159/000111499

[155] Liu Q, Jin W-N, Liu Y, Shi K, Sun H, Zhang F, Zhang C, Gonzales RJ, Sheth KN, La Cava A et al. 2017. "Brain ischemia suppresses immunity in the periphery and brain via different neurogenic innervations." *Immunity*. 46(3):474–487. doi:10.1016/j.immuni.2017.02.015

[156] Shim R, Wong C. 2016. "Ischemia, immunosuppression and infection – Tackling the predicaments of post-stroke complications." *International Journal of Molecular Sciences*. 17(1):64. doi:10.3390/ijms17010064

[157] Radak D, Resanovic I, Isenovic ER. 2014. "Link between oxidative stress and acute brain ischemia." *Angiology*. 65(8):667–676. doi:10.1177/0003319713506516

[158] Dantzer R. 2018. "Neuroimmune interactions: From the brain to the immune system and vice versa." *Physiological Reviews*. 98(1):477–504. doi:10.1152/physrev.00039.2016

[159] Enzmann G, Kargaran S, Engelhardt B. 2018. "Ischemia–reperfusion injury in stroke: Impact of the brain barriers and brain immune privilege on neutrophil function." *Therapeutic Advances in Neurological Disorders*. 11:1–15.

[160] Feng Y, Li Y, Zhang Y, Zhang B-H, Zhao H, Zhao X, Shi F-D, Jin W-N, Zhang X-A. 2021. "miR-1224 contributes to ischemic stroke-mediated natural killer cell dysfunction by targeting Sp1 signaling." *Journal of Neuroinflammation*. 18(1):133. doi:10.1186/s12974-021-02181-4

[161] Chen C, Ai Q-D, Chu S-F, Zhang Z, Chen N-H. 2019. "NK cells in cerebral ischemia." *Biomedicine & Pharmacotherapy*. 109:547–554. doi:10.1016/j.biopha.2018.10.103

[162] Liu Q, Johnson EM, Lam RK, Wang Q, Bo Ye H, Wilson EN, Minhas PS, Liu L, Swarovski MS, Tran S et al. 2019. "Peripheral TREM1 responses to brain and intestinal immunogens amplify stroke severity." *Nature Immunology*. 20(8):1023–1034. doi:10.1038/s41590-019-0421-2

[163] Weinstein JR, Koerner IP, Möller T. 2010. "Microglia in ischemic brain injury." *Future Neurology*. 5(2):227–246. doi:10.2217/fnl.10.1

[164] Kawabori M, Yenari M. 2015. "Inflammatory responses in brain ischemia." *Current Medicinal Chemistry*. 22(10):1258–1277. doi:10.2174/0929867322666150209154036

[165] Schnell L, Fearn S, Klassen H, Schwab ME, Perry VH. 1999. "Acute inflammatory responses to mechanical lesions in the CNS: differences between brain and spinal cord." *European Journal of Neuroscience*.

[166] Turner MD, Nedjai B, Hurst T, Pennington DJ. 2014. "Cytokines and chemokines: At the crossroads of cell signalling and inflammatory disease." *Biochimica et Biophysica Acta (BBA) – Molecular Cell Research*. 1843(11):2563–2582. doi:10.1016/j.bbamcr.2014.05.014

[167] Fabrizi GM, Zanette G. 2015. "Disorders of peripheral nerves." *Prognosis of Neurological Diseases*. 405–444.

[168] Haskó G, Pacher P. 2008. "A2A receptors in inflammation and injury: Lessons learned from transgenic animals." *Journal of Leukocyte Biology*. 83(3):447–455. doi:10.1189/jlb.0607359

[169] Jayaraj RL, Azimullah S, Beiram R, Jalal FY, Rosenberg GA. 2019. "Neuroinflammation: Friend and foe for ischemic stroke." *Journal of Neuroinflammation*. 16(1):142. doi:10.1186/s12974-019-1516-2

[170] Warach S, Latour LL. 2004. "Evidence of reperfusion injury, exacerbated by thrombolytic therapy, in human focal brain ischemia using a novel imaging marker of early blood–brain barrier disruption." *Stroke*. 35(11_suppl_1):2659–2661. doi:10.1161/01.STR.0000144051.32131.09

[171] Overgaard K. 1994. "Thrombolytic therapy in experimental embolic stroke." *Cerebrovascular and brain metabolism reviews*. 6(3):257–286.

[172] Ye L, Cai R, Yang M, Qian J, Hong Z. 2015. "Reduction of the systemic inflammatory induced by acute cerebral infarction through ultra-early thrombolytic therapy." *Experimental and Therapeutic Medicine*. 10(4):1493–1498. doi:10.3892/etm.2015.2672

[173] Wu P, Zhang Z, Wang F, Chen J. 2010. "Natural compounds from traditional medicinal herbs in the treatment of cerebral ischemia/reperfusion injury." *Acta Pharmacologica Sinica*. 31(12):1523–1531. doi:10.1038/aps.2010.186

[174] Abdel-Daim MM, Alkahtani S, Almeer R, Albasher G. 2020. "Alleviation of lead acetate-induced nephrotoxicity by Moringa oleifera extract in rats: Highlighting the antioxidant, anti-inflammatory, and anti-apoptotic activities." *Environmental Science and Pollution Research*. 27(27):33723–33731. doi:10.1007/s11356-020-09643-x

[175] Ghosh N, Ghosh H, Bhat ZA, Mandal V, Bachar SC, Nima ND, Sunday OO, Mandal SC. 2014. "Advances in herbal medicine for treatment of ischemic brain injury." *Natural Product Communications*. 9(7):1045–1055.

[176] Xu M, Wu R-X, Li X-L, Zeng Y-S, Liang J-Y, Fu K, Liang Y, Wang Z. 2022. "Traditional medicine in China for ischemic stroke: Bioactive components, pharmacology, and mechanisms." *Journal of Integrative Neuroscience*. 21(1):026. doi:10.31083/j.jin2101026

[177] Ji X-Y, Tan BK, Zhu Y-Z. 2000. "Salvia miltiorrhiza and ischemic diseases." *Acta Pharmacologica Sinica*. 21(12):1089–1094.

[178] Chen J, Huang Q, Li J, Yao Y, Sun W, Zhang Z, Qi H, Chen Z, Liu J, Zhao D. 2022. "Panax ginseng against myocardial ischemia/reperfusion injury: A review of preclinical evidence and potential mechanisms." *Journal of Ethnopharmacology*. 115715.

[179] Sun L, Jia H, Yu M, Yang Y, Li J, Tian D, Zhang H, Zou Z. 2021. "Salvia miltiorrhiza and Pueraria lobata, two eminent herbs in Xin-Ke-Shu, ameliorate myocardial ischemia partially by modulating the accumulation of free fatty acids in rats." *Phytomedicine*. 89:153620.

[180] Yang S, Wang H, Yang Y, Wang R, Wang Y, Wu C, Du G. 2019. "Baicalein administered in the subacute phase ameliorates ischemia-reperfusion-induced brain injury by reducing neuroinflammation and neuronal damage." *Biomedicine & Pharmacotherapy*. 117:109102.

[181] Suzuki M, Tabuchi M, Ikeda M, Umegaki K, Tomita T. 2004. "Protective effects of green tea catechins on cerebral ischemic damage." *Medical Science Monitor: International Medical Journal of Experimental and Clinical Research*. 10(6):166–174.

[182] Hosseinzadeh H, Parvardeh S, Asl MN, Sadeghnia HR, Ziaee T. 2007. "Effect of thymoquinone and Nigella sativa seeds oil on lipid peroxidation level during global cerebral ischemia-reperfusion injury in rat hippocampus." *Phytomedicine*. 14(9):621–627.

[183] Pan R, Zhou M, Zhong Y, Xie J, Ling S, Tang X, Huang Y, Chen H. 2019. "The combination of Astragalus membranaceus extract and ligustrazine to improve the inflammation in rats with thrombolytic cerebral ischemia." *International Journal of Immunopathology and Pharmacology*. 33:2058738419869055.

[184] Zengyong Q, Jiangwei M, Huajin L. 2011. "Effect of Ligusticum wallichii aqueous extract on oxidative injury and immunity activity in myocardial ischemic reperfusion rats." *International Journal of Molecular Sciences*. 12(3):1991–2006.

[185] Han Y, Chen Y, Zhang Q, Liu B-W, Yang L, Xu Y-H, Zhao Y-H. 2021. "Overview of therapeutic potentiality of Angelica sinensis for ischemic stroke." *Phytomedicine*. 90:153652.

[186] Joshi P, Dhawan V. 2007. "Axillary multiplication of Swertia chirayita (Roxb. Ex Fleming) H. Karst., a critically endangered medicinal herb of temperate Himalayas." *In Vitro Cellular & Developmental Biology – Plant*. 43(6):631–638. doi:10.1007/s11627-007-9065-2

[187] Kim D, Nguyen MD, Dobbin MM, Fischer A, Sananbenesi F, Rodgers JT, Delalle I, Baur JA, Sui G, Armour SM et al. 2007. "SIRT1 deacetylase protects against neurodegeneration in models for Alzheimer's disease and amyotrophic lateral sclerosis." *EMBO Journal*. 26(13):3169–3179. doi:10.1038/sj.emboj.7601758

[188] Leal-Cardoso JH, Fonteles MC. 1999. "Pharmacological effects of essential oils of plants of the northeast of Brazil." *Anais da Academia Brasileira de Ciencias*. 71(2):207–213.

[189] Govindarajan R, Vijayakumar M, Pushpangadan P. 2005. "Antioxidant approach to disease management and the role of 'Rasayana' herbs of Ayurveda." *Journal of Ethnopharmacology*. 99(2):165–178. doi:10.1016/j.jep.2005.02.035

[190] Posadzki P, Watson L, Ernst E. 2013. "Herb-drug interactions: an overview of systematic reviews." *British Journal of Clinical Pharmacology*. 75(3):603–618. doi:10.1111/j.1365-2125.2012.04350.x

[191] Dutta RR, Kumar T, Ingole N. 2022. "Diet and vitiligo: The story so far." *Cureus*. 14(8):e28516. doi:10.7759/cureus.28516

[192] Ingole SR, Rajput SK, Sharma SS. 2008. "Cognition enhancers: Current strategies and future perspectives." *CRIPS*. 9(3):42–48.

[193] Chakravarthi KK, Avadhani R. 2013. "Beneficial effect of aqueous root extract of Glycyrrhiza glabra on learning and memory using different behavioral models: An experimental study." *Journal of Natural Science, Biology, and Medicine*. 4(2):420.

[194] Kshirsagar SN. 2011. "Nootropic activity of dried seed kernels of Caesalpinia crista Linn against scopolamine induced amnesia in mice." *International Journal of PharmTech Research*. 3(1):104–109.

[195] Søholm B. 1998. "Clinical improvement of memory and other cognitive functions by Ginkgo biloba: Review of relevant literature." *Advances in therapy*. 15(1):54–65.

[196] Matthews DG, Caruso M, Murchison CF, Zhu JY, Wright KM, Harris CJ, Gray NE, Quinn JF, Soumyanath A. 2019. "Centella asiatica improves memory and promotes antioxidative signaling in 5XFAD mice." *Antioxidants*. 8(12):630.

[197] Malve HO, Raut SB, Marathe PA, Rege NN. 2014. "Effect of combination of Phyllanthus emblica, Tinospora cordifolia, and Ocimum sanctum on spatial learning and memory in rats." *Journal of Ayurveda and Integrative Medicine*. 5(4):209.

[198] Wattanathorn J, Jittiwat J, Tongun T, Muchimapura S, Ingkaninan K. 2010. "Zingiber officinale mitigates brain damage and improves memory impairment in focal cerebral ischemic rat." *Evidence-Based Complementary and Alternative Medicine*. 2011.

[199] Peth-Nui T, Wattanathorn J, Muchimapura S, Tong-Un T, Piyavhatkul N, Rangseekajee P, Ingkaninan K, Vittaya-Areekul S. 2012. "Effects of 12-week Bacopa monnieri consumption on attention, cognitive processing, working memory, and functions of both cholinergic and monoaminergic systems in healthy elderly volunteers." *Evidence-Based Complementary and Alternative Medicine*. 2012:606424.

[200] Prediger RDS, Fernandes MS, Rial D, Wopereis S, Pereira VS, Bosse TS, Da Silva CB, Carradore RS, Machado MS, Cechinel-Filho V. 2008. "Effects of acute administration of the hydroalcoholic extract of mate tea leaves (Ilex paraguariensis) in animal models of learning and memory." *Journal of Ethnopharmacology*. 120(3):465–473.

[201] Yadav MK, Singh SK, Singh M, Mishra SS, Singh AK, Tripathi JS, Tripathi YB. 2019. "Neuroprotective activity of Evolvulus alsinoides & Centella asiatica ethanolic extracts in scopolamine-induced amnesia in Swiss albino mice." *Open Access Macedonian Journal of Medical Sciences*. 7(7):1059.

[202] Esfandiari E, Ghanadian M, Rashidi B, Mokhtarian A, Vatankhah AM. 2018. "The effects of Acorus calamus L. in preventing memory loss, anxiety, and oxidative stress on lipopolysaccharide-induced neuroinflammation rat models." *International Journal of Preventive Medicine*. 9:85.

[203] Sudhakara G, Ramesh B, Mallaiah P, Sreenivasulu N, Saralakumari D. 2012. "Protective effect of ethanolic extract of Commiphora mukul gum resin against oxidative stress in the brain of streptozotocin induced diabetic wistar male rats." *EXCLI Journal*. 11:576.

[204] Vasudevan M, Parle M. 2007. "Memory enhancing activity of Anwala churna (Emblica officinalis Gaertn.): An Ayurvedic preparation." *Physiology & behavior*. 91(1):46–54.

[205] Tildesley NTJ, Kennedy DO, Perry EK, Ballard CG, Savelev S, Wesnes KA, Scholey AB. 2003. "Salvia lavandulaefolia (Spanish sage) enhances memory in healthy young volunteers." *Pharmacology Biochemistry and Behavior*. 75(3):669–674.

[206] Lee YK, Yuk DY, Kim TI, Kim YH, Kim KT, Kim KH, Lee BJ, Nam S-Y, Hong JT.2009. "Protective effect of the ethanol extract of Magnolia officinalis and 4-O-methylhonokiol on scopolamine-induced memory impairment and the inhibition of acetylcholinesterase activity." *Journal of Natural Medicines*. 63:274–282.

[207] Biessels GJ, Despa F. 2018. "Cognitive decline and dementia in diabetes mellitus: Mechanisms and clinical implications." *Nature Reviews Endocrinology*. 14(10):591–604. doi:10.1038/s41574-018-0048-7

[208] Barnes M, Brannelly T. 2008. "Achieving care and social justice for people with dementia." *Nursing Ethics*. 15(3):384–395. doi:10.1177/0969733007088363

[209] Stephan A, Bieber A, Hopper L, Joyce R, Irving K, Zanetti O, Portolani E, Kerpershoek L, Verhey F, de Vugt M et al. 2018. "Barriers and facilitators to the access to and use of formal dementia care: Findings of a focus group study with people with dementia, informal carers and health and social care professionals in eight European countries." *BMC Geriatrics*. 18(1):131. doi:10.1186/s12877-018-0816-1

[210] Hasna Imami N, Haryono Y, Dwi Sensusiati A, Hamdan M, Badriyah Hidayati H. 2021. "Dementia in Dr. Soetomo General Hospital Surabaya: A synthetic review of its characteristics." *MNJ (Malang Neurology Journal)*. 7(1):12–16. doi:10.21776// ub.mnj.2021.007.01.3

[211] Pujades-Rodriguez M, Assi V, Gonzalez-Izquierdo A, Wilkinson T, Schnier C, Sudlow C, Hemingway H, Whiteley WN. 2018. "The diagnosis, burden and prognosis of dementia: A record-linkage cohort study in England." *PLOS One*. 13(6):e0199026. doi:10.1371/journal.pone.0199026

[212] Wortmann M. 2012. "Dementia: A global health priority – highlights from an ADI and World Health Organization report." *Alzheimer's Research & Therapy*. 4(5):40. doi:10.1186/alzrt143

[213] Dening T, Sandilyan MB. 2015. "Dementia: definitions and types." *Nursing Standard (Royal College of Nursing (Great Britain)*. 29(37):37–42.

[214] Korsnes MS, Winkler AS. 2020. "Global, regional, and national burden of dementia, 1990–2016: Predictions need local calibration." *Neurology*. 94(16):718–719. doi:10.1212/WNL.0000000000009301

[215] Podcasy JL, Epperson CN. 2016. "Considering sex and gender in Alzheimer disease and other dementias." *Dialogues in Clinical Neuroscience*. 18(4):437–446. doi:10.31887/DCNS.2016.18.4/cepperson

[216] Wimo A, Guerchet M, Ali G, Wu Y, Prina AM, Winblad B, Jönsson L, Liu Z, Prince M. 2017. "The worldwide costs of dementia 2015 and comparisons with 2010." *Alzheimer's & Dementia*. 13(1):1–7. doi:10.1016/j.jalz.2016.07.150

[217] Lastri DN, Alwahdy AS. 2020. "Clinical and radiologic approach to probable mixed dementia (vascular dementia and progressive supranuclear palsy)." *MNJ (Malang Neurology Journal)*. 6(1):46–50.

[218] Rizzi L, Rosset I, Roriz-Cruz M. 2014. "Global epidemiology of dementia: Alzheimer's and vascular types." *BioMed Research International*. 2014:1–8. doi:10.1155/2014/ 908915

[219] Sahu PK, Tiwari P, Prusty SK, Subudhi BB. 2018. "Past and present drug development for Alzheimer's disease." *Frontiers in Clinical Drug Research – Alzheimer Disorders*. 7:214–253.

[220] El-Hayek YH, Wiley RE, Khoury CP, Daya RP, Ballard C, Evans AR, Karran M, Molinuevo JL, Norton M, Atri A. 2019. "Tip of the iceberg: Assessing the global socioeconomic costs of Alzheimer's disease and related dementias and strategic

implications for stakeholders." *Journal of Alzheimer's Disease*. 70(2):323–341. doi:10.3233/JAD-190426

[221] James BD, Leurgans SE, Hebert LE, Scherr PA, Yaffe K, Bennett DA. 2014. "Contribution of Alzheimer disease to mortality in the United States." *Neurology*. 82(12):1045–1050.

[222] Alzheimer's Association, Thies W, Bleiler L. 2013. "2013 Alzheimer's disease facts and figures." *Alzheimer's & Dementia*. 9(2):208–245. doi:10.1016/j.jalz.2013.02.003

[223] Bhushan I, Kour M, Kour G, Gupta S, Sharma S, Yadav A. 2018. "Alzheimer's disease: Causes & treatment – A review." *Annals of Biotechnology*. 1(1). doi:10.33582/2637-4927/1002

[224] Wilcock GK. 2003. "Memantine for the treatment of dementia." *The Lancet. Neurology*. 2(8):503–505.

[225] Porsteinsson AP, Grossberg GT, Mintzer J, Olin JT, Memantine MEM-MD-12 Study Group. 2008. "Memantine treatment in patients with mild to moderate Alzheimer's disease already receiving a cholinesterase inhibitor: A randomized, double-blind, placebo-controlled trial." *Current Alzheimer*. 5(1):83–89.

[226] Stowe RM. 1998. "Assessment methods in behavioral neurology and neuropsychiatry." *Neuropsychology*. 439–485.

[227] Twelves D, Perkins KS, Counsell C. 2003. "Systematic review of incidence studies of Parkinson's disease." *Movement Disorders: Official Journal of the Movement Disorder Society*. 18(1):19–31.

[228] Perez-Lloret S, Rey MV, Pavy-Le Traon A, Rascol O. 2013. "Emerging drugs for autonomic dysfunction in Parkinson's disease." *Expert Opinion on Emerging Drugs*. 18(1):39–53.

[229] Soheili M, Khalaji F, Mirhashemi M, Salami M. 2018. "The effect of essential oil of Lavandula angustifolia on amyloid beta polymerization: An in vitro study." *Iranian Journal of Chemistry and Chemical Engineering*. 37(6):201–207.

[230] Adsersen A, Gauguin B, Gudiksen L, Jäger AK. 2006. "Screening of plants used in Danish folk medicine to treat memory dysfunction for acetylcholinesterase inhibitory activity." *Journal of Ethnopharmacology*. 104(3):418–422.

[231] Shi C, Zhao L, Zhu B, Li Q, Yew DT, Yao Z, Xu J. 2009. "Protective effects of Ginkgo biloba extract (EGb761) and its constituents quercetin and ginkgolide B against β-amyloid peptide-induced toxicity in SH-SY5Y cells." *Chemico-Biological Interactions*. 181(1):115–123.

[232] Bastianetto S, Ramassamy C, Dore S, Christen Y, Poirier J, Quirion R. 2000. "The Ginkgo biloba extract (EGb 761) protects hippocampal neurons against cell death induced by β-amyloid." *European Journal of Neuroscience*. 12(6):1882–1890.

[233] Smith JV, Luo Y. 2003. "Elevation of oxidative free radicals in Alzheimer's disease models can be attenuated by Ginkgo biloba extract EGb 761." *Journal of Alzheimer's Disease*. 5(4):287–300.

[234] Pereira RP, Boligon AA, Appel AS, Fachineto R, Ceron CS, Tanus-Santos JE, Athayde ML, Rocha JBT. 2014. "Chemical composition, antioxidant and anticholinesterase activity of Melissa officinalis." *Industrial Crops and Products*. 53:34–45.

[235] Hassanzadeh G, Pasbakhsh P, Akbari M, Shokri S, Ghahremani M, Amin G, Kashani I, Tameh AA. 2011. "Neuroprotective properties of Melissa officinalis L. extract against ecstasy-induced neurotoxicity." *Cell Journal (Yakhteh)*. 13(1):25.

[236] Phung HM, Lee S, Kang KS. 2020. "Protective effects of active compounds from Salviae miltiorrhizae Radix against glutamate-induced HT-22 hippocampal neuronal cell death." *Processes*. 8(8):914.

[237] Zheng M, Liu C, Fan Y, Shi D, Jian W. 2019. "Total glucosides of paeony (TGP) extracted from radix Paeoniae Alba exerts neuroprotective effects in MPTP-induced experimental parkinsonism by regulating the cAMP/PKA/CREB signaling pathway." *Journal of Ethnopharmacology*. 245:112182.

[238] Batarseh YS, Bharate SS, Kumar V, Kumar A, Vishwakarma RA, Bharate SB, Kaddoumi A. 2017. "Crocus sativus extract tightens the blood–brain barrier, reduces amyloid β load and related toxicity in 5XFAD mice." *ACS Chemical Neuroscience*. 8(8):1756–1766.

[239] Ghahghaei A, Bathaie SZ, Kheirkhah H, Bahraminejad E. 2013. "The protective effect of crocin on the amyloid fibril formation of Aβ42 peptide in vitro." *Cellular & Molecular Biology Letters*. 18:328–339.

[240] Choi JG, Kim N, Huh E, Lee H, Oh MH, Park JD, Pyo MK, Oh MS. 2017. "White ginseng protects mouse hippocampal cells against amyloid-beta oligomer toxicity." *Phytotherapy Research*. 31(3):497–506.

[241] Cong W-H, Liu J-X, Xu L. 2007. "Effects of extracts of ginseng and Ginkgo biloba on hippocampal acetylcholine and monoamines in PDAP-pV717I transgenic mice." *Zhongguo Zhong xi yi jie he za zhi Zhongguo Zhongxiyi Jiehe Zazhi [Chinese Journal of Integrated Traditional and Western Medicine]*. 27(9):810–813.

[242] Lee Y-J, Choi D-Y, Yun Y-P, Han SB, Kim HM, Lee K, Choi SH, Yang M-P, Jeon HS, Jeong J-H. 2013. "Ethanol extract of Magnolia officinalis prevents lipopolysaccharide-induced memory deficiency via its antineuroinflammatory and antiamyloidogenic effects." *Phytotherapy Research*. 27(3):438–447.

[243] Lin Y-R, Chen H-H, Ko C-H, Chan M-H. 2006. "Neuroprotective activity of honokiol and magnolol in cerebellar granule cell damage." *European Journal of Pharmacology*. 537(1–3):64–69.

[244] Vaidya ADB, Devasagayam TPA. 2007. "Current status of herbal drugs in India: An overview." *Journal of Clinical Biochemistry and Nutrition*. 41(1):1–11. doi:10.3164/jcbn.2007001

[245] Rashrash M, Schommer JC, Brown LM. 2017. "Prevalence and predictors of herbal medicine use among adults in the United States." *Journal of Patient Experience*. 4(3):108–113. doi:10.1177/2374373517706612

[246] Ardalan M-R, Rafieian-Kopaei M. 2013. "Is the safety of herbal medicines for kidneys under question?" *Journal of Nephropharmacology*. 2013;2(2):11.

[247] Welz AN, Emberger-Klein A, Menrad K. 2018. "Why people use herbal medicine: Insights from a focus-group study in Germany." *BMC Complementary and Alternative Medicine*. 18(1):92. doi:10.1186/s12906-018-2160-6

[248] Kamsu-Foguem B, Foguem C. 2014. "Adverse drug reactions in some African herbal medicine: Literature review and stakeholders' interview." *Integrative Medicine Research*. 3(3):126–132. doi:10.1016/j.imr.2014.05.001

[249] Ssempijja F, Iceland Kasozi K, Daniel Eze E, Tamale A, Ewuzie SA, Matama K, Ekou J, Bogere P, Mujinya R, Musoke GH et al. 2020. "Consumption of raw herbal medicines is associated with major public health risks amongst Ugandans." *Journal of Environmental and Public Health*. 2020:1–10. doi:10.1155/2020/8516105

[250] Daniele C, Mazzanti G, Pittler MH, Ernst E. 2006. "Adverse-event profile of Crataegus Spp.: A systematic review." *Drug Safety*. 29(6):523–535. doi:10.2165/00002018-200629060-00005

[251] Ulbricht C, Isaac R, Milkin T, A. Poole E, Rusie E, M. Grimes Serrano J, Weissner W, C. Windsor R, Woods J. 2010. "An evidence-based systematic review of stevia by the Natural Standard Research Collaboration." *Cardiovascular & Hematological Agents in Medicinal Chemistry*. 8(2):113–127. doi:10.2174/187152510791170960

[252] Daniele C, Thompson Coon J, Pittler MH, Ernst E. 2005. "Vitex agnus castus: A systematic review of adverse events." *Drug Safety*. 28(4):319–332. doi:10.2165/00002018-200528040-00004
[253] Ulbricht C, Abrams TR, Conquer J, Costa D, Serrano JMG, Iovin R, Isaac R, Nguyen Y, Rusie E, Tran D et al. 2010. "An evidence-based systematic review of Umckaloabo (*Pelargonium sidoides*) by the Natural Standard Research Collaboration." *Journal of Dietary Supplements*. 7(3):283–302. doi:10.3109/19390211.2010.507116
[254] Ulbricht C, Abrams TR, Brigham A, Ceurvels J, Clubb J, Curtiss W, Kirkwood CD, Giese N, Hoehn K, Iovin R et al. 2010. "An evidence-based systematic review of rosemary (*Rosmarinus officinalis*) by the Natural Standard Research Collaboration." *Journal of Dietary Supplements*. 7(4):351–413. doi:10.3109/19390211.2010.525049
[255] Coon JT, Ernst E. 2002. "Panax ginseng: A systematic review of adverse effects and drug interactions." *Drug Safety*. 25(5):323–44. doi:10.2165/00002018-200225050-00003
[256] Basch E, Ulbricht C, Basch S, Dalton S, Ernst E, Foppa I, Szapary P, Tiffany N, Orlando CW, Vora M. 2005. "An evidence-based systematic review of echinacea (E. angustifolia DC, E. pallida, E. purpurea) by the Natural Standard Research Collaboration." *Journal Of Herbal Pharmacotherapy*. 5(2):57–88.
[257] Ulbricht C, Conquer J, Costa D, Hamilton W, Higdon ERB, Isaac R, Rusie E, Rychlik I, Serrano JMG, Tanguay-Colucci S et al. 2011. "An evidence-based systematic review of senna (*Cassia senna*) by the Natural Standard Research Collaboration." *Journal of Dietary Supplements*. 8(2):189–238. doi:10.3109/19390211.2011.573186
[258] Ulbricht C, Seamon E, Windsor RC, Armbruester N, Bryan JK, Costa D, Giese N, Gruenwald J, Iovin R, Isaac R. 2011. "An evidence-based systematic review of cinnamon (Cinnamomum spp.) by the Natural Standard Research Collaboration." *Journal of Dietary Supplements*. 8(4):378–454.
[259] Agbabiaka TB, Pittler MH, Wider B, Ernst E. 2009. "Serenoa repens (Saw Palmetto): A systematic review of adverse events." *Drug Safety*. 32(8):637–647. doi:10.2165/00002018-200932080-00003
[260] Agbabiaka TB, Guo R, Ernst E. 2009. "Pelargonium sidoides for acute bronchitis: A systematic review and meta-analysis." *Phytomedicine*. 16(8):798–799.
[261] Ulbricht C, Armstrong J, Basch E, Basch S, Bent S, Dacey C, Dalton S, Foppa I, Giese N, Hammerness P et al. 2008. "An evidence-based systematic review of *Aloe vera* by the Natural Standard Research Collaboration." *Journal of Herbal Pharmacotherapy*. 7(3–4):279–323. doi:10.1080/15228940802153339
[262] Keifer D, Ulbricht C, Abrams TR, Basch E, Giese N, Giles M, Kirkwood CD, Miranda M, Woods J. 2008. "Peppermint (Mentha xpiperita): An evidence-based systematic review by the natural standard research collaboration." *Journal of Herbal Pharmacotherapy*. 7(2):91–143.
[263] Ulbricht C, Basch E, Boon H, Ernst E, Hammerness P, Sollars D, Tsourounis C, Woods J, Bent S. 2005. "Safety review of kava (*Piper methysticum*) by the Natural Standard Research Collaboration." *Expert Opinion on Drug Safety*. 4(4):779–794. doi:10.1517/14740338.4.4.779
[264] Dugoua J-J, Seely D, Perri D, Cooley K, Forelli T, Mills E, Koren G. 2007. "From type 2 diabetes to antioxidant activity: A systematic review of the safety and efficacy of common and cassia cinnamon bark." *Canadian Journal of Physiology and Pharmacology*. 85(9):837–847. doi:10.1139/Y07-080
[265] Boullata JI, Nace AM. 2000. "Safety issues with herbal medicine." *Pharmacotherapy*. 20(3):257–269. doi:10.1592/phco.20.4.257.34886
[266] Almeida JC, Grimsley EW. 1996. "Coma from the health food store: interaction between kava and alprazolam." *Annals of Internal Medicine*. 125(11):940–941.

[267] Wong AH, Smith M, Boon HS. 1998. "Herbal remedies in psychiatric practice." *Archives of General Psychiatry*. 55(11):1033–1044.
[268] Bennet Jr. DA, Phun L, Polk JF, Voglino SA, Zlotnik V, Raffa RB. 1998. "Neuropharmacology of St. John's wort (hypericum)." *Annals of Pharmacology*. 32(11):1201–1208.
[269] Rey JM, Walter G. 1998. "Hypericum perforatum (St John's wort) in depression: Pest or blessing?" *Medical Journal of Australia*. 169(11–12):583–586.
[270] Posadzki P, Watson LK, Ernst E. 2013. "Adverse effects of herbal medicines: An overview of systematic reviews." *Clinical Medicine*. 13(1):7–12. doi:10.7861/clinmedicine.13-1-7
[271] Posadzki P, Watson L, Ernst E. 2013. "Contamination and adulteration of herbal medicinal products (HMPs): An overview of systematic reviews." *European Journal of Clinical Pharmacology*. 69(3):295–307. doi:10.1007/s00228-012-1353-z
[272] Raynor DK, Dickinson R, Knapp P, Long AF, Nicolson DJ. 2011. "Buyer beware? Does the information provided with herbal products available over the counter enable safe use?" *BMC Medicine*. 9:1–9.
[273] Bandaranayake WM. 2006. "Quality control, screening, toxicity, and regulation of herbal drugs." In: *Modern phytomedicine: turning medicinal plants into drugs*. Germany: Wiley-VCH Verlag GmbH & Co. KGaA.; 2006. p. 25–57.
[274] Ekar T, Kreft S. 2019. "Common risks of adulterated and mislabeled herbal preparations." *Food and Chemical Toxicology*. 123:288–297. doi:10.1016/j.fct.2018.10.043
[275] Navarro V, Avula B, Khan I, Verma M, Seeff L, Serrano J, Stolz A, Fontana R, Ahmad J. 2019. "The contents of herbal and dietary supplements implicated in liver injury in the United States are frequently mislabeled." *Hepatology Communications*. 3(6):792–794. doi:10.1002/hep4.1346
[276] Shaban NS, Abdou KA, Hassan NE-HY. 2016. "Impact of toxic heavy metals and pesticide residues in herbal products." *Beni-Suef University Journal of Basic and Applied Sciences*. 5(1):102–106. doi:10.1016/j.bjbas.2015.10.001
[277] Chan K. 2003. "Some aspects of toxic contaminants in herbal medicines." *Chemosphere*. 52(9):1361–1371. doi:10.1016/S0045-6535(03)00471-5
[278] Luo L, Dong L, Huang Q, Ma S, Fantke P, Li J, Jiang J, Fitzgerald M, Yang J, Jia Z et al. 2021. "Detection and risk assessments of multi-pesticides in 1771 cultivated herbal medicines by LC/MS-MS and GC/MS-MS." *Chemosphere*. 262:127477. doi:10.1016/j.chemosphere.2020.127477
[279] Harris ESJ, Cao S, Littlefield BA, Craycroft JA, Scholten R, Kaptchuk T, Fu Y, Wang W, Liu Y, Chen H et al. 2011. "Heavy metal and pesticide content in commonly prescribed individual raw Chinese herbal medicines." *Science of the Total Environment*. 409(20):4297–4305. doi:10.1016/j.scitotenv.2011.07.032
[280] Ernst E. 2002. "Heavy metals in traditional Indian remedies." *European Journal of Clinical Pharmacology*. 57(12):891–896. doi:10.1007/s00228-001-0400-y
[281] Fleshner N, Harvey M, Adomat H, Wood C, Eberding A, Hersey K, Guns E. 2005. "Evidence for contamination of herbal erectile dysfunction products with phosphodiesterase type 5 inhibitors." *Journal of Urology*. 174(2):636–641. doi:10.1097/01.ju.0000165187.31941.cd
[282] Ismail SF, Daud M, Jalil JAbd, Azmi IMAG, Safuan S. 2018. "Protecting consumers from misleading online advertisement for herbal and traditional medicines in Malaysia: Are the laws sufficient?" In: *2018 6th International Conference on Cyber and IT Service Management (CITSM)*. Parapat, Indonesia: IEEE; 2018. p. 1–6. doi:10.1109/CITSM.2018.8674372

[283] Morris CA, Avorn J. 2003. "Internet marketing of herbal products." *JAMA*. 290(11):1505. doi:10.1001/jama.290.11.1505

[284] Rousseaux CG, Schachter H. 2003. "Regulatory issues concerning the safety, efficacy and quality of herbal remedies." *Birth Defects Research Part B: Developmental and Reproductive Toxicology*. 68(6):505–510. doi:10.1002/bdrb.10053

[285] Sahoo N, Manchikanti P, Dey S. 2010. "Herbal drugs: Standards and regulation." *Fitoterapia*. 81(6):462–471. doi:10.1016/j.fitote.2010.02.001

11 Natural Polymeric Nanoparticles for Brain Targeting

Gaurav K. Pandit, Ritesh K. Tiwari, Ashish Kumar, Veer Singh, Gufran Ahmed, Shazia Kazmi, Shaliha Irfan, Vishal Mishra, Anurag Kumar Singh, Snigdha Singh, and Meenakshi Singh

11.1 INTRODUCTION

A significant transformation is unfolding in the realm of therapeutics, which deals with the treatment of diseases and the actions of therapeutic agents on the body. Currently, people are embracing various disciplines that incorporate new advancements and a deeper understanding of the natural principles behind them [1, 2]. This has led to the emergence of innovative therapeutic approaches. A revolution is underway in the field of medicine, driven by various scientific technologies, including the most recent one, nanotechnology, which involves the manipulation of matter at the atomic, molecular, and supramolecular levels [3]. Personalized healthcare is in demand, and to comprehend the unique characteristics of our bodies, sensors are needed both on the body's external surfaces and within its internal spaces [4, 5]. Nanosciences and nanotechnology are leading us towards the development of novel devices, known as nanomachines, which have the potential to revolutionize the field of medicine [6].

Nanotechnology concerns planning and creating designs, gadgets, or frameworks through using iotas and particles at the nanoscale level [4, 7]. Nevertheless, nanotechnology is a relatively recent development in the realm of scientific research, even though the foundation of its fundamental concepts was laid out many years ago. A Japanese researcher, Norio Taniguchi, was quick to utilize this innovation. He characterized the term "nanotechnology" in 1974 as nanotechnology chiefly comprising the handling of partition, union, and misshapening of materials by one iota or one atom [6–8].

The American physicist and Nobel Prize laureate Richard Feynman proposed the idea of nanotechnology in 1959 [9]. In the 1980s, the evolution of this innovation was additionally improved through trial advancement.

The invention of the scanning tunneling microscope in 1981 and the discovery of fullerenes in 1985 introduced further breakthroughs to this field [10, 11]. In the early 2000s, nanotechnology found various commercial applications, although many early explorations primarily focused on bulk uses of nanomaterials rather than

DOI: 10.1201/9781032661964-11

transformative applications. Nanomedicine and nanomaterials can be categorized based on various parameters.

Extensively, they can be characterized into [12]:

1. Nanoparticles
2. Nanoclays
3. Nanoemulsions.

NPNs possess several advantages over synthetic nanoparticles, including biocompatibility, biodegradability, and low toxicity. These attributes make them a promising area of research in the field of nanomedicine. [13].

11.2 NANOPARTICLES

Nanomaterials are materials that have primary parts under 1 miniature meter in something like one aspect. Nanoparticles are strong colloidal particles ranging from 1 to 1,000 nm in size. They are macromolecular materials in which the dynamic fixings are broken up, entangled or exemplified, or retained [14, 15]. The different types of nanomaterials and their application are listed in Table 11.1.

Nanoparticulate matter refers to an assortment of nanoparticles, underscoring their aggregate way of behaving. Nanoparticles are not set in stone by the compound creation, the number of molecules and the substance communication between the particles. They can have customary glasslike, shapeless, or pseudo-close nuclear courses of action [16]. Nanoparticles can be of various kinds depending upon their size, surface, and there properties.

TABLE 11.1
Types of Nanoparticles along with Their Composition and Application

Types of Nanoparticles	Material used	Application
Nanosuspensions and Nanocrystals.	Drug powders are arranged in surfactant arrangement.	Stable framework for controlled conveyance of ineffectively solvent medication
Polymeric nanoparticles	Biodegradable polymer.	Controlled and designated conveyance
Polymeric micelles	Amphiphilic block copolymers.	Controlled and foundational conveyance of water insoluble medications
Strong lipid nanoparticles	Softened lipid scattered in fluid surfactant.	Not so much harmful but rather more steady. Colloidal transporter framework as elective material to polymers.
Attractive nanoparticles.	Attractive Fe2O3, covered with dextran.	Drug focusing on, Symptomatic in medication
Carbon nanotubes.	Metals, semiconductors	Qualities and DNA conveyance

(a) **Carbon based:** These nanoparticles are made up of carbon parts and are largely utilized for reinforcing the material designs. Carbon-based nanoparticles are composed of two materials: carbon nanotubes (CNTs) and fullerenes. The carbon nanotube is a graphene sheet rolled into a cylinder shape and is mostly utilized for underlying support (multiple times more grounded than steel). They are thermally conductive along the length and non-conductive all through the cylinder. Because of their electrical conductivity, structure, high strength, and electron likeness, they have business applications [17, 18].
(b) **Ceramic based:** These are composed of oxides, carbonates, and phosphates, and they exhibit excellent resistance to chemicals and durability. By manipulating specific characteristics of ceramic nanoparticles, such as size, surface area, porosity, and surface-to-volume ratio, they prove to be effective drug delivery agents. These nanoparticles have been successfully employed as drug delivery systems for various diseases, including bacterial infections, glaucoma, cancer, and more[19, 20].
(c) **Metal based:** These nanoparticles are prepared from metals using chemical and electrochemical processes. These nanoparticles have applications in research fields, the location and imaging of biomolecules, and ecological and bioanalytical applications.
(d) **Semiconductor based:** These nanoparticles have properties like numerous metals and non-metals. Its utilizations are in photocatalysis, gadgets, photograph optics, and water parting.
(e) **Polymer based:** These are particles acquired from natural materials. They have applications in drug conveyance and diagnostics. Drug conveyance with polymeric nanoparticles (PNPs) is profoundly biodegradable.

11.2.1 Polymeric Nanoparticles

PNPs are a system of sub-micron colloidal, biocompatible, and preferably biodegradable particles made of synthetic or natural polymers [21, 22]. A suitable drug is usually encapsulated or adhered to the surface of the nanoparticle for the drug's delivery to the specific target. PNPs are effective DNA carriers in gene therapy and are considered efficient drug-delivery systems that help with the controlled release of drugs to a specific target site [23]. A schematic representation of polymeric nanomaterials is shown in Figure 11.1.

PNPs can be classified as nanocapsules and nanospheres based on their structure. A nanocapsule is a hollow system in which the drug is entrapped or encapsulated within an oily or aqueous core surrounded by a polymeric membrane. In contrast, the nanosphere is a matrix system, made of a solid mass of polymeric network in which the drug is uniformly distributed within the core or is surface-bound to the nanosphere. A schematic diagram of PNPs is shown in Figure 11.2.

Furthermore, certain components may also be attached to the surface of the nanoparticle in order to facilitate its passage through biological barriers such as the skin, mucus, blood, and cellular organelles. Biodegradable PNPs are preferred over

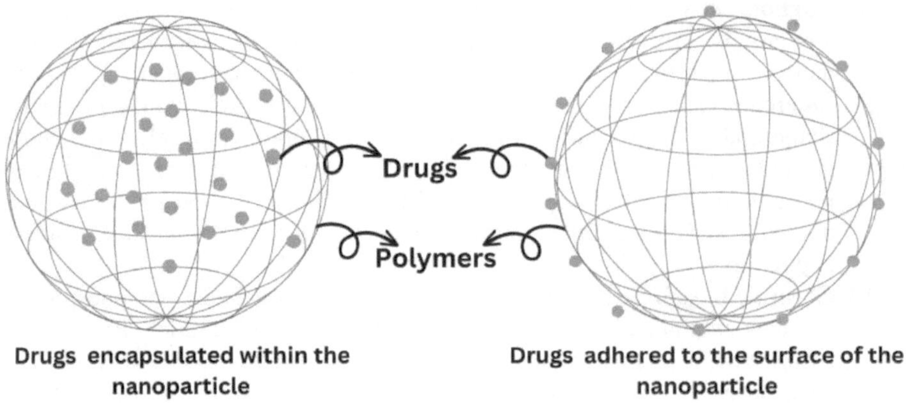

FIGURE 11.1 Schematic representation of polymeric nanoparticles as drug-delivery systems.

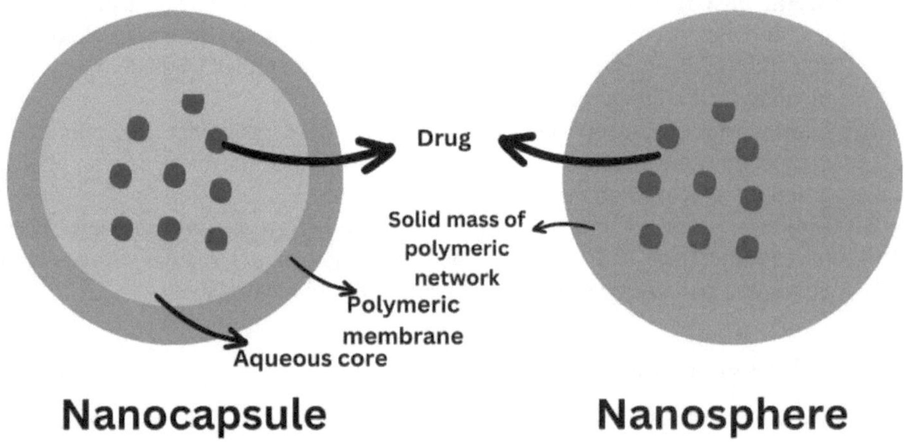

FIGURE 11.2 Schematic representation of nanocapsule and nanosphere.

non-biodegradable nanoparticles made of polymers such as polyacrylamide, polystyrene, and polyacrylates because they are more biocompatible, have a lower risk of toxicity, and degrade into oligomers and monomers in much less time than non-biodegradable ones. Biodegradable PNPs are made up of either synthetic polymers such as poly(D, L-glycolide), co-polymer poly(lactide-co-glycolide), and poly-Ɛ-caprolactone, or natural polymers derived from plants, animals, or microbes such as chitosan, alginate, gelatin, zein, and albumin [24].

PNPs are preferred over other nanocarriers such as liposomes and micelles due to their small size (1 to 1000 nm) increased stability in biological environments, flexibility in modifying their structures according to the requirements of the drug, improved ability to target specific organs or tissues, and low side effects [25, 26].

11.2.1.1 Preparation Techniques of Polymeric Nanoparticles

PNPs are developed to encapsulate molecules, such as proteins and DNA. The encapsulated molecules are released in a controlled manner on the target site through diffusion or erosion of the matrix. There are various techniques used for the development of PNPs depending on the nature of the polymer, the type of molecule to be entrapped in the nanoparticle, convenience, and expense of the approach [27].

(a) **Solvent evaporation:** The solvent evaporation technique was the first technique used for the development of PNPs, specifically nanospheres, from a preformed polymer [28]. This method involves preparing a solution of the polymer in a polar organic solvent such as chloroform, dichloromethane, or ethyl acetate. The drug to be encapsulated is then added to the solution by dissolution or dispersion. Under high-speed homogenization or ultrasonication, the resulting solution is emulsified in an aqueous solution containing a surfactant or emulsifier such as polyvinyl alcohol or polysorbate 80 [29]. The processes of solvent evaporation techniques are shown in Figure 11.3.

    These organic solvents pose toxicological and environmental risks. Therefore, they are removed by evaporating the solvent, either by increasing the temperature under reduced pressure or by continuous magnetic stirring at room temperature. The solidified nanoparticles are then washed and freeze-dried to obtain a fine powder of nanoparticles once the solvent has evaporated [30].

(b) **Nanoprecipitation:** This technique, also known as the solvent displacement method, was developed by Fessi and his colleagues for the development of PNPs of around 175 nm in size. A water-miscible organic solvent containing the polymer and the active molecule, such as drugs, is prepared and then added drop-by-drop to an aqueous solution, which usually contains a surfactant for maintaining the stability of the colloidal suspension, while continuously stirring the mixture. This results in rapid diffusion of the organic solvent in the aqueous solution and the instantaneous formation of small droplets of nanoparticles characterized by a well-defined size as well as a narrow size distribution at the interface of organic solvent and the aqueous phase, following the diffusion of the solvent from the nanodroplet and the precipitation of the polymer in the form of PNPs. To ensure the formation of nanocapsules, the drug is dissolved in oil before its emulsification in the organic polymeric solution. After the formation of the nanoparticles, it is freeze-dried to obtain a fine powder of nanoparticles [31]. The preparation of nanoprecipitation technique is shown in Figure 11.4.

11.2.1.2 Polymeric Nanoparticles for Non-viral Gene Delivery

Gene delivery is a technique used to correct defective genes responsible for disease development by gene augmentation, gene suppression, or gene editing. Successful gene delivery is achieved by the use of appropriate gene carriers that do not induce any immunological response, that easily enter the cell, and integrate the gene at the

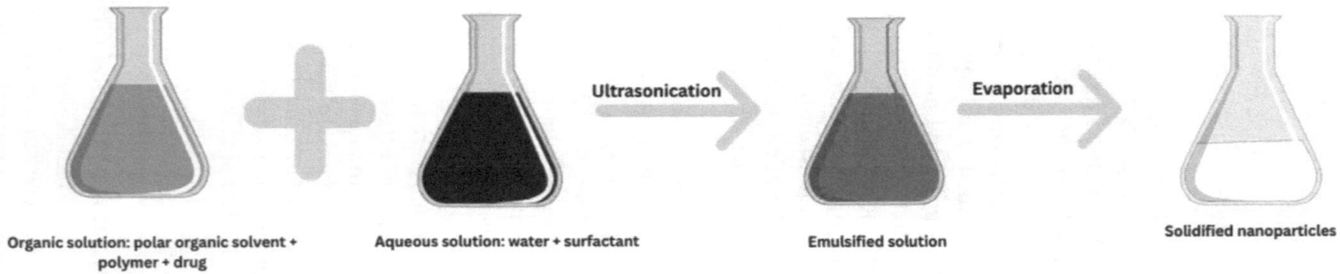

FIGURE 11.3 Schematic representation of solvent evaporation technique.

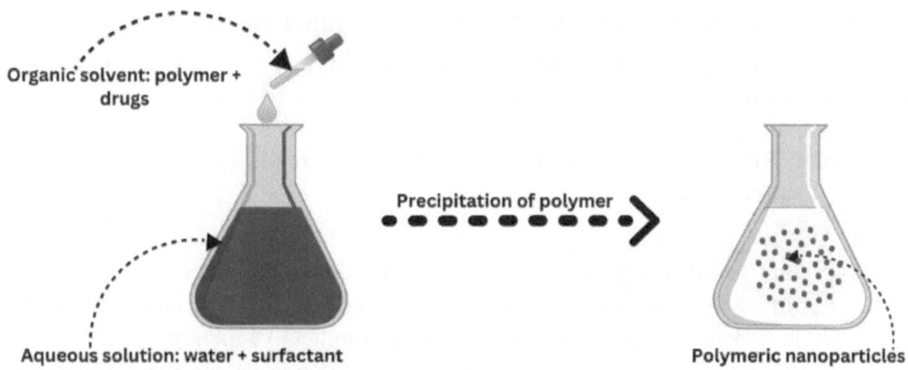

FIGURE 11.4 Schematic representation of nanoprecipitation technique.

desired site. Due to these limitations, non-viral gene carriers have been developed, such as the cationic lipid-based non-viral gene delivery system that was first used in 1987 by Felgner and his colleagues [2].

PNPs are one of the safest and most efficient non-viral gene carriers because of their small size, easy accessibility, biodegradability, biocompatibility, low risk of cytotoxicity, passive targeting by using the enhanced permeability and retention (EPR) effect, flexibility in modifications to achieve the desired therapeutic efficacy, protection against enzymatic degradation, and ease of elimination. The condensed genetic material can be incorporated with the polymer to develop polyplex nanoparticles or solid PNPs [2, 3]. Polyplex nanoparticles are the most common PNPs that are formed when the cationic polymers are conjugated with the condensed genetic material through electrostatic forces. The most commonly used cationic nanoparticle is the Food and Drug Administration-approved poly(lactic-*co*-glycolic acid) cationic nanoparticle because of its stable structure and its ability to protect genetic material from degradation during *in vivo* gene therapy. Because of the positive charge present on the cationic polymers, they easily conjugate with the negatively charged genetic material, and also because of the positive charge, they can easily cross the cell membrane for gene delivery. However, these charges also have their disadvantages, like toxicity, and as a result, most polyplex nanoparticles cannot be used in *in vivo* gene therapy [31, 4].

The general mechanism of gene delivery by means of polyplexes and nanoparticles is quite simple. The first step is the cellular uptake of the nanoparticle by endocytosis and its entrapment in the endosome. However, the nanoparticle must escape the endosome to avoid degradation by the lysosome. After its escape, the nanoparticle will release the genetic material into the cytoplasm, where it will be transported into the nucleus by transport proteins, get incorporated at the target site, and express the desired product [32].

11.2.1.3 Natural Polymeric Nanoparticles for Human Health

Normal PNPs enjoy the upperhand over manufactured nanoparticles in a few ways, including biocompatibility, biodegradability, and low poisonousness, which make them a promising area of exploration in the field of nanomedicine.

Normal PNPs can be classified into a few categories in view of their creation and construction, including:

a) Protein-based nanoparticles: These nanoparticles are made out of normally occurring proteins, like egg whites, gelatin, and casein, and can be utilized for drug conveyance, designated treatment, and indicative imaging.
b) Carbohydrate-based nanoparticles: These nanoparticles are made up of normally occurring carbs, like starch, cellulose, and chitosan, and can be utilized for drug conveyance, designated treatment, and tissue designing.
c) Lipid-based nanoparticles: These nanoparticles are comprised of normally occurring lipids, like phospholipids and liposomes, and can be utilized for drug conveyance, designated treatment, and symptomatic imaging.
d) Nucleic acid-based nanoparticles: These nanoparticles are comprised of normally occurring nucleic acids, like DNA and RNA, and can be utilized for quality treatment and indicative imaging.
e) Plant-based nanoparticles: These nanoparticles are extracted from plant sources, like leaves, stems, and seeds, and can be utilized for drug conveyance, designated treatment, and demonstrative imaging. This classification provides a general overview of the types of natural polymeric nanoparticles (NPNs) that are being used and researched in the field of nanomedicine. The exact composition and structure of these nanoparticles can vary depending on the specific application and the requirements of the therapeutic agent being delivered [33].

11.2.1.4 Potential Applications of Polymeric Nanoparticles in Improving Human Health

(a) Drug Conveyance: Normal PNPs can exemplify and transport various restorative specialists, like medications and qualities, to specific target locales in the body. These nanoparticles can protect therapeutic agents from degradation, thereby enhancing their stability and efficacy. Moreover, normal polymeric nanoparticles can be intended to specifically target sick cells, lessening the symptoms of conventional medication conveyance techniques [31].
(b) Diagnostic Imaging: Normal PNPs can be functionalized with imaging specialists, like difference specialists and fluorescent colours, to upgrade the perceivability of sicknesses and issues in symptomatic imaging. This can prompt early location and further developed treatment results [31].
(c) Targeted Treatment: Normal PNPs can be designed to specifically target ailing cells, tissues, and organs, consequently decreasing the adverse consequence of conventional treatment techniques on solid cells. This can bring about better restorative results and decreased incidental effects [31].

(d) Tissue Designing: Normal PNPs can be utilized in combination with other biomaterials to make platforms for tissue designing and regenerative medication. These platforms can give a steady and defensive climate for the development and recovery of tissues and organs [31].

11.3 BLOOD–BRAIN BARRIER

The BBB is a particular arrangement of vessels and cells that act as a hurdle to foreign matter between the circulating blood and the central nervous system (CNS), which incorporates the brain and spinal cord. The BBB is framed by close intersections between the cells that line the veins in the brain, which prevent most substances in the blood, including possibly unsafe particles, from crossing into the CNS [34, 35].The primary function of the BBB is to protect the delicate and highly sensitive tissue of the brain and spinal cord by preventing the passage of potentially harmful substances and maintaining the appropriate chemical environment within the CNS. This protective barrier also regulates the entry of essential substances, such as oxygen, glucose, and neurotransmitters, into the brain, ensuring they are delivered in the correct quantities and at the right times .

The BBB comprises several distinct cell types, including endothelial cells, pericytes, astrocytes, and neurons, each of which plays a specific role in preserving the integrity of the barrier. The tight junctions between the endothelial cells create a hurdale that effectively prevents most substances from crossing the BBB. Pericytes, found on the outer surface of blood vessels, provide structural support and help regulate blood flow. Astrocytes, the most abundant type of glial cells in the brain, contribute to maintaining the proper chemical environment within the CNS and can also influence BBB function [35].

The BBB permits tight control of substances between the blood and the brain. These properties can be arranged into actual vehicle and metabolic classifications:

- The cerebrum endothelial cells are kept intact by close intersections which fill in as actual obstructions, preventing the development of substances in spaces between cells.
- They regulate the passage of ions and specific substances through specialized carriers, which are two types:
  (i) Efflux Carriers utilize cell energy to move substances against their fixation slope. They transport lipophilic atoms which have latently diffused through cell film back to the blood.
  (ii) Supplement Carriers work with the development of supplements like glucose and fundamental amino acids into the brain down their concentration gradient.

Not all areas of the brain have a BBB-like model; some brain structures are engaged with hormonal control and require better admittance to foundational blood, so they can recognize changes in circling signals.

While the BBB gives significant security to the CNS, it likewise presents a test for the treatment of neurological problems, as many medications cannot enter the BBB to arrive at their objective site in the brain. Researchers are exploring various methods to overcome the BBB, such as the use of drugs or other compounds that can temporarily disrupt the barrier to allow for the delivery of therapeutic agents, or the utilization of nanoparticle-based drug delivery systems capable of penetrating the BBB (Daniel et al., 2020). The BBB is an intricate and sophisticated system that plays a crucial role in protecting the CNS and maintaining its proper function. Further investigation into the structure and function of the BBB is required to gain a better understanding of its role in health and disease, and to develop more effective approaches for treating neurological disorders [36].

11.4 POLYMERIC NANOPARTICLES FOR BRAIN TARGETING

The brain is a complex organ composed of various regions and cell types, each with distinct functions. Comprehending the structure of the brain and the characteristics of specific areas and cells is essential for devising strategies for targeting the brain effectively [37].

The primary areas of the brain include:

- Frontal cortex: The biggest area of the brain, it is responsible for cognizant ideas, insight, and development. It is separated into two hemispheres (left and right) that are associated by a heap of strands called the corpus callosum.
- Brainstem: Interfaces the spinal column to the rest of the brain and controls imperative capabilities, for example, pulse and relaxation.
- Cerebellum: Directs development and equilibrium.
- Hippocampus: Assumes a critical part in memory and spatial route.
- Basal ganglia: Manages wilful development and is engaged with development problems, like Parkinson's disease.
- Thalamus: Serves as a transfer place for tangible data and assumes a part in cognition and rest.
- Nerve centre: Manages the autonomic sensory system and controls functions like appetite, thirst, and internal heat level.

Focusing on unambiguous locales or cells in the brain can be accomplished through utilizing different strategies, including;

- Attractive reverberation imaging (X-ray): Comprises painless imaging of the brain and can be utilized to distinguish explicit districts and cells in the cerebrum.
- Positron outflow tomography (PET): Utilizes radioactive tracers to image explicit locales or cells in the brain.
- Optical imaging: Uses fluorescent colours or hereditarily encoded fluorescent proteins to picture explicit areas or cells in the brain.
- Microinjection: Includes the immediate infusion of restorative specialists into explicit areas or cells in the brain.

11.4.1 Brain Targeting

Cerebrum focusing is a vital part of treating neurological problems, like Alzheimer's disease, Parkinson's disease, and different sclerosis, among others. The brain is safeguarded by the BBB, which restricts the passage of most medications into the cerebrum, making it challenging to treat these problems. Thus, there is a developing requirement for successful and designated drug conveyance frameworks that can sidestep the BBB and convey remedial specialists straightforwardly to the cerebrum [38].

PNPs are a promising answer for designated drug conveyance to the brain. PNPs are nanoscale drug conveyance frameworks made out of a polymeric material that can epitomize medications and target explicit tissues in the body, including the cerebrum. PNPs offer a few benefits over regular medication conveyance techniques, like expanded soundness, designated conveyance, and controlled arrival of medications [38].

Notwithstanding their true capacity as medication conveyance vehicles, PNPs additionally offer a few exceptional highlights that make them especially appropriate for cerebrum focusing on. For instance, PNPs can be intended to take advantage of the BBB's regular vehicle systems, for example, receptor-intervened transport, to expand the effectiveness of medication conveyance to the brain. PNPs can likewise be functionalized with explicit focusing on moieties, like antibodies or peptides, to specifically tie to synapses or tissues and to work on the particularity of medication conveyance.

In spite of these benefits, the improvement of PNPs for cerebrum focusing remains a difficult undertaking. A few variables, like the size and security of PNPs, the similarity of the polymeric materials with drugs, and the capacity of PNPs to target explicit synapses and tissues, should be painstakingly viewed as part of the plan and combination of these nanoscale frameworks. Taking everything into account, cerebrum focusing with PNPs can possibly improve the treatment of neurological problems by working on the conveyance of medications to the brain and diminishing the symptoms of regular medication conveyance strategies. Further exploration is expected to lead to complete understanding of the capability of PNPs for brain focusing, including the advancement of a PNP plan, blend, and focusing, as well as improvement of additional viable and explicit medications for the treatment of neurological problems [39].

11.4.2 Methods for Brain Targeting by Polymeric Nanoparticles

There are a few strategies that have been created to accomplish brain focusing through utilizing PNPs. The absolute most regularly utilized strategies incorporate

(a) Passive targeting: This technique exploits the improved porousness and maintenance (EPR) impact, which alludes to the propensity of macromolecules and nanoscale particles to gather in cancers and other strange tissues due to their cracked vasculature. PNPs can latently focus on the cerebrum by crossing the brainBBB through the EPR impact and through aggregating in cerebrum tissues [40].

(b) Active targeting: This technique includes the functionalization of PNPs with explicit focusing on moieties, like antibodies, peptides, or little atoms, to tie to explicit cells or tissues in the cerebrum specifically. This can work on the particularity of medication conveyance to the brain and decrease the harmfulness of medications to different tissues in the body.
(c) pH-sensitive PNPs: This strategy depends on the pH distinction between the blood and the mbrain. PNPs can be intended to be pH-delicate and discharge drugs in light of the acidic climate of the brain, consequently expanding the productivity of medication conveyance to the cerebrum.
(d) Transcytosis-intervened focusing on: This strategy includes the utilization of PNPs that can be taken up by cerebrum endothelial cells through a cycle known as transcytosis, in which particles are assimilated by the cells and afterward move across the BBB. This permits PNPs to sidestep the BBB and enter the brain without being limited by the BBB's tight intersections.
(e) Magnetically directed PNPs: This strategy includes the functionalization of PNPs with attractive materials, like iron oxide, to consider the attractive direction of PNPs to the cerebrum. This can be achieved by applying an outside attractive field to draw in PNPs to the brain.

These are the absolute most ordinarily involved techniques for brain focusing on utilizing PNPs. The decision on technique relies upon a few variables, including the sort of illness being dealt with, the medication being conveyed, and the particular requirements of the objective tissue or cells.

PNPs have been shown extraordinarily likely in the conveyance of medications to the cerebrum for the treatment of different brain issues like Alzheimer's, Parkinson's, and epilepsy. The PNPs can embody the medications and shield them from debasement, taking into account the controlled arrival of the medications over a lengthy period. PNPs can likewise be utilized for quality treatment in the cerebrum, conveying remedial qualities straightforwardly to the site of injury or sickness. This approach has shown promising outcomes in the treatment of neurodegenerative illnesses, brain cancers, and stroke [39, 40].

PNPs can likewise be functionalized with imaging agents for use in attractive reverberation imaging (X-ray) or positron emission tomography (PET) filters. This is considered harmless imaging of the brain, working with the early location of neurodegenerative illnesses like Alzheimer's and Parkinson's. PNPs can be utilized to convey mitigating specialists explicitly to the cerebrum, diminishing the fundamental incidental effects related with customary foundational conveyance strategies. This approach has shown promising outcomes in the treatment of neuroinflammatory conditions like different sclerosis. PNPs can likewise be utilized to convey immature microorganisms to the cerebrum, giving another helpful choice in the treatment of neurodegenerative illnesses, stroke, and brain injuries. This approach has shown promising outcomes in animal studies and is a promising area for future exploration [39, 40].

11.5 CHALLENGES AND LIMITATIONS OF BRAIN TARGETING BY NANOPARTICLES

Brain targeting by nanoparticles is a promising methodology in the field of nanomedicine for conveying medications, diagnostics, and other restorative specialists to the focal sensory system (CNS). Nonetheless, it faces a few difficulties and restrictions, including [39]:

(a) Blood–Brain Barrier: The BBB is a semi-porous film that isolates the circulatory system from the cerebrum and is a significant hindrance in conveying nanoparticles to the CNS.
(b) Size and Surface Charge: The size and surface charge of nanoparticles can influence their capacity to cross the BBB and their circulation inside the CNS.
(c) Poisonousness: The harmfulness of nanoparticles, both to the brain and different organs, is a significant concern and requires further examination to guarantee their protected use in people. (Nanotoxicology centres around determining the antagonistic impacts of nanomaterials on human well-being and the climate).
(d) Biodistribution: The distribution of nanoparticles within the CNS and the ability to precisely target specific brain regions continue to be challenging.
(e) Administrative Endorsement: The administrative endorsement process for nanoparticle-based cerebrum focusing on advancements is intricate and requires broad preclinical and clinical testing to show well-being and adequacy.

These difficulties and constraints feature the requirement to proceed with innovative work to overcome the obstructions and work on the adequacy of a nanoparticle-based brain focusing on advancements.

11.6 CURRENT PROGRESS ON BRAIN TARGETING BY POLYMERIC NANOPARTICLES

PNPs stand out as a promising medication conveyance framework for brain focusing because of their capacity to cross the BBB. Researchers are investigating different systems to upgrade the BBB porousness of PNPs, for example, surface adjustment with explicit peptides or medications that can expand the vehicle of PNPs across the BBB. Also, PNPs with boosts responsive, like pH-delicate or focused on explicit receptors on the BBB, are being created to work on the particularity and proficiency of brain focusing. Nonetheless, there are still challenges to overcome, such as enhancing the stability and biocompatibility of PNPs, as well as reducing their toxicity and side effects. Nevertheless, recent advancements in the field have demonstrated promising results for the use of PNPs in brain drug delivery, and ongoing research is focused on improving their design and performance [37–40].

11.7 CONCLUSION AND FUTURE PERSPECTIVE

NPNs have emerged as a promising approach for targeting the brain due to their biocompatibility and their ability to encapsulate various therapeutic substances. In contrast to synthetic polymers, these nanoparticles offer several advantages, such as being derived from natural sources and having diverse structures, which leads to improved biodegradability and reduced toxicity. Research has demonstrated that NPNs can effectively traverse the BBB and reach the brain, making them a viable option for delivering drugs to treat various neurological disorders, including Alzheimer's, Parkinson's, and epilepsy. Some commonly used natural polymers for brain targeting include chitosan, gelatin, and alginate.

However, the use of NPNs for brain targeting still faces challenges, including optimizing particle size, surface charge, and stability. Moreover, the BBB is a complex and dynamic barrier, and a more comprehensive understanding of the mechanisms by which nanoparticles penetrate the BBB is needed to enhance their effectiveness. NPNs hold promise as drug delivery vehicles for brain targeting, but further research is required to fully unlock their potential. The development of efficient and safe brain targeting systems using these nanoparticles has the potential to revolutionize the treatment of neurological disorders

ACKNOWLEDGEMENTS

The authors are thankful to the Patna University, Patna for necessary support of the present research work.

REFERENCES

[1] Sophie Laurent, Delphine Forge, Marc Port, Alain Roch, Caroline Robic, Luce Vander Elst, Robert N. Muller. 2008. "Magnetic Iron Oxide Nanoparticles: Synthesis, Stabilization, Vectorization, Physicochemical Characterizations, and Biological Applications". *Chem Rev.* (June). doi: 10.1021/cr068445e

[2] Veer Singh, Jyoti Singh, Nidhi Singh et al. 2022. "Simultaneous Removal of Ternary Heavy Metal Ions by a Newly Isolated *Microbacterium Paraoxydans* Strain VSVM IIT(BHU) from Coal Washery Effluent". *BioMetals.* (December). doi: 10.1007/s10534-022-00476-4

[3] Veer Singh, Jyoti Singh, Vishal Mishra. 2021. "Development of a Cost-Effective, Recyclable and Viable Metal Ion Doped Adsorbent for Simultaneous Adsorption and Reduction of Toxic Cr (VI) Ions". *Journal of Environmental Chemical Engineering* 9 105124. doi: 10.1016/j.jece.2021.105124

[4] Jitendra N. Tiwari, Rajanish N. Tiwari, Kwang S. Kim. 2012. "Zero-Dimensional, One-Dimensional, Two-Dimensional and Three-Dimensional Nanostructured Materials for Advanced Electrochemical Energy Devices". *Progress in Materials Science* 57 (May). doi: 10.1016/j.pmatsci..2011.08.003

[5] Veer Singh and Vishal Mishra. 2021. "Sustainable Reduction of Cr (VI) and its Elemental Mapping on Chitosan Coated Citrus Limetta Peels Biomass in Synthetic Wastewater". *Separation Science and Technology.* 57 (October). doi: 10.1080/01496395.2021.1993921

[6] Erik C. Dreaden, Alaaldin M. Alkilany, Xiaohua Huang, Catherine J. Murphy, Mustafa A. El-Sayed. 2012. "The Golden Age: Gold Nanoparticles for Biomedicine". *Chem Soc Rev*. (April). doi: 10.1039/c1cs15237h

[7] Alina Astefanei, Oscar Núñez, Maria Teresa Galceran. 2015. "Characterisation and Determination of Fullerenes: A Critical Review". *Anal Chim Acta* 882 (July). doi: 10.1016/j.aca.2015.03.025

[8] M. Lamberti, P. Pedata, N. Sannolo, S. Porto, A. De Rosa, M. Caraglia M. 2015. "Carbon Nanotubes: Properties, Biomedical Applications, Advantages and Risks in Patients and Occupationally-Exposed Workers". *Int J Immunopathol Pharmacol*. (March). doi: 10.1177/0394632015572559

[9] Ahmad Aqel, Kholoud M.M. Abou El-Nour, Reda A.A. Ammar, Abdulrahman Al-Warthan. 2012. "Carbon Nanotubes, Science and Technology Part (I) Structure, Synthesis and Characterisation". *Arab J Chem* 5 (January). doi: 10.1016/j.arabjc.2010.08.022

[10] Wolfgang Sigmund, Junhan Yuh, Hyun Park, Vasana Maneeratana, Georgios Pyrgiotakis, Amit Daga, Joshua Taylor, Juan C. Nino. 2006. "Processing and Structure Relationships in Electrospinning of Ceramic Fiber Systems". *J Am Ceram Soc*. (January). doi: 10.1111/j.1551-2916.2005.00807.x

[11] Shindu C. Thomas, Harshita, Pawan Kumar Mishra, Sushama Talegaonkar. 2015. "Ceramic Nanoparticles: Fabrication Methods and Applications in Drug Delivery". *Curr Pharm Des*. (October). doi: 10.2174/1381612821666151027153246

[12] Shahid Ali, Ibrahim Khan, Safyan Akram Khan, Manzar Sohail, Ahmed, Riaz Ahmed, Ateequr Rehman, Muhammad Shahid Ansari, Mohamed Ali Morsy. 2017. "Electrocatalytic Performance of Ni@Pt Core–Shell Nanoparticles Supported on Carbon Nanotubes for Methanol Oxidation Reaction". *J Electroanal Chem* 795 (June). doi: 10.1016/j.jelechem.2017.04.040

[13] Vivek K. Chaturvedi, Sachchida Nand Rai, NazishTabassum, Navneet Yadav, Veer Singh, Raghvendra A. Bohara, Mohan P. Singh. "Rapid Eco-friendly Synthesis, Characterization, and Cytotoxic Study of Trimetallic Stable Nanomedicine: A Potential Material for Biomedical Applications" *Biochemistry and Biophysics Reports* 24 (2020) 100812. https://doi.org/10.1016/j.bbrep.2020.100812

[14] Takashi Hisatomi, Jun Kubota, Kazunari Domen. 2014. "Recent Advances in Semiconductors for Photocatalytic and Photoelectrochemical Water Splitting". *Chem Soc Rev*. (November). doi: 10.1039/c3cs60378d

[15] Singh V., M. P. Singh, Vishal Mishra. 2020. "Bioremediation of Toxic Metal Ions from Coal Washery Effluent". *Desalination and Water Treatment* 197 (September). doi: 10.5004/dwt.2020.25996

[16] Muhammad Mansha, Ibrahim Khan, Nisar Ullah, Qurashi. 2017. "Synthesis, Characterization and Visible-Light-Driven Photoelectrochemical Hydrogen Evolution Reaction of Carbazole-Containing Conjugated Polymers". *Int J Hydrogen Energy* 42 (April). doi: 10.1016/j.ijhydene.2017.02.053

[17] Veer Singh, Priyanka Yadav, Vishal Mishra. 2020. "Recent Advances on Classification, Properties, Synthesis, and Characterization of Nanomaterials". In: Srivastava N., Srivastava M., Mishra P., Gupta V.K. (eds). Green Synthesis of Nanomaterials for Bioenergy Applications. John Wiley & Sons. pp.83–97. ISBN:9781119576785

[18] Veer Singh, Vipul Kumar Yadav, Vishal Mishra. 2020. "Nanotechnology: An Application in Biofuel Production". In: Srivastava M., Srivastava N., Mishra P., Gupta V. (eds) Nanomaterials in Biofuels Research. Clean Energy Production Technologies. Springer., Singapore. doi: 10.1007/978-981-13-9333-4_6

[19] Azam Bolhassani, Shabnam Javanzad, Tayebeh Saleh, Mehrdad Hashemi, Mohammad Reza Aghasadeghi, Seyed Mehi Sadat. 2014. "Polymeric Nanoparticles". *Hum Vaccin Immunother.* (February). doi: 10.4161/hv.26796

[20] Belén Begines, Tamara Ortiz, María Pérez-Aranda, Guillermo Martínez et al. 2020. "Polymeric Nanoparticles for Drug Delivery: Recent Developments and Future Prospects". *Nanomaterials* (July). doi: 10.3390/nano10071403

[21] Schiela R. Schaffazick, Adriana R. Pohlmann, Teresa Dalla-Costa, Sílvia S Guterres. 2003. "Freeze-Drying Polymeric Colloidal Suspensions: Nanocapsules, Nanospheres and Nanodispersion. A Comparative Study". *Eur. J. Pharm. Biopharm* (November). doi: 10.1016/s0939-6411(03)00139-5

[22] Veer Singh, Nidhi Singh, Sachchida Nand Rai, Ashish Kumar, Anurag Kumar Singh, Mohan P. Singh, Ansuman Sahoo, Shashank Shekhar, Emanuel Vamanu, Vishal Mishra. 2023. "Heavy Metal Contamination in the Aquatic Ecosystem: Toxicity and its Remediation using Eco-Friendly Approaches". *Toxics* 11 (February). doi: 10.3390/toxics11020147

[23] Sílvia S. Guterres, Marta P. Alves, Adriana R. Pohlmann. 2007. "Polymeric Nanoparticles, Nanospheres and Nanocapsules for Cutaneous Applications". *Drug Target Insights* (July). doi: 10.1177/117739280700200002

[24] K.S. Soppimath, T.M. Aminabhavi, A.R. Kulkarni, W.E. Rudzinski. 2001. "Biodegradable Polymeric Nanoparticles as Drug Delivery Devices". *J. Control. Release* (January). doi: 10.1016/s0168-3659(00)00339-4

[25] Aleksandra Zielińska, Filipa Carreiró, Ana M. Oliveira, Andreia Neves, Bárbara Pires et al. 2020. "Polymeric Nanoparticles: Production, Characterization, Toxicology, and Ecotoxicology". *Molecules* (August). doi: 10.3390/molecules25163731

[26] Nidhi Singh, Sachchida Rai, Veer Singh, Mohan P. Singh. 2020. "Molecular Characterization, Pathogen-Host Interaction Pathway and In Silico Approaches for Vaccine Design against COVID-19". *Journal of Chemical Neuroanatomy* 110 (December). doi: 10.1016/j.jchemneu.2020.101874

[27] Catarina Pinto Reis, Ronald J. Neufeld, Antonio J. Ribeiro, Francisco Veiga. 2006. "Nanoencapsulation I. Methods for Preparation of Drug-Loaded Polymeric Nanoparticles". *Nanomedicine* (March). doi: 10.1016/j.nano.2005.12.003

[28] Stéphanie Desgouilles, Christine Vauthier, Didier Bazile, Joël Vacus, Jean-Louis Grossiord, Michel Veillard, Patrick Couvreur. 2003. "The Design of Nanoparticles Obtained by Solvent Evaporation: A Comprehensive Study". *Langmuir* (October). doi: 10.1021/la034999q

[29] Sarvesh Bohrey, Vibha Chourasiya, Archana Pandey. 2016. "Polymeric Nanoparticles Containing Diazepam: Preparation, Optimization, Characterization, In-Vitro Drug Release and Release Kinetic Study". *Nano Converg* (March). doi: 10.1186/s40580-016-0061-2

[30] Claudia Janeth Martínez Rivas, Mohamad Tarhini, Waisudin Badri, Karim Miladi, Hélène Greige-Gerges, Qand Agha Nazari, Sergio Arturo Galindo Rodríguez, Rocío Álvarez Román, Hatem Fessi, Abdelhamid Elaissari. 2017. "Nanoprecipitation Process: From Encapsulation to Drug Delivery". *Int. J. Pharm* (October). doi: 10.1016/j.ijpharm.2017.08.064

[31] Veer Singh, Nidhi Singh, Manisha Verma, Rashmi Kamal, Ritesh Tiwari, Mahesh Sanjay Chivate, Sachchida Nand Rai, Ashish Kumar, Anupama Singh, Mohan P. Singh, Emanuel Vamanu, and Vishal Mishra. "Hexavalent-Chromium-Induced Oxidative Stress and the Protective Role of Antioxidants against Cellular Toxicity". *Antioxidants* 12 (2022) 2375. https://doi.org/10.3390/antiox11122375.

[32] T. Govender, S. Stolnik, M.C. Garnett, L. Illum, S.S. Davis. 1999. "PLGA Nanoparticles Prepared by Nanoprecipitation: Drug Loading And Release Studies of a Water Soluble Drug". *Journal of Controlled Release* (February). doi: 10.1016/s0168-3659(98)00116-3

[33] P.L. Felgner, T.R. Gadek, M. Holm, R. Roman, H.W. Chan, M. Wenz et al. 1987. "Lipofection: A Highly Efficient, Lipid-Mediated DNA-Transfection Procedure". *Proc Natl Acad Sci USA* (November). doi: 10.1073/pnas.84.21.7413

[34] Jacob A. Poliskey, Samuel T. Crowley, Raghu Ramanathan, Christopher W. White, Basil Mathew, Kevin G. Rice. 2018. "Metabolically Stabilized Double-Stranded mRNA Polyplexes". *Gene Ther* (October). doi: 10.1038/s41434-018-0038-3

[35] Cinzia M. Bellettato, Maurizio Scarpa. 2018. "Possible Strategies to Cross the Blood–Brain Barrier". *Italian J Pediatrics* (November). doi: 10.1186/s13052-018-0563-0

[36] Daniel Gonzalez-Carter, Xueying Liu, Theofilus A. Tockary, Anjaneyulu Dirisala et al. 2020. "Targeting Nanoparticles to The Brain by Exploiting the Blood–Brain Barrier Impermeability to Selectively Label the Brain Endothelium". *Proc Natl Acad Sci USA* (August). doi: 10.1073/pnas.2002016117

[37] Mantosh Kumar Satapathy, Ting-Lin Yen, Jing-Shiun Jan, Ruei-Dun Tang et al. 2021. "Solid Lipid Nanoparticles (Slns): An Advanced Drug Delivery System Targeting the Brain through BBB". *Pharmaceutics* (July). doi: 10.3390/pharmaceutics13081183

[38] Jyoti Ahlawat, Gileydis Guillama Barroso, Shima Masoudi Asil, Melinda Alvarado et al. 2020. "Nanocarriers as Potential Drug Delivery Candidates for Overcoming the Blood–Brain Barrier: Challenges and Possibilities". *ACS Omega* 5 (June). doi: 10.1021/acsomega.0c01592

[39] Sonia M. Lombardo, Marc Schneider, Akif E. Türeli, Nazende Günday Türeli. 2020. "Key for Crossing the BBB with Nanoparticles: The Rational Design". *Beilstein J Nanotechnology* (June). doi: 10.3762/bjnano.11.72

[40] Ambra Del Grosso, Marianna Galliani, Lucia Angella, Melissa Santi et al. 2019. "Brain-Targeted Enzyme-Loaded Nanoparticles: A Breach Through the Blood–Brain Barrier for Enzyme Replacement Therapy in Krabbe Disease". *Sci Adv* 5 (November). doi: 10.1126/sciadv.aax7462

12 Herbal Drug-Loaded Nanoparticles for the Treatment of Neurodegenerative Diseases

Soumya Katiyar, Shikha Kumari, Abhay Dev Tripathi, Ritika Singh, Pradeep K. Srivastava, and Abha Mishra

12.1 INTRODUCTION

Neurological disorders (NDs) are characterized by alterations in the structure or functioning of the nervous system (or neurons). This long-term damage over time can impair reasoning, mobility, learning, perception, and memory. The most common kinds of NDs include Alzheimer's disease (AD); Parkinson's disease (PD); Friedreich ataxia (FA); diabetic neuropathy; multiple sclerosis (MS); Huntington's disease (HD); spinal muscular atrophy (SMA); and amyotrophic lateral sclerosis (ALS). In current history, the global growth in the proportion of the elderly population has increased the prevalence of neurological illnesses [1]. According to a thorough analysis of the worldwide burden of illnesses, traumas, and adverse outcomes published in 2016, 276 million individuals worldwide suffer from a neurological impairment, and around 9 million people die from NDs per year. The cause of NDs is unknown; nevertheless, they appear to be the result of a combination of events that cause neuronal degeneration. A confluence of variables, including ageing, mitochondrial malfunction, increased ROS production, and/or environmental exposures (e.g. effects of toxic metals, harmful chemicals, pesticides, electromagnetic interference), may be involved in the development of NDs [2–4]. Despite numerous research studies and considerable improvement, promising options for early detection and treatment techniques for these disorders remain limited. Additionally, most existing therapies are symptomatic and incapable of enhancing one's life quality or delaying or ameliorating harm. Perhaps the most significant barrier to ND diagnosis is the existence of the blood–brain barrier, or BBB, which precludes the preponderance of medications and diagnostic agents from penetrating the brain and producing collateral adverse effects [5]. In order to shield the brain's parenchyma against being exposed to possibly toxic compounds transported by circulation, the BBB acts as a barrier here

 DOI: 10.1201/9781032661964-12

between the bloodstream and the central nervous system (CNS) [6]. Nowadays, the monitoring and therapeutic options for brain illnesses are frequently dependent on vascular lesions and BBB leakiness. Hence, continued attempts have been undertaken to build methods that enhance medication transit through the BBB.

Nanomedicine is the use of nanoscale technology in the medical sector for medicinal, monitoring, and preventative procedures. Identifying and treating several diseases, such as malignancies, cardiovascular conditions, and neurological problems, may be made possible through nanotechnology-based technological advances. Among the numerous mechanisms for the delivery of therapeutics to the CNS, nanotechnology-based medicine and particularly targeted administration of NP systems are gaining some traction [5, 7–8]. While NPs have numerous benefits from the regulated distribution of medications, there are constraints to their employment in clinics. The difficulties associated with the industrial scalability of their manufacture and difficult regulatory requirements are indeed notable among these [9]. Nonetheless, clinical studies to examine the treatment effectiveness of different nanotechnology-based devices for ND disorders have already begun. Through the use of therapeutic drug-loaded NPs, it is possible to enhance the pharmacodynamics and bioavailability of medications, strengthen therapeutic effectiveness, augment immunomodulatory responses, and assist the entry of therapeutic components into the brain. NPs' multipurpose and adaptive designs make them suitable for the administration of medications to the brain. Nevertheless, a number of aspects, such as the chemical nature, hydrophobicity, structure, size, and charge, to name a few, should always be taken into account prior to being employed. An ideal NP would have cytocompatibility, non-toxicity, and the ability to bind and deliver drugs or treatments, among other favourable characteristics. It can pass across the BBB and regulate drug release for a prolonged time as it does not break down fast *in vivo*. Given all of these traits, NPs are particularly successful in breaching the BBB [10–11].

A multitude of synthetic medications (such as donepezil, memantine, triheptanoin, levodopa etc.) have demonstrated efficacy in the management of a number of prevalent NDs, such as PD, HD, AD, and many other neurodegenerative conditions [12]. Synthetic medication usage is connected with a number of negative impacts, rendering them unsuitable for routine medical care. The scientific community has taken a cautious approach to the use of herbal drugs because they have fewer side effects and have economic viability compared to these manufactured medications' negative consequences [13]. Herbal drugs or phytochemicals are potentially effective therapeutic medications due to their potent antioxidant, anti-cholinesterase, anti-inflammatory, and anti-amyloid capabilities [14–15]. Nevertheless, a limited effective dose and dosage standardization and low water solubility, penetration, and bioavailability have limited the implementation of biologically active phytochemicals in medical research. Scientists have worked extremely hard to develop cutting-edge methods for better medication delivery to resolve these issues. This situation has led to the incredible development of nanotechnology to effectively deliver herbal drugs that produce full beneficial health effects [16]. Hence, this chapter focuses on the potential role of various herbal drugs used to control and treat NDs, together with the application of cutting-edge nanotechnology to overcome their medicinal shortcomings.

12.2 MEDICINAL PLANTS FOR NEURODEGENERATIVE DISEASES (NDS)

Neurodegenerative diseases (NDs), which include PD, AD, motor neuron disease and so on, are some of the most common progressive degenerative diseases. These diseases cause neurons to lose their function and die off in the end. Many NDs are more likely to happen as people get older [17–18]. The number of NDs rises slowly as people age [19]. In the case of brain injury, stroke, cerebral or subarachnoid haemorrhage, and head injury, neurons are rapidly injured and frequently die [20]. Still, progressive neurodegeneration in contrast, is a long-term disorder in which some populations of neurons in the brain experience a neurodegenerative problem that often commences progressively and worsens over time due to several factors [19]. Now it is important to find and develop new drugs to cure NDs with better safety and effectiveness profiles. The therapeutic efficacy of medicinal plants like ashwagandha, *S. hydrangea*, *Baccopa monnieri*, Aloe vera, *Saussurea pulvinata*, *Zingiber officinale*, Ginkgo biloba, *Knema laurina*, *Curcuma longa*, *Centella asiatica*, and *Azadirachta indica*, as well as their phytocompounds like flavonoids, celastrol, alkaloids, trehalose, terpenes, lycopene, sesamol, and curcumin, have been receiving significant attention as a potential option for the effective management and treatment of NDs. In-depth discussion of a few medicinal plants is provided below.

12.2.1 *Zingiber officinale* (Ginger)

Zingiber officinale (*Z. officinale*) is a perennial herb that belongs to the *Zingiberaceae* family. It is recognized for its medical properties as well as its usage as a spice and ingredient for flavouring meals and beverages. The pharmacological effects of ginger and its bioactive components, including gingerol, terpenes, shogaol, and many more, have been studied recently [21]. As a result, many studies have shown that ginger can help one avoid conditions including coronary heart disease, diabetes, osteoarthritis, gastrointestinal malfunction, respiratory illnesses, and NDs. Typically, neuronal inflammation, mitochondrial dysfunction, and protein misfolding define neurodegenerative disorders, which lead to neurological impairment, synaptic failure, and neuronal loss. In particular, gingerols, a bioactive component of ginger, have demonstrated anti-oxidant, anti-amyloidogenic, anti-inflammatory, and immunomodulatory properties, and anti-cholinesterase effects beneficial for NDs treatment without side effects in comparison to the available synthetic drugs [22–23].

12.2.2 Aloe vera

Aloe vera (A. vera) is grown for its edible and medicinal properties. It is a succulent perennial plant that stays green year after year. Aloe vera alone has been shown to reduce depolarization and neuronal death by preventing the development of ROS inside cells and increasing the production of calcium (Ca2+) [24]. Indications like this point to the possibility that aloe vera is a suitable and efficient substitute treatment for cerebrovascular diseases [25–26].

12.2.3 *Azadirachta indica* (Neem)

Brain post-ischemic reperfusion and hypoperfusion were reported to be protected by *Azadirachta indica* (*A. indica*), and the plant was also discovered to have a preventative effect against cisplatin-generated neurotoxicity in rats [27]. Extracts of *A. indica*, which are anti-oxidative and anti-apoptotic, have been reported to be neuroprotective in the treatment of PD-induced functional impairment [28]. Standardized *A. indica* leaf extract has been shown to have neuroprotective effects in rats with partial sciatic nerve injury [29].

12.2.4 *Withania somnifera* (Ashwagandha)

Withania somnifera, called Ashwagandha, is a foremost therapeutic plant used in Ayurveda, which is an associated plant of the *Solanaceae* family. This plant has hairy covers and grows perennially. From different parts of the plant, scientists have been able to isolate and identify a wide range of chemical substances, such as steroidal lactones, alkaloids, flavonoids, tannins, withanolides, and a plethora of sitoindosides [30]. Treatments with an extract of *Withania somnifera* lowered oxidative stress and improved catecholamine content [31] in a study using a rat model for PD. *In vivo* mice models with PD showed better behaviour after administering Withania somnifera root extract [32].

12.2.5 *Curcuma longa* (Turmeric)

Since the beginning of time, the *Zingiberaceae* family plant *Curcuma longa L.* has been significant to Indian tradition. The well-known turmeric spice is derived from the root of this medicinal plant, the benefits of which encompass multiple culinary dishes, colours, pharmaceuticals, religious rituals, and conventional medicine [33]. According to the latest published findings, the phytochemical constituents of *C. longa*, such as curcumin, terpenoids, flavonoids, and so on, have a wide range of medicinal attributes, which include anti-inflammatory, anti-oxidant activity, anti-diabetic, and antitumoral, along with neuro- and hepatoprotective activity [34–35]. Moreover, curcumin intervenes in the neuroprotective mechanisms linked to neurodegeneration by reducing oxidative stress and regulating the inflammatory cascade [36–37].

12.3 COMMON PLANT-DERIVED BIOACTIVES FOR NDS

Current studies on a large range of herbal medicinal plants have revealed that their separated pure components or crude extracts offer superior curative capabilities to the complete plant as an option for the management of NDs. These qualities are mostly owing to the availability of phytonutrients generated by plants as secondary bioactive metabolites, such as polyphenols, tannins, alkaloids, and terpenoids, and many others. Epidemiological research, and *in vivo* (both animal and human) clinical trials all provide credible indications that phytonutrients or polyphenols can alleviate a variety of inflammation-related diseases. The primary actions of polyphenolic compounds include their well-known anti-oxidant properties, suppression of intracellular kinase action, anti-inflammatory properties, ability to couple to receptors at the cell surface, and ability to alter the functioning of cell membranes.

12.3.1 Curcumin

Common characteristics of neurodegenerative disorders of ageing include protein aggregation, oxidative damage, and inflammation. The benefits of curcumin as a neuro-protective drug include its anti-oxidant, anti-inflammatory, as well anti-protein-aggregate capabilities [38]. Due to its pluripotency, long antiquity of practice, oral safety, and significant low cost, curcumin has become a good option for treating several neurological illnesses for which there are currently inadequate treatments [39]. Ageing, PD, head traumas, HD, and stroke are a few examples that are mentioned [40]. Contrary to what is widely believed, curcumin's poor bioavailability inhibits therapeutic usefulness outside the colon. There is a plethora of animal model evidence demonstrating it is extremely effective against a variety of neurodisease types [41].

12.3.2 Berberine

Berberine, which alleviates rotenone-induced cytotoxicity in SH-SY5Y cells through antioxidant properties and stimulation of the PI3K/Akt signalling cascade, is neuroprotective through the upregulation of the Nrf2 gene. This finding was made possible by the discovery that berberine is neuroprotective [40]. Berberine has neuroprotective effects in animal models of AD that have come into the frame of knowledge through several studies. NPs of berberine have been found to have a neuroprotective role against LPS-induced neurodegenerative alterations [42]. By inhibiting the provocation of inflammatory cytokines, berberine can provide neuroprotection to patients suffering from localized cerebral ischemia. Berberine has also been proven to have a protective effect against the spoiled intrinsic feature of the CA1 neurons that were generated by Aβ neurotoxicity. There are numerous different mechanisms by which berberine protects neurons, and some of these mechanisms have just recently been examined [43]. According to the authors, it is a possible option for treating neurodegenerative illnesses.

12.3.3 Quercetin

Based on their chemical structure, flavonoids (secondary metabolites) can be categorized into six distinct groups: flavanols, flavanones, flavones, flavonols, iso-flavonoids, and anthocyanidins. Targeting numerous pathways at once, they have shown significant potential to halt the advances in NDs and may even slow them down. Flavonoids have the potential to pass the BBB, suggesting they may be useful in preventing neurodegenerative ailments [44].

Some of the most frequent flavonoids in food plants are quercetin and its related compounds. It is a type of flavonoid called flavonols, and it is a very important type of polyphenol. Daily quercetin consumption should be between 10 and 16 milligrams. To experience the health benefits of quercetin, one should take 1gm/day [44–45].

It has been shown to have a variety of positive impacts on human health, including being anti-cancerous, anti-inflammatory, anti-oxidant, and several other beneficial properties, such as a neuroprotective role. The neuroprotective beneficial role of quercetin has been documented in several investigational studies of *in vivo* and *in vitro* cell line and animal models respectively for NDs such as cognitive deficits, ischemia, traumatic damage, PD, HD, and so on [44, 46–49].

12.3.4 Lycopene

Tomatoes, watermelons, and red pomelo are just a few of the many fruits and vegetables that constitute the carotenoids known as lycopene (Lyc) [50–51]. There is a high concentration of lycopene in red tomatoes, and this structure is preserved even after cooking. Recent years have seen a surge in interest in research into the medicinal potential of carotenoids, notably in lycopene, because of their efficacy and protection in treating human diseases. Studies have revealed that Lycopene has a wide range of beneficial effects on human health and acts against several diseases, like protecting against cardiovascular disease and preventing the growth of cancers like breast and prostate [52–53]. Reports have also revealed that lycopene has an anti-inflammatory role in the treatment of intestines of rats and the lungs of mice [53]. Findings suggest that Lyc protects Leydig cells via regulating the Nrf2 pathway in hypoxic-ischemic (HI) disease, which has an anti-inflammatory and antioxidant effect [54–55].

12.3.5 Thymoquinone

Plants are the world's greatest producer of chemical compounds; thus, they naturally play a role in the traditional medicine of human health [56]. *Nigella sativa* comes from the *Ranunculaceae* family. It is also known as nutmeg flower, fennel flower, and black cumin. Black caraway seeds, habbatusawda, and Kalonji seeds [57] are some of the other names for *N sativa* [57]. People call it a medicinal plant with religious uses, and Habatul Baraka is called "the Blessed Seed" and "the cure for all diseases except death" (Prophetic hadith) [57–58]. Black cumin oil has several beneficial compounds, including tocopherols, polyunsaturated fatty acids, phytosterols, thymoquinone (TQ), 4-terpineol, and carvacrol. Thymoquinone, the major component of *N. sativa* seeds, is also prevalently found in many other medicinal plants like Monarda and Juniperus [59]. Thymoquinone, the plant's principal active ingredient, has shown potential in the prevention of a wide range of conditions, including those related to the cardiovascular system, the excretory system, and the respiratory system [58, 60–62]. Furthermore, thymoquinone is known to have anti-inflammatory, antioxidant, anti-cancerous, anti-bacterial, and anti-mutagenic effects [61, 63–68]. Oral administration of chrysin to hyper-ammonia rats dramatically recovered brain ammonia, water content, and the manifestations of glutamine synthetase (GS), TNF-alpha, IL 1, IL-6, and glial fibrillary acidic protein (GFAP), revealing that thymoquinone could be an effective therapeutic treatment for preventing brain ammonia accumulation. Chrysin synergistically reduces the neuro-inflammatory process and boosts the synthesis of astrocytic proteins and decreases ammonia levels. Studies suggest that TQ effectively counters the neuroinflammation caused by hyper-ammonia and works as a neuroprotective agent [69].

12.3.6 Ferulic Acid

Polyphenols are regularly found in plant products such as fruits, vegetables, coffee, tea, and olive oil. Polyphenols offer a range of protective benefits and protection in against UV radiation and microbial infections [70–71]. Polyphenols promote human health, which is possible due to their antioxidant effect, immune system regulation, maintenance of endothelial function, and control of gut microflora [72]. In particular, it has been shown that natural phenolic acids, particularly caffeic acid and chlorogenic acid, which are highly copious in fruits and vegetables, can inhibit the accumulation of proteins involved in NDs marked by cognitive decline. AD is one example of this condition. This beneficial quality might be attributable due to the significant anti-oxidant and anti-inflammatory action exhibited by these compounds [71]. In recent times, one of the significant phenolic acids known as ferulic acid has been used as a candidate for a neuroprotective agent. In fact, it has been proven to prevent oligomer accumulation and display anti-inflammatory, anti-apoptotic, and antioxidant actions. These activities appear to alleviate AD pathogenesis by slowing neurodegeneration in a number of different brain regions [73].

12.4 NEUROPROTECTIVE ROLE OF BIOACTIVE COMPOUNDS (PHYTOCHEMICALS) FOR ND TREATMENT

Numerous plants and plant-based foods contain phytochemicals, often in synergistic combinations. According to their chemical make-up and function, the bulk of phytochemicals may be classified into a few primary groups. There are several compounds, including carbohydrates, lipids, steroids, polyphenols, terpenes, alkaloids, and a few more substances containing nitrogen, as shown in Figure 12.1, have demonstrated a significant role in NDs treatment and are briefly discussed below.

12.4.1 Polyphenols

Polyphenols, which constitute a huge part of plant secondary metabolites, can range in complexity from simple phenols associated with hydroxyl groups attached to the aromatic ring to the extremely complex polymeric components found in tannins and lignins. Polyphenols, according to their chemical composition, play a significant role in the treatment of many diseases by reducing inflammation and preventing cell damage. Flavonoids, the largest bioactive subgroup of polyphenols with over 6,000 members, are the primary antioxidant family. Prominent flavonoids including apigenin, luteolin [74], flavanols like epigallocatechin-3-gallate (EGCG) [75], flavonols including quercetin (QC) and kaempferol [76–77], isoflavones (daidzein and genistein) [78–79], flavanones (such as naringenin and hesperetin) [80](67), and anthocyanins are the most well-known flavonoids that have significant medical and nutritional benefits, particularly neuroprotective qualities.

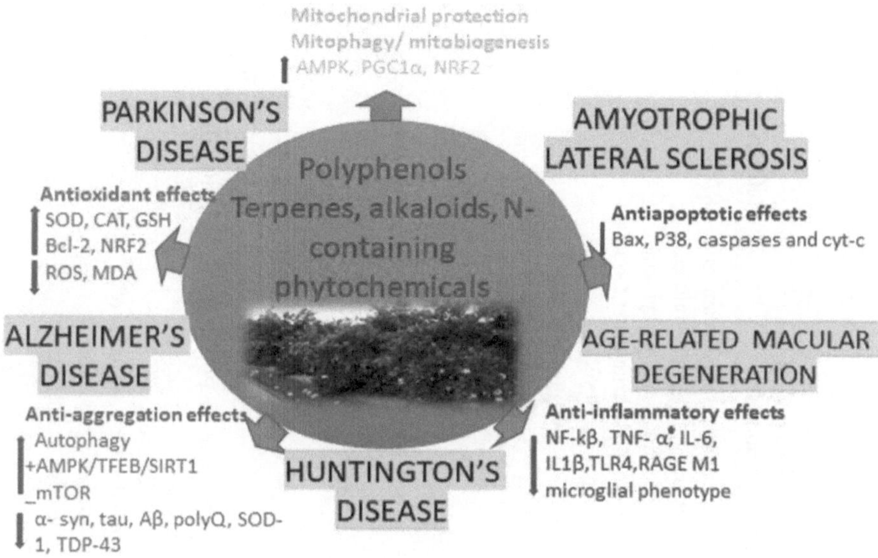

FIGURE 12.1 Potent roles of bioactive compounds against NDs.

12.4.2 Alkaloids

Alkaloids are organic, naturally occurring substances that have nitrogen atoms in them. Alkaloids can be classified into several categories according to their precursor molecule, biological sources, and pharmacokinetics. More frequently, heterocyclic alkaloids have a nitrogen atom in the cyclic ring. A number of isoquinoline alkaloids, including berberine (*Berberis vulgaris*) [81], morphine (*Papaver somniferum*) [82], salsoline (*Salsola oppositifolia*), and galantamine (*Galanthus nivalis*) [83], have been shown to have beneficial effects on NDs.

12.4.3 Terpenoids

Isoprene units are the fundamental building blocks of the unsaturated chemical compounds known as terpenoids. There is evidence that Ginkgolides A, B, and C, in addition to organic acids and flavonoid glycosides, are present in Ginkgo biloba, which has been reported to have a positive impact on NDs [84]. It has been hypothesized that the neuroprotective properties of *Nigella sativa* are caused by its primary component, which is a monoterpene known as thymoquinone (TQ). The monoterpene thymol, which comes from *Thymus vulgaris*, is another neuroprotective compound [85]. It is quite likely that GABA-mediated modulation of synaptic transmission is responsible for the neuroprotective effect of thymol [86]. However, there are many phytochemicals; therefore, this chapter will focus on the effects of small groups that protect the brain and related NDs, which are illustrated in Table 12.1.

TABLE 12.1
Important Phytochemicals that Protect the Brain from Related NDs

Name of the plant source	Bioactive compounds	Structure	Neuroprotective role of bioactive compounds	References
1. Curcuma longa	Curcumin	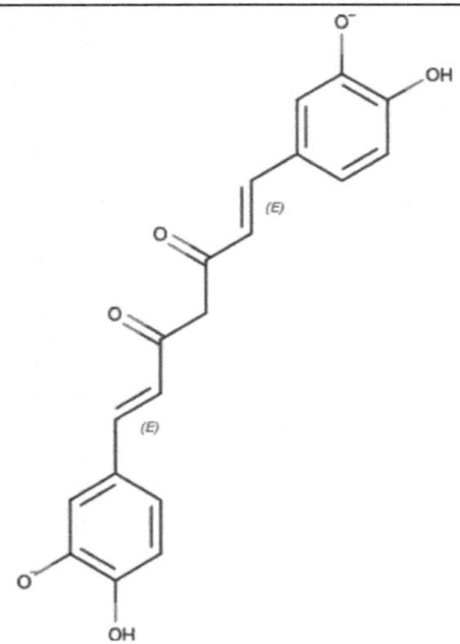	1. Anti-inflammatory, antioxidant, and anti-protein-aggregate capabilities 2. Decrease proinflammatory cytokine and prevent total nitrite generation 3. Prevent a reduced level of dopamine and tyrosine hydroxylase immunological action	[87–89]
2. Berberis aristate	Berberine	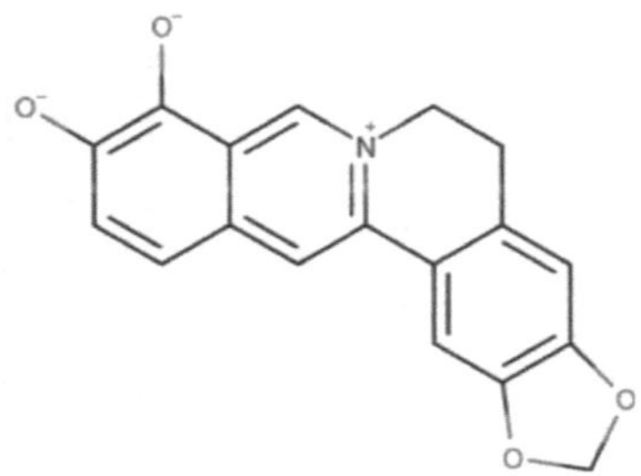	1. Activation of the PI3K/Akt signalling for upregulation of the Nrf2 gene 2. Inhibiting the production of inflammatory cytokines 3. Protective against Aβ neurotoxicity	[90–91]

3. Red wine, berries, green tea, apples, and onions	Quercetin (flavonoids)	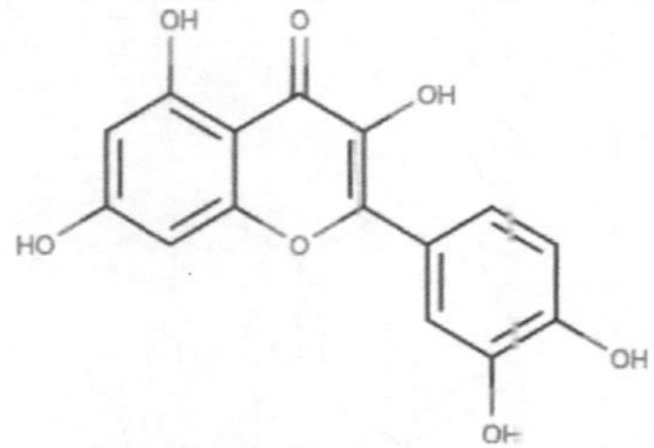	1. AChE inhibition 2. Act as an anti-oxidant and anti-amyloidogenic 3. GSK3β inhibition	[92–94]
4. Tomatoes, watermelons, red pomelo, etc.	Lycopene	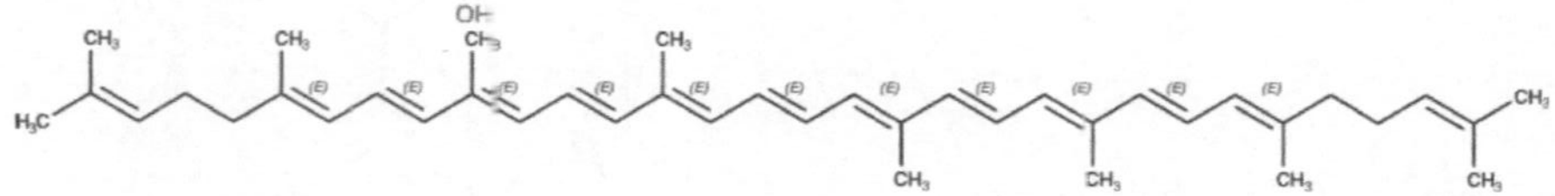	1. Lycopene protects Leydig cells via regulating the Nrf2 pathway in HI disease, 2. Lycopene has an anti-inflammatory as well antioxidant effect	[55, 95]

(*Continued*)

TABLE 12.1 (Continued)
Important Phytochemicals that Protect the Brain from Related NDs

Name of the plant source	Bioactive compounds	Structure	Neuroprotective role of bioactive compounds	References
5. Nigella sativa	Thymoquinone	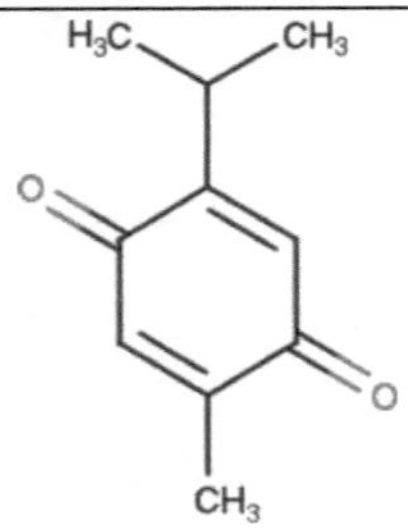	1. Prevent cardiovascular, excretory, and respiratory system disorders 2. TQ inhibits inflammatory mediators PGE2, NO, IL-1β, and TNF- α 3. Act as an anti-depression agent 4. Act against epilepsy disorder	[96–98]
6. Spinach, blueberry, grapes, pepper, turnip, cucumber, parsley, tomatoes, red beet, radish carrots, etc.	Ferulic acid	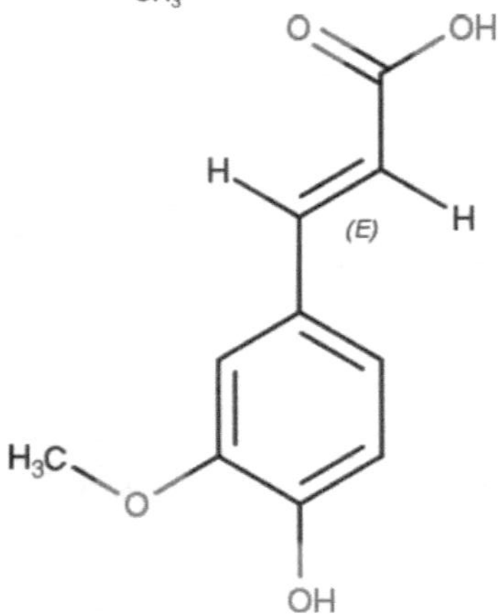	1. Neuroprotective approach against AD 2. Acts as an anti-inflammatory and anti-oxidant agent	[99–100]

12.5 ROLE OF NANOCARRIER-BASED STRATEGIES FOR NDS

Simple colloidal NPs are known as "nanocarriers" (NCs), and they are frequently utilized to deliver medicinal and chemical agents towards a specific target [101]. According to Peer et al., NCs vary among spectra of size between 1 to 100 nm [102]. But NCs that are used in therapeutic applications should be less than 200 nm in size because of the smaller size of the microcapillaries of the body [103]. Since these nanocarriers are inactive and typically regarded as a safe medium, they offer good biocompatibility. With the prolonged release of medication, these nanocarriers will have a larger circulation time and will bypass the endosome-lysosome process [104]. NCs' physical and chemical characteristics, like their size, shape, and composition, can be changed in order to enhance their activity and minimize side effects [105]. Although many different types of NCs are manufactured, only a select number possess a remarkable ability to deliver medicine in the desired location. According to Mishra et al., NCs have several distinctive characteristics like improved pharmacokinetics and biodistribution, enhanced stability, superior solubility, decreased toxicity, and targeted drug delivery [106]. Organic, inorganic, and hybrid NCs are the three major types of NCs that are used for drug-delivery applications. Multiple nanocarrier-based delivery techniques are addressed more thoroughly below and shown schematically in Figure 12.2.

12.5.1 Inorganic Nanocarriers

Inorganic NCs, due to their simplicity in crossing the BBB and building up in the brain, are metal NPs that have attracted a lot of attention [107–108]. For effective brain targeting, their many features, including size, surface alterations, and stability,

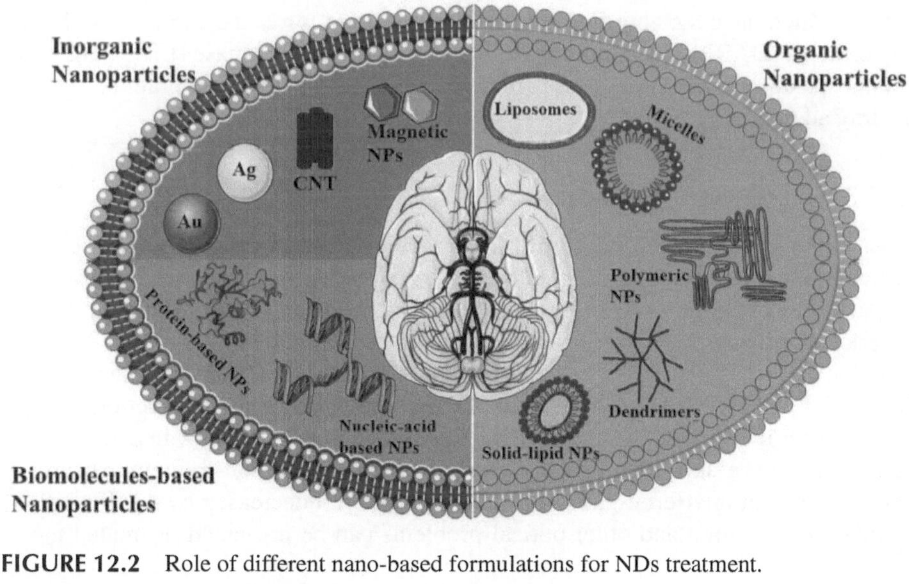

FIGURE 12.2 Role of different nano-based formulations for NDs treatment.

can be easily modified [108]. For improved medication delivery to the CNS, metal NPss are frequently functionalized with a variety of brain-targeted ligands, including antibodies, proteins, and small molecules. The imaging and diagnostic uses of these NPs are also well known [109–110]. Gold, silver, and cerium NPs have been the most successfully used metallic NPs for CNS administration [107] .

12.5.2 Gold-based Nanocarriers

Over the past century, gold NPs have captivated scientists' attention, and they have been widely utilized for biomedical and theranostic purposes. Due to their versatility, gold NPs (Au-NPs) are widely utilized in the field of drug delivery, imaging, and therapeutics systems [111]. AuNPs are notable for their tunable nanomaterial qualities like porosity or optical responsiveness as well as their relatively larger surface area that facilitates the coalition of various targeted ligands. Low toxicity, biocompatibility, anti-bacterial, higher (Z) atomic number, higher (μ_a) X-ray absorption coefficient, simplicity of synthesis, and cost-effectiveness are further noteworthy characteristics [112–113]. AuNPs, as well as other synthetic NP-based delivery systems, however, exhibit lower selectivity when it comes to targeting cells since they lack distinctive moieties that distinguish between targeted and non-targeted sites [114] . The BBB can be crossed by AuNPs with a diameter of less than 50 nm, according to research [115]. Additionally, because tumour cells have a perforated vascular system, PEGylated AuNPs coupled with TNF (tumour necrosis factor) can discharge via these infected cells [116]. Numerous AuNP species were thoroughly investigated for delivery of siRNA [117–118]. They include cationic quaternary ammonium- or branching PEI-functionalized AuNPs, cationic lipid bilayer-coated AuNPS, and oligonucleotide-modified AuNPs. It has also been discovered that gold nanorods possess a greater possibility for siRNA delivery to specific cells or tissues [119]. A research team developed gold nanorod-DARPP-32 siRNA complexes (nano plexes), which have the ability to selectively target and lower the expression of specific proteins (DARPP-32) like extracellular signal-regulated kinase (ERK), and protein phosphatase 1 (PP-1) in the dopaminergic signalling pathway in brain tissues for the drug addiction treatment.

12.5.3 Silver-based Nanocarriers

Silver NPs (AgNPs) are widely utilized in several areas of chemistry, physics and medicine like catalysis, optical, electrical, and photothermal properties, treatments, diagnosis, and immunoassays [120–122]. AgNPs are widely popular for their antibacterial or anticancer properties, according to numerous studies [123–124]. Contrary to its ionic form, silver when utilized in NP form shows lessened cellular toxicity. Undoubtedly, AgNPs' better antibacterial capabilities aid in the production of free radicals from the surface of Ag [124]. AgNPs not only work well against germs, but also seem to have anti-inflammatory characteristics. Interleukin-6, tumour necrosis factor-alpha, and interferon-gamma production were all decreased by AgNPs [125]. Macular degeneration and other optical problems can be prevented or treated more effectively with AgNPs [126–127]. The growth factor that makes endothelial cells more permeable is inhibited by AgNPs. Subsequently, they also reduced the onset of degenerative disorders related to the eyes and, in certain cases, might also improve sharp-sightedness by reducing this permeability [128]. It was reported in one of the studies conducted by Daniel et al. that intracellular Ag_2S generation segregates silver ions released from silver NPs; it also dramatically decreased their toxicity and, consequently, lowered microglial inflammation and associated neurotoxicity [129]. Thus, AgNPs can be a suitable NP for the treatment of brain inflammation and related neurotoxicity.

12.5.4 Carbon-based Nanocarriers

Carbon nanotubes (CNTs) are a highly sought-after choice for several biological applications like biosensors for DNA and protein detection, diagnostic tools used in differentiating distinct proteins from serum samples, and carriers for delivering medication molecules, protein, or vaccines [130]. The value of the CNT-based drug-delivery therapy has greatly increased due to its biocompatibility and supporting substrate. Through attachment to the outer walls of nanotubes, the drugs can be administered to particular targets [131]. Bioactive molecules including proteins, peptides, nucleic acids (NAs), and medicinal compounds, can be used to functionalize them. One of the key benefits for using carbon nanotubes in the treatment of cancer is the many covalent functionalizations on their sidewalls or tips. According to this idea, treating inflammatory diseases like Parkinson's, Huntington's, ALS, and AD can help prevent tissue damage by coating healthy tissues with complement proteins or using NPs.

12.5.5 Magnetic Nanocarriers

Widder, Senyi, and colleagues fostered the idea of comprehending magnetic micro- and nanoparticles and using them as a medication delivery mechanism in the late 1970s [132][94, 95]. For biological applications, such particles that have superparamagnetism at room temperature are typically chosen. Magnetic NPs possess several biological and medical uses because of their higher field irreversibility, saturation field, superparamagnetism, and additional anisotropy [133]. These characteristics result from the surface effects and narrowness and limitation in size that determine the magnetic behaviour of single NPs [134]. Due to the applied magnetic field, magnetic NPs allow for the systematic delivery of medication to a precise target place within the human body while remaining eventually localised. The fundamental concept is that medicinal substances are encapsulated or linked to a magnetic microcarrier. By functionalizing the polymer or metal coating, cytotoxic medicines or therapeutic DNA for targeted treatment is added to address a genetic abnormality.

12.5.6 Organic Nanocarriers

Organic NPs such as lipid NPs, liposomes, dendrimers, polymeric NPs, micelles, and viral NPs are examples of organic nanocarriers (ONCs). ONCs may merge with several spectra of medicines as well as ligands used in drug delivery, and they have a very flexible nature with low toxicity. In terms of ONCs, the improved permeability and retention effect of micelles and liposomes allows for drug accumulation at the appropriate spot [135]. The first generation of nanocarriers is basic excipients known as polymeric nanocarriers and liposome-mediated drug delivery [16].

12.5.7 Lipid-based Nanocarriers

Small molecules, vaccines, peptides, small and long.For instance, the medication doxorubicin in stealth liposomes had a lower dispersion in plasma and a higher concentration in healthy cells than the drug in solution (Wang et al. 2012). Temperature response liposomes, a type of programmable switch nanocarrier, are said to improve local medication release (Rosenblum et al. 2018)

12.5.8 Polymeric Nanocarriers

Colloidal, solid NPs made from any biodegradable polymer, are known as polymeric NPs [136–137]. Nanospheres are a matrix type that encloses the molecules of the drug inside the polymeric matrix, whereas nanocapsules are a reservoir type that dissolves or disperses the drug molecules in the polymer's core. Both varieties can chemically combine or adsorb the medication to their exterior [138]. The biodegradation of the polymeric nanocarriers inside the human body results in monomers that are readily broken down through metabolic pathways [139]. Synthetic polymers like poly(lactic-co-glycolic acid), PEG, PGA, and PCL, and natural polymers like chitosan, gelatin and albumin, and so on, can both be used to make polymeric nanocarriers [140]. These nanocarriers possess enhanced stability, drug payload, half-life in systemic circulation, and longer drug release when compared to other nanocarriers. To target malignant cells, an anticancer medication like doxorubicin is confined inside polymeric nanocarriers. Physiochemical changes to the polymeric source can improve the regulated release of the medication. Additionally, the manufacturing of polymeric NPs for targeted drug administration using stimuli-sensitive polymers has advanced. When internal or external environmental stimuli (low pH, redox, enzyme) are present, these intelligent polymers release drugs (temperature, light, ultrasound, magnetic and electric field). Scalability, toxicity/biocompatibility, and stimuli sensitivity are design hurdles for smart polymers. Extrinsic stimuli, on the other hand, present difficulties like stimuli supplying compliance, tissue penetration, and localization, whereas intrinsic stimuli face variations between clinical and preclinical models [141–142].

12.5.9 Dendrimers

Dendrimers are the highest ramification nanoscale polymers [143]. In recent years, scientists have created a wide variety of dendrimers, and novel dendrimer types are still being created and processed. Such extensively branched polymers are considered desirable drug carriers due to their ordered three-dimensional architecture and wide surface functionalities [144–145]. Drug molecules may be affixed to the surface groups of dendrimers or incorporated therein. On the dendrimer surface, various functional groups can accommodate pharmaceuticals and medicinal compounds with ease [146–147]. Dendrimers are one type of nanocarrier-based DDS that has shown considerable potential in the treatment of numerous CNS illnesses. These nanocarriers have shown promising properties for administering CNS medications, including low immunogenicity and toxicity and improved solubility of drugs, stability, and permeability. Additionally, dendrimers exhibit higher effective paracellular and transcellular transport through the BBB, which qualifies them as good carriers for delivering drugs inside the brain [148]. In order to improve the delivery of water-insoluble medications to the brain, researchers looked at the possibility of PAMAM dendrimer for intranasal efficacy of the antipsychotic medicine haloperidol [149–150]. They discovered that the dendrimer-based formulation increased the water solubility of haloperidol. Drug-dendrimer interaction mostly occurs through the creation of chemical and physical bonds. This dendrimer can be utilised for vaccine delivery, gene delivery, medication delivery, antiviral delivery, and magnetic resonance imaging scanning [151].

12.5.10 Protein Nanocarriers

Protein nanocarriers are safer than synthetic polymers and therefore they are frequently employed in medical formulations. Protein's amphiphilicity makes it the perfect material for creating NPs and enables improved interactions between the medication and solvent [152]. The benefits of protein NPs include biocompatibility, non-antigenicity, and biodegradability. These NPs can be made safely without the use of harmful chemicals or organic solvents under modest conditions. Furthermore, protein-based NPs' specified fundamental structure allows for surface alterations, enabling covalent attachment of medicines and targeting ligands [153].

12.5.11 Solid Lipid Nanocarriers

Over the first decade of the 1990s, solid lipid nanocarriers have proven a successful method of delivering lipophilic drugs. The melted solid lipids are dispersed in water to create solid lipid nanocarriers, which are then stabilised by the addition of emulsifiers by micro-emulsification or high-pressure homogenization [154–155]. Solid lipid nanocarriers are often prepared using the solid form of lipids at room temperature, such as free fatty alcohol or acids, steroids or waxes, and mono-, di-, or triglycerides [156]. According to the circumstances and make-up of the solid lipid's creation, the drug molecules may be incorporated into the matrix, shell, or core of the substance. Due to its adaptability, this solid lipid nanocarrier can get around the limitations of traditional chemotherapy. Ionic and hydrophilic anticancer medications can now be added to lipophilic anticancer agents using solid lipid nanocarriers. As an effective source for oral medication delivery, a polymer-lipid hybrid nanocarrier, for instance, has been investigated [157]. For the treatment of ocular illnesses, for the regulated release of active medicines [155], and for the targeted medication delivery of anticancer agents, numerous studies on solid lipid nanocarriers have been conducted [158–159].

12.5.12 Hybrid Nanocarriers

Recently, hybrid NPs have been created as nanocarriers that combine the benefits of current systems with well-known features to create lipid-polymer NPs and solid liposomal NPs. The core and corona structure, which make up the essential components of hybrid NPs, are made of at least two distinct materials. Typically, the protective membrane, which resembles a liposome or micelle, is created by coating the metallic and polymeric core with one or more lipid layers [160]. When organic or inorganic NPs are combined with another molecular or macromolecular entity, new systems with numerous or synergistic features are created. Inflammatory macrophages are the target of lipid-latex (LiLa) hybrid NPs, which were reported by Vaishali Bagalkot and colleagues. The lipids provided targeting capabilities and colloidal stability, and the latex core served as a model hydrophobic polymeric template. LiLa was coated with phosphatidylserine (PtdSer) and the oxidized cholesterol ester product cholesterol-9-carboxynonanoate to target inflammatory macrophages (9-CCN). These lipids are effectively phagocytosed by macrophages, which are frequently referred to as "eat-me" signals [161]. Protein-polymer hybrid NPs for cancer medication delivery have been reported by Ge et al. It has also been examined how bovine serum albumin (BSA)-poly(methyl methacrylate) (PMMA) conjugates self-assemble hybrid protein-polymer NPs [162].

12.6 HERBAL DRUG-LOADED NANOFORMULATIONS FOR NEURODEGENERATIVE DISEASES (NDS) TREATMENT

The mechanism of drug delivery enables the active pharmacological component to be delivered, resulting in the anticipated therapeutic outcome. Traditional medication delivery methods (tablets, capsules, syrups, ointments, etc.) have poor bioavailability and inconsistent plasma drug levels, which make it difficult for them to provide sustained release. Without an effective distribution method, the entire therapeutic procedure can be unsuccessful. To achieve optimal efficacy and safety, the medicine must also be administered at a precise controlled rate and at the intended spot [163]. So, a different approach to solving these urgent issues might be to adopt novel drug-delivery techniques that target treatments to specific body regions [164]. As a result, nanotechnology significantly influences current medication formulations, their regulated drug release profile, and their successful delivery [165]. A number of serious ailments, including cancer, diabetes, cardiovascular, inflammatory, and microbial illnesses, are currently being treated with natural chemicals. This is mainly because herbal medicines have unique advantages such as low cost, significant medicinal effectiveness, and less toxicity and adverse effects [110]. Recent studies have concentrated on creating formulations for plant extracts to safely distribute them as well as to increase their therapeutic efficacy, as summarized in Table 12.2. Plant extract-loaded NPs are designed to help people get over biological barriers, boost the bioavailability of phytochemicals that are poorly water-soluble, encapsulate mixtures of diverse phytochemicals, deliver phytochemicals to specific organs with low toxicity, and more [166]. Citrus fruits and vegetables include the polyphenol quercetin, a member of the flavonoid family with antioxidant effects. Polymeric micelles were

TABLE 12.2
Different Herbal Bioactive Compounds and Their Effect on Neurodegenerative Diseases

NDs	Herbal drug (bioactive compounds)	Nanocarrier (NPs)	NPs size (nm)	Biological study (*in vitro* and *in vivo* study of NPs)	Key findings	References
1. Alzheimer's Disease	a. Curcumin b. Quercetin c. Piperine	a. PLGA-PEG b. Nano-quercetin c. Chitosan	a. 50–250 b. <300 c. 248.50	a. HT22 cells, APP/PS1 Mice b. Albino Wister Rat c. Male Wister Rat	a. NPs made of PLGA-PEG-B6/Cur show promise as an Alzheimer's disease (AD) therapy. b. A preventative approach against the advancement of AD was demonstrated in rats treated with NQC, who displayed extra distinct findings in comparison to the quercetin group. c. The anti-apoptosis and anti-inflammatory properties of PIP have been reported as another mechanism for its actions in AD.	[175–177]
2. Parkinson's Disease	a. Curcumin+ piperine b. Quercetin (QNE)	Glyceryl monooleate b. Capmul MCM NF oil and cremophor RH 40	a. 93 b. 50	a. PD mouse model b. Bristol wild-type strain (C. elegans), MIA PaCa-2 strain	a. In-vivo research shown that constructed dual drug loaded NPs could pass the bloodbrain barrier, reverse the motor coordination deficit caused by rotenone, and stop the degradation of dopaminergic neurons in a PD mouse model. b. In the C. elegans model of PD, QNE demonstrated enhanced solubility, targetability, and neuro-protective benefits.	[178–179]
3. Huntington Disease (HD)	a. Curcumin	a. Hyaluron	a. 150–500	a. Mouse (STHdh111/111)	a. In an *in vitro* model of HD nanoparticles encapsulated with curcumin infiltrate the cells and lessen their vulnerability to apoptosis.	[180]
4. Friedreich ataxia	a. Curcumin	a. Silk fibroin	a. 150	a. Mouse (FRDA transgenic mice YG8R and control mice Y47)	a. According to this study, oxidative stress was reduced and iron was removed from the heart. Also, it enhanced the synthesis of iron-sulfur clusters, which counteracts the lack of FXN to enhance the shape and functionality of mitochondria in FRDA illness.	[181]
5. Prion disease	a. Curcumin	a. Poly-ε-caprolactone/ F68	a. 149	a. MIO-M1 and SH-SY5Y cells	a. Spinocerebellar ataxias and other neurological illnesses might benefit from the use of curcumin-loaded nanoparticles as an alternative therapy.	[182]

employed to transport quercetin in a study by Dian et al. [167], and the findings revealed that these micelles could give continuous release for up to 10 days *in vitro,* with continuous plasma level and increased full accessibility of the medication under *in vivo* conditions. The most researched nanostructures are liposomes, which have been employed in a number of formulations to carry natural compounds like resveratrol [168]. One of the studies performed by Karthik et al. showed that delivering rivastigmine liposomes through the intranasal route might be a newer approach for the treatment of AD [169]. In a recent study after three days of treatment, curcumin-loaded exosomes, which were derived from mouse embryonic stem cells and given nasally to ischemia-damaged mice, were dispersed throughout the entire brain and improved the neurological score. Additionally, the therapy increased the tight (claudin-5 and occludin) and adherent (VE-cadherin) junction proteins of the vascular endothelium (VE), showing that merging the potentials of embryonic stem cell (ESCs) exosomes and curcumin can help with neurovascular recovery after ischemia-reperfusion damage in mice [170]. For the treatment of cancer, liposomal curcumin formulations have been created [171]. Curcumin was encapsulated in liposomes using several techniques, and Cheng et al. [172] evaluated the results and found that the approach that depended on pH produced stable products with good encapsulation efficiency and bioaccessibility which might be used to treat cancer. Thus, it can be claimed that naturally found bioactive constituents (or herbal drugs) with controlled release systems show themselves as significant instruments for improving their bioactivity and minimizing their limits by providing novel possibilities for the management of chronic and fatal disorders [173]. According to BBC Research, the global market for herbal pharmaceuticals has expanded at a compound annual growth rate (CAGR) of 6.15% from $29.4 billion in 2017 to around $39.6 billion in 2022 [174].

12.7 CONCLUSION AND FUTURE PERSPECTIVE

ND illnesses are becoming more prevalent, which is a significant social and economic healthcare issue throughout the globe and is mostly caused by ageing populations and a shortage of impactful treatments. Additionally, the CNS is well known to be firmly protected by a number of barriers. Hence, in order for a suitable medicine to reach the CNS, it must basically cross the BBB. Since there is currently no treatment, ND is expensive for the health sector and also for the families of sufferers. The majority of herbal drugs include both anti-inflammatory and antioxidant effects; therefore, looking into alternate sources for ND treatment can lead to herbal remedies. Despite the fact that there are many drug-delivery methods that have been devised and established, herbal drug-based nanostructures stand out for having benefits including being safe, non-toxic, economical, simple to expand, and for offering NPs with controllable shapes and sizes. Irrespective of the availability of intriguing herbal compounds, their limited transport to the brain in therapeutically useful quantities prevents them from realizing their detailed clinical significance. Hence, among the most difficult tasks facing modern neurological research is identifying clinically viable entry sites from the bloodstream to the brain. Studies investigating neuro-pharmaceuticals are attempting to comprehend both the receptor-assisted and adsorptive transcytosis mechanisms in addition to all the physical and chemical characteristics that are unique to neuropharmaceuticals. This may result in novel treatments that have a greater chance of being successful at penetrating the BBB. According to the data presented here, herbal drug-loaded nanostructures have the potential to modify neurobiological knowledge and restorative approaches and may be utilized to potentially make important pledges for the significant emergence of nano-enhanced herbal products for the management of NDs. Owing to these NPs' innate biodegradability, cytocompatibility, ease of clearance, and low toxicity, they are acceptable for use in the administration of medication. Therefore, it can be inferred that nano-formulated herbal drugs offer an extensive source of chemically, structurally, and functionally varied compounds for novel therapeutic and curative usage in NDs.

ACKNOWLEDGEMENTS

The authors are thankful to the School of Biochemical Engineering, IIT (BHU) Varanasi, for providing technical support. This work was financially supported by the CSIR JRF/SRF, India, under the CSIR NET/JRF Ph.D. program, for providing a fellowship to author Soumya Katiyar during the tenure of this study.

REFERENCES

1. Karthivashan G, Ganesan P, Park S-Y, Kim J-S, Choi D-K. Therapeutic strategies and nano-drug delivery applications in management of ageing Alzheimer's disease. *Drug Delivery*. 2018;25(1):307–20.
2. Niedzielska E, Smaga I, Gawlik M, Moniczewski A, Stankowicz P, Pera J et al. Oxidative stress in neurodegenerative diseases. *Molecular Neurobiology*. 2016;53:4094–125.
3. Hou Y, Dan X, Babbar M, Wei Y, Hasselbalch SG, Croteau DL et al. Ageing as a risk factor for neurodegenerative disease. *Nature Reviews Neurology*. 2019;15(10):565–81.
4. Chin-Chan M, Navarro-Yepes J, Quintanilla-Vega B. Environmental pollutants as risk factors for neurodegenerative disorders: Alzheimer and Parkinson diseases. *Frontiers in Cellular Neuroscience*. 2015;9:124.
5. Zhang W, Mehta A, Tong Z, Esser L, Voelcker NH. Development of polymeric nanoparticles for blood–brain barrier transfer – strategies and challenges. *Advanced Science*. 2021;8(10):2003937.
6. Rhea EM, Banks WA. Role of the blood–brain barrier in central nervous system insulin resistance. *Frontiers in Neuroscience*. 2019;13:521.
7. Satapathy MK, Yen T-L, Jan J-S, Tang R-D, Wang J-Y, Taliyan R et al. Solid lipid nanoparticles (SLNs): an advanced drug delivery system targeting brain through BBB. *Pharmaceutics*. 2021;13(8):1183.
8. Akel H, Ismail R, Csoka I. Progress and perspectives of brain-targeting lipid-based nanosystems via the nasal route in Alzheimer's disease. *European Journal of Pharmaceutics and Biopharmaceutics*. 2020;148:38–53.
9. Cano A, Turowski P, Ettcheto M, Duskey JT, Tosi G, Sánchez-López E et al. Nanomedicine-based technologies and novel biomarkers for the diagnosis and treatment of Alzheimer's disease: From current to future challenges. *Journal of Nanobiotechnology*. 2021;19(1):122.

10. Ding S, Khan AI, Cai X, Song Y, Lyu Z, Du D et al. Overcoming blood–brain barrier transport: Advances in nanoparticle-based drug delivery strategies. *Materials Today*. 2020;37:112–25.
11. Teleanu DM, Negut I, Grumezescu V, Grumezescu AM, Teleanu RI. Nanomaterials for drug delivery to the central nervous system. *Nanomaterials*. 2019;9(3):371.
12. Rasool M, Malik A, Qureshi MS, Manan A, Pushparaj PN, Asif M et al. Recent updates in the treatment of neurodegenerative disorders using natural compounds. *Evidence-Based Complementary and Alternative Medicine*. 2014;2014.
13. Bansal R, Singh R. Exploring the potential of natural and synthetic neuroprotective steroids against neurodegenerative disorders: A literature review. *Medicinal Research Reviews*. 2018;38(4):1126–58.
14. Yadav DK. Potential therapeutic strategies of phytochemicals in neurodegenerative disorders. *Current Topics in Medicinal Chemistry*. 2021;21(31):2814–38.
15. Naoi M, Shamoto-Nagai M, Maruyama W. Neuroprotection of multifunctional phytochemicals as novel therapeutic strategy for neurodegenerative disorders: Antiapoptotic and antiamyloidogenic activities by modulation of cellular signal pathways. *Future Neurology*. 2019;14(1):FNL9.
16. Niu X, Chen J, Gao J. Nanocarriers as a powerful vehicle to overcome blood–brain barrier in treating neurodegenerative diseases: Focus on recent advances. *Asian Journal of Pharmaceutical Sciences*. 2019;14(5):480–96.
17. Ciccocioppo F, Bologna G, Ercolino E, Pierdomenico L, Simeone P, Lanuti P et al. Neurodegenerative diseases as proteinopathies-driven immune disorders. *Neural Regeneration Research*. 2020;15(5):850.
18. Xu X-L, Li S, Zhang R, Le W-D. Neuroprotective effects of naturally sourced bioactive polysaccharides: An update. *Neural Regeneration Research*. 2022;17(9):1907.
19. Gao H-M, Hong J-S. Why neurodegenerative diseases are progressive: uncontrolled inflammation drives disease progression. *Trends in Immunology*. 2008;29(8):357–65.
20. Allan SM, Rothwell NJ. Cytokines and acute neurodegeneration. *Nature Reviews Neuroscience*. 2001;2(10):734–44.
21. Ha SK, Moon E, Ju MS, Kim DH, Ryu JH, Oh MS et al. 6-Shogaol, a ginger product, modulates neuroinflammation: a new approach to neuroprotection. *Neuropharmacology*. 2012;63(2):211–23.
22. Zhang F, Zhang J-G, Yang W, Xu P, Xiao Y-L, Zhang H-T. 6-Gingerol attenuates LPS-induced neuroinflammation and cognitive impairment partially via suppressing astrocyte overactivation. *Biomedicine & Pharmacotherapy*. 2018;107:1523–29.
23. Kim C-Y, Seo Y, Lee C, Park GH, Jang J-H. Neuroprotective effect and molecular mechanism of [6]-gingerol against scopolamine-induced amnesia in C57BL/6 mice. *Evidence-based Complementary and Alternative Medicine: eCAM*. 2018;2018.
24. Tabatabaei SRF, Ghaderi S, Bahrami-Tapehebur M, Farbood Y, Rashno M. Aloe vera gel improves behavioral deficits and oxidative status in streptozotocin-induced diabetic rats. *Biomedicine & Pharmacotherapy*. 2017;96:279–90.
25. Lal UR, Lal S. Bioactive molecules from Indian medicinal plants as possible candidates for the management of neurodegenerative disorders. Bioactive Compounds in Nutraceutical and Functional Food for Good Human Health. 2020.
26. Chang R, Zhou R, Qi X, Wang J, Wu F, Yang W et al. Protective effects of aloin on oxygen and glucose deprivation-induced injury in PC12 cells. *Brain Research Bulletin*. 2016;121:75–83.
27. Xiang X, Wu L, Mao L, Liu Y. Anti-oxidative and anti-apoptotic neuroprotective effects of Azadirachta indica in Parkinson-induced functional damage. *Molecular Medicine Reports*. 2018;17(6):7959–65.

28. Kandhare AD, Mukherjee AA, Bodhankar SL. Neuroprotective effect of Azadirachta indica standardized extract in partial sciatic nerve injury in rats: Evidence from anti-inflammatory, antioxidant and anti-apoptotic studies. *EXCLI journal*. 2017;16:546.
29. Moneim AEA. Azadirachta indica attenuates cisplatin-induced neurotoxicity in rats. *Indian Journal of Pharmacology*. 2014;46(3):316.
30. Mirjalili MH, Moyano E, Bonfill M, Cusido RM, Palazón J. Steroidal lactones from Withania somnifera, an ancient plant for novel medicine. *Molecules*. 2009;14(7):2373–93.
31. Ahmad M, Saleem S, Ahmad AS, Ansari MA, Yousuf S, Hoda MN et al. Neuroprotective effects of Withania somnifera on 6-hydroxydopamine induced Parkinsonism in rats. *Human & Experimental Toxicology*. 2005;24(3):137–47.
32. Sankar SR, Manivasagam T, Krishnamurti A, Ramanathan M. The neuroprotective effect of Withania somnifera root extract in MPTP-intoxicated mice: An analysis of behavioral and biochemical variables. *Cellular & Molecular Biology Letters*. 2007;12:473–81.
33. Gupta SC, Sung B, Kim JH, Prasad S, Li S, Aggarwal BB. Multitargeting by turmeric, the golden spice: From kitchen to clinic. *Molecular Nutrition & Food Research*. 2013;57(9):1510–28.
34. SHL Kim D, Y Kim J, Han Y. Curcuminoids in neurodegenerative diseases. *Recent Patents on CNS Drug Discovery (Discontinued)*. 2012;7(3):184–204.
35. Gezici S. A study on Turmeric (Curcuma longa L.): Multifunctional agents for the management of oxidative damage, neurodegeneration and cancer. *Current Research in Pharmaceutical Sciences*. 2019.
36. Berry A, Collacchi B, Masella R, Varì R, Cirulli F. Curcuma Longa, the "Golden Spice" to Counteract Neuroinflammaging and Cognitive Decline – What Have We Learned and What Needs to Be Done. *Nutrients*. 2021;13(5):1519.
37. Satpathy L, Parida S. Neuroprotective Role of Curcumin against Benzo [a] pyrene-Induced Neurodegeneration in Zebrafish. *Biointerface Research in Applied Chemistry*. 2021;12:7311–20.
38. Ghosh S, Banerjee S, Sil PC. The beneficial role of curcumin on inflammation, diabetes and neurodegenerative disease: A recent update. *Food and Chemical Toxicology*. 2015;83:111–24.
39. Aggarwal BB, Harikumar KB. Potential therapeutic effects of curcumin, the anti-inflammatory agent, against neurodegenerative, cardiovascular, pulmonary, metabolic, autoimmune and neoplastic diseases. *International Journal of Biochemistry & Cell Biology*. 2009;41(1):40–59.
40. Huang L, Chen C, Zhang X, Li X, Chen Z, Yang C et al. Neuroprotective effect of curcumin against cerebral ischemia-reperfusion via mediating autophagy and inflammation. *Journal of Molecular Neuroscience*. 2018;64:129–39.
41. Forouzanfar F, Read MI, Barreto GE, Sahebkar A. Neuroprotective effects of curcumin through autophagy modulation. *IUBMB Life*. 2020;72(4):652–64.
42. Soudi SA, Nounou MI, Sheweita SA, Ghareeb DA, Younis LK, El-Khordagui LK. Protective effect of surface-modified berberine nanoparticles against LPS-induced neurodegenerative changes: a preclinical study. *Drug Delivery and Translational Research*. 2019;9:906–19.
43. Lin X, Zhang N. Berberine: Pathways to protect neurons. *Phytotherapy Research*. 2018;32(8):1501–10.
44. Khan H, Ullah H, Aschner M, Cheang WS, Akkol EK. Neuroprotective effects of quercetin in Alzheimer's disease. *Biomolecules*. 2019;10(1):59.

45. Kawabata K, Mukai R, Ishisaka A. Quercetin and related polyphenols: new insights and implications for their bioactivity and bioavailability. *Food & Function*. 2015;6(5):1399–417.
46. Rishitha N, Muthuraman A. Therapeutic evaluation of solid lipid nanoparticle of quercetin in pentylenetetrazole induced cognitive impairment of zebrafish. *Life Sciences*. 2018;199:80–7.
47. Li X, Wang H, Gao Y, Li L, Tang C, Wen G et al. Protective effects of quercetin on mitochondrial biogenesis in experimental traumatic brain injury via the Nrf2 signaling pathway. *PLoS One*. 2016;11(10):e0164237.
48. El-Horany HE, El-latif RNA, ElBatsh MM, Emam MN. Ameliorative effect of quercetin on neurochemical and behavioral deficits in rotenone rat model of Parkinson's disease: modulating autophagy (quercetin on experimental Parkinson's disease). *Journal of Biochemical and Molecular Toxicology*. 2016;30(7):360–9.
49. Sandhir R, Mehrotra A. Quercetin supplementation is effective in improving mitochondrial dysfunctions induced by 3-nitropropionic acid: implications in Huntington's disease. *Biochimica et Biophysica Acta (BBA) – Molecular Basis of Disease*. 2013;1832(3):421–30.
50. Condori MAV, Chagman GJP, Barriga-Sanchez M, Vilchez LFV, Ursetta S, Pérez AG et al. Effect of tomato (Solanum lycopersicum L.) lycopene-rich extract on the kinetics of rancidity and shelf-life of linseed (Linum usitatissimum L.) oil. *Food Chemistry*. 2020;302:125327.
51. Olson JA, Krinsky NI. Introduction: The colorful, fascinating world of the carotenoids: Important physiologic modulators. *FASEB Journal*. 1995;9(15):1547–50.
52. Frei B. Cardiovascular disease and nutrient antioxidants: role of low-density lipoprotein oxidation. *Critical Reviews in Food Science & Nutrition*. 1995;35(1–2):83–98.
53. Qi WJ, Sheng WS, Peng C, Xiaodong M, Yao TZ. Investigating into anti-cancer potential of lycopene: Molecular targets. *Biomedicine & Pharmacotherapy*. 2021;138:111546.
54. Zhao Y, Li M-Z, Shen Y, Lin J, Wang H-R, Talukder M et al. Lycopene prevents DEHP-induced Leydig cell damage with the Nrf2 antioxidant signaling pathway in mice. *Journal of Agricultural and Food Chemistry*. 2019;68(7):2031–40.
55. Fu C, Zheng Y, Zhu J, Chen B, Lin W, Lin K et al. Lycopene exerts neuroprotective effects after hypoxic–ischemic brain injury in neonatal rats via the nuclear factor erythroid-2 related factor 2/nuclear factor-κ-gene binding pathway. *Frontiers in Pharmacology*. 2020;11:585898.
56. Dubick MA. Historical perspectives on the use of herbal preparations to promote health. *Journal of Nutrition*. 1986;116(7):1348–54.
57. Qidwai W, Hamza HB, Qureshi R, Gilani A. Effectiveness, safety, and tolerability of powdered Nigella sativa (kalonji) seed in capsules on serum lipid levels, blood sugar, blood pressure, and body weight in adults: results of a randomized, double-blind controlled trial. *Journal of Alternative and Complementary Medicine*. 2009;15(6):639–44.
58. Ahmad A, Husain A, Mujeeb M, Khan SA, Najmi AK, Siddique NA et al. A review on therapeutic potential of Nigella sativa: A miracle herb. *Asian Pacific Journal of Tropical Biomedicine*. 2013;3(5):337–52.
59. Taborsky J, Kunt M, Kloucek P, Lachman J, Zeleny V, Kokoska L. Identification of potential sources of thymoquinone and related compounds in Asteraceae, Cupressaceae, Lamiaceae, and Ranunculaceae families. *Central European Journal of Chemistry*. 2012;10:1899–906.
60. Cobourne-Duval MK, Taka E, Mendonca P, Bauer D, Soliman KF. The antioxidant effects of thymoquinone in activated BV-2 murine microglial cells. *Neurochemical Research*. 2016;41:3227–38.

61. Su X, Ren Y, Yu N, Kong L, Kang J. Thymoquinone inhibits inflammation, neoangiogenesis and vascular remodeling in asthma mice. *International Immunopharmacology*. 2016;38:70–80.
62. Ali BH, Al Za'abi M, Shalaby A, Manoj P, Waly MI, Yasin J et al. The effect of thymoquinone treatment on the combined renal and pulmonary toxicity of cisplatin and diesel exhaust particles. *Experimental Biology and Medicine*. 2015;240(12):1698–707.
63. Velagapudi R, El-Bakoush A, Lepiarz I, Ogunrinade F, Olajide OA. AMPK and SIRT1 activation contribute to inhibition of neuroinflammation by thymoquinone in BV2 microglia. *Molecular and Cellular Biochemistry*. 2017;435:149–62.
64. Elsherbiny NM, Maysarah NM, El-Sherbiny M, Al-Gayyar MM. Renal protective effects of thymoquinone against sodium nitrite-induced chronic toxicity in rats: Impact on inflammation and apoptosis. *Life Sciences*. 2017;180:1–8.
65. Velagapudi R, Kumar A, Bhatia HS, El-Bakoush A, Lepiarz I, Fiebich BL et al. Inhibition of neuroinflammation by thymoquinone requires activation of Nrf2/ARE signalling. *International Immunopharmacology*. 2017;48:17–29.
66. Mostofa A, Hossain MK, Basak D, Bin Sayeed MS. Thymoquinone as a potential adjuvant therapy for cancer treatment: evidence from preclinical studies. *Frontiers in Pharmacology*. 2017;8:295.
67. Rifaioglu MM, Nacar A, Yuksel R, Yonden Z, Karcioglu M, Zorba OU et al. Antioxidative and anti-inflammatory effect of thymoquinone in an acute Pseudomonas prostatitis rat model. *Urologia Internationalis*. 2013;91(4):474–81.
68. Inci M, Davarci M, Motor S, Yalcinkaya F, Nacar E, Aydin M et al. Anti-inflammatory and antioxidant activity of thymoquinone in a rat model of acute bacterial prostatitis. *Human & Experimental Toxicology*. 2013;32(4):354–61.
69. Farkhondeh T, Samarghandian S, Shahri AMP, Samini F. The neuroprotective effects of thymoquinone: A review. *Dose-Response*. 2018;16(2):1559325818761455.
70. Caruso G, Torrisi SA, Mogavero MP, Currenti W, Castellano S, Godos J et al. Polyphenols and neuroprotection: Therapeutic implications for cognitive decline. *Pharmacology & Therapeutics*. 2022;232:108013.
71. Sova M, Saso L. Natural sources, pharmacokinetics, biological activities and health benefits of hydroxycinnamic acids and their metabolites. *Nutrients*. 2020;12(8):2190.
72. van der Merwe M. Gut microbiome changes induced by a diet rich in fruits and vegetables. *International Journal of Food Sciences and Nutrition*. 2021;72(5):665–9.
73. Di Giacomo S, Percaccio E, Gullì M, Romano A, Vitalone A, Mazzanti G et al. Recent Advances in the Neuroprotective Properties of Ferulic Acid in Alzheimer's Disease: A Narrative Review. *Nutrients*. 2022;14(18):3709.
74. Patil SP, Jain PD, Sancheti JS, Ghumatkar PJ, Tambe R, Sathaye S. RETRACTED: Neuroprotective and neurotrophic effects of Apigenin and Luteolin in MPTP induced parkinsonism in mice. Elsevier; 2014.
75. Singh NA, Mandal AKA, Khan ZA. Potential neuroprotective properties of epigallocatechin-3-gallate (EGCG). *Nutrition Journal*. 2015;15:1–17.
76. Lagoa R, Lopez-Sanchez C, Samhan-Arias A, Ganan C, Garcia-Martinez V, Gutiérrez-Merino C. Kaempferol protects against rat striatal degeneration induced by 3-nitropropionic acid. *Journal of Neurochemistry*. 2009; 111(2):473–87.
77. Barreca D, Bellocco E, DOnofrio G, Fazel Nabavi S, Daglia M, Rastrelli L et al. Neuroprotective effects of quercetin: from chemistry to medicine. *CNS & Neurological Disorders-Drug Targets (Formerly Current Drug Targets-CNS & Neurological Disorders)*. 2016;15(8):964–75.
78. Qian Y, Guan T, Huang M, Cao L, Li Y, Cheng H et al. Neuroprotection by the soy isoflavone, genistein, via inhibition of mitochondria-dependent apoptosis pathways

and reactive oxygen induced-NF-κB activation in a cerebral ischemia mouse model. *Neurochemistry International*. 2012;60(8):759–67.

79. Aras AB, Guven M, Akman T, Ozkan A, Sen HM, Duz U et al. Neuroprotective effects of daidzein on focal cerebral ischemia injury in rats. *Neural Regeneration Research*. 2015;10(1):146.
80. Cirmi S, Ferlazzo N, Lombardo GE, Ventura-Spagnolo E, Gangemi S, Calapai G et al. Neurodegenerative diseases: might citrus flavonoids play a protective role? *Molecules*. 2016;21(10):1312.
81. Jiang W, Li S, Li X. Therapeutic potential of berberine against neurodegenerative diseases. *Science China Life Sciences*. 2015;58:564–9.
82. Wang B, Su C-J, Liu T-T, Zhou Y, Feng Y, Huang Y et al. The neuroprotection of low-dose morphine in cellular and animal models of Parkinson's disease through ameliorating endoplasmic reticulum (ER) stress and activating autophagy. *Frontiers in Molecular Neuroscience*. 2018;11:120.
83. Pagliosa L, Monteiro S, Silva K, De Andrade J, Dutilh J, Bastida J et al. Effect of isoquinoline alkaloids from two Hippeastrum species on in vitro acetylcholinesterase activity. *Phytomedicine*. 2010;17(8–9):698–701.
84. Shi C, Liu J, Wu F, Yew DT. Ginkgo biloba extract in Alzheimer's disease: from action mechanisms to medical practice. *International Journal of Molecular Sciences*. 2010;11(1):107–23.
85. Deng X-Y, Li H-Y, Chen J-J, Li R-P, Qu R, Fu Q et al. Thymol produces an antidepressant-like effect in a chronic unpredictable mild stress model of depression in mice. *Behavioural Brain Research*. 2015;291:12–9.
86. Delgado Marin L, Sanchez-Borzone M, A Garcia D. Comparative antioxidant properties of some GABAergic phenols and related compounds, determined for homogeneous and membrane systems. *Medicinal Chemistry*. 2011;7(4):317–24.
87. Ojha RP, Rastogi M, Devi BP, Agrawal A, Dubey G. Neuroprotective effect of curcuminoids against inflammation-mediated dopaminergic neurodegeneration in the MPTP model of Parkinson's disease. *Journal of Neuroimmune Pharmacology*. 2012;7:609–18.
88. Mohd Sairazi NS, Sirajudeen K. Natural products and their bioactive compounds: neuroprotective potentials against neurodegenerative diseases. *Evidence-Based Complementary and Alternative Medicine*. 2020;2020.
89. Nascimento CP, Ferreira LO, Silva ALMd, Silva ABNd, Rodrigues JCM, Teixeira LL et al. A Combination of Curcuma longa and Diazepam Attenuates Seizures and Subsequent Hippocampal Neurodegeneration. *Frontiers in Cellular Neuroscience*. 2022;16:291.
90. Qin S, Tang H, Li W, Gong Y, Li S, Huang J et al. AMPK and its activator berberine in the treatment of neurodegenerative diseases. *Current Pharmaceutical Design*. 2020;26(39):5054-66.
91. Lin L, Li C, Zhang D, Yuan M, Chen C-h, Li M. Synergic effects of berberine and curcumin on improving cognitive function in an Alzheimer's disease mouse model. *Neurochemical Research*. 2020;45:1130–41.
92. Islam MS, Quispe C, Hossain R, Islam MT, Al-Harrasi A, Al-Rawahi A et al. Neuropharmacological effects of quercetin: a literature-based review. *Frontiers in Pharmacology*. 2021;12:665031.
93. Yammine A, Zarrouk A, Nury T, Vejux A, Latruffe N, Vervandier-Fasseur D et al. Prevention by dietary polyphenols (resveratrol, quercetin, apigenin) against 7-ketocholesterol-induced oxiapoptophagy in neuronal N2a cells: Potential interest for the treatment of neurodegenerative and age-related diseases. *Cells*. 2020;9(11):2346.

94. Suganthy N, Devi KP, Nabavi SF, Braidy N, Nabavi SM. Bioactive effects of quercetin in the central nervous system: Focusing on the mechanisms of actions. *Biomedicine & Pharmacotherapy*. 2016;84:892–908.
95. Saini RK, Rengasamy KR, Mahomoodally FM, Keum Y-S. Protective effects of lycopene in cancer, cardiovascular, and neurodegenerative diseases: An update on epidemiological and mechanistic perspectives. *Pharmacological Research.* 2020;155:104730.
96. Samarghandian S, Farkhondeh T, Samini F. A review on possible therapeutic effect of Nigella sativa and thymoquinone in neurodegenerative diseases. *CNS & Neurological Disorders-Drug Targets (Formerly Current Drug Targets-CNS & Neurological Disorders).* 2018;17(6):412–20.
97. Ardah MT, Merghani MM, Haque ME. Thymoquinone prevents neurodegeneration against MPTP in vivo and modulates α-synuclein aggregation in vitro. *Neurochemistry International*. 2019;128:115–26.
98. Dariani S, Baluchnejadmojarad T, Roghani M. Thymoquinone attenuates astrogliosis, neurodegeneration, mossy fiber sprouting, and oxidative stress in a model of temporal lobe epilepsy. *Journal of Molecular Neuroscience*. 2013;51:679–86.
99. Mori T, Koyama N, Tan J, Segawa T, Maeda M, Town T. Combination therapy with octyl gallate and ferulic acid improves cognition and neurodegeneration in a transgenic mouse model of Alzheimer's disease. *Journal of Biological Chemistry*. 2017;292(27):11310–25.
100. Singh S, Arthur R, Upadhayay S, Kumar P. Ferulic acid ameliorates neurodegeneration via the Nrf2/ARE signalling pathway: A Review. *Pharmacological Research-Modern Chinese Medicine*. 2022:100190.
101. Qian C, Decker EA, Xiao H, McClements DJ. Nanoemulsion delivery systems: Influence of carrier oil on β-carotene bioaccessibility. *Food Chemistry*. 2012;135(3):1440–7.
102. Peer D, Karp JM, Hong S, Farokhzad OC, Margalit R, Langer R. Nanocarriers as an emerging platform for cancer therapy. *Nature Nanotechnology*. 2007;2(12):751–60.
103. Singh R, Lillard Jr JW. Nanoparticle-based targeted drug delivery. *Experimental and Molecular Pathology*. 2009;86(3):215–23.
104. Kingsley JD, Dou H, Morehead J, Rabinow B, Gendelman HE, Destache CJ. Nanotechnology: a focus on nanoparticles as a drug delivery system. *Journal of Neuroimmune Pharmacology*. 2006;1:340–50.
105. Sun M, Qu S, Hao Z, Ji W, Jing P, Zhang H et al. Towards efficient solid-state photoluminescence based on carbon-nanodots and starch composites. *Nanoscale*. 2014;6(21):13076–81.
106. Mishra B, Patel BB, Tiwari S. Colloidal nanocarriers: a review on formulation technology, types and applications toward targeted drug delivery. *Nanomedicine: Nanotechnology, Biology and Medicine*. 2010;6(1):9–24.
107. Persidsky Y, Ramirez SH, Haorah J, Kanmogne GD. Blood–brain barrier: structural components and function under physiologic and pathologic conditions. *Journal of Neuroimmune Pharmacology*. 2006;1:223–36.
108. Pinheiro RG, Coutinho AJ, Pinheiro M, Neves AR. Nanoparticles for targeted brain drug delivery: what do we know? *International Journal of Molecular Sciences*. 2021;22(21):11654.
109. Baetke SC, Lammers T, Kiessling F. Applications of nanoparticles for diagnosis and therapy of cancer. *British Journal of Radiology*. 2015;88(1054):20150207.
110. Patra JK, Das G, Fraceto LF, Campos EVR, Rodriguez-Torres MdP, Acosta-Torres LS et al. Nano based drug delivery systems: recent developments and future prospects. *Journal of Nanobiotechnology*. 2018;16(1):1–33.

111. Eltanameli B, Sneed K, Pathak Y. Nanomedicine and Nano Formulations for Neurodegenerative Diseases. *Biomedical Journal of Scientific & Technical Research.* 2022;42(2):33387–96.
112. Milan J, Niemczyk K, Kus-Liśkiewicz M. Treasure on the Earth – Gold Nanoparticles and Their Biomedical Applications. *Materials.* 2022;15(9):3355.
113. Khan SS, Ullah I, Zada S, Ahmad A, Ahmad W, Xu H et al. Functionalization of Se-Te Nanorods with Au Nanoparticles for Enhanced Anti-Bacterial and Anti-Cancer Activities. *Materials.* 2022;15(14):4813.
114. Aghaie T, Jazayeri MH, Manian M, Khani L, Erfani M, Rezayi M et al. Gold nanoparticle and polyethylene glycol in neural regeneration in the treatment of neurodegenerative diseases. *Journal of Cellular Biochemistry.* 2019;120(3):2749–55.
115. Báez DF, Gallardo-Toledo E, Oyarzún MP, Araya E, Kogan MJ. The influence of size and chemical composition of silver and gold nanoparticles on in vivo toxicity with potential applications to central nervous system diseases. *International Journal of Nanomedicine.* 2021;16:2187.
116. Xie J, Shen Z, Anraku Y, Kataoka K, Chen X. Nanomaterial-based blood–brain-barrier (BBB) crossing strategies. *Biomaterials.* 2019;224:119491.
117. Mishra N, Ashique S, Garg A, Rai VK, Dua K, Goyal A et al. Role of siRNA-based nanocarriers for the treatment of neurodegenerative diseases. *Drug Discovery Today.* 2022.
118. Shyam R, Ren Y, Lee J, Braunstein KE, Mao H-Q, Wong PC. Intraventricular delivery of siRNA nanoparticles to the central nervous system. *Molecular Therapy-Nucleic Acids.* 2015;4:e242.
119. Bonoiu AC, Bergey EJ, Ding H, Hu R, Kumar R, Yong K-T et al. Gold nanorod–siRNA induces efficient in vivo gene silencing in the rat hippocampus. *Nanomedicine.* 2011;6(4):617–30.
120. Austin LA, Mackey MA, Dreaden EC, El-Sayed MA. The optical, photothermal, and facile surface chemical properties of gold and silver nanoparticles in biodiagnostics, therapy, and drug delivery. *Archives of Toxicology.* 2014;88:1391–417.
121. Huy TQ, Huyen P, Le A-T, Tonezzer M. Recent advances of silver nanoparticles in cancer diagnosis and treatment. *Anti-Cancer Agents in Medicinal Chemistry (Formerly Current Medicinal Chemistry-Anti-Cancer Agents).* 2020;20(11):1276–87.
122. Khan AM, Korzeniowska B, Gorshkov V, Tahir M, Schrøder H, Skytte L et al. Silver nanoparticle-induced expression of proteins related to oxidative stress and neurodegeneration in an in vitro human blood–brain barrier model. *Nanotoxicology.* 2019;13(2):221–39.
123. Takáč P, Michalková R, Čižmáriková M, Bedlovičová Z, Balážová Ľ, Takáčová G. The Role of Silver Nanoparticles in the Diagnosis and Treatment of Cancer: Are There Any Perspectives for the Future? *Life.* 2023;13(2):466.
124. Khalandi B, Asadi N, Milani M, Davaran S, Abadi AJN, Abasi E et al. A review on potential role of silver nanoparticles and possible mechanisms of their actions on bacteria. *Drug Research.* 2017;11(02):70–6.
125. Liu X, Hao W, Lok C-N, Wang YC, Zhang R, Wong KK. Dendrimer encapsulation enhances anti-inflammatory efficacy of silver nanoparticles. *Journal of Pediatric Surgery.* 2014;49(12):1846–51.
126. Rapalli VK, Gorantla S, Waghule T, Mahmood A, Singh PP, Dubey SK et al. Nanotherapies for the treatment of age-related macular degeneration (AMD) disease: Recent advancements and challenges. *Recent Patents on Drug Delivery & Formulation.* 2019;13(4):283–90.

127. Sheikpranbabu S, Kalishwaralal K, Lee K-j, Vaidyanathan R, Eom SH, Gurunathan S. The inhibition of advanced glycation end-products-induced retinal vascular permeability by silver nanoparticles. *Biomaterials*. 2010;31(8):2260–71.
128. Morris B, Imrie F, Armbrecht A-M, Dhillon B. Age-related macular degeneration and recent developments: new hope for old eyes? *Postgraduate Medical Journal*. 2007;83(979):301–7.
129. Gonzalez-Carter DA, Leo BF, Ruenraroengsak P, Chen S, Goode AE, Theodorou IG et al. Silver nanoparticles reduce brain inflammation and related neurotoxicity through induction of H2S-synthesizing enzymes. *Scientific Reports*. 2017;7(1):42871.
130. Zare H, Ahmadi S, Ghasemi A, Ghanbari M, Rabiee N, Bagherzadeh M et al. Carbon nanotubes: Smart drug/gene delivery carriers. *International Journal of Nanomedicine*. 2021;16:1681.
131. Zhang W, Zhang Z, Zhang Y. The application of carbon nanotubes in target drug delivery systems for cancer therapies. *Nanoscale Research Letters*. 2011;6(1):1–22.
132. McBain SC, Yiu HH, Dobson J. Magnetic nanoparticles for gene and drug delivery. *International Journal of Nanomedicine*. 2008;3(2):169–80.
133. Dai R, Hang Y, Liu Q, Zhang S, Wang L, Pan Y et al. Improved neural differentiation of stem cells mediated by magnetic nanoparticle-based biophysical stimulation. *Journal of Materials Chemistry B*. 2019;7(26):4161–8.
134. Vio V, Jose Marchant M, Araya E, J Kogan M. Metal nanoparticles for the treatment and diagnosis of neurodegenerative brain diseases. *Current Pharmaceutical Design*. 2017;23(13):1916–26.
135. López-Dávila V, Seifalian AM, Loizidou M. Organic nanocarriers for cancer drug delivery. *Current Opinion in Pharmacology*. 2012;12(4):414–9.
136. Ashique S, Afzal O, Yasmin S, Hussain A, Altamimi MA, Webster TJ et al. Strategic nanocarriers to control neurodegenerative disorders: concept, challenges, and future perspective. *International Journal of Pharmaceutics*. 2023:122614.
137. Bamrungsap S, Zhao Z, Chen T, Wang L, Li C, Fu T et al. Nanotechnology in therapeutics: a focus on nanoparticles as a drug delivery system. *Nanomedicine*. 2012;7(8):1253–71.
138. Prabhu RH, Patravale VB, Joshi MD. Polymeric nanoparticles for targeted treatment in oncology: current insights. *International Journal of Nanomedicine*. 2015;10:1001.
139. Ahlawat J, Henriquez G, Narayan M. Enhancing the delivery of chemotherapeutics: role of biodegradable polymeric nanoparticles. *Molecules*. 2018;23(9):2157.
140. Bishop CJ, Kozielski KL, Green JJ. Exploring the role of polymer structure on intracellular nucleic acid delivery via polymeric nanoparticles. *Journal of Controlled Release*. 2015;219:488–99.
141. Vissers C, Ming G-l, Song H. Nanoparticle technology and stem cell therapy team up against neurodegenerative disorders. *Advanced Drug Delivery Reviews*. 2019;148:239–51.
142. Handa M, Singh A, Flora SJS, Shukla R. Stimuli-responsive Polymeric Nanosystems for Therapeutic Applications. *Current Pharmaceutical Design*. 2022;28(11):910–21.
143. Pérez-Carrión MD, Posadas I. Dendrimers in Neurodegenerative Diseases. *Processes*. 2023;11(2):319.
144. Ortega MÁ, Guzmán Merino A, Fraile-Martínez O, Recio-Ruiz J, Pekarek L, G. Guijarro L et al. Dendrimers and dendritic materials: From laboratory to medical practice in infectious diseases. *Pharmaceutics*. 2020;12(9):874.
145. Rajani C, Borisa P, Karanwad T, Borade Y, Patel V, Rajpoot K et al. *Cancer-targeted chemotherapy: emerging role of the folate anchored dendrimer as drug delivery*

nanocarrier. In: *Pharmaceutical Applications of Dendrimers*. Elsevier; 2020. pp. 151–98

146. Kannan R, Nance E, Kannan S, Tomalia DA. Emerging concepts in dendrimer-based nanomedicine: from design principles to clinical applications. *Journal of Internal Medicine*. 2014;276(6):579–617.
147. Moorthy H, Govindaraju T. Dendrimer architectonics to treat cancer and neurodegenerative diseases with implications in theranostics and personalized medicine. *ACS Applied Bio Materials*. 2021;4(2):1115–39.
148. Liu C, Zhao Z, Gao H, Rostami I, You Q, Jia X et al. Enhanced blood–brain-barrier penetrability and tumor-targeting efficiency by peptide-functionalized poly (amidoamine) dendrimer for the therapy of gliomas. *Nanotheranostics*. 2019;3(4):311.
149. Santos SD, Xavier M, Leite DM, Moreira DA, Custódio B, Torrado M et al. PAMAM dendrimers: blood–brain barrier transport and neuronal uptake after focal brain ischemia. *Journal of Controlled Release*. 2018;291:65–79.
150. Wang G, Babazadeh A, Shi B. Intrinsically Fluorescent PAMAM Dendrimer as Drug carrier and Nanoprobe: Bioimaging and Neuron protection Study. *Macquarie Neurodegeneration Meeting* 20192019.
151. Kalomiraki M, Thermos K, Chaniotakis NA. Dendrimers as tunable vectors of drug delivery systems and biomedical and ocular applications. *International Journal of Nanomedicine*. 2016;11:1.
152. Verma D, Gulati N, Kaul S, Mukherjee S, Nagaich U. Protein based nanostructures for drug delivery. *Journal of Pharmaceutics*. 2018;2018.
153. Delfi M, Sartorius R, Ashrafizadeh M, Sharifi E, Zhang Y, De Berardinis P et al. Self-assembled peptide and protein nanostructures for anti-cancer therapy: Targeted delivery, stimuli-responsive devices and immunotherapy. *Nano Today*. 2021;38:101119.
154. Malam Y, Loizidou M, Seifalian AM. Liposomes and nanoparticles: nanosized vehicles for drug delivery in cancer. *Trends in Pharmacological Sciences*. 2009;30(11):592–9.
155. Müller RH, Mäder K, Gohla S. Solid lipid nanoparticles (SLN) for controlled drug delivery–a review of the state of the art. *European Journal of Pharmaceutics and Biopharmaceutics*. 2000;50(1):161–77.
156. Üner M, Yener G. Importance of solid lipid nanoparticles (SLN) in various administration routes and future perspectives. *International Journal of Nanomedicine*. 2007;2(3):289–300.
157. Hallan SS, Kaur P, Kaur V, Mishra N, Vaidya B. Lipid polymer hybrid as emerging tool in anocarriers for oral drug delivery. *Artificial Cells, Nanomedicine, and Biotechnology*. 2016;44(1):334–49.
158. Bondì ML, Botto C, Amore E, Emma MR, Augello G, Craparo EF et al. Lipid nanocarriers containing sorafenib inhibit colonies formation in human hepatocarcinoma cells. *International Journal of Pharmaceutics*. 2015;493(1–2):75–85.
159. Stella B, Peira E, Dianzani C, Gallarate M, Battaglia L, Gigliotti CL et al. Development and characterization of solid lipid nanoparticles loaded with a highly active doxorubicin derivative. *Nanomaterials*. 2018;8(2):110.
160. Akbarzadeh A, Rezaei-Sadabady R, Davaran S, Joo SW, Zarghami N, Hanifehpour Y et al. Liposome: classification, preparation, and applications. *Nanoscale Research Letters*. 2013;8(1):1–9.
161. Li W. Eat-me signals: Keys to molecular phagocyte biology and "Appetite" control. *Journal of Cellular Physiology*. 2012;227(4):1291–7.
162. Ge J, Lei J, Zare RN. Bovine serum albumin–poly (methyl methacrylate) nanoparticles: An example of frustrated phase separation. *Nano Letters*. 2011;11(6):2551–4.

163. Adepu S, Ramakrishna S. Controlled drug delivery systems: current status and future directions. *Molecules*. 2021;26(19):5905.
164. Briggs F, Browne D, Asuri P. Role of polymer concentration and crosslinking density on release rates of small molecule drugs. *International Journal of Molecular Sciences*. 2022;23(8):4118.
165. Mitchell MJ, Billingsley MM, Haley RM, Wechsler ME, Peppas NA, Langer R. Engineering precision nanoparticles for drug delivery. *Nature Reviews Drug Discovery*. 2021;20(2):101–24.
166. Husni P, Ramadhania ZM. Plant extract loaded nanoparticles. *Indonas J Pharm*. 2021;3:38–49.
167. Dian L, Yu E, Chen X, Wen X, Zhang Z, Qin L et al. Enhancing oral bioavailability of quercetin using novel soluplus polymeric micelles. *Nanoscale Research Letters*. 2014;9(1):1–11.
168. Bonechi C, Martini S, Ciani L, Lamponi S, Rebmann H, Rossi C et al. Using liposomes as carriers for polyphenolic compounds: the case of trans-resveratrol. *PLoS One*. 2012;7(8): e41438.
169. Arumugam K, Sundararajan Subramanian G, Rajan Mallayasamy S, Kumar Averineni R, Sreenivasa Reddy M, Udupa N. A study of rivastigmine liposomes for delivery into the brain through the intranasal route. *Acta Pharmaceutica*. 2008;58(3):287–97.
170. Kalani A, Kamat P, Chaturvedi P, Tyagi S, Tyagi N. Curcumin-primed exosomes mitigate endothelial cell dysfunction during hyperhomocysteinemia. *Life Sciences*. 2014;107(1–2):1–7.
171. Wei X, Senanayake TH, Bohling A, Vinogradov SV. Targeted nanogel conjugate for improved stability and cellular permeability of curcumin: synthesis, pharmacokinetics, and tumor growth inhibition. *Molecular Pharmaceutics*. 2014;11(9):3112–22.
172. Cheng C, Peng S, Li Z, Zou L, Liu W, Liu C. Improved bioavailability of curcumin in liposomes prepared using a pH-driven, organic solvent-free, easily scalable process. *RSC Advances*. 2017;7(42):25978–86.
173. Bilia AR, Guccione C, Isacchi B, Righeschi C, Firenzuoli F, Bergonzi MC. Essential oils loaded in nanosystems: A developing strategy for a successful therapeutic approach. *Evidence-Based Complementary and Alternative Medicine*. 2014;2014.
174. Bobo D, Robinson KJ, Islam J, Thurecht KJ, Corrie SR. Nanoparticle-based medicines: A review of FDA-approved materials and clinical trials to date. *Pharmaceutical Research*. 2016;33:2373–87.
175. Fan S, Zheng Y, Liu X, Fang W, Chen X, Liao W et al. Curcumin-loaded PLGA-PEG nanoparticles conjugated with B6 peptide for potential use in Alzheimer's disease. *Drug Delivery*. 2018;25(1):1091–102.
176. Palle S, Neerati P. Quercetin nanoparticles attenuates scopolamine induced spatial memory deficits and pathological damages in rats. *Bulletin of Faculty of Pharmacy, Cairo University*. 2017;55(1):101–6.
177. Elnaggar YS, Etman SM, Abdelmonsif DA, Abdallah OY. Intranasal piperine-loaded chitosan nanoparticles as brain-targeted therapy in Alzheimer's disease: Optimization, biological efficacy, and potential toxicity. *Journal of Pharmaceutical Sciences*. 2015;104(10):3544–56.
178. Kundu P, Das M, Tripathy K, Sahoo SK. Delivery of dual drug loaded lipid based nanoparticles across the blood–brain barrier impart enhanced neuroprotection in a rotenone induced mouse model of Parkinson's disease. *ACS Chemical Neuroscience*. 2016;7(12):1658–70.
179. Das SS, Sarkar A, Chabattula SC, Verma PRP, Nazir A, Gupta PK et al. Food-grade quercetin-loaded nanoemulsion ameliorates effects associated with

parkinson's disease and cancer: Studies employing a transgenic c. elegans model and human cancer cell lines. *Antioxidants*. 2022;11(7):1378.
180. Pepe G, Calce E, Verdoliva V, Saviano M, Maglione V, Di Pardo A et al. Curcumin-loaded nanoparticles based on amphiphilic hyaluronan-conjugate explored as targeting delivery system for neurodegenerative disorders. *International Journal of Molecular Sciences*. 2020;21(22):8846.
181. Xu L, Sun Z, Xing Z, Liu Y, Zhao H, Tang Z et al. Cur@ SF NPs alleviate Friedreich's ataxia in a mouse model through synergistic iron chelation and antioxidation. *Journal of Nanobiotechnology*. 2022;20(1):1–15.
182. Del Prado-Audelo M, Magaña J, Mejía-Contreras B, Borbolla-Jiménez F, Giraldo-Gomez D, Piña-Barba M et al. In vitro cell uptake evaluation of curcumin-loaded PCL/F68 nanoparticles for potential application in neuronal diseases. *Journal of Drug Delivery Science and Technology*. 2019;52:905–14.

13 Neuropharmacological Potential of Ayurvedic Nanomedicines

Pankaj Kumar

13.1 INTRODUCTION

The complex anatomical and pathophysiological features of the brain make it particularly challenging to comprehend and manage neurological diseases. Despite recent rapid drug discovery, there continues to be a substantial rate of failure in the efficient management of neurological illnesses. On the other hand, a severe public health hazard has arisen as a result of the significant rise in neurological diseases over the past few decades. It is the second most frequent cause of death worldwide [1]. The global burden of brain illnesses is so large that it will affect approximately 100 million Americans, with a projected cost of $800 billion (including $37 billion for epilepsy, $86 billion for traumatic brain injury (TBI), and $110 billion for stroke) [2]. The bitter truth is that conventional therapies are largely symptomatic-centric rather than addressing the underlying aetiology or pathogenesis of the disease. In addition, the severe acute respiratory syndrome coronavirus-2 (SARS-CoV-2) epidemic of the novel coronavirus disease 2019 (Covid-19) may bring about new difficulties and contribute to an increase in the worldwide burden of central nervous system (CNS) disorders. As the ability of SARS-CoV-2 to target the nervous system has now been established [3], it is believed that approximately 40% of Covid-19 patients experience CNS-related problems, including encephalitis, an increased risk of stroke, and damage brought on by hypoxic condition [4–6]. The effects of SARS-CoV-2 infections during pregnancy are another mystery. One major explanation for the origin of abnormal developmental disorders of the brain such as autism or schizophrenia posits certain viral infections during pregnancy may activate the mother's immune system, potentially disrupting physiological mechanisms necessary for typical neurodevelopment [7,8]. The aforementioned examples highlight how the field of brain disorders and their aetiologies and processes are continually changing and how new research approaches may require coordinated efforts.

The currently prescribed modified chemical interventions are associated with an inadequate pharmaco-therapeutic profile with various psycho-somatic complications including psychedelic impairments, agitation, and other behavioural issues [9–11]. A major hindrance to the effectiveness of therapeutic interventions is the blood–brain barrier (BBB), which restricts the efficient transfer of many chemically modified synthetic drugs from the blood to the brain milieu. This makes it difficult to effectively

DOI: 10.1201/9781032661964-13

treat CNS illnesses [12–14]. However, nanoparticles with a diameter between 10 and 100 nm can cross the BBB by varying degrees [15,16]. *Bhasmas* (herbo-mineral-metallic compounds) and *Rasa sindoor* (red-HgS), on the other hand, are Ayurvedic nanomedicines that show a unique set of special characteristics, including *Rasayana* (immune regulation and anti-aging efficiency), *Yogavahi* (targeted drug distribution), *Alpamatra* (recommended in small doses ranging from 15 to 250 mg/day), *Rasibhava* (quickly and easily absorbable, adaptable, assimilable, and non-poisonous), *Shigravyapi* (distributes quickly and act rapidly), and *Agnideepana* (enhances cellular metabolism at multiple level and acts as catalyst). These characteristics are developed by opting herbal derivative-based modus operandi during a pharmaceutical procedure [17,18]. Being biocompatible, nontoxic, and nonantigenic by nature, these nanomedicines can also be used for selective, targeted, or controlled drug administration [19,20]. In this section, we will address the potential neuro-therapeutic impacts of Ayurvedic nanomedicines.

13.2 BLOOD–BRAIN BARRIER: ANATOMICAL AND PHYSIOLOGICAL PERSPECTIVE

The human brain is the most complicated and vital organ, which produces serious health consequences when it becomes diseased. While brain disorders are becoming more prevalent, there are currently no effective treatments. The challenge of getting medications to their intended target components in the brain is one of the main causes of the significant failure rates in the development of drugs for the brain. The desired pharmacological effect can only be achieved when the drugs penetrate the BBB sufficiently and interact with target cellular component of the brain.

The BBB is regarded as the most important component of the neurovascular unit (NVU) [21]. The NVU, which is made up of endothelial cells (ECs), neurons, pericytes (PCs), glial cells, and the extracellular matrix, is critical for the CNS microenvironment's integrity. The effective functioning of the NVU relies on efficient communication between its various parts. The BBB, on the other hand, is formed by ECs that are tightly packed within the capillaries [22]. PCs, vascular smooth muscle cells (VSMCs), and ECs have cell-specific surface proteins, ion channels, pump proteins, specific bioreceptors, and transport proteins that maintain BBB integrity and establish the equilibrium of substances by transcellular or paracellular transport [22]. The BBB is a semi-permeable multicellular complex, communicating the blood and the brain tissue (Figure 13.1). This complex is supported by complicated intercommunication and the arrangement of endothelial cells, astroglia, pericytes, and perivascular mast cells [23–25]. The BBB blocks the entry of infections, blood cells, and neurotoxic plasma components into the brain [26]. Moreover, the BBB precisely controls molecular entry and exit from the CNS, ensuring that the neuronal milieu's chemical composition is carefully regulated and suitable for neuronal activity [27,28]. The transfers occur between the two compartments, allowing only specific types of molecules or ions to do so by simple diffusion, facilitated diffusion, passive transport, or active transport. This ultimately brings about the maintenance of homeostatic equilibrium for neuronal functions, protecting the CNS from

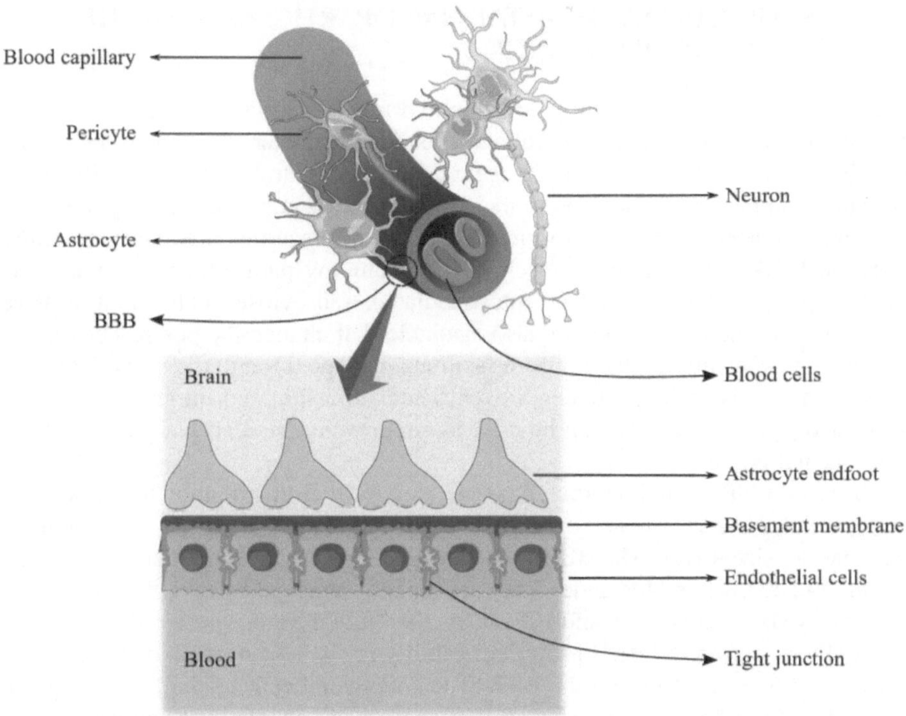

FIGURE 13.1 Structural illustration of blood–brain barrier.

xenobiotic assaults, coordinating communication between the regulatory and structural components, and providing nutritional support to the brain. In disease states, the BBB breaks down and dysfunction results in leakages of potentially harmful blood products into the CNS, cellular infiltration, and abnormal molecule transport and clearance, which is connected to cerebral blood flow reductions and dysregulation [29–32] and contributes to neurological impairments [26–28].

The inherent resistivity of the BBB is governed by the uninterrupted covering of endothelial cells interconnected through tight junctions (TJs), adherent junctions (AJs), and gap junctions (GJs) that restrict paracellular transport [33] and exhibit little pinocytotic activity [34,35], although limited transcellular transport does occur. However, among the junctions that give the BBB increased trans-endothelial resistance, TJs are the essential part of the BBB's make-up [33]. Furthermore, the BBB's endothelial cells serve as a few additional transport pathways (such as fenestra, trans endothelial channels, and pinocytotic vesicles) and express high concentrations of active efflux transport proteins, such as P-glycoprotein (P-gp, MDR-1 or ABCB1) and breast cancer resistance protein (BCRP, ABCG2) [36,37]. The most difficult aspect is creating a vehicle that is physiologically efficient and can transport medications through the BBB with ease. These vectors, which attach to a particular receptor at the BBB and traverse it via transcytosis, can acquire a specific form of intracellular entity or other tailored formulations like nanoparticles.

13.3 INTERACTIONS OF METAL NANOPARTICLES WITH THE BLOOD–BRAIN BARRIER

Nanoparticles (NPs) are a cutting-edge method for breaching the BBB and are rich in a diverse range of unique physical and chemical characteristics that allow for the selective delivery of the therapeutic agent within the neural tissue [38]. NPs are a particularly appealing choice due to their small size, dynamic functioning, low toxicity, and managed release of drug method [39–41]. Once there, NPs can naturally cross the BBB via a variety of mechanisms, including paracellular transport, carrier transport, adsorptive- and receptor-mediated transcytosis. Other non-invasive techniques, on the other hand, are also available that change the pharmacodynamic characteristics by altering the drugs to facilitate passage through the BBB. Transient BBB integrity disruption, intracerebroventricular infusion, and intrathecal infusion are invasive procedures that can be used to circumvent the BBB but are still in the experimental phase.

The size of NPs is an important characteristic for their distribution to the targeted tissue, cellular absorption, and capacity to reach target proteins, since even chemical reactions are size driven. The BBB has the least permeability for particles larger than 200 nm [42,43], while NPs under 5 nm are quickly removed by renal filtration [44]. NPs having sizes between 10 and 100 nm are therefore the most preferred for targeted drug delivery across the BBB [45]. Permeability is also determined by electrostatic interactions between NPs and the BBB. The endothelial cells of the BBB are given a high density of anionic surface charges by negatively charged proteoglycans. As a result, positively charged particles are suitable for adsorptive-mediated transcytosis throughout the BBB because they electrostatically interact favourably with endothelial cell membranes [46]. Neutral particles, on the other hand, are approximately 100 times less accessible than positively charged NPs [47]. The plasma membranes of the BBB endothelial cell 'layer can passively absorb small lipophilic cationic NPs in to the brain' [48]. This spontaneous but seldom occurring process occurs at the BBB, but due to their small size, NPs can take advantage of it. NPs loaded with enhanced cationic charge density show increased diffusion capacity [49]. Particularly gold nanoparticles have been demonstrated to passively diffuse through endothelial cells of the BBB [50]. The distinctive physico-chemical characteristic imparted to NPs can also lead to targeting the specific carrier transporters, such as glucose for activating the glucose transporter [51]. Active transcytosis of NPs across endothelial cell plasma membranes via adsorptive or receptor-mediated processes is a common transport route at the BBB [52]. Positively charged NPs may internalize through charge-dependent manner. This occurs when charged molecules/particles engage electrostatically with the oppositely charged cell membrane and incorporate via adsorption-mediated transcytosis [53]. Such interplays induce the cell membrane of endothelium to invaginate and form intracellular vesicle. Caveolae contribute in adsorptive-mediated endocytosis (AMT) of extracellular molecules and receptor trafficking, while clathrin-coated pits participate in the majority of receptor-mediated transcytosis (RMT) [54]. AMT is frequently associated with electrostatic communication between positively charged NPs and the negatively charged plasma membrane

The binding of NPs to specific receptors on the luminal side of endothelial cells facilitates endocytosis via RMT. Similar to AMT, the vesicle-based intracellular transport system is generated by the inward folding of the cell membrane, and the NP is carried to the basolateral surface [55]. NPs can be targeted to specific brain tissues based on surface characteristics by binding to receptors on the apical surface of BBB endothelial cells as well as target tissue, including cancer cells [56–58]. Bioinspired designed homologous NPs easily bind to the cell surface and produce a desired cell response [38,59,60].

13.4 AYURVEDIC NANOMEDICINES CAN EFFECTIVELY MANAGE SEVERAL NEUROLOGICAL DISEASES

Additional to the botanical category, there is another medicinal class based on metals and minerals mentioned in the Indian traditional medicine, Ayurveda [59,61]. The Ayurvedic nanomedicines are metal nanopowder (also called as *bhasma*) and are considered the most potent formulation with the least adverse effect when administered in the recommended dose [62–66]. When any classical pharmaceutical method is opted for, the surface of *bhasma* NPs (BNPs) spontaneously develops a corona of several trace elements of varying degrees of thickness around the metallic core [67]. The corona has very high pharmacological significance as it has distinctive physico-chemical characteristics. Moreover, the core has its own pharmacotherapeutic significance. This means that no additional surface-related modifications are required in the BNPs as is the case in conventional synthetic drugs for promoting therapeutic effects. The versatile functionalities of *bhasmas* are the result of a series of steps in a tedious well-defined pharmaceutical process, called *bhavana*. It is a special technique of drug preparation in ayurveda which involves levigation or wet grinding of single/compound powdered medications with liquid derivatives, that is, juice/decoction/solution of plant, animal, or mineral origin [68]. In simple words, it is a technique used in drug manufacturing to imbue the substance with the properties of liquid media. The end result of the *bhavana* process is the transformation of the solid inorganic material into a nanosized bio-assimilable organometallic/organomineral complex with a rich trace element composition and distinctive surface chemical properties. BNP as a vehicle, on the other hand, is a novel strategy for improved and efficient drug delivery to targeted tissue and is still in the experimental phase. The pharmacological aspects of Ayurvedic nanomedicines can be outlined as follows:

13.4.1 Multielemental Composition and Nanocrystalline Structure

BNPs are packed with a chemical cocktail of several constituent metals that are produced as a result of treating botanical derivatives during pharmaceutical processes. BNPs can serve as a source of different metal ions in the cellular environment despite their limited solubility. One per cent of a person's body is made up of alkali metals and alkaline earth cations (Na^+, K^+, Mg^{2+}, and Ca^{2+}), yet numerous additional metal ions, particularly transition metal ions like copper, zinc, iron, manganese, and cobalt, which are essential to many biological processes but make up less than 0.01% of the body, are also needed in trace amounts. Most frequently, these transition metal ions are found attached to biomolecules. A metalloenzyme, for instance, is made up of metal ion-protein complexes, with the metal ion serving as the essential component in the active site. The bonding might be as loose or easily interchangeable as in zinc carboxypeptidase, or as rigid as iron to haemoglobin. A biological process that is regulated by metal ions is quickly reversible and also extremely reactive to cause alterations at the molecular scale. When an enzyme attaches to a metal ion, changes in the structural organisation take place concurrently with the reactivity of the nearby metal ions. The best illustration of this phenomenon is when apoenzymes are activated by metal ions. The auxiliary groups that are linked to metal ions bring about additional biochemical alterations. Due to their high reactivity, metal ions are thus involved across all biological processes, including the production of DNA, RNA, and proteins and intermediate reactions [69]. Metal chelation biomolecules can limit virus-derived enzymes in diseased cells by combining with metal ions at their active sites [70]. Moreover, the toxicity of NPs and the pattern of interactions between cellular functional machineries are also influenced by the crystal structure. According to Zhang et al., metal nanoparticles can modify their crystalline structure following contact with water or other dispersion media [71]. They stated that when water is present, ZnS NPs undergo a crystal structure rearrangement that makes them more organised and structurally similar to a solid piece of ZnS [72]. This explains why some NPs have a toxic nature while some do not exhibit toxicity despite having identical particle size and chemical composition. Thus, it can be postulated that *bhasma* nano-crystallites might alter surface-related characteristics and crystalline-specific chemical behaviour (including the mechanism of interaction with interacting biological proteins/receptors) in the cellular media from its expected natural structural organization. Broad scientific investigations are required for the authentication of this statement. It explains why, despite having equal particle sizes and elemental composition, certain NPs are hazardous in comparison to others. Therefore, it can be hypothesised that *bhasma* nano-crystallites may be distinguished from their expected natural structural organisation in terms of surface-related properties and crystalline-specific chemical behaviour in a water-rich biological milieu. The verification of this argument requires extensive scientific research.

13.4.2 Size and Shape Factor

The size and geometry of NPs significantly determine cellular import and responses, gene expression, and bloodstream circulation time. Cellular receptors are typically 10–50nm in size, whereas proteins are 50–100nm in size. Nuclear pores range in size from 9 to 12nm. Because of the multi-element pathway and varying nano-size, they are compatible with a wide range of receptors, proteins, enzymes, and so on. These interactions may affect a pathway by engaging with several regulatory agents at multiple levels in a multistage pathway at the same time, or by interacting with regulators at distinct pathways, resulting in a single altered outcome. Several studies using modern analytical tools such as XRD, SEM, and TEM have revealed that the formulation is a heterogeneous mixture containing nanoparticles as groups of irregularly shaped flakes [73]; some have polyhedral particles [74]; a few have a spherical geometry [75]; some have unusual morphologies [76]); and some have a cocktail of spherical, elliptical, and elongated shapes [77]. BNPs' varied surface architecture provides extra advantages. They have planes with facets of different atom density. The design of NPs with equal surface areas matters because planes with high atom density facets facilitate reactivity [78]. These distinctive crystalline morphologies with different corners, edges, and other electrochemically active surface sites, as well as an incredibly high surface area, allow *bhasma* to interface fundamental regulatory biomolecules of cellular pathways to produce a specific output. A subtle change in NP size could lead to substantially diverse cell response levels [79,80]. Furthermore, the majority of studies have shown that non-spherical NPs have lower cellular internalisation than spherical NPs [81]. Additionally, such NPs have a longer blood circulation half-life duration [81].

13.4.3 Effect of Surface Charge

The ion-specific electrostatic interaction of metal NPs has a substantial impact at nano/bio interfaces [82–86]. The negative membrane potentials of cell membranes can exhibit electrostatic interactions more efficiently with cationic NPs, leading to a faster rate of intake of positively charged NPs in diverse cell types [87–91]. Cationic NPs are reported to be more active than neutral or anionic NPs [92]. The surface charge density of NPs substantially influences their cellular internalisation, aggregation tendency, reactivity, and cytotoxic properties [93,94]. The surface charge density is largely size dependent, with smaller NPs (10nm) exhibiting a significant increase in surface charge density as compared to large particles [95]. Many electropositive metals constituents are packed into the diversely sized and shaped metal *bhasma* nanocrystallites. The BNPs can be thought of as a huge collection of different-sized nano crystallites with a high surface charge density. Few positively charged particles can escape the endosomal system of cellular internalisation; therefore, these NPs can either be taken up by different types of cells by an endocytotic mechanism or can escape this process and become located directly in the cytosol [96,97]. Certain *bhasma* NPs may be internally absorbed directly because of high surface charge properties. This allows them to engage with specific intracellular receptors and trigger rapid cell-type-specific actions.

13.4.4 Effect of Dissolution

Bhasmas' multi-element structure produces dissolving effects based on the parent metal/mineral types. The interplay of *bhasmas* with target cells may behave as a localized source of metal ions that discontinuously release ions; however, toxicological tests of *bhasmas* show no harmful signs at the therapeutic dose and, in some cases, are considerably safer when administered with a dose factor larger than the prescribed dose [98,99]. The hypothesis that the *bhasma* delivers ions gently in a bid to avoid metal poisoning may help explain these findings. It is possible that the *bhasma*'s size and shape have a significant impact on the kinetics of dissolution. This is only a hypothesis; thus, further research is required. According to Slavin et al., NPs' surface morphology has a substantial impact on their activity, and a rougher surface causes NPs to dissolve more quickly. Furthermore, faster dissolution is facilitated by smaller NPs' higher surface area-to-volume ratio [78]. The *bhasma* dispersion does, however, appear to be element-dependent. For instance, Cu-NPs produced 253-fold more ions compared to Ag-NP, which is probably because Cu seems to be more susceptible to oxidation. Notwithstanding ion production, Ag-NPs even have stronger antimicrobial properties than Cu-NPs [78]. The excessive generation of metallic ions might be hazardous. Furthermore, cytotoxicity occurs in the following order: ions > micro > nano [100]. From the perspective of toxic apprehension, nano- and micromaterials reverse the above pattern. The bulk of experimental research, however, reveals no or low toxicity of various *bhasmas*. That could be because the majority of *bhasma* particles exist in nano form in biological territory, while a tiny proportion of *bhasma* particles become ionised and become a potential source of metal ions. Further, in-depth research is necessary for a thorough explanation. Additionally, the homeostasis mechanism that has developed for the essential elements does not apply to non-essential elements like Ag. This encourages Ag to remain in the cellular milieu for an extended period of time at low concentrations, allowing it to continue performing its metabolic role [78]. Being components of the biological system, Ag, Au, Hg, Sn, Pb, and several other elements are also regularly detected in *bhasma*, either as the primary component or in residues from medicinal herbs. From this, it can be inferred that Ayurvedic *bhasma*s' sustained therapeutic impact may be brought on by avoiding intracellular homeostasis systems. Further research is needed to confirm this.

13.4.5 Contribution of Hydrophobicity

The surface hydrophobicity of NPs influences their biodistribution. Hydrophobic coatings allow the particle to evade phagocytosis and have a longer half-life in circulation [101–103]. Prolonged circulating NPs can be employed to target the tumour [104], spleen [105,106], and site of acutely wounded tissue where vasodilation can accelerate the deposition of hydrophobic NPs, depending on their size. *Bhasma* nanocrystalline particles are largely insoluble in water-based media, including biological media. Through hydrophobic interactions, the hydrophobic feature of *bhasma* metal NPs may increase penetration into cell membranes and nuclear pores [107–109]. Its ease of cellular penetration may favour *bhasma* metal NPs in cytoplasmic pharmacodynamic alterations.

The ancient use of several Ayurvedic nanomedicines for treating different neurological illnesses is being decoded in terms of molecular biology [110,111]. Several types of drug dose forms, including *Chyawanprash*, have also pronounced biomolecular explanation in this context [112,113]. The therapeutic approach in ayurveda is highly patient oriented and offers a well-elaborated, strategic, personalised treatment protocol for curing a disease as the Ayurvedic system of medicine firmly advocates that each patient has a unique, characteristic phenotype-based human constitution [114]. In general, herbal and metal-based ayurvedic nanomedicines reduce oxidative changes and inflammation-related neuro-glial changes, as observed clinically [115–118]. Thus, the neuroprotective capabilities of ayurvedic medicines are produced due to imparting the antioxidant potential and checking the inflammatory activities at various pathological strata [119–121]. The most frequently prescribed formulation for a variety of medical conditions is *Swarna bhasma*, which is only prescribed with a certain adjuvant (vehicle) (Table 13.1). The diversified pharmacological effects of *Swarna bhasma* in multiple health conditions are impregnated by classically defined pharmaceutical methods of incineration (Table 13.2).

The gold preparation, *Swarna bhasma* (SB), and the silver preparation, *Rajat bhasma* (RB), are frequently recommended in dementia, neurodegeneration and promote nootropic functions [133]. SB were found to restore the restraint stress-induced elevation in the levels of brain catecholamines (norepinephrine, epinephrine, and dopamine), 5-HT, and plasma corticosterone for therapeutic benefits [134,135]. Zinc preparation, *Yashad bhasma* [136], as well as *Rajat bhasma* was reported to be effective in Parkinson's disease [133,134]. *Rasasindura* is composed of single-phase α-HgS nanoparticles (size ~24 nm), free of Hg^0 or organic molecules [137]. In fly models of Huntington's and Alzheimer's diseases, it prevented neurodegeneration (Figure 13.2). It suppressed apoptosis, reduced the build-up of inclusion bodies and heat shock proteins, increased levels of heterogeneous nuclear ribonucleoproteins and cAMP response element binding protein, and simultaneously enhanced the ubiquitin-proteasomal system for better protein clearance in the affected cells [138]. Ayurvedic nanomedicines can therefore effectively manage CNS diseases of primary or secondary origin [139,140]. Besides these, a newer strategy involves repurposing traditional herbo-mineral/metal/ mineral drugs for managing brain-related disorders with better clinical output [38,141,142].

13.5 CONCLUSION

The chemical architecture and surface-related characteristics of naturally synthesised *bhasmas* are extremely distinctive. Even a tiny amount after crossing the BBB can produce significant dynamic metabolic alterations by carrying out multiple pathway regulatory and modulatory functions. Many of the *bhasmas* examined so far have tremendous medicinal potentials based on traditional knowledge, but only a small number of them have had their scientific advantages thoroughly evaluated. Despite this lack of research, the low cost, and the reduced toxicity compared to more expensive and unreliable synthetic drugs, ayurvedic nanomedicines provide a great alternative to effectively managing neurological diseases and providing a solid foundation for the development of newer and safer drugs.

TABLE 13.1
List of Vehicle Drugs Recommended along with Swarna bhasma Mentioned in Classical Ayurvedic Texts

Disease conditions/ health purposes	Vehicle for SB	References
Burning sensation	Bile of fish	[122], [123], [124]
Aphrodisiac	*Elipta prostrata Linn.* [*Asteraceae*]	[122–124]
General weakness, Phthisis	Cow's milk	[122–124]
Eye diseases	*Boerhavia diffusa* Linn. [*Nyctaginaceae*]	[122–124]
Rejuvenation	Cow's ghee/clarified butter	[122–124]
Old age-related diseases	Cow's ghee/clarified butter	[122–124]
Debilities developed due to chronic diseases like tuberculosis	Cow's milk	[122,124]
Schizophrenia	Dried form of *Zingiber officinale* Linn. [*Zingiberaceae*]; *Syzygium aromaticum* Linn. [*Myrtaceae*], *Piper nigrum* Linn. [*Piperaceae*]	[122,124]
Chronic fever	*Abhraka bhasma* (fine ash of calcined mica) along with honey	[122]
Malabsorption disorders (IBS, IBD, Tropical spruce disease)	*Rasaparpari* (cubic and hexagonal crystallite of mercury sulphide)	[122]
Acute and Chronic Jaundice	*Guduchi satva* (a starchy extract obtained from stem of *Tinospora cordifolia* Linn. [*Menispermaceae*]	[122]
Tuberculosis	*Abhraka bhasma, Rasasindura* and *mukta pisti* (very fine paste of pearl)	[122]
Potentiation of uterus	Powder of *Gymnema lactiferum* Linn. [*Apocynaceae*] and *Smilax china* Linn. [*Smilacaceae*]	[122]
Chronic syphilis	*Rasa puspa* (a mercurial preparation) along with blood purifying herbs*	[122]
Acute or Chronic condition of hyperacidity	Powder of fruits of *Phyllanthus emblica* Linn. [*Euphorbiaceae*]	[122]
Epilepsy and Hysteria	*Rasasindura, Abhraka bhasma*, powder of *Clitoria ternatea* Linn. [*Fabaceae*]	[122]
Parkinsonism	Decoction of *Sida cordifolia* Linn. [*Malvaceae*]	[122]
Swelling in testicles	Mixture of *kallali*# with equal proportionated mercury sulphur preparation) and powder of *Boerhaavia diffusa* Linn. [*cryophyllales*] along with cow's urine	[122]

TABLE 13.1 (Continued)
List of Vehicle Drugs Recommended along with Swarna bhasma Mentioned in Classical Ayurvedic Texts

Disease conditions/ health purposes	Vehicle for SB	References
	or, Mixture of powder of *Curcuma longa* Linn. and *Boerhaavia diffusa* Linn. along with juice of *Zingiber officinale* Linn.	
For pleasant and euphonious sound	*Raisins* (dehydrated or dried form of grapes), powder of *Piper longum* Linn. [*Piperaceae*], powder of *Myrica negi* Linn. [*Myricaceae*] and powder of *Glycorrhiza glabra* Linn. [*Fabaceae*]	[122]
Improve beauty of women	Blood purifying herbs and hemopoietic herbs¶	[122]
Ominous sign of near death	Powder of *Phyllanthus emblica* Linn. triturated with decoction of bark/skin of *Senegalia catechu* Linn.	[122]
Improving intellect	Powder of *Acorus calmus* Linn., *Tinospora cordifolia*, dry form of *zingiber officinale* Linn. and *Asparagus racemosus* Linn.	[122]
For generalized strengthening, rejuvenation and beautification	Decoction of *Phyllanthus emblica* Linn., *Desmodium gangeticum*, dried form of *Zingiber officinale* Linn. and *Boerhavia diffusa* Linn.	[122]
Uterine fecundity	Powder of *Mesua ferrea* Linn.	[122]
Lactogenesis in nursing women	Herbs of *kakolyadi gana* †	[122]
Bone disorders	*Khand* (a brown powder obtained from the processing of sugarcane juice)	[122]
Nephrotic disorders	*Swarna bhasma*, *Abhraka bhasma* and *Lauha bhasma* in the ratio of 1:1:3 along with decoction of *Crataeva nurvala* Linn. [*Caparaceae*]	[122]
Uterine swelling with associated complications	*Shilajit* (mineral pitch; a sticky, brown-black substance primarily obtained from between the mountain rocks of Himalayan range), *Lauha bhasma* and *Silver bhasma* along with decoction of *Dashmool* plants (formulation of 10 specific medicinal herbs)	[122]

(*Continued*)

TABLE 13.1 (Continued)
List of Vehicle Drugs Recommended along with Swarna bhasma Mentioned in Classical Ayurvedic Texts

Disease conditions/ health purposes	Vehicle for SB	References
Improvement in memory	*Vacha* (Sweet flag – *Acorus calmus* Linn.)	[123]
Luster of body	Saffron (*Crocus sativus* Linn.)	[123]
Antidote to poison	*Nirvisa* (*Aconitum heterophyllum* Linn.)	[123]
Hyperacidity	Gooseberry powder	[122]
Chronic fever	*Abhraka bhasma* (incinerated mica) with honey	[122]

Notes:

* Blood-purifying herbs are group of detoxicant herbs claiming antiseptic, anti-inflammatory, and antioxidant properties which are very commonly recommended for rashes, acne, allergic irritation, and other skin disorders. It includes *Azadirachta indica* (Family: *Meliaceae*), *Glycyrrhiza glabra* (Family: *Fabaeceae*), *Tinospora cordifolia* (Family: *Menispermaceae*), *Rubia cordifolia* (Family: *Rubiaceae*), *Curcuma longa* (Family: *Zingiberaceae*) etc.

Kajjali is a chemical mixture of mercury, sulphur, and compound HgS, obtained after result of continuous trituration of bio-purified mercury and sulphur.

¶ Hemopoietic herbs are groups of drugs which include *iron bhasma, copper bhasma, abhraka bhasma, Cordeauxia edulis* (family: *Fabaceae*), *Achyranthes aspera* (family: *Amaranthaceae*), and many more.

† *kakolyadi gana* are includes *Roscoea procera* (family: *Zingiberaceae*), *Lilium polphyllum* (family: *Aliaceae*), *Malaxis acuminata* (family: *Orchidaceae*) etc.

TABLE 13.2
Summary of the Material Required in Different Methodologies for the Preparation of Swarna Bhasma

Methods (Serial number)	Ingredients which are treated for incineration and trituration		References
	Metallic ingredients	Herbal ingredients	
1.	Gold (purified), Mercury-*bhasma* or kajjali	*Citrus medica* Linn. [*Rutaceae*]	[125], [126]
2.	Gold (purified), *Rasa sindura*[¥] or *kajjali*, Cinnabar (HgS)	*Citrus medica* Linn. [*Rutaceae*]	[125]
3.	Gold (purified), mercury purified, Sulphur purified	*Citrus medica* Linn. [*Rutaceae*]	[127]
4.	Gold (purified), lead purified, sulphur purified	*Citrus medica* Linn. [*Rutaceae*]	[127]
5.	Gold (purified), *kajjali*	*Bauhinia variegate* Linn. [*Leguminosae*]	[127]

TABLE 13.2 (Continued)
Summary of the Material Required in Different Methodologies for the Preparation of Swarna Bhasma

Methods (Serial number)	Ingredients which are treated for incineration and trituration		
	Metallic ingredients	Herbal ingredients	References
6.	Gold (purified), *kajjali*, realgar (As_2S_2)	*Gloriosa superba* Linn. [*Colchicaceae*], *Tridax procumbens* Linn. [*Asteraceae*]	[127], [126], [128]
7.	Gold (purified), *Rasa sindura*	*Calotropis procera* Linn. [*Apocynaceae*], or *Citrus medica* Linn. [*Rutaceae*]	[129]
8.	Gold (purified), *Rasa sindura*, *Hingula** (HgS)	*Citrus medica* Linn. [*Rutaceae*]	[127], [130]
9.	Gold (purified), Mercury(purified), *Hingula* (purified), Sulphur (purified), Realgar (purified), Ammonium chloride (NH_4Cl)	*Citrus medica* Linn. [*Rutaceae*]	[131]
10.	Gold (purified), Mercury (purified), Realgar (purified), *Rasa sindura*, Copper pyrite ($Cu_2S.Fe_2S_3$)	Citrus medica Linn. [Rutaceae]	[131]
11.	Gold (purified), Mercury(purified)	*Citrus medica* Linn. [*Rutaceae*]	[131]
12.	Gold (purified), Mercury(purified), Sulphur (purified), Lime stone ($CaCO_3$)	*Citrus medica* Linn. [*Rutaceae*], *Bauhinia variegate* Linn. [*Caesalpiniaceae*]	[131]
13.	Gold (purified), *Hingula* (purified)	Ferula asafoetida Linn. [Umbelliferae], Euphorbia nerifolia Linn. [Euphorbiaceae]	[131]
14.	Gold (purified), *Lauha parpati*, *Hingula*	*Citrus medica* Linn. [*Rutaceae*]	[126]
15.	Gold (purified)	*Cordia dichotomy* Linn. [*Boraginaceae*], *Bauhinia variegate* Linn. [*Caesalpiniaceae*]	[126]

(Continued)

TABLE 13.2 (Continued)
Summary of the Material Required in Different Methodologies for the Preparation of Swarna Bhasma

Methods (Serial number)	Ingredients which are treated for incineration and trituration		
	Metallic ingredients	Herbal ingredients	References
16.	Gold (purified), Mercury(purified), Galena (PbS)	-	[130]
17.	Gold (purified), Mercury (purified), Realgar (purified), Red lead (Vermillion)	*Euphorbia neriifolia* Linn. [*Euphorbiaceae*], *Citrus medica* Linn. [*Rutaceae*]	[130]
18.	Gold (purified), Sulphur	Excreta of pigeon or chicken	[130]
19.	Gold (purified), *kajjali*	*Citrus medica* Linn. [*Rutaceae*]	[128], [129]
20.	Gold (purified), Iron pyrite, Lead (purified)	*Calotropis procera* Linn. [*Apocynaceae*]	[128], [129]
21.	Gold (purified), Mercury (purified), Lead (purified)	-	[128], [129]
22.	Gold (purified), Mercury (purified), *Hingula* (purified), Rasa sindura, Realgar (purified)	*Ferula asafoetida* Linn. [*Umbeliferrae*], *Bauhinia variegate* Linn. [*Caesalpiniaceae*]	[128], [129]
23.	Gold (purified), Realgar (purified), *Rasa sindura*	Calotropis procera Linn. [Apocynaceae]	[128], [129]
24.	Gold (purified), Stibnite (Sb_2S_3)	*Eclipta alba* Linn. [*Compositae*]	[128], [129]
25.	Gold (purified), Mercury (purified), Sulphur (purified)	-	[132]
26.	Gold (purified), White Arsenic powder	Juice of *Bauhinia variegate* Linn., Leaf juice of Tulsi – *Ocimum sanctum*	[132]

Notes:
Ψ *Rasa sindura* is mercury-based ayurvedic formulation that contains rejuvenating properties.
ɹ *Hingula* is chemically mercury sulphides and is ore of mercury.

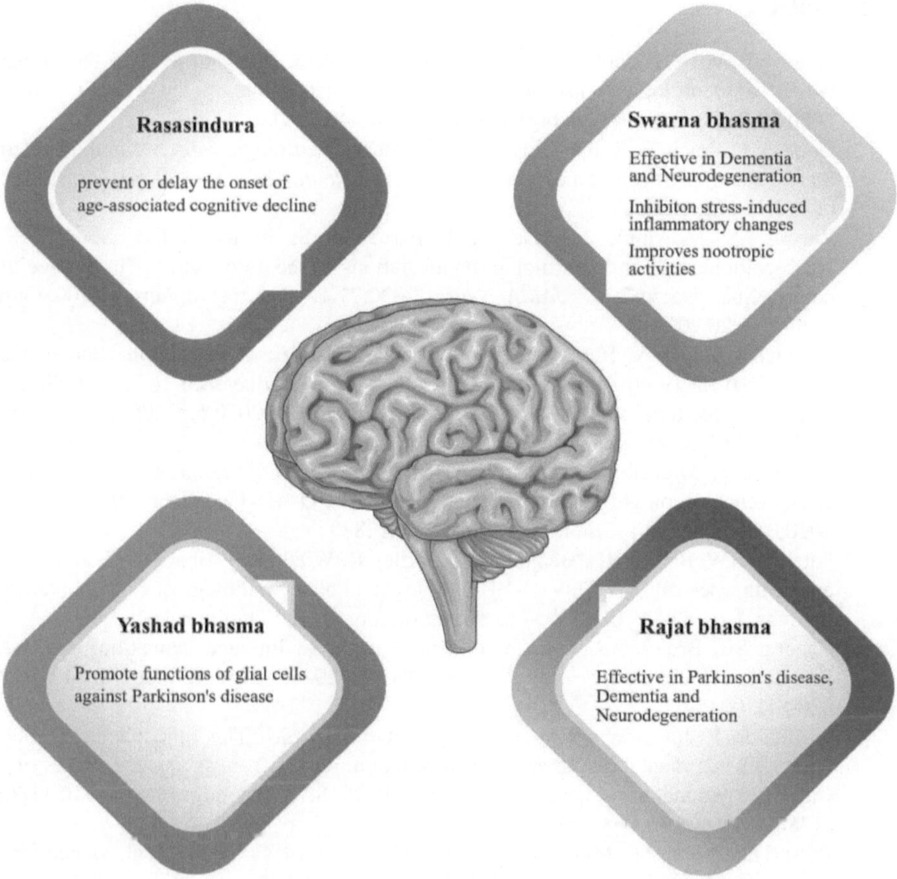

FIGURE 13.2 Therapeutic effects of ayurvedic nanomedicines in neurological disorders.

13.6 ABBREVIATIONS

BBB	Blood–Brain Barrier
Covid-19	Coronavirus disease 2019
CNS	Central Nervous System
NVU	Neurovascular unit
EC	Endothelial cells
NPs	Nanoparticles
AMT	Adsorptive-mediated endocytosis
RMT	Receptor-mediated transcytosis

REFERENCES

[1] Feigin VL, Vos T, Nichols E, Owolabi MO, Carroll WM, Dichgans M et al. The global burden of neurological disorders: translating evidence into policy. *Lancet Neurol* 2020;19:255–65. https://doi.org/10.1016/S1474-4422(19)30411-9

[2] Gooch CL, Pracht E, Borenstein AR. The burden of neurological disease in the United States: a summary report and call to action. *Ann Neurol* 2017;81:479–84. https://doi.org/10.1002/ana.24897

[3] Zubair AS, McAlpine LS, Gardin T, Farhadian S, Kuruvilla DE, Spudich S. Neuropathogenesis and neurologic manifestations of the coronaviruses in the age of coronavirus disease 2019. *JAMA Neurol* 2020;77:1018. https://doi.org/10.1001/jamaneurol.2020.2065

[4] Fridman I, Lucas N, Henke D, Zigler CK. Association between public knowledge about COVID-19, trust in information sources, and adherence to social distancing: cross-sectional survey. *JMIR Public Health Surveill* 2020;6:e22060. https://doi.org/10.2196/22060

[5] Kantonen J, Mahzabin S, Mäyränpää MI, Tynninen O, Paetau A, Andersson N et al. Neuropathologic features of four autopsied COVID-19 patients. *Brain Pathol* 2020;30:1012–6. https://doi.org/10.1111/bpa.12889

[6] Paterson RW, Brown RL, Benjamin L, Nortley R, Wiethoff S, Bharucha T et al. The emerging spectrum of COVID-19 neurology: clinical, radiological and laboratory findings. *Brain* 2020;143:3104–20. https://doi.org/10.1093/brain/awaa240

[7] Canetta SE, Brown AS. Prenatal infection, maternal immune activation, and risk for schizophrenia. *Transl Neurosci* 2012;3:320–7. https://doi.org/10.2478/s13380-012-0045-6

[8] Lombardo P, Jones W, Wang L, Shen X, Goldner EM. The fundamental association between mental health and life satisfaction: results from successive waves of a Canadian national survey. *BMC Public Health* 2018;18:342. https://doi.org/10.1186/s12889-018-5235-x

[9] Passeri E, Elkhoury K, Morsink M, Broersen K, Linder M, Tamayol A et al. Alzheimer's disease: treatment strategies and their limitations. *Int J Mol Sci* 2022;23. https://doi.org/10.3390/ijms232213954

[10] Perucca E. The pharmacological treatment of epilepsy: recent advances and future perspectives. *Acta Epileptologica* 2021;3:22. https://doi.org/10.1186/s42494-021-00055-z

[11] Rahman MM, Islam MR, Supti FA, Dhar PS, Shohag S, Ferdous J et al. Exploring the therapeutic effect of neurotrophins and neuropeptides in neurodegenerative diseases: at a glance. *Mol Neurobiol* 2023. https://doi.org/10.1007/s12035-023-03328-5

[12] Pardridge WM. The blood–brain barrier: bottleneck in brain drug development. *NeuroRx* 2005;2:3–14. https://doi.org/10.1602/neurorx.2.1.3

[13] Abbott NJ. Blood–brain barrier structure and function and the challenges for CNS drug delivery. *J Inherit Metab Dis* 2013;36:437–49. https://doi.org/10.1007/s10545-013-9608-0

[14] Pulgar VM. Transcytosis to cross the blood brain barrier, new advancements and challenges. *Front Neurosci* 2019;12. https://doi.org/10.3389/fnins.2018.01019

[15] Ohta S, Kikuchi E, Ishijima A, Azuma T, Sakuma I, Ito T. Investigating the optimum size of nanoparticles for their delivery into the brain assisted by focused ultrasound-induced blood–brain barrier opening. *Sci Rep* 2020;10:18220. https://doi.org/10.1038/s41598-020-75253-9

[16] Saraiva C, Praça C, Ferreira R, Santos T, Ferreira L, Bernardino L. Nanoparticle-mediated brain drug delivery: overcoming blood–brain barrier to treat neurodegenerative diseases. *J Control Release* 2016;235:34–47. https://doi.org/10.1016/j.jconrel.2016.05.044
[17] Sharma R, Bedarkar P, Timalsina D, Chaudhary A, Prajapati PK. Bhavana, an ayurvedic pharmaceutical method and a versatile drug delivery platform to prepare potentiated micro-nano-sized drugs: core concept and its current relevance. *Bioinorg Chem Appl* 2022;2022:1–15. https://doi.org/10.1155/2022/1685393
[18] Sharma R, Bolleddu R, Maji JK, Ruknuddin G, Prajapati PK. In-vitro α-amylase, α-glucosidase inhibitory activities and in-vivo anti-hyperglycemic potential of different dosage forms of guduchi (tinospora cordifolia [Willd.] Miers) prepared with ayurvedic bhavana process. *Front Pharmacol* 2021;12:642300. https://doi.org/10.3389/fphar.2021.642300
[19] Sharma R, Prajapati PK. Nanotechnology in medicine: leads from Ayurveda. *J Pharm Bioallied Sci* 2016;8:80–1. https://doi.org/10.4103/0975-7406.171730
[20] Kabra A, Sharma R, Kabra R, Baghel US. Emerging and alternative therapies for Parkinson disease: an updated review. *Curr Pharm Des* 2018;24:2573–82. https://doi.org/10.2174/1381612824666180820150150
[21] Saint-Pol J, Gosselet F, Duban-Deweer S, Pottiez G, Karamanos Y. Targeting and crossing the blood–brain barrier with extracellular vesicles. *Cells* 2020;9. https://doi.org/10.3390/cells9040851
[22] Sweeney MD, Zhao Z, Montagne A, Nelson AR, Zlokovic B v. Blood–brain barrier: from physiology to disease and back. *Physiol Rev* 2019;99:21–78. https://doi.org/10.1152/physrev.00050.2017
[23] Aird WC. Phenotypic heterogeneity of the endothelium: II. Representative vascular beds. *Circ Res* 2007;100:174–90. https://doi.org/10.1161/01.RES.0000255690.03436.ae
[24] Aird WC. Phenotypic heterogeneity of the endothelium: I. Structure, function, and mechanisms. *Circ Res* 2007;100:158–73. https://doi.org/10.1161/01.RES.0000255691.76142.4a
[25] Anderson JM, van Itallie CM. Physiology and function of the tight junction. *Cold Spring Harb Perspect Biol* 2009;1:a002584. https://doi.org/10.1101/cshperspect.a002584
[26] Montagne A, Zhao Z, Zlokovic B v. Alzheimer's disease: a matter of blood–brain barrier dysfunction? *J Exp Med* 2017;214:3151–69. https://doi.org/10.1084/jem.20171406
[27] Zhao Z, Nelson AR, Betsholtz C, Zlokovic B v. Establishment and dysfunction of the blood–brain barrier. *Cell* 2015;163:1064–78. https://doi.org/10.1016/j.cell.2015.10.067
[28] Zlokovic B v. Neurovascular pathways to neurodegeneration in Alzheimer's disease and other disorders. *Nat Rev Neurosci* 2011;12:723–38. https://doi.org/10.1038/nrn3114
[29] Iadecola C. The pathobiology of vascular dementia. *Neuron* 2013;80:844–66. https://doi.org/10.1016/j.neuron.2013.10.008
[30] Iadecola C. The neurovascular unit coming of age: a journey through neurovascular coupling in health and disease. *Neuron* 2017;96:17–42. https://doi.org/10.1016/j.neuron.2017.07.030
[31] Iadecola C. Neurovascular regulation in the normal brain and in Alzheimer's disease. *Nat Rev Neurosci* 2004;5:347–60. https://doi.org/10.1038/nrn1387

[32] Kisler K, Nelson AR, Montagne A, Zlokovic B v. Cerebral blood flow regulation and neurovascular dysfunction in Alzheimer disease. *Nat Rev Neurosci* 2017;18:419–34. https://doi.org/10.1038/nrn.2017.48
[33] Zhou Y, Peng Z, Seven ES, Leblanc RM. Crossing the blood–brain barrier with nanoparticles. *J Control Release* 2018;270:290–303. https://doi.org/10.1016/j.jconrel.2017.12.015
[34] He Q, Liu J, Liang J, Liu X, Li W, Liu Z et al. Towards improvements for penetrating the blood–brain barrier-recent progress from a material and pharmaceutical perspective. *Cells* 2018;7. https://doi.org/10.3390/cells7040024
[35] Redzic Z. Molecular biology of the blood–brain and the blood–cerebrospinal fluid barriers: similarities and differences. *Fluids Barriers CNS* 2011;8:3. https://doi.org/10.1186/2045-8118-8-3
[36] Pardridge WM. Drug targeting to the brain. *Pharm Res* 2007;24:1733–44. https://doi.org/10.1007/s11095-007-9324-2
[37] Pardridge WM. CNS drug design based on principles of blood–brain barrier transport. *J Neurochem* 1998;70:1781–92. https://doi.org/10.1046/j.1471-4159.1998.70051781.x
[38] Chouke PB, Shrirame T, Potbhare AK, Mondal A, Chaudhary AR, Mondal S et al. Bioinspired metal/metal oxide nanoparticles: a road map to potential applications. *Mater Today Adv* 2022;16:100314. https://doi.org/10.1016/j.mtadv.2022.100314
[39] Bhardwaj K, Chopra C, Bhardwaj P, Dhanjal DS, Singh R, Najda A et al. Biogenic metallic nanoparticles from seed extracts: characteristics, *Properties, and Applications. J Nanomater* 2022;2022:1–22. https://doi.org/10.1155/2022/2271278
[40] Rhaman MdM, Islam MdR, Akash S, Mim M, Noor Alam Md, Nepovimova E et al. Exploring the role of nanomedicines for the therapeutic approach of central nervous system dysfunction: at a glance. *Front Cell Dev Biol* 2022;10:989471. https://doi.org/10.3389/fcell.2022.989471
[41] Aborode AT, Fajemisin EA, Obadawo B, Alexiou A, Mukerjee N, Ghosh S et al. Advancements in cutting-edge cancer treatments using nanotechnology. *Int J Surg* 2023. https://doi.org/10.1097/JS9.0000000000000079
[42] Sonavane G, Tomoda K, Makino K. Biodistribution of colloidal gold nanoparticles after intravenous administration: effect of particle size. *Colloids Surf B Biointerfaces* 2008;66:274–80. https://doi.org/10.1016/j.colsurfb.2008.07.004
[43] Kulkarni SA, Feng S-S. Effects of particle size and surface modification on cellular uptake and biodistribution of polymeric nanoparticles for drug delivery. *Pharm Res* 2013;30:2512–22. https://doi.org/10.1007/s11095-012-0958-3
[44] Zhang W, Mehta A, Tong Z, Esser L, Voelcker NH. Development of polymeric nanoparticles for blood–brain barrier transfer – strategies and challenges. *Adv Sci (Weinh)* 2021;8:2003937. https://doi.org/10.1002/advs.202003937
[45] Saraiva C, Praça C, Ferreira R, Santos T, Ferreira L, Bernardino L. Nanoparticle-mediated brain drug delivery: Overcoming blood–brain barrier to treat neurodegenerative diseases. *J Control Release* 2016;235:34–47. https://doi.org/10.1016/j.jconrel.2016.05.044
[46] Ribeiro MMB, Domingues MM, Freire JM, Santos NC, Castanho MARB. Translocating the blood–brain barrier using electrostatics. *Front Cell Neurosci* 2012;6:44. https://doi.org/10.3389/fncel.2012.00044
[47] Zhang L, Fan J, Li G, Yin Z, Fu BM. Transcellular model for neutral and charged nanoparticles across an in vitro blood–brain barrier. *Cardiovasc Eng Technol* 2020;11:607–20. https://doi.org/10.1007/s13239-020-00496-6
[48] Bellettato CM, Scarpa M. Possible strategies to cross the blood–brain barrier. *Ital J Pediatr* 2018;44:131. https://doi.org/10.1186/s13052-018-0563-0

[49] Masserini M. Nanoparticles for brain drug delivery. *ISRN Biochem* 2013;2013:238428. https://doi.org/10.1155/2013/238428

[50] Male D, Gromnicova R, McQuaid C. Gold nanoparticles for imaging and drug transport to the CNS. *Int Rev Neurobiol* 2016;130:155–98. https://doi.org/10.1016/bs.irn.2016.05.003

[51] Kou L, Bhutia YD, Yao Q, He Z, Sun J, Ganapathy V. Transporter-guided delivery of nanoparticles to improve drug permeation across cellular barriers and drug exposure to selective cell types. *Front Pharmacol* 2018;9:27. https://doi.org/10.3389/fphar.2018.00027

[52] Pulgar VM. Transcytosis to cross the blood brain barrier, new advancements and challenges. *Front Neurosci* 2018;12:1019. https://doi.org/10.3389/fnins.2018.01019

[53] Hervé F, Ghinea N, Scherrmann J-M. CNS delivery via adsorptive transcytosis. *AAPS J* 2008;10:455–72. https://doi.org/10.1208/s12248-008-9055-2

[54] Elkin SR, Lakoduk AM, Schmid SL. Endocytic pathways and endosomal trafficking: a primer. *Wien Med Wochenschr* 2016;166:196–204. https://doi.org/10.1007/s10354-016-0432-7

[55] Jones AR, Shusta EV. Blood–brain barrier transport of therapeutics via receptor-mediation. *Pharm Res* 2007;24:1759–71. https://doi.org/10.1007/s11095-007-9379-0

[56] Kratz F, Beyer U. Serum proteins as drug carriers of anticancer agents: a review. *Drug Deliv* 1998;5:281–99. https://doi.org/10.3109/10717549809065759

[57] Dehouck B, Fenart L, Dehouck MP, Pierce A, Torpier G, Cecchelli R. A new function for the LDL receptor: Transcytosis of LDL across the blood–brain barrier. *J Cell Biol* 1997;138:877–89. https://doi.org/10.1083/jcb.138.4.877

[58] Zhao Y, Li D, Zhao J, Song J, Zhao Y. The role of the low-density lipoprotein receptor-related protein 1 (LRP-1) in regulating blood–brain barrier integrity. *Rev Neurosci* 2016;27:623–34. https://doi.org/10.1515/revneuro-2015-0069

[59] Chaudhary RG, Sonkusare V, Bhusari G, Mondal A, Potbhare A, Juneja H et al. Preparation of mesoporous ThO2 nanoparticles: influence of calcination on morphology and visible-light-driven photocatalytic degradation of indigo carmine and methylene blue. *Environ Res* 2023:115363. https://doi.org/10.1016/j.envres.2023.115363

[60] Tamboli QY, Patange SM, Mohanta YK, Sharma R, Zakde KR. Green synthesis of cobalt ferrite nanoparticles: *an emerging material for environmental and biomedical applications. J Nanomater* 2023;2023:1–15. https://doi.org/10.1155/2023/9770212

[61] Sharma R, Singla RK, Banerjee S, Sinha B, Shen B, Sharma R. Role of shankhpushpi (Convolvulus pluricaulis) in neurological disorders: an umbrella review covering evidence from ethnopharmacology to clinical studies. *Neurosci Biobehav Rev* 2022;140:104795. https://doi.org/10.1016/j.neubiorev.2022.104795

[62] Sharma R, Hazra J, Prajapati PK. Knowledge and awareness of pharmacovigilance among ayurveda physicians in Himachal Pradesh. *Anc Sci Life* 2017;36:234–5. https://doi.org/10.4103/asl.ASL_41_17

[63] Kumar A, Nair AGC, Reddy AVR, Garg AN. Bhasmas: unique ayurvedic metallic-herbal preparations, chemical characterization. *Biol Trace Elem Res* 2006;109:231–54. https://doi.org/10.1385/bter:109:3:231

[64] Jha CB, Bhattacharya B, Narang KK. Bhasmas as natural nanorobots: the biorelevant metal complex. *J Trad Nat Med* 2015;1:2–9.

[65] Liu J, Zhang F, Ravikanth V, Olajide OA, Li C, Wei L-X. Chemical Compositions of metals in bhasmas and Tibetan zuotai are a major determinant of their therapeutic effects and toxicity. *Evid Based Complement Alternat Med* 2019;2019:1697804. https://doi.org/10.1155/2019/1697804

[66] Pal D, Sahu CK, Haldar A. Bhasma: the ancient Indian nanomedicine. *J Adv Pharm Technol Res* 2014;5:4–12. https://doi.org/10.4103/2231-4040.126980
[67] Biswas S, Dhumal R, Selkar N, Bhagat S, Chawda M, Thakur K et al. Physicochemical characterization of Suvarna bhasma, its toxicity profiling in rat and behavioural assessment in zebrafish model. *J Ethnopharmacol* 2020;249:112388. https://doi.org/10.1016/j.jep.2019.112388
[68] Sharma R, Bedarkar P, Timalsina D, Chaudhary A, Prajapati PK. Bhavana, an ayurvedic pharmaceutical method and a versatile drug delivery platform to prepare potentiated micro-nano-sized drugs: core concept and its current relevance. *Bioinorg Chem Appl* 2022;2022:1685393. https://doi.org/10.1155/2022/1685393
[69] Williams RJP. Role of transition metal ions in biological processes. *Royal Institute of Chemistry, Reviews* 1968;1:13. https://doi.org/10.1039/rr9680100013
[70] Hutchinson DW. Metal chelators as potential antiviral agents. *Antiviral Res* 1985;5:193–205. https://doi.org/10.1016/0166-3542(85)90024-5
[71] Zhang H, Gilbert B, Huang F, Banfield JF. Water-driven structure transformation in nanoparticles at room temperature. *Nature* 2003;424:1025–9. https://doi.org/10.1038/nature01845
[72] Gatoo MA, Naseem S, Arfat MY, Mahmood Dar A, Qasim K, Zubair S. Physicochemical properties of nanomaterials: implication in associated toxic manifestations. *Biomed Res Int* 2014;2014. https://doi.org/10.1155/2014/498420
[73] Rugmini RK, Sridurga CH, K vs. analytical study of tamra bhasma. *International Ayurvedic Medical Journal* 2018;2:107–17.
[74] B S. Analytical study of yashada bhasma (zinc based ayurvedic metallic preparation) with reference to ancient and modern parameters. *J Allergy Ther* 2012;S1:1–7. https://doi.org/10.4172/scientificreports.582
[75] Chandran S, Patgiri B, Bedarkar P, Gokarna RA, Shukla VJ. Particle size estimation and elemental analysis of yashada bhasma. *International Journal of Green Pharmacy* 2017;11:S765–73.
[76] Beaudet D, Badilescu S, Kuruvinashetti K, Sohrabi Kashani A, Jaunky D, Ouellette S et al. Comparative study on cellular entry of incinerated ancient gold particles (Swarna bhasma) and chemically synthesized gold particles. *Sci Rep* 2017;7:10678. https://doi.org/10.1038/s41598-017-10872-3
[77] Sharma R, Bhatt A, Thakur M. Physicochemical characterization and antibacterial activity of Rajata bhasma and silver nanoparticle. *Ayu* n.d.;37:71–5. https://doi.org/10.4103/ayu.AYU_167_15
[78] Slavin YN, Asnis J, Häfeli UO, Bach H. Metal nanoparticles: understanding the mechanisms behind antibacterial activity. *J Nanobiotechnology* 2017;15:65. https://doi.org/10.1186/s12951-017-0308-z
[79] Pan Y, Neuss S, Leifert A, Fischler M, Wen F, Simon U et al. Size-dependent cytotoxicity of gold nanoparticles. *Small* 2007;3:1941–9. https://doi.org/10.1002/smll.200700378
[80] Yen HJ, Hsu SH, Tsai CL. Cytotoxicity and immunological response of gold and silver nanoparticles of different sizes. *Small* 2009;5:1553–61. https://doi.org/10.1002/smll.200900126
[81] Mathaes R, Winter G, Besheer A, Engert J. Non-spherical micro- and nanoparticles: fabrication, characterization and drug delivery applications. *Expert Opin Drug Deliv* 2015;12:481–92. https://doi.org/10.1517/17425247.2015.963055
[82] Attwood SJ, Kershaw R, Uddin S, Bishop SM, Welland ME. Understanding how charge and hydrophobicity influence globular protein adsorption to alkanethiol and

material surfaces. *J Mater Chem B* 2019;7:2349–61. https://doi.org/10.1039/c9tb00168a
[83] Walker DA, Kowalczyk B, de la Cruz MO, Grzybowski BA. Electrostatics at the nanoscale. *Nanoscale* 2011;3:1316–44. https://doi.org/10.1039/c0nr00698j
[84] Netz RR, Andelman D. Neutral and charged polymers at interfaces. *Phys Rep* 2003;380:1–95. https://doi.org/10.1016/S0370-1573(03)00118-2
[85] Zdrali E, Okur HI, Roke S. Specific ion effects at the interface of nanometer-sized droplets in water: structure and stability. *Journal of Physical Chemistry C* 2019;123:16621–30. https://doi.org/10.1021/acs.jpcc.9b01001
[86] Liang D, Dahal U, Zhang YK, Lochbaum C, Ray D, Hamers RJ et al. Interfacial water and ion distribution determine: ζ potential and binding affinity of nanoparticles to biomolecules. *Nanoscale* 2020;12:18106–23. https://doi.org/10.1039/d0nr03792c
[87] Murphy CJ, Gole AM, Stone JW, Sisco PN, Alkilany AM, Goldsmith EC et al. Gold nanoparticles in biology: beyond toxicity to cellular imaging. *Acc Chem Res* 2008;41:1721–30. https://doi.org/10.1021/ar800035u
[88] Albanese A, Chan WCW. Effect of gold nanoparticle aggregation on cell uptake and toxicity. *ACS Nano* 2011;5:5478–89. https://doi.org/10.1021/nn2007496
[89] Hauck TS, Ghazani AA, Chan WCW. Assessing the effect of surface chemistry on gold nanorod uptake, toxicity, and gene expression in mammalian cells. *Small* 2008;4:153–9. https://doi.org/10.1002/smll.200700217
[90] Goodman CM, McCusker CD, Yilmaz T, Rotello VM. Toxicity of gold nanoparticles functionalized with cationic and anionic side chains. *Bioconjug Chem* n.d.;15:897–900. https://doi.org/10.1021/bc049951i
[91] Li Z, Lei Z, Zhang J, Liu D, Wang Z. Effects of size, shape, surface charge and functionalization on cytotoxicity of gold nanoparticles. *Nano Life* 2015;05:1540003. https://doi.org/10.1142/s1793984415400036
[92] Adabi M, Naghibzadeh M, Adabi M, Zarrinfard MA, Esnaashari SS, Seifalian AM et al. Biocompatibility and nanostructured materials: applications in nanomedicine. *Artif Cells Nanomed Biotechnol* 2017;45:833–42. https://doi.org/10.1080/21691401.2016.1178134
[93] Jiang J, Oberdörster G, Biswas P. Characterization of size, surface charge, and agglomeration state of nanoparticle dispersions for toxicological studies. *Journal of Nanoparticle Research* 2009;11:77–89. https://doi.org/10.1007/s11051-008-9446-4
[94] Wang N, Hsu C, Zhu L, Tseng S, Hsu JP. Influence of metal oxide nanoparticles concentration on their zeta potential. *J Colloid Interface Sci* 2013;407:22–8. https://doi.org/10.1016/j.jcis.2013.05.058
[95] Abbas Z, Labbez C, Nordholm S, Ahlberg E. Size-dependent surface charging of nanoparticles. *Journal of Physical Chemistry C* 2008;112:5715–23. https://doi.org/10.1021/jp709667u
[96] Guo S, Huang L. Nanoparticles escaping RES and endosome: challenges for siRNA delivery for cancer therapy. *J Nanomater* 2011;2011:1–12. https://doi.org/10.1155/2011/742895
[97] Yang Y, Gao N, Hu Y, Jia C, Chou T, Du H et al. Gold nanoparticle-enhanced photodynamic therapy: effects of surface charge and mitochondrial targeting. *Ther Deliv* 2015;6:307–21. https://doi.org/10.4155/tde.14.115
[98] Joshi N, Dash M, Dwivedi L, Khilnani G. Toxicity study of Lauha bhasma (calcined iron) in albino rats. *Anc Sci Life* 2016;35:159. https://doi.org/10.4103/0257-7941.179870

[99] Chaudhari SY, Nariya MB, Galib R, Prajapati PK. Acute and subchronic toxicity study of Tamra bhasma (incinerated copper) prepared with and without Amritikarana. *J Ayurveda Integr Med* 2016;7:23–9. https://doi.org/10.1016/j.jaim.2015.11.001

[100] Petrarca C, Clemente E, Amato V, Pedata P, Sabbioni E, Bernardini G et al. Engineered metal based nanoparticles and innate immunity. *Clin Mol Allergy* 2015;13:13. https://doi.org/10.1186/s12948-015-0020-1

[101] Otsuka H, Nagasaki Y, Kataoka K. PEGylated nanoparticles for biological and pharmaceutical applications. *Adv Drug Deliv Rev* 2003;55:403–19. https://doi.org/10.1016/s0169-409x(02)00226-0

[102] Storm G, Belliot SO, Daemen T, Lasic DD. Surface modification of nanoparticles to oppose uptake by the mononuclear phagocyte system. *Adv Drug Deliv Rev* 1995;17:31–48. https://doi.org/10.1016/0169-409X(95)00039-A

[103] Torchilin VP, Trubetskoy VS. Which polymers can make nanoparticulate drug carriers long-circulating? *Adv Drug Deliv Rev* 1995;16:141–55. https://doi.org/10.1016/0169-409X(95)00022-Y

[104] Jindal AB. The effect of particle shape on cellular interaction and drug delivery applications of micro- and nanoparticles. *Int J Pharm* 2017;532:450–65. https://doi.org/10.1016/j.ijpharm.2017.09.028

[105] Klibanov AL, Maruyama K, Beckerleg AM, Torchilin VP, Huang L. Activity of amphipathic poly(ethylene glycol) 5000 to prolong the circulation time of liposomes depends on the liposome size and is unfavorable for immunoliposome binding to target. *Biochim Biophys Acta* 1991;1062:142–8. https://doi.org/10.1016/0005-2736(91)90385-1

[106] Peracchia MT, Fattal E, Desmaële D, Besnard M, Noël JP, Gomis JM et al. Stealth PEGylated polycyanoacrylate nanoparticles for intravenous administration and splenic targeting. *J Control Release* 1999;60:121–8. https://doi.org/10.1016/s0168-3659(99)00063-2

[107] Cheng L-C, Jiang X, Wang J, Chen C, Liu R-S. Nano-bio effects: interaction of nanomaterials with cells. *Nanoscale* 2013;5:3547–69. https://doi.org/10.1039/c3nr34276j

[108] Braakhuis HM, Park MVDZ, Gosens I, de Jong WH, Cassee FR. Physicochemical characteristics of nanomaterials that affect pulmonary inflammation. *Part Fibre Toxicol* 2014;11. https://doi.org/10.1186/1743-8977-11-18

[109] Naim B, Zbaida D, Dagan S, Kapon R, Reich Z. Cargo surface hydrophobicity is sufficient to overcome the nuclear pore complex selectivity barrier. *EMBO J* 2009;28:2697–705. https://doi.org/10.1038/emboj.2009.225

[110] Sharma R, Martins N. Telomeres, DNA damage and ageing: potential leads from Ayurvedic Rasayana (anti-ageing) drugs. *J Clin Med* 2020;9:2544. https://doi.org/10.3390/jcm9082544

[111] Sharma R, Kuca K, Nepovimova E, Kabra A, Rao MM, Prajapati PK. Traditional Ayurvedic and herbal remedies for Alzheimer's disease: from bench to bedside. *Expert Rev Neurother* 2019;19:359–74. https://doi.org/10.1080/14737175.2019.1596803

[112] Sharma R, Kakodkar P, Kabra A, Prajapati PK. Golden Ager Chyawanprash with meager evidential base from human clinical trials. *Evidence-Based Complementary and Alternative Medicine* 2022;2022:1–6. https://doi.org/10.1155/2022/9106415

[113] Kakodkar P, Sharma R, Dubewar AP. Classical vs commercial: is the "efficacy" of chyawanprash lost when tradition is replaced by modernization? *J Ayurveda Integr Med* 2021;12:751–2. https://doi.org/10.1016/j.jaim.2021.08.014

[114] Golubnitschaja O, Kinkorova J, Costigliola V. Predictive, preventive and personalised medicine as the hardcore of "Horizon 2020": EPMA position paper. *EPMA J* 2014;5:6. https://doi.org/10.1186/1878-5085-5-6
[115] Rahman MM, Islam MR, Yamin M, Islam MM, Sarker MT, Meem AFK et al. Emerging role of neuron-glia in neurological disorders: at a glance. *Oxid Med Cell Longev* 2022;2022:3201644. https://doi.org/10.1155/2022/3201644
[116] Shohag S, Akhter S, Islam S, Sarker T, Sifat MK, Rahman MM et al. Perspectives on the molecular mediators of oxidative stress and antioxidant strategies in the context of neuroprotection and neurolongevity: *an extensive review. Oxid Med Cell Longev* 2022;2022:7743705. https://doi.org/10.1155/2022/7743705
[117] Sharma R, Jadhav M, Choudhary N, Kumar A, Rauf A, Gundamaraju R et al. Deciphering the impact and mechanism of Trikatu, a spices-based formulation on alcoholic liver disease employing network pharmacology analysis and in vivo validation. *Front Nutr* 2022;9:1063118. https://doi.org/10.3389/fnut.2022.1063118
[118] Rahman MM, Wang X, Islam MR, Akash S, Supti FA, Mitu MI et al. Multifunctional role of natural products for the treatment of Parkinson's disease: at a glance. *Front Pharmacol* 2022;13:976385. https://doi.org/10.3389/fphar.2022.976385
[119] Sharma R, Kabra A, Rao MM, Prajapati PK. Herbal and holistic solutions for neurodegenerative and depressive disorders: leads from Ayurveda. *Curr Pharm Des* 2018;24:2597–608. https://doi.org/10.2174/1381612824666180821165741
[120] Rahman MM, Islam MR, Mim SA, Sultana N, Chellappan DK, Dua K et al. Insights into the promising prospect of G protein and GPCR-mediated signaling in neuropathophysiology and its therapeutic regulation. *Oxid Med Cell Longev* 2022;2022:8425640. https://doi.org/10.1155/2022/8425640
[121] Emran T bin, Islam F, Nath N, Sutradhar H, Das R, Mitra S et al. Naringin and naringenin polyphenols in neurological diseases: understandings from a therapeutic viewpoint. *Life (Basel)* 2022;13. https://doi.org/10.3390/life13010099
[122] Sharma S. Rasa Tarangini. 11th ed. New Delhi: Motilal banarsidas, Bungalow Road; 1979.
[123] Bhudeb Mookerjee. Rasa-jala Nidhi. 2nd ed. Varanasi: Srigokul mudranalaya; 1984.
[124] Dattram chaubey. Brihat Rasarajasunder. 3rd ed. Varanasi: Chaukhamba orientalia; 2000.
[125] Siddhinandanmishra. Rasaratnasamucchya. Varanasi: Chaukhamba orientalia; 2017.
[126] Mishra S. Rasaprakasha Sudhakar. Varanasi: Chaukhamba orientalia; 2009.
[127] Tripathi B. Sarangadhara- Samhita. Varanasi: Chaukhamba Sanskrit Bhavan; 2006.
[128] Duttram chaubey. Brihatrajasunder. Varanasi: Chaukhamba orientalia; 2000.
[129] Ramprasad. Rasendrapuran. Mumbai: Krishnadas; 1983.
[130] Mishra S. Rasendra-Chudamani. Varanasi: Chaukhamba orientalia; 2017.
[131] Kasinath. Rasatarangini. New Delhi: Motilal banarsidas, Bungalow Road; 2009.
[132] Anonymous. Part-1. The Ayurvedic Formulary of India, Delhi: Ministry of Health and Family Welfare, Govt. of India; 2003, pp. 246–47.
[133] Sharma R, Kuca K, Nepovimova E, Kabra A, Rao MM, Prajapati PK. Traditional Ayurvedic and herbal remedies for Alzheimer's disease: from bench to bedside. *Expert Rev Neurother* 2019;19:359–74. https://doi.org/10.1080/14737175.2019.1596803
[134] Ekka D, Dubey S, Dhruw DS. Effect of Rajat bhasma with Smritisagar Rasa in Parkinson. *Journal of Ayurveda and Integrated Medical Sciences (JAIMS)* 2017;2. https://doi.org/10.21760/jaims.v2i4.9341
[135] Shah ZA, Gilani RA, Sharma P, Vohora SB. Attenuation of stress-elicited brain catecholamines, serotonin and plasma corticosterone levels by calcined gold

preparations used in Indian system of medicine. *Basic Clin Pharmacol Toxicol* 2005;96:469–74. https://doi.org/10.1111/j.1742-7843.2005.pto_10.x
[136] Patgiri B, Galib R, Prasanth D. A review through therapeutic attributes of Yashada bhasma: a review through therapeutic attributes of Yashada bhasma. *International Journal of Pharmaceutical & Biological Archives* 2016;7:6–11.
[137] Ramanan N, Lahiri D, Rajput P, Varma RC, Arun A, Muraleedharan TS et al. Investigating structural aspects to understand the putative/claimed non-toxicity of the Hg-based Ayurvedic drug Rasasindura using XAFS. *J Synchrotron Radiat* 2015;22:1233–41. https://doi.org/10.1107/S1600577515012473
[138] Verma B, Sinha P, Ganesh S. Ayurvedic formulations amalaki rasayana and rasa sindoor improve age-associated memory deficits in mice by modulating dendritic spine densities. *J Ayurveda Integr Med* 2022;13:100636. https://doi.org/10.1016/j.jaim.2022.100636
[139] Rhaman MM, Islam MR, Akash S, Mim M, Noor Alam M, Nepovimova E et al. Exploring the role of nanomedicines for the therapeutic approach of central nervous system dysfunction: at a glance. *Front Cell Dev Biol* 2022;10:989471. https://doi.org/10.3389/fcell.2022.989471
[140] Rauf A, Abu-Izneid T, Khalil AA, Hafeez N, Olatunde A, Rahman MdM et al. Nanoparticles in clinical trials of COVID-19: an update. *International Journal of Surgery* 2022;104:106818. https://doi.org/10.1016/j.ijsu.2022.106818
[141] Mukerjee N, Al-Khafaji K, Maitra S, Suhail Wadi J, Sachdeva P, Ghosh A et al. Recognizing novel drugs against Keap1 in Alzheimer's disease using machine learning grounded computational studies. *Front Mol Neurosci* 2022;15:1036552. https://doi.org/10.3389/fnmol.2022.1036552
[142] Varghese R, Patel P, Kumar D, Sharma R. Monkeypox and drug repurposing: seven potential antivirals to combat the viral disease. *Rev Environ Health* 2023. https://doi.org/10.1515/reveh-2023-0001

14 Insights into Progressive Perspectives of Solid Lipid Nanoparticles in Brain Targeting

Debarshi Kar Mahapatra, Ratiram G. Choudhary, Kanhaiya M. Dadure, Animeshchandra G. M. Haldar, and Rohit Sharma

14.1 INTRODUCTION

The chronic neurological conditions that affect a significant portion of the population worldwide and are to blame for a great deal of suffering and death include epilepsy, Alzheimer's disease (AD), Huntington's disease (HD), neuromuscular disease, brain tumors/cancers, multiple sclerosis (MS), neurodegeneration, and Parkinson's disease (PD) [1]. Central nervous system (CNS)-related disorders often include an imbalance in neurological function, which ultimately causes the death of neurons [2,3,4]. Many processes contribute to various neuropathologies. Misfolded proteins, mitochondrial malfunction, a lack of neurotrophic factor synthesis, a depletion of endogenous antioxidant enzyme activity, a lack of neurotrophins, and occasionally problems at the genetic and molecular levels all contribute to CNS illnesses. This makes it difficult to identify a definitive therapeutic plan for CNS disorders. The blood–brain barrier (BBB) is an additional critical factor as a barrier that these medications must overcome [5]. Hence, the pharmacokinetic effectiveness of currently available medicines is disheartening for treating neurological illnesses. In order to create drugs and carrier systems that can effectively transport the medicine to the brain region with minimal side effects, a better comprehension of the BBB is necessary. As of yet, less effective therapy options have been discovered for neurodegenerative illnesses [6]. Meanwhile, innovative drug-delivery techniques like polymer-based nano-carrier-mediated administering drugs have emerged as a first-line clinical treatment approach for evading the obstacles posed by the BBB. While polymeric nano-formulations have shown promise in the clinic, their broad usage has been limited by a lack of safe polymers and their expensive cost [7]. A newer, cheaper carrier of medicine – solid lipid nanoparticles (SLNs) – may pass through the BBB for treating neurological disorders in a benign, acceptable, and efficient manner. Because the functionality and effectiveness of SLNs are dependent on their unique physico-chemical properties, and synthetic procedures, it is critical to have an understanding of the innovative manufacturing techniques. Over time, improved lipid NPs have made up for the

DOI: 10.1201/9781032661964-14

drawbacks of older SLNs [8]. To improve and ensure efficient delivery of medications to the brain, scientists have developed second-generation nano lipid carriers (NLCs) that are essentially improved SLNs. These NLCs are able to circumvent problems associated with the former technology, such as drug spillage and the abrupt exposure of pharmacologically active constituents. Drugs that are designed to be delivered to the brain through SLNs may be able to bypass the BBB and have greater bioavailability as a result.

As SLNs and their variations may one day be used to treat neurological illnesses with reduced toxicity and adverse effects, it is crucial that their characteristics and the BBB are well investigated.

14.2 BLOOD–BRAIN BARRIER

The BBB, together with the choroid plexus and cerebrospinal fluid (CSF), serve as metabolic and anatomical barriers at the interface of the brain tissue and the vascular supply. The BBB protects the CNS tissue from being exposed to the vascularly circulating components directly [9]. Specialized lining cells of the blood vessels, specialized glial cells and their connections among them and brain cells, supporting the acellular layer underlyng the endothelial cells, junctions between the endothelial cells, and pericytes are the primary components of the BBB [10,11,12]. Tight junctions and the metabolic barrier provide the physical barriers through which chemicals are carefully regulated in their entry into the brain through the BBB (various enzymes). A complex barrier unit is formed by endothelial cell adhesion molecules, pericytes, smooth muscle cells, astrocytes, microglia, and so on. [13,14,15,16], these cell types are important to the BBB's functioning. Endothelial cells and pericytes are rich in transporters, receptors, and channels to facilitate the carrier- or receptor-mediated transport across the BBB [17]. The BBB serves as a transport and secretory interface [18] to the brain and neuro-regulatory organizations in addition to its other functions as a physical barrier. It is the BBB's job to prevent neurotoxic chemicals from entering the brain while also facilitating the controlled and specialized transit of a number of components involved in neurological function from serum [5]. ATP-driven carrier proteins, transporter proteins, and ectoenzymes are all part of the capillary endothelial plasma membrane, which determine the selective transport of nutrients and medicines across the BBB [19]. Neurological illnesses are treated with a wide variety of medications, however, only a subset of these therapies is effective when given systemically due to the BBB's unique microvasculature.

Drug-related physicochemical parameters, including molecular weight (below 400 Da), shape (spherical), size (nano meter range), ionization (physiological pH), and lipophilicity, have a role in drug penetration of the BBB [20, 21].

The management of BBB transport as well as neuronal functions such as brain proliferation and degeneration are essential to the CNS's special function. Hence, the BBB is a fascinating target for designing sophisticated technologically advanced biocompatible drugs. Current clinical biomedical research focuses on developing more advanced drugs, carriers, and smaller molecules in order to better understand the BBB and treat neurological diseases.

14.3 BRAIN DRUG-DELIVERY STRATEGIES

Historically, several methods have been discovered to successfully transport therapeutic chemicals to the brain, where they may be used to manage neurological problems (Figure 14.1). Drugs may be administered locally to the brain, via a catheter, or directly during and after invasive surgical procedures. This method of administration involves implanting drug-loaded polymeric biodegradable polymers for prolonged release of the medication to a particular spot in the brain [22,23]. Whilst very successful in animal models for delivering medication formulation to the brain, local delivery is among the most intrusive administration ways and will thus be ineffective for treating actual human patients (with their varying physiology). Hence, less intrusive drug-delivery methods that maintain pharmacological action over time are required. The intranasal method of drug administration is also promising since it allows the medication to traverse through the BBB and enter the brain unimpeded [24,25,26]. The drug's active ingredient is delivered to the brain after being loaded onto a nanocarrier device that travels via the nasal cavity [27,28,29]. However, the variability in the released dosage at the target location caused by the specialized nasal epithelium and its interaction with the medication [22,30] makes the intranasal route less than optimal. The systemic delivery pathway has been the most researched and is generally accepted as the best way to get the medicine to the brain. However, this method of medicine administration faces a huge obstacle from the BBB. To overcome this barrier, it is necessary to build NPs that are both safe and porous enough

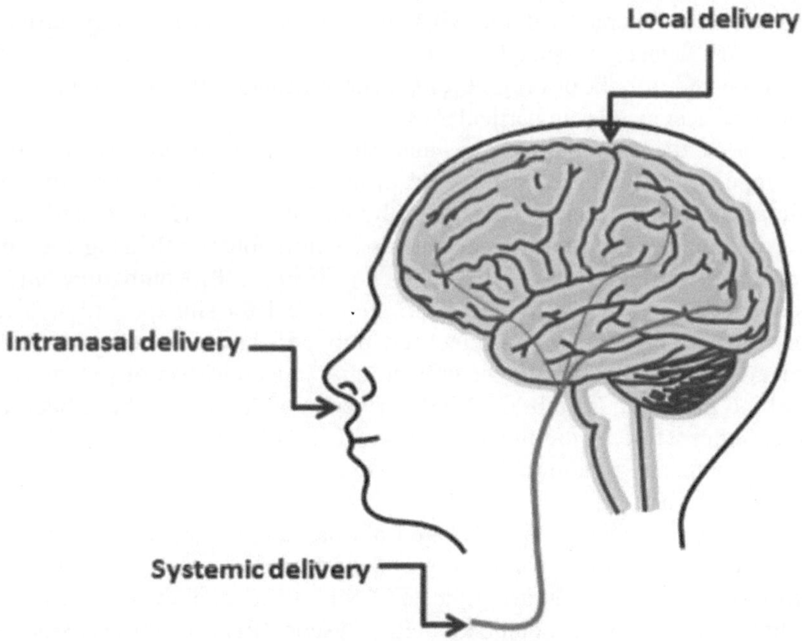

FIGURE 14.1 Transport of therapeutic chemicals to the brain.

to penetrate the BBB [31]. The BBB may be made more permeable in a number of ways, for example, by injecting hyperosmolar mannitol [32], which causes reversible transient structural alterations, or by using high energy soundwaves as a physical activation [33,34]. Neurotoxins were able to enter the brain when the BBB was compromised, causing extensive damage [31]. Hence, cutting-edge medication modification tactics may be useful in the treatment of neurological illnesses to improve pharmaceuticals' capacity to cross the BBB and reduce the risk of neuronal dysfunction caused by BBB disruption. NPs made of lipids can cross the BBB without causing any harm [35].

14.4 OVERVIEW OF SLNS AS NEWLY DESIGNED CNS DRUG-DELIVERY SYSTEM

Although there are various methods for administering medications, the desired outcome has not yet been attained because of concerns with toxicity, low absorption, and lack of targeted approaches. Many of them currently rely on trial-and-error techniques and are not entirely complete. Tricking enables the administration of therapeutic molecules that have been altered with carrier molecules like liposomes or nanoparticles, the receptors encourage cellular internalization, and the ligands promote the targeted drug response [36].

In the framework of a membrane-bound carrier-based delivery system, re-engineering the active drug that may cross the BBB is of interest. According to research, small lipophilic molecules, defined as those with a molecular weight of less than 400 Da, can easily pass through the BBB endothelium [17]. Hence, lipid nanoparticles may interact with the BBB and its components as a drug carrier molecule, allowing them to cross the BBB because of their size and characteristics. These will be discussed in light of drug development in general [36] and with a focus on CNS-oriented therapeutics in particular [37].

Because of their distinctive size and physicochemical properties, NPs can be developed for efficient and targeted drug delivery. Furthermore, the target-specific action of NPs can be redesigned by beautifying surface-related capabilities to traverse several anatomical barriers, continuously releasing therapeutic substance and maintaining particle size consistency. Biocompatible and biodegradable polymeric NPs, in particular, are critical for site-specific medication delivery [38]. To present, only a select few polymers have been cleared for usage in clinical settings. Another factor preventing widespread use of polymeric NPs is their high price [7]. Membrane lipid-derived vehicle systems have been found as a great alternative in the manufacturing of lipophilic medications. SLNs are achieving popularity as a global drug-delivery method for a wide range of therapeutic applications [39].

The primary components of SLNs are lipid-based biomolecules, making them a novel kind of biocompatible nanocarrier system. Because of their hydrophobic lipid core, SLNs may carry both hydrophilic and lipophilic medicines [40,41]. Their role in the breakdown of the reticuloendothelial system (RES) of the BBB is critical [42,43,44]. Because of its solid lipid composition, this colloidal nano-carrier was intended as a preferable alternative to polymeric NPs and liposomes for protecting active drugs against biochemical breakdown [45]. In contrast to polymeric NPs, their biocompatibility is higher and their systemic toxicity is lower since they are generated largely from a biological lipid emulsion system rather than chemical solvents [46]. The combination of lipids, newly adopted pharmaceuticals, and additional components in a specific ratio results in a unique physicochemical status that allows for an extensive diffusion route and regulated drug release in drug-containing SLNs [47,48,49]. Studies in rats have demonstrated that administering drug-loaded SLNs may improve the drug characteristics within the animal body [50]. SLNs may be economically sterilized and lyophilized at cheap cost and require only low costs for raw ingredients. They also have great physico-chemical stability. These benefits make SLNs a good option for mass industrial manufacturing [51,52]. Furthermore, SLNs serve as an ideal drug delivery system with a number of important characteristic features, including maximum drug bioavailability upon administration [53,54], specific tissue targeting [55,56], controlled release kinetics [57,58], minimal immune response [59,60], the ability to deliver conventional pharmaceutical formulations and biomolecules [61,62], sufficient drug loading capacity [63,64], good patient compliance [65,66], and cost effectiveness [67,68], which potentially render it superior and distinct from polymeric drug-delivery systems.

14.4.1 Drug Stabilization by SLNs

Although some pharmaceutical formulations can cross the BBB, they have minimal *in vivo* effectiveness due to chemical instability, fast clearance, and reduced half-life [69,70]. Camptothecin, an anticancer medicine, may traverse the BBB and be used in the treatment of glioblastoma [71,72], however, it is not stable enough for use in clinical procedures. To improve brain targeting effectiveness, however, SLN changes have been included into the formulation to maintain a physiological pH while also maintaining a constant size, charge, and pharmacokinetics [49,73,74,75].

14.4.2 SLNs Show Improved Drug Bioavailability

Encapsulating in SLNs may improve the bioavailability of numerous lipophilic oral formulations used in the management of neurological diseases. Based on the efflux mechanism, BBB-active drug efflux transporters may increase drug permeability to the brain location [76]. Surface medication to SLNs can achieve a high brain-targeting efficacy for CNS diseases [77]. The antipsychotic medicines clozapine and nitrendipine were made more bioavailable in this way: (1) a greater gradient of concentration at BBB due to increased SLN load, stimulating the enhanced movement across the barrier endothelium; and (2) a decrease in RES adsorption onto SLNs in the plasma due to surface modification with Pluronic F-68. Another study found that surface PEGylation, which may prevent RES absorption, and increased the medication's plasma half-life [78].

14.5 ENHANCED BBB PERMEABILITY OF DRUGS BY SLNS

When it comes to encapsulating and transporting various pharmacological molecules, SLNs and their variants provide a far superior carrier system. Doxorubicin, an anticancer medication that is hydrophilic and hence cannot cross the BBB, has significant side effects including acute toxicity and cardiomyopathy. If it can get to where it has to go, those problems will be solved. Through specified laboratory techniques, researchers were able to demonstrate that doxorubicin could be integrated into SLNs. As compared to free doxorubicin, RES treatment resulted in reduced drug load in the liver, heart, and kidneys of rats, and greater concentrations in the brain [79]. When doxorubicin-loaded SLNs were administered intravenously to rats, it was shown to enhance both drug plasma circulation and drug availability in the brain. the governing body [57]. Research on the amyotrophic lateral sclerosis (ALS) medication riluzole found that it was more effectively delivered in the brain tissue designed by SLN formulation [80]. The SLN formulation of paclitaxel (anticancer treatment) stabilized with Brij 78 showed improved brain drug distribution, most likely due to activation of the P-gp-efflux mechanism [81].

Learning how the BBB may be traversed by biological and pharmaceutically active components is essential. To get a feel for how active pharmaceutical components, transported by a carrier system, may counter the BBB and reach within the CNS tissue, a short description of the transport processes of each route is provided. Although numerous methods have been discovered to nonspecifically break through the BBB and enable pharmaceutical medicines access to the brain, there is a risk that circulating poisons will be able to reach the brain tissue from the blood and cause severe neuropathological changes. The BBB must be preserved while an optimum and safe method is developed to increase drug permeability to the brain in a targeted and extended-release manner. Biomaterials developed recently, such as SLNs, have great promise in the context of a BBB-targeted drug-delivery approach for the management of neurological diseases.

14.5.1 Paracellular Pathway and Passive Transmembrane Diffusion

Paracellular routes rely heavily on the tight connections between endothelial cells, which enable only hydrophilic molecules to pass. Lipophilic nano-sized molecules (having molecular weight less than 400 Da) may undertake diffusion through an alternate transcellular channel [82]. In addition, BBB endothelial cells decrease pinocytic activity, which prevents active chemicals from accessing the brain [83,84,85].

14.5.2 Protein-mediated Transport

The transporter proteins transfer chemicals with a certain molecular weight and charge to specific locations in the brain. The endothelial cells have these on both their luminal and basolateral surfaces. Size- and stereo-selective translocation of diverse biomolecules [84,86,87] and their substrates [88] is facilitated by transporters such as GLUT-1, which transports both cations and anions, and large neutral amino acid transporters (LAT), which transport neutral amino acids. Breast cancer resistance proteins (BCRP/ABCG2), multidrug resistance-associated proteins (MRP1, 2, 4, and 5, ABCC), and P-glycoproteins (P-gp or ABCB1, MDR1 gene product) are all examples of efflux-mediated proteins that can be used to transport pharmacologically active molecules and their derivatives across the BBB [84].

14.5.3 Receptor-mediated Transcytosis (RMT)

Upon activating endothelial cells of the BBB, the RMT mode of transport allows the passage of endogenous substances through it [89]. This mechanism is a potentially useful route for medication delivery across the BBB. Endocytosis, intracellular vesicular trafficking, and exocytosis are the stages involved in this process [90]. During this process, elements bind to their specific receptors of the BBB's endothelial cells. After this, vesicles for intracellular transport of receptor-ligand complexes are constructed. Vesicles are generated, and exocytosis is used to transport the ligand from the cell's apical surface to the basolateral side [90, 91, 92]. Clathrin-coated pits, caveolae, and macropinocytosis vesicles are the endocytic vesicles that play a significant part in this process. Most internalization mechanisms regulated by receptors like TfR or insulin receptors entail clathrin-coated pits [89,90]. Hence, RMT is influenced by the receptor ligand binding type and the internalization method (clathrin-mediated or caveolae) [89].

Adsorptive mediated transcytosis (AMT) (4) is an additional critical BBB-crossing mechanism that does not need the participation of plasma membrane receptors. Therefore, compared to SLNs, the AMT's binding affinity is low, its binding ability is great, and its transcytosis efficiency [93,94]. The fundamental mechanism of AMT lies in the electrostatic interactions between positively charged proteins and the negatively charged luminal membrane [95,96].

14.6 METHODS TO IMPROVE SLNS FOR BRAIN DRUG DELIVERY

The quality of SLNs may be enhanced by adjusting a number of defining characteristics. Because of nano pharmacological advances, even hydrophilic drugs that can be loaded with SLNs [41,49,73,97] may pass the BBB. Yet, the pharmacological activity and therapeutic effectiveness of such medications may be subpar because of their pharmacokinetic restrictions. This is because the RES plays a role in their detection. Several studies have investigated methods for addressing the limitations of SLNs.

14.6.1 Particle Size

The therapeutic impact and clearance from the body that result from SLN drug administration are mostly influenced by particle size. SLNs must be either small or extremely flexible in order to pass through the interendothelial cell slits (IES) during the splenic filtration process [98,99]. Slits in endothelial cells range in size from around 200 to 500 nm [98]. The particle size of the SLNs should be modified so that it does not surpass 200 nm in order to prolong blood circulation and the drug's interaction with the BBB for as long as possible. As a result, drugs will be able to permeate the brain's barrier more effectively. If the SLNs are sufficiently big, they may be distorted to escape IES filtering.

14.6.2 Surface Coating with Hydrophilic Polymers/Surfactants

Since the liver is so efficient at clearing out toxins, the half-life of drugs containing colloidal nano-particles is drastically shortened by their widespread use in RES-mediated active detection. Opsonization is crucial to the drug clearance process as a whole. Preventing RES from recognizing the drug's components may boost its effectiveness [100]. SLNs can be altered by impregnating them with the proper surfactant or hydrophilic drugs to prevent them from being ingested by the body's defense mechanisms. Opsonization can be prevented and the blood circulation time and consequently the bioavailability, can be increased by safeguarding the hydrophobic nature of the drug-containing nanoparticle [101]. SLNs coated with polyethylene glycol (PEG) showed positive results in avoiding unfavorable interactions with the biological components due to their hydrophilic nature, carbon-chain stability, neutral behavior, and absence of reactive groups. Furthermore, coating SLNs with PEGs in the molecular weight range of 2000–5000 can reduce plasma protein adsorption. The clearance by the reticuloendothelial system (RES) is also delayed in proportion to the thickness of the PEG coating. Consequently, this results in improved resistance to the reticuloendothelial system, enhancing the nanoparticle's ability to evade rapid clearance[41,102,103]. Drug bioavailability is dramatically improved when the paclitaxel-SLN formulation is coated on hydrophilic molecules like Brij 78, Poloxamer F68, and Brij 68, and administered intravenously through injection as opposed to just taking the medicine orally [97]. The pharmacological activity of SLNs coated with polysorbate (20, 60, 80) was increased because they were easily transported across the BBB through endocytosis caused by the apolipoprotein [103,104]. The BBB can be traversed by unfunctionalized doxorubicin and pristine SLNs, according to another research study. In contrast to pure SLNs, stealth SLNs were shown to be superior in transporting doxorubicin to the brain. In the case of SLN-doxorubicin stealth, better outcomes were seen in a dose-dependent manner, leading to an adequate circulation duration [57,105,106,107].

14.6.3 Use of Ligands

The addition of ligands improves SLN selectivity, transforming it into a prolonged-circulating delivery agent and acting as a tracking device that has a preferentially binding tendency to cell-specific receptors, and peptide with ligand-conjugated SLNs, medication retention at the BBB is increased [60,108,109]. Another study [110] found that liposome-like particles linked to sterically stabilized oppositely charged albumin interact more favorably with brain endothelial cells and concentrate more densely within brain cells.

14.6.4 SLN and Arginine-glycine-aspartic (RGD) Conjugation

When doxorubicin-SLN is combined with arginine-glycine-aspartic (RGD), its *in vitro* anticancer activity and *in vivo* cytotoxicity are increased compared to non-targeted SLN [111]. Drugs given to the brain via RGD-conjugated SLNs easily pass through the BBB. A docetaxel-functionalized SLN formulation was demonstrated to promote cytotoxicity and receptor-based endocytosis permeability to the BBB [112]. This was accomplished by targeting the LDL-receptor-related protein-1 (LRP1), which is excessively expressed at the BBB. Some methods for binding a targeting ligand to an SLN focus on adjoining the fatty acid component of the NP to the $-NH_2$ group of the ligand [113], others on linking the $-NH_2$ group of a phospholipid to the –COOH group of the ligand [114], and still others on linking the $-NH_2$ group of the chitosan coating to the –COOH group of the ligand [115]. Any of these things might improve SLN medication transport through the BBB and into the brain.

14.7 SLNS' DIFFERENT MODELS

The relative abundance of drug components within SLN formulations results in a variety of patterns. The following are some SLN models:

14.7.1 Enrichment of Model Shell by Drugs

A homogenization technique is required for development of this type of SLN variant. As a result, when the resulting dispersion is cooled, the phospholipid content crystallizes in the central region at a specific temperature, so that the medications lie on the outer shell. When the lipid recrystallizes without the drug present, a solid core of lipid is prepared. The great peripheral area of the outer layer causes a fast burst release of drug particles in these SLNs [116,117]. The burst release of pharmaceuticals can be adjusted by exchanging microscopic medications for larger ones, such as lipid microparticles, depending on the surfactants-related properties [118]. Bursts may be controlled, and drug release time extended, by using surfactants at lower concentrations during SLN production.

14.7.2 Enrichment of Model Core by Drugs

The SLN model shown here has the active substance localized in the center, surrounded by a lipid bilayer. This particular SLN evolves through a series of stages. The medication is initially dissolved in the lipid, which leads to solubility at the critical level and the beginning of the formation of a drug lipid emulsion. After that, the mixture is chilled out, and the active ingredient of the drug migrates to the middle where it becomes supersaturated. When this version of SLNs forms, the medication precipitates before the lipid crystallizes, and thus it is concentrated in the lipid's inner core. Fick's rule of diffusion and the lipid membrane properties govern drug release in this SLN model [43].

14.7.3 Homogeneous Matrix Model

The solid solution model is another name for this framework. The medicine in the lipid may be dispersed throughout the lipid, or it may be present as amorphous clusters. This SLN is made by combining the medication with the lipid in a cold homogenization procedure. This sort of SLN is formed due to the drug's robust molecular interactions with the lipid. This form of SLN is often formulated by encapsulating lipophilic medicines in a lipid matrix, as opposed to using surfactants. Since the drug particles are so firmly dispersed at the molecular level in the colloidal matrix, the release profile is stretched out in these SLN formulations [116].

14.8 SYNTHESIS PROCEDURES FOR SLN

The standard and well-accepted modus operandi and materials are owned by the following [119, 120, 121]. The size, shape, and chemical composition of drug-entrapped SLNs all contribute to their biological activity upon administration. Any necessary adjustments may be made to these formulae. Several methods have been developed throughout the years in an effort to produce natural diversity in the physical forms/dimension of SLNs.

14.8.1 High-speed Ultrasonic Homogenization

Historically, SLN [122,170] suspension has been made by high-shear homogenization. High-speed/high-shear homogenization is used in melt emulsification to create SLNs [123,169,171]. Time, stirring speed, and chilling environment are only a few of the many variables that affect the final SLNs' physico-chemical and electrical characteristics, as well as poly-dispersity index. This technique is used to create Ex-Witepsol W35 SLN dispersions [124,172]. The quality of the dispersion may be compromised if microparticle production occurs during this process. To get beyond the restrictions of high-shear homogenization, SLNs may be generated by ultrasonication [120,125,170,173] in a straightforward, evaluable approach. This method's main benefit is that it requires nothing in the way of high-tech tools. Metal contamination and the potential for the particles to become physically unstable during storage are two potential drawbacks. Thus, high-speed ultrasonication may guarantee the creation of high-quality biocompatible SLNs [126,174].

14.8.2 Hot Homogenization

When lipids are heated to temperatures over their melting points, a process known as hot homogenization occurs, resulting in an emulsion [127]. The aqueous emulsion is created by melting a pre-emulsion (containing the medication and lipid combination) in a high-shear mixer. The resulting lipid SLNs crystallize when the mixture is cooled [128]. The emulsion size and qualities of finished SLNs are determined by the components of the pre-emulsion and the surfactant used. This is typically how microparticles are produced [129]. Nevertheless, the viscosity of the lipid phase decreases with increasing processing temperature, resulting in smaller particle sizes

[130,175]. The deterioration of the medication and carrier material due to high temperatures is a potential drawback of this method [131,176].

14.8.3 Cold Homogenization

By using dry ice or liquid nitrogen, medicines and lipids may be cooled to a controlled temperature and pressure for cold homogenization [132,176]. Then, lipid microparticles between 50 and 100 mm in size are obtained by grinding the solid drug-lipid core using a ball or mortar mill. Lipid fragility caused by rapid cooling might be a drawback of this method. Nonetheless, it is preferable to hot homogenization since it generates SLNs of diverse size range [133,177].

14.8.4 Solvent Emulsification/Evaporation Technique for SLN Preparation

The procedure entails using an appropriate organic solvent to create a homogeneous lipid solution. When the lipid solution has been homogenized, water is added to create an o/w coarse emulsion [134]. The solution combination with bigger globules is then homogenized under high pressure to create a nano-emulsion. After overnight stirring, the organic solvent may be removed, leaving behind the SLNs in the nano-emulsion. The resulting SLNs have 25 nm particle size [135,178].

14.8.5 SLN Preparations Based on Micro-emulsions

The solid lipid melts are produced using indirect heating in this procedure. Once the solid lipid melts, an aqueous solution of surfactant, and a co-surfactant is prepared [136]. Microemulsions may be generated spontaneously by aqueous-lipid solutions. The creation of SLN by the diluting of microemulsions was pioneered by Gasco and colleagues [137,144]. For instance, when using more lipophilic solvents, bigger SLNs may be generated, but when using hydrophilic co-solvents, tiny and uniform particles can be formed [138,179].

14.8.6 Utilizing Supercritical Fluid to Prepare SLNs

Unlike more typical methods, this one enables particle-based generation of SLNs from gas-saturated solutions (GSS). GSS is first used to liquefy lipids [139]. At room temperature and pressure, the lipid melts and GSS can be dissolved in the supercritical fluid (SCF). When sprayed with an atomizer, the SCF evaporates fast, leaving behind fine, dry SLNs. The fundamental supremacy of this process is that it produces nano-sized SLN powder without the need for any solvents [140,180,181]. Ex-SLN is a solvent that can be created by carbon dioxide (99.99%) and is used in Rapid Expansion of Supercritical Carbon Dioxide Solutions (RESS). [141,182].

14.8.7 Spray-drying Method

This strategy is seldom utilized nowadays. If you need to convert an aqueous SLN solution into a pharmaceutical, you may use an alternative, cost-effective lyophilization approach [142]. The high temperature, shear pressures, and partial melting of the particle all contribute to the fundamental restriction of this technique, which is particle aggregation [129,143]. This technique can only be used on lipids having a melting point higher than 70°C [144,183,184].

14.8.8 Double-emulsion Method

This double-emulsion technique, in which the basic step is solvent emulsification–evaporation, can be utilized to load hydrophilic drugs onto SLNs in general [145,185]. The drug is encased in a stabilizing ingredient during this technique to prevent it from partitioning to the water phase of the w/o/w double emulsion [146]. However, because the SLNs it produces are frequently bigger, surface-related synthesis changes might be necessary [147,186].

14.9 OPPORTUNITIES FOR CNS DISORDERS USING SLNS

Most pharmacological formulations fail to treat effectively the CNS-related pathologies because of being incapable to overcome the BBB. Because of this, SLNs are now recognized as a viable rational biological technique for enhancing medicine administration [148]. Recently, SLNs as a vehicle agent has focused on carrying drugs beyond the BBB. SLNs seems a novel intelligent way for nervous system-related medicaments with desirable advantages including nano dimension [149,150], tissue-specific delivery (via receptor-mediated transcytosis) [151,152], stability [153,154], capability to avoid the phagocytes [155,156], prolonged circulation time [157,158], sustained and controlled release [159,160], and broad safe use [161,162], biodegradability [163,164], and biocompatibility [165,166]. SLN manufacturing is both scalable and cost-effective [167,187].

Drug-loaded SLN carriers have been found to have a greater tendency to accumulate and greater target-specific activity in the brain than in other organs after intravenous injection [49,168]. It is possible to administer SLNs orally, inhalantly, or intravenously [169,188] to reach the neuronal locations, making them a novel delivery strategy for encapsulating active drugs to counter the CNS illnesses. The neuropathologies are then corrected by SLNs' intervention in the abnormal signaling pathways and the metabolism. Many potential uses for SLNs including medicines for treating CNS diseases have been proposed [189,190]. Drug-loaded SLNs have shown promise in treating a wide range of CNS conditions, including AD, PD, HD, MS, brain tumors and cancer, epilepsy, ischemic stroke, and other neurodegenerative diseases [191,192] (Table 14.1).

TABLE 14.1
Physiological Role of SLNs against Various Neuropathological Conditions

CNS Disorders	SLNs	Functions	Model
Alzheimer's Disease	Curcumin	Full reversal of aluminium-induced brain damage	In vivo
	Galantamine	bBtter medication distribution and increased bioavailability	In vitro
	Quercetin	Reversal of neural tissue damage	In vivo
	Piperine	Avoid BBB permeability	In vivo
	Sesamol	Oxidative-nitrergic stress was reduced, and acetylcholinesterase activity was decreased	In vivo
Epilepsy	Carbamazepine	Anticonvulsant effect	In vitro
	Clonazepam	Improved permeability of the blood–brain barrier	In vivo
	Diazepam	Massive and extended release was seen, and the encapsulation effectiveness was good	In vitro
	Raloxifene	Enhanced absorption from lymphatics, greater oral bioavailability and physical stability	In vivo
Huntington's Disease	Curcumin	the improvement of mitochondrial anomalies	In vivo
	Rosmarinic acid	improve the effectiveness of intranasal delivery for brain targeting and treat behavioural issues related to HD	In vivo
Multiple Sclerosis	Riluzole	increased ability to distribute the drug to the brain and less random biodistribution	In vivo
Neurodegeneration	Curcumin	Therapeutically effective	In vivo
	Idebenone	Enhancing delivery to the brain and lowering cytotoxicity and oxidative stress in rat cerebral cortex astrocytes	In vitro
	Luteolin	Enhance the compound's pharmacokinetics and bioavailability	In vitro

(*Continued*)

TABLE 14.1 (Continued)
Physiological Role of SLNs against Various Neuropathological Conditions

CNS Disorders	SLNs	Functions	Model
Parkinson's Disease	Apomorphine	Oral administration to increase bioavailability	In vitro
	Bromocriptine	stabilise plasma levels and lengthen the half-life and concentration of CNS medications	In vivo
	Levodopa	Higher physical stability and trapping effectiveness	In vitro
	Ropinirole	Alternate delivery methods using intranasal formulations	In vitro
	Rotigotine	Oral inhalation improvement	In vitro
Stroke	Curcumin	Acetylcholinesterase, the mitochondrial enzyme complex, the oxidative and nitrosative stress response, and physiological parameters have all been lessened	In vitro
	Daidzein	Increased cerebral circulation, decreased cerebrovascular immunity, and brain targeting have a protective impact on people who have undergone ischemia-reperfusion.	In vitro
	Vinpocetine	Using brain targeting and sustained release, treat chronic cerebral vascular ischemia or stroke	In vitro
Tumor	Camptothecin	Increased drug density in brain and blood flow	In vivo
	Doxorubicin	Increased bioavailability when targeting tumours	In vivo
	Etoposide	Increased inhibition of glioma cell lines' proliferative potential	In vitro
	Paclitaxel	Increased bioavailability when targeting tumours	In vitro

14.9.1 Optimizing SLNs for Alzheimer's Disease

Alzheimer's disease (AD) is one of the neurodegenerative conditions that primarily affect the elderly. The gradual deterioration and final loss of cognitive skills, such as memory and behavior, are its defining characteristics [193, 218]. Cholinesterase inhibitor development forms the basis of its therapies [219]. Food and Drug Administration-approved acetylcholinesterase inhibitors for treating different stages of AD include donepezil, galantamine, and rivastigmine [195, 220]. One of the main drawbacks of these medications is that the necessary drug percentage cannot be attained at the location of the neuronal tissues [196,197]. The major reason for this is because the medications cannot cross the BBB, reducing their pharmacological efficacy. Better neuroprotection can be achieved at higher medication concentrations [201]. The existing medications have been put into SLNs for further extraordinary effectiveness in managing AD [221,222]. According to *in vitro* research findings, donepezil (an anti-medicine for AD) enhanced drug transport and a preferred release strategy in CMEC/D3 brain endothelial cells and human SH-SY5Y neuronal cells [207,223]. Galantamine hydrobromide SLNs are among the most effective anti-AD medications [192,208]. Tween 80 was used as a surfactant in a solvent emulsification–diffusion synthesis to create this drug combination. The synthesized SLN has a polydispersity index (PDI of 0.432), a Z-potential of 14.83 mV, and a particle size of 772 nm. Piperine loaded in SLN was also investigated *in vivo* by Yusuf et al. [194] as an anti-AD drug. This SLN is created using the solvent emulsification–diffusion approach employing Polysorbate-80 as a coating for selective brain distribution and glycerol monostearate as an exemplary solid lipid. Kakkar et al. conducted research on curcumin compounded with Compritol® 888, Polysorbate-80, and soy lecithin. This was used in the microemulsification approach to [198] aluminum-induced AD. The AD treatment technique is enhanced by the SLN's capacity to overcome the drug's poor bioavailability, reactivity at physiological pH, fast metabolism, and renal clearance [216,224,225,226].

14.9.2 Optimizing SLNs for Parkinson's Disease

Parkinson's disease (PD) is the most common neurophysiological deficit condition. Depression, tremor, and bradykinesia are some of the psychological and physical illness symptoms that come with aging [210,228]. The pathogenic process includes the loss of dopaminergic neurons brought on by mitochondrial dysfunction, oxidative stress, and protein misfolding. Thus far, the dopaminergic receptor-targeting medication levodopa has shown to be the most successful strategy against the Parkinson's disease [229,230,231. The BBB may be traversed by levodopa. There is a decrease in treatment effectiveness due to the inadequate bioavailability of the necessary drugs [232,233]. In order to circumvent these problems, microemulsion technology has recently been used to create SLN drug-delivery systems that encapsulate levodopa [199,211]. Bromocriptine loaded in SLNs proved effective for treating PD, as discovered by Esposito et al. [200] in order to enhance brain concentrations of drugs and half-life. Several dopaminergic agonists have demonstrated promise in *in vitro*, *ex vivo*, and *in vivo* rat models of PD, including oral apomorphine and intranasal ropinirole [202, 203].

14.9.3 Optimizing SLNs for Huntington's Disease

Dementia, schizophrenia, bipolar disorders, depression, chorea, abnormal body movements, oculomotor apraxia, athetosis, and sometimes suicidal tendencies are just some of the neurological disturbances and phenotypes associated with Huntington's disease (HD) [212,234]. HD is incurable due to a lack of effective treatments [235,236]. Because of the BBB's peculiar nature as a barrier to drug-crossing and targeting, HD therapy plans continue to fall short of their goals [213]. Because of their ability to penetrate the BBB and reach the target location in the CNS, the medication candidates for HD may be delivered via advanced SLN drug carriers, leading to improved therapeutic action. The anti-inflammatory chemical curcumin, which has shown encouraging outcomes in *in vivo* trials for the treatment of HD [203,214], is one such candidate. It has been demonstrated that this SLN can repair mitochondrial dysfunctions and oxidative stress-related neuronal loss in the HD brain. Bhatt et al. examined the neuroprotective benefits of a rosmarinic-acid-loaded SLN carrier for HD [204]. They were successful in *in vivo* animal models by minimizing oxidation-induced stress in HD.

14.9.4 Optimizing SLNs for Multiple Sclerosis

In persons with MS, the protective coatings of nerve fibers in the CNS are damaged and deactivated [237]. Thus, serious physical, behavioral, and psychiatric issues emerge from a breakdown in signal transmission in the brain [238,239,240]. Poor drug bioavailability and plasma concentration lead to diminished pharmacological effect for numerous medications [227]. Several MS medications have had their effectiveness boosted by the latest SLN-based drug-delivery approach. Microemulsion-synthesized riluzole-loaded SLNs (average diameter 88, PDI 0.27 nm) showed improved drug delivery to the brain in *in vivo* research. More drug availability across the brain increases the medication's neuroprotective properties in the rats of MS and ALS [241].

14.9.5 Optimizing SLNs for Brain Tumor and Cancer

There are many different types of benign and malignant brain tumors, with glioblastoma being the most common and carrying a significant risk of recurrence if not treated well. The poor therapeutic effectiveness of anticancer medicines is mostly due to their inefficient translocation through the BBB [242,243]. Targeted delivery of an anticancer medicine without harming healthy cells is made possible by a revolutionary nano-drug carrier technology [244]. Several other medications and drug modifications, including etoposide SLN [205] and paclitaxel SLN [206], have been studied for their potential to treat glioblastoma. The results from *in vitro* experiments showed that they were more effective than the free medication at inhibiting the growth of glioma cell lines. Cationic solid lipid nanoparticles (CASLNs) functionalized with an antibody against epidermal growth factor receptor (EGFR) were used in another investigation. Malignant glioblastoma cells were shown to be the focus of the specific SLN's anti-proliferative action [245]. Research afterward examined the effects of SLN composites containing doxorubicin, etoposide, and other drugs on human brain microvascular endothelial cells (HBMEC), human U87 malignant glioma cells (glioma cells), and human astrocytes using *in vitro* studies. According to the findings, SLNs are safe to use and may even slow the growth of cancer cells. This may be due to the fact that drug-loaded SLNs are able to enter the BBB, which bodes well for their therapeutic use in the future treatment of various types of glioblastoma [245,246,247,248,249]. The anticancer medication edelfosine was loaded onto SLNs and then evaluated on a C6 glioma cell line and C6 glioma xenograft tumor, the outcomes were promising in both cases. An anti-proliferative activity was shown by greater deposits in brain tissue and a considerable decline in tumor growth [250]. The nanoparticles were internalized, according to internalization studies conducted *in vitro* and *in vivo*, improving the therapeutic efficiency of the drug's ability to penetrate the BBB [251]. In order to increase drug penetrability through BBB, another study examined SLNs functionalized with a targeting moiety and loaded with resveratrol [252], indicating their natural potential to passively target the brain (hCMEC/D3 cell monolayer *in vitro* BBB model). Fatty acid coacervation-made SLNs containing paclitaxel and bevacizumab were reported to traverse the BBB [253].

14.9.6 Optimizing SLNs for Epilepsy

Epilepsy is a CNS illness that causes partial or widespread seizures due to an overstimulation of the brain's electrical circuitry [254]. In this pathology, the BBB limits the extent of medicine that gets to the target region in the brain and so reduces the effectiveness of the therapy. SLN has demonstrated potential for overcoming the current shortcomings in the therapeutic management of epilepsy [255], entering the ranks of conventional and recently found drug-delivery systems. The anticonvulsant impact of SLNs loaded with carbamazepine has been demonstrated to be superior to that of nanoemulsions loaded carbamazepine [209], according to recent studies. Equally convincing evidence showed that both muscimol- and amiloride-loaded SLNs effectively control focal seizures in animal models through an improved and more effective drug release compared with the drug administered alone, according to equally strong data [256, 257].

14.9.7 Optimizing SLNs in Ischemic Stroke

When brain tissue suddenly stops receiving blood and oxygen, neurological function suddenly ceases, and irreversible impairment results [258]. Ischemic strokes occur in several forms, including lacunar, cardioembolic, cryptogenic, and hemorrhagic [259]. There is currently no curative treatment for this brain abnormality, despite its devastating effects on people all over the globe. The damage to brain tissue following an ischemic stroke is also progressive. Hypoxia is the initial cause of ischemic stroke, which is followed by secondary effects such severe brain tissue inflammation, reactive oxygen species (ROS) generation, glutamate excitotoxicity, and so on. Neuronal cell loss and related diseases, such as brain edema and BBB impairment, develop over time [260,261,262]. Reducing proinflammatory effects and promoting neuroprotection [263] should be the primary focus of therapy. Due to the low medication bioavailability across the BBB, conventional therapeutic methods are ineffective. Stroke care presents significant challenges that might be ameliorated with the use of a cutting-edge nano-drug-delivery technique [264]. One contemporary nanotechnological method investigating possible medication formulations for ischemic stroke therapies is SLN carrier-based drug delivery. Primary research showed that high-shear homogenization-produced SLNs loaded with vincristine and temozolomide had a deep, prolonged release, which bodes well for their potential human use as a regulated delivery method [265]. Curcumin-loaded SLNs (an antioxidant) have also attracted attention for their potential application in stroke therapy [266]. Inhibiting acetylcholinesterase levels and increasing glutathione (GSH), superoxide dismutase (SOD), and catalase levels are only some of the therapeutic effects that SLN-encapsulated curcumin has been shown to have in this research. The corrective capabilities of encapsulated baicalin with enhanced bioavailability and stability were discovered in a separate investigation examining the effects of SLNs containing baicalin on ischemic stroke [267]. Regarding the therapy of chronic cerebral vascular ischemia [215], vinpocetine loaded in a specific SLN formulation may be superior to free vinpocetine due to its higher bioavailability and longer half-life. Low-density lipoprotein (LDL) receptors in the BBB may recognize resveratrol-loaded SLN that has been surface modified (with apolipoprotein E: ApoE). Hence, improved BBB permeability was observed with this functionalized SLN drug carrier in an *in vitro* cell model [268]. Neurobehavioral impairments were dramatically ameliorated by ferulic acid (FA)-loaded NLC in ischemia rat models, with increased bioavailability and decreased oxidative stress [269].

14.9.8 Optimizing SLN for Other Neurodegenerative Diseases

Most neurodegenerative illnesses have a common feature: oxidative stress, which causes the malfunction and eventual death of neuronal cells [270]. Free radicals generated by ROS may be neutralized with the help of powerful antioxidants like glutathione (GSH), lipoic acid (LA), carnosine, and caffeic acid [222,271]. With improved stability and hydrophilicity [272], SLNs encapsulating LA have been shown to be useful for the topical distribution of LA as an anti-aging agent [273]. Lipoyl-memantine (LA-MEM codrug)-loaded SLNs were shown to be a novel method, with the added benefit of being stable in stomach and intestinal fluid models. This facilitated better stability, solubility, and absorption. This indicates that even at high concentrations, they are able to traverse the BBB. In addition, hydrolysis resulted in the release of LA and MEM, which demonstrated therapeutic activity while being completely safe and nontoxic [273]. Idebenone is another popular anti-oxidant medication that can be effectively delivered to the brain by SLNs [152,228]. *In vitro* analysis of rat cerebral cortex astrocyte primary cultures demonstrated that idebenone-loaded SLNs suppressed 2,2′-azobis-(2-amidinopropane) dihydrochloride (APPH)-induced

LDH release and reactive oxygen species (ROS) generation. Idebenone-loaded SLNs might pass through the BBB and boost a drug's bioavailability in the brain [217]. Hot-microemulsion SLNs loaded with synthetic luteolin (LU, 5, 7, 30, 40-tetrahydroxyflavone) have been found to reduce oxidation-induced damage in animal models when used to treat neurodegenerative diseases. Interestingly, SLNs loaded with grape extract and resveratrol, a natural polyphenolic flavonoid that promotes the rapid recovery of unhealthy neurons [274,275], have shown promise in the treatment of PD and AD, both of which are linked to severe neurodegeneration.

This chapter focused on the therapeutic assessment of several different types of drug-loaded SLNs with potential for use in the future clinical treatment of various neurological illnesses. Moreover, intriguing is the fact that SLN formulations have shown efficacy in both *in vitro* and *in vivo* BBB-crossing scenarios. However, only a small number of them have received clinical approval for BBB crossing in the treatment of neurological illnesses [276,277], with the exception of those used to treat cardiac diseases and a small number of malignancies. No adequate clinical trial of a medication containing SLN for neurological diseases has been conducted. Nevertheless, the clinical trial showed [278] that ingestion of SLNs loaded with melatonin was sufficient to achieve improved therapeutic ranges even in the initial phase of severe disease with a favorable pharmacokinetic profile, compared to mere melatonin. There may be pharmacokinetic benefits to encapsulation into lipid nano vectors. When applied topically, transdermal melatonin therapy has the potential to restore circadian rhythms in critically sick patients by mimicking the natural pattern of melatonin blood levels. Another key unfavorable conclusion found in preclinical research was that the pharmacokinetic characteristics of the SLN-loaded medication varied across various animal models when it crossed the BBB. Different brain microenvironments in the animal models may account for the discrepancy in medication effectiveness findings. To predict the pharmacological activity and drug absorption of the SLNs, it is desirable to assess their bioavailability in animal models whose neurophysiology is extremely comparable to that of humans. As a result, there is a greater likelihood that the SLNs may be clinically approved and then commercialized for the treatment of neurological disorders by targeting the BBB.

14.10 CONCLUSIONS

The medical community has a formidable challenge when attempting to treat CNS illnesses. The BBB acts as a barrier for most of the therapeutic medications, which is problematic since the incidence of mortality and morbidity associated with complicated neuro-pathologies and the reasons underlying the illnesses are still open questions. There has been significant development in our knowledge of the BBB as a possible target for brain medication delivery thanks to recent scientific research. It is crucial to take into account the BBB as both a physical barrier and a specific therapeutic target when figuring out how to deliver medications to the CNS with the goal of treating neuropathologies. One of the lipid-based enhanced nano-drug-delivery vehicles that aims to get over the BBB's restrictions is SLNs and their alterations as a unique therapy strategy. Their pharmacological efficacy has been shown to increase.

In addition, their one-of-a-kind physicochemical makeup allows them to transport the drug's active ingredients in a targeted and regulated fashion, with reduced toxicity. Fewer side effects, an extended half-life, and the possibility for enhanced drug passage over the BBB are some of the therapeutic advantages of SLNs for effective brain medicine delivery. The drawbacks of SLNs include its inadequate drug-loading efficiency, the more complicated physical nature of lipid components, and chemical stability concerns during dosing and repository steps. Due to their limitations, SLNs must be further developed to become the ideal CNS medicine delivery technology for countering the broadest spectrum of neurological disorders. Although it is true that present SLN techniques are unable to effectively treat neurological illnesses, recent technology advances and a deeper comprehension of the BBB dependent transport mechanism provide optimism for the future of this innovative treatment approach. Further obstacles that must be surmounted before SLNs may be used in clinical settings include standardizing the modified synthetic methods, optimizing the sterilizing process, scaling up production operations, and fixing present stability difficulties.

REFERENCES

1. Sharma R., Kabra A., Rao M.M, Prajapati P.K. Herbal and holistic solutions for neurodegenerative and depressive disorders: Leads from Ayurveda. *Curr. Pharm. Des.* 2018, 27(3): 2597–2608. doi: 10.2174/1381612824666180821165741
2. Sharma R., Kuca K., Nepovimova E., Kabra A., Rao M.M., Prajapati P.K. Traditional Ayurvedic and herbal remedies for Alzheimer's disease from bench to bedside. *Expert Rev. Neurother.* 2019, 19: 359–374. doi: 10.1080/14737175.2019.1596803
3. Sharma R., Garg N., Verma D., Rathi P., Sharma V., Kuca K., Prajapati P.K. Indian medicinal plants as drug leads in neurodegenerative disorders. In *Nutraceuticals in Brain Health and Beyond* 2021 Jan 1 (pp. 31–45). Academic Press. doi: 10.1016/B978-0-12-820593-8.00004-5
4. Sharma R., Singla R.K., Banerjee S., Sinha B., Shen B., Sharma R. Role of Shankhpushpi (Convolvulus pluricaulis) in neurological disorders: An umbrella review covering evidence from ethnopharmacology to clinical studies. *Neurosci Biobehav Rev.* 2022 Sep,140:104795. doi: 10.1016/j.neubiorev.2022.104795. Epub 2022 Jul 22. PMID: 35878793.
5. Patel, M., Souto, E.B., Singh, K.K. Advances in brain drug targeting and delivery: Limitations and challenges of solid lipid nanoparticles. *Expert Opin. Drug Deliv.* 2013, *10*, 889–905.
6. Barchet, T.M., Amiji, M.M. Challenges and opportunities in CNS delivery of therapeutics for neurodegenerative diseases. *Expert Opin. Drug Deliv.* 2009, *6*, 211–225.
7. Scheffel, U., Rhodes, B.A., Natarajan, T., Wagner, H.N. Albumin microspheres for study of the reticuloendothelial system. *J. Nucl. Med.* 1972, *13*, 498–503.
8. Sawant; K.K., Dodiya, S.S. Recent advances and patents on solid lipid nanoparticles. *Recent Pat. Drug Deliv. Formul.* 2008, *2*, 120–135.
9. Begley, D.J. Delivery of therapeutic agents to the central nervous system: The problems and the possibilities. *Pharmacol. Ther.* 2004, *104*, 29–45.

10. Cecchelli, R., Berezowski, V., Lundquist, S., Culot, M., Renftel, M., Dehouck, M.-P., Fenart, L. Modelling of the blood–brain barrier in drug discovery and development. *Nat. Rev. Drug Discov.* 2007, *6*, 650–661.
11. Zhou, J., Atsina, K.-B., Himes, B.T., Strohbehn, G.W., Saltzman, W.M. Novel delivery strategies for glioblastoma. *Cancer J.* 2012, *18*, 89–99.
12. Newton, H.B. Advances in strategies to improve drug delivery to brain tumors. *Expert Rev. Neurother.* 2006, *6*, 1495–1509.
13. Harris, J.J., Jolivet, R., Attwell, D. Synaptic energy use and supply. *Neuron* 2012, *75*, 762–777.
14. Iadecola, C., Yaffe, K., Biller, J., Bratzke, L.C., Faraci, F.M., Gorelick, P.B., Gulati, M., Kamel, H., Knopman, D.S., Launer, L.J. Impact of hypertension on cognitive function: A scientific statement from the American Heart Association. *Hypertension* 2016, *68*, e67–e94.
15. Zlokovic, B.V. The blood–brain barrier in health and chronic neurodegenerative disorders. *Neuron* 2008, *57*, 178–201.
16. Zlokovic, B.V. Neurovascular pathways to neurodegeneration in Alzheimer's disease and other disorders. *Nat. Rev. Neurosci.* 2011, *12*, 723–738.
17. Pardridge, W.M. Drug transport across the blood–brain barrier. *J. Cereb. Blood Flow Metab.* 2012, *32*, 1959–1972.
18. Abbott, N.J. Astrocyte–endothelial interactions and blood–brain barrier permeability. *J. Anat.* 2002, *200*, 523–534.
19. Pardridge, W.M. Molecular biology of the blood–brain barrier. *Mol. Biotechnol.* 2005, *30*, 57–69.
20. Levin, V.A. Relationship of octanol/water partition coefficient and molecular weight to rat brain capillary permeability. *J. Med. Chem.* 1980, *23*, 682–684.
21. Van De Waterbeemd, H., Smith, D.A ., Beaumont, K., Walker, D.K. Property-based design: Optimization of drug absorption and pharmacokinetics. *J. Med. Chem.* 2001, *44*, 1313–1333.
22. Patel, M.M., Goyal, B.R., Bhadada, S.V., Bhatt, J.S., Amin, A.F. Getting into the brain. *CNS Drugs* 2009, *23*, 35–58.
23. Chaichana, K.L., Pinheiro, L., Brem, H. Delivery of local therapeutics to the brain: Working toward advancing treatment for malignant gliomas. *Ther. Deliv.* 2015, *6*, 353–369.
24. Erdő, F., Bors, L.A., Farkas, D., Bajza, Á., Gizurarson, S. Evaluation of intranasal delivery route of drug administration for brain targeting. *Brain Res. Bull.* 2018, *143*, 155–170.
25. Agrawal, M., Saraf, S., Saraf, S., Antimisiaris, S.G., Chougule, M.B., Shoyele, S.A., Alexander, A. Nose-to-brain drug delivery: An update on clinical challenges and progress towards approval of anti-Alzheimer drugs. *J. Control. Release* 2018, *281*, 139–177.
26. Pires, P.C., Santos, A.O. Nanosystems in nose-to-brain drug delivery: A review of non-clinical brain targeting studies. *J. Control. Release* 2018, *270*, 89–100.
27. Mistry, A., Stolnik, S., Illum, L. Nanoparticles for direct nose-to-brain delivery of drugs. *Int. J. Pharm.* 2009, *379*, 146–157.
28. Bourganis, V., Kammona, O., Alexopoulos, A., Kiparissides, C. Recent advances in carrier mediated nose-to-brain delivery of pharmaceutics. *Eur. J. Pharm. Biopharm.* 2018, *128*, 337–362.
29. Gänger, S., Schindowski, K. Tailoring formulations for intranasal nose-to-brain delivery: A review on architecture, physico-chemical characteristics and mucociliary clearance of the nasal olfactory mucosa. *Pharmaceutics* 2018, *10*, 116.

30. Lochhead, J.J., Thorne, R.G. Intranasal delivery of biologics to the central nervous system. *Adv. Drug Deliv. Rev.* 2012, *64*, 614–628.
31. Posadas, I., Monteagudo, S., Ceña, V. Nanoparticles for brain-specific drug and genetic material delivery, imaging and diagnosis. *Nanomedicine* 2016, *11*, 833–849.
32. Blanchette, M., Fortin, D. Blood–brain barrier disruption in the treatment of brain tumors. In *The Blood–Brain and Other Neural Barriers*, Springer: Berlin/Heidelberg, Germany, 2011, pp. 447–463.
33. Etame, A.B., Diaz, R.J., O'Reilly, M.A., Smith, C.A., Mainprize, T.G., Hynynen, K., Rutka, J.T. Enhanced delivery of gold nanoparticles with therapeutic potential into the brain using MRI-guided focused ultrasound. *Nanomed. Nanotechnol. Biol. Med.* 2012, *8*, 1133–1142.
34. Bing, K.F., Howles, G.P., Qi, Y., Palmeri, M.L., Nightingale, K.R. Blood–brain barrier (BBB) disruption using a diagnostic ultrasound scanner and Definity® in mice. *Ultrasound Med. Biol.* 2009, *35*, 1298–1308.
35. Tapeinos, C., Battaglini, M., Ciofani, G. Advances in the design of solid lipid nanoparticles and nanostructured lipid carriers for targeting brain diseases. *J. Control. Release* 2017, *264*, 306–332.
36. Anthony, D.P., Hegde, M.M., Shetty, S.S., Rafic, T., Mutalik, S., Rao, B.S. Targeting receptor-ligand chemistry for drug delivery across blood–brain barrier in brain diseases. *Life Sci.* 2021, *274*, 119326.
37. Alavijeh, M.S., Chishty, M., Qaiser, M.Z., Palmer, A.M. Drug metabolism and pharmacokinetics, the blood–brain barrier, and central nervous system drug discovery. *NeuroRx* 2005, *2*, 554–571.
38. Rakotoarisoa, M., Angelova, A. Amphiphilic nanocarrier systems for curcumin delivery in neurodegenerative disorders. *Medicines* 2018, *5*, 126.
39. Jumaa, M., Müller, B.W. Lipid emulsions as a novel system to reduce the hemolytic activity of lytic agents: Mechanism of the protective effect. *Eur. J. Pharm. Sci.* 2000, *9*, 285–290.
40. Kaur, I.P., Bhandari, R., Bhandari, S., Kakkar, V. Potential of solid lipid nanoparticles in brain targeting. *J. Control. Release* 2008, *127*, 97–109.
41. Chen, D.-B., Yang, T.-Z., Lu, W.-L., Zhang, Q. In vitro and in vivo study of two types of long-circulating solid lipid nanoparticles containing paclitaxel. *Chem. Pharm. Bull.* 2001, *49*, 1444–1447.
42. Pardeshi, C., Rajput, P., Belgamwar, V., Tekade, A., Patil, G., Chaudhary, K., Sonje, A. Solid lipid based nanocarriers: An overview. *Acta Pharm.* 2012, *62*, 433–472.
43. Müller, R.H., Mäder, K., Gohla, S. Solid lipid nanoparticles (SLN) for controlled drug delivery – A review of the state of the art. *Eur. J. Pharm. Biopharm.* 2000, *50*, 161–177.
44. Freitas, C., Müller, R.H. Effect of light and temperature on zeta potential and physical stability in solid lipid nanoparticle (SLN™) dispersions. *Int. J. Pharm.* 1998, *168*, 221–229.
45. Mukherjee, S., Ray, S., Thakur, R. Solid lipid nanoparticles: A modern formulation approach in drug delivery system. *Indian J. Pharm. Sci.* 2009, *71*, 349.
46. Tabatt, K., Kneuer, C., Sameti, M., Olbrich, C., Müller, R.H., Lehr, C.-M., Bakowsky, U. Transfection with different colloidal systems: Comparison of solid lipid nanoparticles and liposomes. *J. Control. Release* 2004, *97*, 321–332.
47. Hamdani, J., Moës, A.J., Amighi, K. Physical and thermal characterisation of Precirol® and Compritol® as lipophilic glycerides used for the preparation of controlled-release matrix pellets. *Int. J. Pharm.* 2003, *260*, 47–57.

48. Mosallaei, N., Jaafari, M.R., Hanafi-Bojd, M.Y., Golmohammadzadeh, S., Malaekeh-Nikouei, B. Docetaxel-loaded solid lipid nanoparticles: Preparation, characterization, in vitro, and in vivo evaluations. *J. Pharm. Sci.* 2013, *102*, 1994–2004.
49. Yang, S.C., Lu, L.F., Cai, Y., Zhu, J.B., Liang, B.W., Yang, C.Z. Body distribution in mice of intravenously injected camptothecin solid lipid nanoparticles and targeting effect on brain. *J. Control. Release* 1999, *59*, 299–307.
50. Manjunath, K., Venkateswarlu, V. Pharmacokinetics, tissue distribution and bioavailability of clozapine solid lipid nanoparticles after intravenous and intraduodenal administration. *J. Control. Release* 2005, *107*, 215–228.
51. Gohla, S., Dingler, A. Scaling up feasibility of the production of solid lipid nanoparticles (SLN). *Die Pharm.* 2001, *56*, 61–63.
52. Sathali, A.H., Ekambaram, P., Priyanka, K. Solid lipid nanoparticles: A review. *Sci. Revs. Chem. Commun* 2012, *2*, 80–102.
53. Reddy, A., Parthiban, S., Vikneswari, A., Senthilkumar, G. A modern review on solid lipid nanoparticles as novel controlled drug delivery system. *Int. J. Res. Pharm. Nano Sci.* 2014, *3*, 313–325.
54. Garud, A., Singh, D., Garud, N. Solid lipid nanoparticles (SLN): Method, characterization and applications. *Int. Curr. Pharm. J.* 2012, *1*, 384–393.
55. Schwarz, C. Solid lipid nanoparticles (SLN) for controlled drug delivery II. Drug incorporation and physicochemical characterization. *J. Microencapsul.* 1999, *16*, 205–213.
56. Freitas, C., Müller, R. Correlation between long-term stability of solid lipid nanoparticles (SLN™) and crystallinity of the lipid phase. *Eur. J. Pharm. Biopharm.* 1999, *47*, 125–132.
57. Fundarò, A., Cavalli, R., Bargoni, A., Vighetto, D., Zara, G.P., Gasco, M.R. Non-stealth and stealth solid lipid nanoparticles (SLN) carrying doxorubicin: Pharmacokinetics and tissue distribution after iv administration to rats. *Pharmacol. Res.* 2000, *42*, 337–343.
58. Reddy, J.S., Venkateswarlu, V. Novel delivery systems for drug targeting to the brain. *Drugs Future* 2004, *29*, 63–83.
59. Baek, J.-S., Cho, C.-W. Surface modification of solid lipid nanoparticles for oral delivery of curcumin: Improvement of bioavailability through enhanced cellular uptake, and lymphatic uptake. *Eur. J. Pharm. Biopharm.* 2017, *117*, 132–140.
60. Lockman, P.R., Oyewumi, M.O., Koziara, J.M., Roder, K.E., Mumper, R.J., Allen, D.D. Brain uptake of thiamine-coated nanoparticles. *J. Control. Release* 2003, *93*, 271–282.
61. Dingler, A. Feste Lipid-Nanopartikel als Kolloidale Wirkstoffträgersysteme zur Dermalen Applikation. Ph.D. Thesis, Freie Universität Berlin, Berlin, Germany, 1998.
62. Müller, R., Mehnert, W., Lucks, J.-S., Schwarz, C., Zur Mühlen, A. Solid lipid nanoparticles (SLN): An alternative colloidal carrier system for controlled drug delivery. *Eur. J. Pharm. Biopharm.* 1995, *41*, 62–69.
63. zur Mühlen, A., Schwarz, C., Mehnert, W. Solid lipid nanoparticles (SLN) for controlled drug delivery–drug release and release mechanism. *Eur. J. Pharm. Biopharm.* 1998, *45*, 149–155.
64. Sun, J., Bi, C., Chan, H.M., Sun, S., Zhang, Q., Zheng, Y. Curcumin-loaded solid lipid nanoparticles have prolonged in vitro antitumour activity, cellular uptake and improved in vivo bioavailability. *Colloids Surf. B Biointerfaces* 2013, *111*, 367–375.
65. Huang, X., Chen, Y.-J., Peng, D.-Y., Li, Q.-L., Wang, X.-S., Wang, D.-L., Chen, W.-D. Solid lipid nanoparticles as delivery systems for Gambogenic acid. *Colloids Surf. B Biointerfaces* 2013, *102*, 391–397.

66. Jain, V., Gupta, A., Pawar, V.K., Asthana, S., Jaiswal, A.K., Dube, A., Chourasia, M.K. Chitosan-assisted immunotherapy for intervention of experimental leishmaniasis via amphotericin B-loaded solid lipid nanoparticles. *Appl. Biochem. Biotechnol.* 2014, *174*, 1309–1330.
67. Rawat, M.K., Jain, A., Singh, S. Studies on binary lipid matrix based solid lipid nanoparticles of repaglinide: In vitro and in vivo evaluation. *J. Pharm. Sci.* 2011, *100*, 2366–2378.
68. Westesen, K., Bunjes, H., Koch, M. Physicochemical characterization of lipid nanoparticles and evaluation of their drug loading capacity and sustained release potential. *J. Control. Release* 1997, *48*, 223–236.
69. Westesen, K., Siekmann, B., Koch, M.H. Investigations on the physical state of lipid nanoparticles by synchrotron radiation X-ray diffraction. *Int. J. Pharm.* 1993, *93*, 189–199.
70. Di, L., Kerns, E.H., Hong, Y., Chen, H. Development and application of high throughput plasma stability assay for drug discovery. *Int. J. Pharm.* 2005, *297*, 110–119.
71. Djuzenova, C.S., Güttler, T., Berger, S., Katzer, A., Flentje, M. Differential response of human glioblastoma cell lines to combined camptothecin and ionizing radiation treatment. *Cancer Biol. Ther.* 2008, *7*, 364–373.
72. Tsai, T., Lee, C., Yeh, P. Effect of P-glycoprotein modulators on the pharmacokinetics of camptothecin using microdialysis. *Br. J. Pharmacol.* 2001, *134*, 1245–1252.
73. Yang, S., Zhu, J., Lu, Y., Liang, B., Yang, C. Body distribution of camptothecin solid lipid nanoparticles after oral administration. *Pharm. Res.* 1999, *16*, 751–757.
74. Martins, S.M., Sarmento, B., Nunes, C., Lúcio, M., Reis, S., Ferreira, D.C. Brain targeting effect of camptothecin-loaded solid lipid nanoparticles in rat after intravenous administration. *Eur. J. Pharm. Biopharm.* 2013, *85*, 488–502.
75. Martins, S., Tho, I., Reimold, I., Fricker, G., Souto, E., Ferreira, D., Brandl, M. Brain delivery of camptothecin by means of solid lipid nanoparticles: Formulation design, in vitro and in vivo studies. *Int. J. Pharm.* 2012, *439*, 49–62.
76. Manjunath, K., Venkateswarlu, V. Pharmacokinetics, tissue distribution and bioavailability of nitrendipine solid lipid nanoparticles after intravenous and intraduodenal administration. *J. Drug Target.* 2006, *14*, 632–645.
77. Wang, J.-X., Sun, X., Zhang, Z.-R. Enhanced brain targeting by synthesis of 3′, 5′ -dioctanoyl-5-fluoro-2′ -deoxyuridine and incorporation into solid lipid nanoparticles. *Eur. J. Pharm. Biopharm.* 2002, *54*, 285–290.
78. Madan, J., Pandey, R.S., Jain, V., Katare, O.P., Chandra, R., Katyal, A. Poly (ethylene)-glycol conjugated solid lipid nanoparticles of noscapine improve biological half-life, brain delivery and efficacy in glioblastoma cells. *Nanomed. Nanotechnol. Biol. Med.* 2013, *9*, 492–503.
79. Zara, G.P., Cavalli, R., Fundarò, A., Bargoni, A., Caputo, O., Gasco, M.R. Pharmacokinetics of doxorubicin incorporated in solid lipid nanospheres (SLN). *Pharmacol. Res.* 1999, *40*, 281–286.
80. Bondì, M.L., Craparo, E.F., Giammona, G., Drago, F. Brain-targeted solid lipid nanoparticles containing riluzole: Preparation, characterization and biodistribution. *Nanomedicine* 2010, *5*, 25–32.
81. Koziara, J.M., Lockman, P.R., Allen, D.D., Mumper, R.J. Paclitaxel nanoparticles for the potential treatment of brain tumors. *J. Control. Release* 2004, *99*, 259–269.
82. Sweeney, M.D., Sagare, A.P., Zlokovic, B.V. Blood–brain barrier breakdown in Alzheimer disease and other neurodegenerative disorders. *Nat. Rev. Neurol.* 2018, *14*, 133–150.

83. Abbott, N.J., Rönnbäck, L., Hansson, E. Astrocyte-endothelial interactions at the blood–brain barrier. *Nat. Rev. Neurosci.* 2006, *7*, 41–53.
84. Sanchez-Covarrubias, L., Slosky, L.M., Thompson, B.J., Davis, T.P., Ronaldson, P.T. Transporters at CNS barrier sites: Obstacles or opportunities for drug delivery? *Curr. Pharm. Des.* 2014, *20*, 1422–1449.
85. Ballabh, P., Braun, A., Nedergaard, M. The blood–brain barrier: An overview: Structure, regulation, and clinical implications. *Neurobiol. Dis.* 2004, *16*, 1–13.
86. Banks, W.A., Owen, J.B., Erickson, M.A. Insulin in the brain: There and back again. *Pharmacol. Ther.* 2012, *136*, 82–93.
87. Boado, R.J., Li, J.Y., Nagaya, M., Zhang, C., Pardridge, W.M. Selective expression of the large neutral amino acid transporter at the blood–brain barrier. *Proc. Natl. Acad. Sci. USA* 1999, *96*, 12079–12084.
88. Zhang, Z., Zhan, C. Receptor-mediated transportation through BBB. In *Brain Targeted Drug Delivery System*, Elsevier: Amsterdam, The Netherlands, 2019, pp. 105–128.
89. Villaseñor, R., Lampe, J., Schwaninger, M., Collin, L. Intracellular transport and regulation of transcytosis across the blood–brain barrier. *Cell. Mol. Life Sci.* 2019, *76*, 1081–1092.
90. Pulgar, V.M. Transcytosis to cross the blood brain barrier, new advancements and challenges. *Front. Neurosci.* 2019, *12*, 1019.
91. Jones, A.R., Shusta, E.V. Blood–brain barrier transport of therapeutics via receptor-mediation. *Pharm. Res.* 2007, *24*, 1759–1771.
92. Preston, J.E., Abbott, N.J., Begley, D.J. Transcytosis of macromolecules at the blood–brain barrier. *Adv. Pharmacol.* 1995, *71*, 147–163.
93. Hervé, F., Ghinea, N., Scherrmann, J.-M. CNS delivery via adsorptive transcytosis. *AAPS J.* 2008, *10*, 455–472.
94. Lu, W. Adsorptive-mediated brain delivery systems. *Curr. Pharm. Biotechnol.* 2012, *13*, 2340–2348.
95. Zhu, X., Jin, K., Huang, Y., Pang, Z. Brain drug delivery by adsorption-mediated transcytosis. In *Brain Targeted Drug Delivery System*, Elsevier: Amsterdam, The Netherlands, 2019, pp. 159–183.
96. Bickel, U., Yoshikawa, T., Pardridge, W.M. Pardridge, Delivery of peptides and proteins through the blood–brain barrier. *Adv. Drug Deliv. Rev.* 1993, *10*, 205–245.
97. Cavalli, R., Caputo, O., Gasco, M.R. Preparation and characterization of solid lipid nanospheres containing paclitaxel. *Eur. J. Pharm. Sci.* 2000, *10*, 305–309.
98. Chen, L.-T., Weiss, L. The role of the sinus wall in the passage of erythrocytes through the spleen. *Blood* 1973, *41*, 529–537.
99. Moghimi, S.M., Porter, C., Muir, I., Illum, L., Davis, S. Non-phagocytic uptake of intravenously injected microspheres in rat spleen: Influence of particle size and hydrophilic coating. *Biochem. Biophys. Res. Commun.* 1991, *177*, 861–866.
100. Jain, N. *Advances in Controlled and Novel Drug Delivery*, CBS Publishers & Distributors: New Delhi, India, 2008.
101. Olivier, J.-C. Drug transport to brain with targeted nanoparticles. *NeuroRx* 2005, *2*, 108–119.
102. Oyewumi, M.O., Yokel, R.A., Jay, M., Coakley, T., Mumper, R.J. Comparison of cell uptake, biodistribution and tumor retention of folate-coated and PEG-coated gadolinium nanoparticles in tumor-bearing mice. *J. Control. Release* 2004, *95*, 613–626.
103. Kreuter, J. Nanoparticulate systems for brain delivery of drugs. *Adv. Drug Deliv. Rev.* 2001, *47*, 65–81.

104. Alyautdin, R.N., Petrov, V.E., Langer, K., Berthold, A., Kharkevich, D.A., Kreuter, J. Delivery of loperamide across the blood–brain barrier with polysorbate 80-coated polybutylcyanoacrylate nanoparticles. *Pharm. Res.* 1997, *14*, 325–328.
105. Zara, G.P., Cavalli, R., Bargoni, A., Fundarò, A., Vighetto, D., Gasco, M.R. Intravenous administration to rabbits of non-stealth and stealth doxorubicin-loaded solid lipid nanoparticles at increasing concentrations of stealth agent: Pharmacokinetics and distribution of doxorubicin in brain and other tissues. *J. Drug Target.* 2002, *10*, 327–335.
106. Carmona-Ribeiro, A.M., Barbassa, L., De Melo, L.D. Antimicrobial biomimetics. In *Biomimetic Based Applications,* IntechOpen: London, UK, 2011.
107. Bargoni, A., Cavalli, R., Zara, G.P., Fundarò, A., Caputo, O., Gasco, M.R. Transmucosal transport of tobramycin incorporated in solid lipid nanoparticles (SLN) after duodenal administration to rats. Part II – Tissue distribution. *Pharmacol. Res.* 2001, *43*, 497–502.
108. Pardridge, W.M. Drug and gene targeting to the brain with molecular Trojan horses. *Nat. Rev. Drug Discov.* 2002, *1*, 131–139.
109. Tiwari, S.B., Amiji, M.M. A review of nanocarrier-based CNS delivery systems. *Curr. Drug Deliv.* 2006, *3*, 219–232.
110. Thöle, M., Nobmann, S., Huwyler, J., Bartmann, A., Fricker, G. Uptake of cationized albumin coupled liposomes by cultured porcine brain microvessel endothelial cells and intact brain capillaries. *J. Drug Target* 2002, *10*, 337–344.
111. Zheng, G., Zheng, M., Yang, B., Fu, H., Li, Y. Improving breast cancer therapy using doxorubicin loaded solid lipid nanoparticles: Synthesis of a novel arginine-glycine-aspartic tripeptide conjugated, pH sensitive lipid and evaluation of the nanomedicine in vitro and in vivo. *Biomed. Pharmacother.* 2019, *116*, 109006.
112. Kadari, A., Pooja, D., Gora, R.H., Gudem, S., Kolapalli, V.R.M., Kulhari, H., Sistla, R. Design of multifunctional peptide collaborated and docetaxel loaded lipid nanoparticles for antiglioma therapy. *Eur. J. Pharm. Biopharm.* 2018, *132*, 168–179.
113. Siddhartha, V.T., Pindiprolu, S.K.S., Chintamaneni, P.K., Tummala, S., Nandha Kumar, S. RAGE receptor targeted bioconjuguate lipid nanoparticles of diallyl disulfide for improved apoptotic activity in triple negative breast cancer: In vitro studies. *Artif. Cells Nanomed. Biotechnol.* 2018, *46*, 387–397.
114. Rajpoot, K., Jain, S.K. Oral delivery of pH-responsive alginate microbeads incorporating folic acid-grafted solid lipid nanoparticles exhibits enhanced targeting effect against colorectal cancer: A dual-targeted approach. *Int. J. Biol. Macromol.* 2020, *151*, 830–844.
115. Kumar, C.S., Thangam, R., Mary, S.A., Kannan, P.R., Arun, G., Madhan, B. Targeted delivery and apoptosis induction of trans-resveratrol-ferulic acid loaded chitosan coated folic acid conjugate solid lipid nanoparticles in colon cancer cells. *Carbohydr. Polym.* 2020, *231*, 115682.
116. Müller, R., Schwarz, C., Zur Mühlen, A., Mehnert, W. Incorporation of lipophilic drugs and drug release profiles of solid lipid nanoparticles (SLN). *Proceedings of International Symposium on Controlled Release of Bioactive Materials, Nice*, France, 27–30 June 1994, pp. 146–147.
117. Zur Mühlen, A., Mehnert, W. Drug release and release mechanism of prednisolone loaded solid lipid nanoparticles. *Pharmazie* 1998, *53*, 552–555.
118. Schwarz, C., Mehnert, W., Lucks, J., Müller, R. Solid lipid nanoparticles (SLN) for controlled drug delivery. I. Production, characterization and sterilization. *J. Control. Release* 1994, *30*, 83–96.

119. Battaglia, L., Gallarate, M., Panciani, P.P., Ugazio, E., Sapino, S., Peira, E., Chirio, D. Techniques for the preparation of solid lipid nano and microparticles. *Appl. Nanotechnol. Drug Deliv.* 2014, *1*, 51–75.
120. Mehnert, W., Mäder, K. Solid lipid nanoparticles: Production, characterization and applications. *Adv. Drug Deliv. Rev.* 2012, *64*, 83–101.
121. Mishra, V., Bansal, K.K., Verma, A., Yadav, N., Thakur, S., Sudhakar, K., Rosenholm, J.M. Solid lipid nanoparticles: Emerging colloidal nano drug delivery systems. *Pharmaceutics* 2018, *10*, 191.
122. Battaglia, L., Trotta, M., Cavalli, R. Method for the Preparation of Solid Micro and Nanoparticles. *WIPO Patent WO2008149215*, 11 December 2008.
123. Battaglia, L., Gallarate, M., Cavalli, R., Trotta, M. Solid lipid nanoparticles produced through a coacervation method. *J. Microencapsul.* 2010, *27*, 78–85.
124. Bianco, M., Gallarate, M., Trotta, M., Battaglia, L. Amphotericin B loaded SLN prepared with the coacervation technique. *J. Drug Deliv. Sci. Technol.* 2010, *20*, 187–191.
125. Chirio, D., Gallarate, M., Peira, E., Battaglia, L., Serpe, L., Trotta, M. Formulation of curcumin-loaded solid lipid nanoparticles produced by fatty acids coacervation technique. *J. Microencapsul.* 2011, *28*, 537–548.
126. Del Curto, M., Chicco, D., D'antonio, M., Ciolli, V., Dannan, H., D'urso, S., Neuteboom, B., Pompili, S., Schiesaro, S., Esposito, P. Lipid microparticles as sustained release system for a GnRH antagonist (Antide). *J. Control. Release* 2003, *89*, 297–310.
127. Trotta, M., Cavalli, R., Trotta, C., Bussano, R., Costa, L. Electrospray technique for solid lipid-based particle production. *Drug Dev. Ind. Pharm.* 2010, *36*, 431–438.
128. Bussano, R., Chirio, D., Costa, L., Turci, F., Trotta, M. Preparation and characterization of insulin-loaded lipid-based microspheres generated by electrospray. *J. Dispers. Sci. Technol.* 2011, *32*, 1524–1530.
129. Byrappa, K., Ohara, S., Adschiri, T. Nanoparticles synthesis using supercritical fluid technology–towards biomedical applications. *Adv. Drug Deliv. Rev.* 2008, *60*, 299–327.
130. Müller, R., Petersen, R., Hommoss, A., Pardeike, J. Nanostructured lipid carriers (NLC) in cosmetic dermal products. *Adv. Drug Deliv. Rev.* 2007, *59*, 522–530.
131. Müller, R.H., Jenning, V., Mader, K., Lippacher, A. Lipid Particles on the Basis of Mixtures of Liquid and Solid Lipids and Method for Producing Same. US Patent US 8663692, 4 March 2014.
132. Dingler, A., Gohla, S. Production of solid lipid nanoparticles (SLN): Scaling up feasibilities. *J. Microencapsul.* 2002, *19*, 11–16.
133. Zhang, S.-h., Shen, S.-c., Chen, Z., Yun, J.-x., Yao, K.-j., Chen, B.-b., Chen, J.-z. Preparation of solid lipid nanoparticles in co-flowing microchannels. *Chem. Eng. J.* 2008, *144*, 324–328.
134. Bodmeier, R., Wang, J., Bhagwatwar, H. Process and formulation variables in the preparation of wax microparticles by a melt dispersion technique. I. Oil-in-water technique for water-insoluble drugs. *J. Microencapsul.* 1992, *9*, 89–98.
135. Bodmeier, R., Wang, J., Bhagwatwar, H. Process and formulation variables in the preparation of wax microparticles by a melt dispersion technique. II. W/O/W multiple emulsion technique for water-soluble drugs. *J. Microencapsul.* 1992, *9*, 99–107.
136. Charcosset, C., El-Harati, A., Fessi, H. Preparation of solid lipid nanoparticles using a membrane contactor. *J. Control. Release* 2005, *108*, 112–120.

137. Ahmed El-Harati, A., Charcosset, C., Fessi, H. Influence of the formulation for solid lipid nanoparticles prepared with a membrane contactor. *Pharm. Dev. Technol.* 2006, *11*, 153–157.
138. Mumper, R.J., Jay, M. Microemulsions as Precursors to Solid Nanoparticles. US Patent US 7153525, 26 December 2006.
139. Koziara, J., Oh, J., Akers, W., Ferraris, S., Mumper, R. Blood compatibility of cetyl alcohol/polysorbate-based nanoparticles. *Pharm. Res.* 2005, *22*, 1821–1828.
140. Oyewumi, M.O., Mumper, R.J. Influence of formulation parameters on gadolinium entrapment and tumor cell uptake using folate-coated nanoparticles. *Int. J. Pharm.* 2003, *251*, 85–97.
141. Hoar, T., Schulman, J. Transparent water-in-oil dispersions: The oleopathic hydro-micelle. *Nature* 1943, *152*, 102–103.
142. Attwood, D. Colloidal drug delivery systems. *Drugs Pharm. Sci.* 1994, *66*, 31–71.
143. Kreilgaard, M. Influence of microemulsions on cutaneous drug delivery. *Adv. Drug Deliv. Rev.* 2002, *54*, S77–S98.
144. Gasco, M.R. Method for Producing Solid Lipid Microspheres Having a Narrow Size Distribution. US Patent US5250236, 5 October 1993.
145. Morel, S., Terreno, E., Ugazio, E., Aime, S., Gasco, M.R. NMR relaxometric investigations of solid lipid nanoparticles (SLN) containing gadolinium (III) complexes. *Eur. J. Pharm. Biopharm.* 1998, *45*, 157–163.
146. Peira, E., Marzola, P., Podio, V., Aime, S., Sbarbati, A., Gasco, M.R. In vitro and in vivo study of solid lipid nanoparticles loaded with superparamagnetic iron oxide. *J. Drug Target.* 2003, *11*, 19–24.
147. Salmaso, S., Elvassore, N., Bertucco, A., Caliceti, P. Production of solid lipid submicron particles for protein delivery using a novel supercritical gas-assisted melting atomization process. *J. Pharm. Sci.* 2009, *98*, 640–650.
148. Vezzù, K., Borin, D., Bertucco, A., Bersani, S., Salmaso, S., Caliceti, P. Production of lipid microparticles containing bioactive molecules functionalized with PEG. *J. Supercrit. Fluids* 2010, *54*, 328–334.
149. Bertucco, A., Caliceti, P., Elvassore, N. Process for the Production of Nanoparticles. WIPO Patent WO2007028421, 15 March 2007.
150. Shinoda, K., Saito, H. The stability of O/W type emulsions as functions of temperature and the HLB of emulsifiers: The emulsification by PIT-method. *J. Colloid Interface Sci.* 1969, *30*, 258–263.
151. Huynh, N.T., Passirani, C., Saulnier, P., Benoît, J.-P. Lipid nanocapsules: A new platform for nanomedicine. *Int. J. Pharm.* 2009, *379*, 201–209.
152. Montenegro, L., Campisi, A., Sarpietro, M.G., Carbone, C., Acquaviva, R., Raciti, G., Puglisi, G. In vitro evaluation of idebenone-loaded solid lipid nanoparticles for drug delivery to the brain. *Drug Dev. Ind. Pharm.* 2011, *37*, 737–746.
153. Berton, A., Piel, G., Evrard, B. Powdered lipid nano and microparticles: Production and applications. *Recent Pat. Drug Deliv. Formul.* 2011, *5*, 188–200.
154. Siekmann, B., Westesen, K. Investigations on solid lipid nanoparticles prepared by precipitation in o/w emulsions. *Eur. J. Pharm. Biopharm.* 1996, *42*, 104–109.
155. Trotta, M., Debernardi, F., Caputo, O. Preparation of solid lipid nanoparticles by a solvent emulsification–diffusion technique. *Int. J. Pharm.* 2003, *257*, 153–160.
156. Garcıa-Fuentes, M., Torres, D., Alonso, M. Design of lipid nanoparticles for the oral delivery of hydrophilic macromolecules. *Colloids Surf. B Biointerfaces* 2003, *27*, 159–168.

157. Gallarate, M., Trotta, M., Battaglia, L., Chirio, D. Preparation of solid lipid nanoparticles from W/O/W emulsions: Preliminary studies on insulin encapsulation. *J. Microencapsul.* 2009, *26*, 394–402.
158. Schubert, M., Müller-Goymann, C. Solvent injection as a new approach for manufacturing lipid nanoparticles – evaluation of the method and process parameters. *Eur. J. Pharm. Biopharm.* 2003, *55*, 125–131.
159. Hu, F., Yuan, H., Zhang, H., Fang, M. Preparation of solid lipid nanoparticles with clobetasol propionate by a novel solvent diffusion method in aqueous system and physicochemical characterization. *Int. J. Pharm.* 2002, *239*, 121–128.
160. Rodriguez, L., Cini, M., Cavallari, C., Motta, G. Apparatus and Method for Preparing Solid Forms with Controlled Release of the Active Ingredient. Australian Patent AU693539B2, 7 February 1998.
161. Passerini, N., Qi, S., Albertini, B., Grassi, M., Rodriguez, L., Craig, D.Q. Solid lipid microparticles produced by spray congealing: Influence of the atomizer on microparticle characteristics and mathematical modeling of the drug release. *J. Pharm. Sci.* 2010, *99*, 916–931.
162. Killeen, M. Spray drying and spray congealing of pharmaceuticals. In *Encyclopedia of Pharmaceutical Technology*, Swarbrick, J., Boylan, J.C., Eds., PharmaceuTech, Inc., Informa Healthcare, Inc.: New York, NY, USA, 2000.
163. Pilcer, G., Amighi, K. Formulation strategy and use of excipients in pulmonary drug delivery. *Int. J. Pharm.* 2010, *392*, 1–19.
164. Sebti, T., Amighi, K. Preparation and in vitro evaluation of lipidic carriers and fillers for inhalation. *Eur. J. Pharm. Biopharm.* 2006, *63*, 51–58.
165. Chattopadhyay, P., Shekunov, B.Y., Seitzinger, J.S., Huff, R.W. Particles from Supercritical Fluid Extraction of Emulsion. WIPO Patent WO2004004862A1, 15 January 2004.
166. Chattopadhyay, P., Shekunov, B.Y., Yim, D., Cipolla, D., Boyd, B., Farr, S. Production of solid lipid nanoparticle suspensions using supercritical fluid extraction of emulsions (SFEE) for pulmonary delivery using the AERx system. *Adv. Drug Deliv. Rev.* 2007, *59*, 444–453.
167. Carlotti, M.E., Sapino, S., Trotta, M., Battaglia, L., Vione, D., Pelizzetti, E. Photostability and stability over time of retinyl palmitate in an O/W emulsion and in SLN introduced in the emulsion. *J. Dispers. Sci. Technol.* 2005, *26*, 125–138.
168. Hou, D., Xie, C., Huang, K., Zhu, C. The production and characteristics of solid lipid nanoparticles (SLNs). *Biomaterials* 2003, *24*, 1781–1785.
169. Corrias, F., Lai, F. New methods for lipid nanoparticles preparation. *Recent Pat. Drug Deliv. Formul.* 2011, *5*, 201–213.
170. Speiser, P. Lipidnanopellets als Trägersystem für Arzneimittel zur peroralen Anwendung. European Patent 167825, 8 August 1990.
171. Ahlin, P., Kristl, J., Smid-Korbar, J. Optimization of procedure parameters and physical stability of solid lipid nanoparticles in dispersions. *Acta Pharm.* 1998, *48*, 259–267.
172. Olbrich, C., Gessner, A., Kayser, O., Müller, R.H. Lipid-drug-conjugate (LDC) nanoparticles as novel carrier system for the hydrophilic antitrypanosomal drug diminazenediaceturate. *J. Drug Target.* 2002, *10*, 387–396.
173. Eldem, T., Speiser, P., Hincal, A. Optimization of spray-dried and-congealed lipid micropellets and characterization of their surface morphology by scanning electron microscopy. *Pharm. Res.* 1991, *8*, 47–54.
174. Tan, M.-e., He, C.-h., Jiang, W., Zeng, C., Yu, N., Huang, W., Gao, Z.-g., Xing, J.-g. Development of solid lipid nanoparticles containing total flavonoid extract

from Dracocephalum moldavica L. and their therapeutic effect against myocardial ischemia–reperfusion injury in rats. *Int. J. Nanomed.* 2017, *12*, 3253.
175. Lander, R., Manger, W., Scouloudis, M., Ku, A., Davis, C., Lee, A. Gaulin homogenization: A mechanistic study. *Biotechnol. Prog.* 2000, *16*, 80–85.
176. Müller, R.H., Benita, S., Bohm, B. *Emulsions and Nanosuspensions for the Formulation of Poorly Soluble Drugs*, CRC Press: Boca Raton, FL, USA, 1998.
177. zur Muhlen, A. Feste Lipid Nanopartikel mit Prolongierter Wirkstoffliberation: Herstellung, Langzeitstabilität, Charakterisierung, Freisetzungsverhalten und Mechanismen. Ph.D. Thesis, Free University of Berlin, Berlin, Germany, 1996.
178. Sjöström, B., Bergenståhl, B. Preparation of submicron drug particles in lecithin-stabilized ow emulsions: I. Model studies of the precipitation of cholesteryl acetate. *Int. J. Pharm.* 1992, *84*, 107–116.
179. Cavalli, R., Marengo, E., Rodriguez, L., Gasco, M.R. Effects of some experimental factors on the production process of solid lipid nanoparticles. *Eur. J. Pharm. Biopharm.* 1996, *42*, 110–115.
180. Chen, Y., Jin, R., Zhou, Y., Zeng, J., Zhang, H., Feng, Q. Preparation of solid lipid nanoparticles loaded with Xionggui powder-supercritical carbon dioxide fluid extraction and their evaluation in vitro release. *Zhongguo Zhongyao Zazhi China J. Chin. Mater. Med.* 2006, *31*, 376–379.
181. Meyer, W. Wettkampf und Spiel in den Miniaturen der Manessischen Liederhandschrift. *Stadion* 1988, *14*, 1–48.
182. Gosselin, P., Thibert, R., Preda, M., McMullen, J. Polymorphic properties of micronized carbamazepine produced by RESS. *Int. J. Pharm.* 2003, *252*, 225–233.
183. Freitas, C., Müller, R.H. Spray-drying of solid lipid nanoparticles (SLNTM). *Eur. J. Pharm. Biopharm.* 1998, *46*, 145–151.
184. Sguizzato, M., Esposito, E., Drechsler, M., Gallerani, E., Gavioli, R., Mariani, P., Carducci, F., Cortesi, R., Bergamini, P. Nafion®-containing solid lipid nanoparticles as a tool for anticancer PT Delivery: Preliminary studies. *J. Chem.* 2017, *2017*.
185. Cortesi, R., Esposito, E., Luca, G., Nastruzzi, C. Production of lipospheres as carriers for bioactive compounds. *Biomaterials* 2002, *23*, 2283–2294.
186. Heurtault, B., Saulnier, P., Benoit, J.-P., Proust, J.-E., Pech, B., Richard, J. Lipid Nanocapsules, Preparation Process and Use as Medicine. US Patent US8057823B2, 15 November 2011.
187. Mori, N., Sheth, N., Mendapara, V., Ashara, K., Paun, J. SLN brain targeting drug delivery for CNS: A novel approach. *Int. Res. J. Pharm* 2014, *5*, 658–662.
188. Battaglia, L., Serpe, L., Foglietta, F., Muntoni, E., Gallarate, M., Del Pozo Rodriguez, A., Solinis, M.A. Application of lipid nanoparticles to ocular drug delivery. *Expert Opin. Drug Deliv.* 2016, *13*, 1743–1757.
189. Vakilinezhad, M.A., Amini, A., Javar, H.A., Zarandi, B.F.B.a.B., Montaseri, H., Dinarvand, R. Nicotinamide loaded functionalized solid lipid nanoparticles improves cognition in Alzheimer's disease animal model by reducing Tau hyperphosphorylation. *DARU J. Pharm. Sci.* 2018, *26*, 165–177.
190. Saini, S., Sharma, T., Jain, A., Kaur, H., Katare, O., Singh, B. Systematically designed chitosan-coated solid lipid nanoparticles of ferulic acid for effective management of Alzheimer's disease: A preclinical evidence. *Colloids Surf. B Biointerfaces* 2021, *205*, 111838.
191. Misra, S., Kuhad, A., Kaur, I., Chopra, K. Neuroprotective potential of solid lipid nanoparticles of sesamol: Possible brain targeting strategy. *Alzheimers Dement.* 2012, *8*, P 199.

192. Nelluri, S., Felix, J., Sathesh, K. Formulation and evaluation of galantamine nanoparticles for neurological disorders. *Int. J. Pharm. Chem. Biol. Sci.* 2015, *5*, 63–70.
193. Dhawan, S., Kapil, R., Singh, B. Formulation development and systematic optimization of solid lipid nanoparticles of quercetin for improved brain delivery. *J. Pharm. Pharmacol.* 2011, *63*, 342–351.
194. Yusuf, M., Khan, M., Khan, R.A., Ahmed, B. Preparation, characterization, in vivo and biochemical evaluation of brain targeted Piperine solid lipid nanoparticles in an experimentally induced Alzheimer's disease model. *J. Drug Target.* 2013, *21*, 300–311.
195. Orlando, A., Re, F., Sesana, S., Rivolta, I., Panariti, A., Brambilla, D., Nicolas, J., Couvreur, P., Andrieux, K., Masserini, M. Effect of nanoparticles binding β-amyloid peptide on nitric oxide production by cultured endothelial cells and macrophages. *Int. J. Nanomed.* 2013, *8*, 1335.
196. Picone, P., Bondi, M.L., Picone, P., Bondi, M.L., Montana, G., Bruno, A., Pitarresi, G., Giammona, G., Di Carlo, M. Ferulic acid inhibits oxidative stress and cell death induced by Ab oligomers: Improved delivery by solid lipid nanoparticles. *Free Radic. Res.* 2009, *43*, 1133–1145.
197. Smith, A., Giunta, B., Bickford, P.C., Fountain, M., Tan, J., Shytle, R.D. Nanolipidic particles improve the bioavailability and α-secretase inducing ability of epigallocatechin-3-gallate (EGCG) for the treatment of Alzheimer's disease. *Int. J. Pharm.* 2010, *389*, 207–212.
198. Kakkar, V., Kaur, I.P. Evaluating potential of curcumin loaded solid lipid nanoparticles in aluminium induced behavioural, biochemical and histopathological alterations in mice brain. *Food Chem. Toxicol.* 2011, *49*, 2906–2913.
199. Zhan, S.M., Hou, D.Z., Ping, Q.N., Xu, Y. Preparation and entrapment efficiency determination of solid lipid nanoparticles loaded levodopa. *Chin. J. Hosp. Pharm.* 2010, *14*, 1171–1175.
200. Esposito, E., Fantin, M., Marti, M., Drechsler, M., Paccamiccio, L., Mariani, P., Sivieri, E., Lain, F., Menegatti, E., Morari, M. Solid lipid nanoparticles as delivery systems for bromocriptine. *Pharm. Res.* 2008, *25*, 1521–1530.
201. Tsai, M.-J., Huang, Y.-B., Wu, P.-C., Fu, Y.-S., Kao, Y.-R., Fang, J.-Y., Tsai, Y.-H. Oral apomorphine delivery from solid lipid nanoparticles with different monostearate emulsifiers: Pharmacokinetic and behavioral evaluations. *J. Pharm. Sci.* 2011, *100*, 547–557.
202. Pardeshi, C.V., Rajput, P.V., Belgamwar, V.S., Tekade, A.R., Surana, S.J. Novel surface modified solid lipid nanoparticles as intranasal carriers for ropinirole hydrochloride: Application of factorial design approach. *Drug Deliv.* 2013, *20*, 47–56.
203. Sandhir, R., Yadav, A., Mehrotra, A., Sunkaria, A., Singh, A., Sharma, S. Curcumin nanoparticles attenuate neurochemical and neurobehavioral deficits in experimental model of Huntington's disease. *Neuromolecular Med.* 2014, *16*, 106–118.
204. Bhatt, R., Singh, D., Prakash, A., Mishra, N. Development, characterization and nasal delivery of rosmarinic acid-loaded solid lipid nanoparticles for the effective management of Huntington's disease. *Drug Deliv.* 2015, *22*, 931–939.
205. des Rieux, A., Fievez, V., Garinot, M., Schneider, Y.-J., Préat, V. Nanoparticles as potential oral delivery systems of proteins and vaccines: A mechanistic approach. *J. Control. Release* 2006, *116*, 1–27.
206. Garcion, E., Lamprecht, A., Heurtault, B., Paillard, A., Aubert-Pouessel, A., Denizot, B., Menei, P., Benoît, J.-P. A new generation of anticancer, drug-loaded, colloidal

vectors reverses multidrug resistance in glioma and reduces tumor progression in rats. *Mol. Cancer Ther.* 2006, *5*, 1710–1722.

207. Blasi, P., Giovagnoli, S., Schoubben, A., Ricci, M., Rossi, C. Solid lipid nanoparticles for targeted brain drug delivery. *Adv. Drug Deliv. Rev.* 2007, *59*, 454–477.
208. Wong, H.L., Wu, X.Y., Bendayan, R. Nanotechnological advances for the delivery of CNS therapeutics. *Adv. Drug Deliv. Rev.* 2012, *64*, 686–700.
209. Samia, O., Hanan, R., Kamal, E.T. Carbamazepine mucoadhesive nanoemulgel (MNEG) as brain targeting delivery system via the olfactory mucosa. *Drug Deliv.* 2012, *19*, 58–67.
210. Abdelbary, G., Fahmy, R.H. Diazepam-loaded solid lipid nanoparticles: Design and characterization. *Aaps Pharmscitech.* 2009, *10*, 211–219.
211. Leyva-Gómez, G., González-Trujano, M.E., López-Ruiz, E., Couraud, P.-O., Weksler, B., Romero, I., Miller, F., Delie, F., Allémann, E., Quintanar-Guerrero, D. Nanoparticle formulation improves the anticonvulsant effect of clonazepam on the pentylenetetrazole-induced seizures: Behavior and electroencephalogram. *J. Pharm. Sci.* 2014, *103*, 2509–2519.
212. Tran, T.H., Ramasamy, T., Cho, H.J., Kim, Y.I., Poudel, B.K., Choi, H.-G., Yong, C.S., Kim, J.O. Formulation and optimization of raloxifene-loaded solid lipid nanoparticles to enhance oral bioavailability. *J. Nanosci. Nanotechnol.* 2014, *14*, 4820–4831.
213. Vickers, N.J. Animal communication: When I'm calling you, will you answer too? *Curr. Biol.* 2017, *27*, R713–R715.
214. Gao, Y., Gu, W., Chen, L., Xu, Z., Li, Y. The role of daidzein-loaded sterically stabilized solid lipid nanoparticles in therapy for cardio-cerebrovascular diseases. *Biomaterials* 2008, *29*, 4129–4136.
215. Morsi, N.M., Ghorab, D.M., Badie, H.A. Brain targeted solid lipid nanoparticles for brain ischemia: Preparation and in vitro characterization. *Pharm. Dev. Technol.* 2013, *18*, 736–744.
216. Frautschy, S.A., Cole, G.M. Bioavailable Curcuminoid Formulations for Treating Alzheimer's Disease and Other Age-Related Disorders. US Patent US20090324703A1, 24 November 2015.
217. Dang, H., Meng, M.H.W., Zhao, H., Iqbal, J., Dai, R., Deng, Y., Lv, F. Luteolin-loaded solid lipid nanoparticles synthesis, characterization, & improvement of bioavailability, pharmacokinetics in vitro and vivo studies. *J. Nanoparticle Res.* 2014, *16*, 1–10.
218. Burlá, C., Rego, G., Nunes, R. Alzheimer, dementia and the living will: A proposal. *Med. Health Care Philos.* 2014, *17*, 389–395.
219. Saykin, A.J., Wishart, H.A., Rabin, L.A., Flashman, L.A., McHugh, T.L., Mamourian, A.C., Santulli, R.B. Cholinergic enhancement of frontal lobe activity in mild cognitive impairment. *Brain* 2004, *127*, 1574–1583.
220. Yiannopoulou, K., Papageorgiou, S. Current and future treatments for Alzheimer's disease. *Ther. Adv. Neurol. Disord.* 2013, *6*, 19–33.
221. Cacciatore, I., Baldassarre, L., Fornasari, E., Cornacchia, C., Di Stefano, A., Sozio, P., Cerasa, L.S., Fontana, A., Fulle, S., Di Filippo, E.S. (R)-α-Lipoyl-Glycyl-L-Prolyl-L-Glutamyl Dimethyl Ester codrug as a multifunctional agent with potential neuroprotective activities. *ChemMedChem* 2012, *7*, 2021–2029.
222. Sozio, P., D'Aurizio, E., Iannitelli, A., Cataldi, A., Zara, S., Cantalamessa, F., Nasuti, C., Di Stefano, A. Ibuprofen and lipoic acid diamides as potential codrugs with neuroprotective activity. *Arch. Der Pharm. Int. J. Pharm. Med. Chem.* 2010, *343*, 133–142.

223. Topal, G.R., Mészáros, M., Porkoláb, G., Szecskó, A., Polgár, T.F., Siklós, L., Deli, M.A., Veszelka, S., Bozkir, A. ApoE-targeting increases the transfer of solid lipid nanoparticles with donepezil cargo across a culture model of the blood–brain barrier. *Pharmaceutics* 2021, *13*, 38.
224. Wang, J., Zhu, R., Sun, D., Sun, X., Geng, Z., Liu, H., Wang, S.-L. Intracellular uptake of curcumin-loaded solid lipid nanoparticles exhibit anti-inflammatory activities superior to those of curcumin through the NF-κB signaling pathway. *J. Biomed. Nanotechnol.* 2015, *11*, 403–415.
225. Wang, J., Wang, H., Zhu, R., Liu, Q., Fei, J., Wang, S. Anti-inflammatory activity of curcumin-loaded solid lipid nanoparticles in IL-1β transgenic mice subjected to the lipopolysaccharide-induced sepsis. *Biomaterials* 2015, *53*, 475–483.
226. Gaur, P.K., Mishra, S., Verma, A., Verma, N. Ceramide–palmitic acid complex based Curcumin solid lipid nanoparticles for transdermal delivery: Pharmacokinetic and pharmacodynamic study. *J. Exp. Nanosci.* 2016, *11*, 38–53.
227. Rajput, A. Frequency and cause of Parkinson's disease. *Can. J. Neurol. Sci.* 1992, *19*, 103–107.
228. Cacciatore, I., Ciulla, M., Fornasari, E., Marinelli, L., Di Stefano, A. Solid lipid nanoparticles as a drug delivery system for the treatment of neurodegenerative diseases. *Expert Opin. Drug Deliv.* 2016, *13*, 1121–1131.
229. Sozio, P., Iannitelli, A., Cerasa, L.S., Cacciatore, I., Cornacchia, C., Giorgioni, G., Ricciutelli, M., Nasuti, C., Cantalamessa, F., Di Stefano, A. New L-dopa codrugs as potential antiparkinson agents. *Arch. Der Pharm. Int. J. Pharm. Med. Chem.* 2008, *341*, 412–417.
230. Minelli, A., Conte, C., Cacciatore, I., Cornacchia, C., Pinnen, F. Molecular mechanism underlying the cerebral effect of Gly-Pro-Glu tripeptide bound to L-dopa in a Parkinson's animal model. *Amino Acids* 2012, *43*, 1359–1367.
231. Minelli, A., Conte, C., Prudenzi, E., Cacciatore, I., Cornacchia, C., Taha, E., Pinnen, F. N-Acetyl-L-Methionyl-L-Dopa-Methyl Ester as a dual acting drug that relieves L-dopa-induced oxidative toxicity. *Free Radic Biol. Med.* 2010, *49*, 31–39.
232. Jankovic, J., Stacy, M. Medical management of levodopa-associated motor complications in patients with Parkinson's disease. *CNS Drugs* 2007, *21*, 677–692.
233. Cingolani, G.M., Di Stefano, A., Mosciatti, B., Napolitani, F., Giorgioni, G., Ricciutelli, M., Claudi, F. Synthesis of L-(+)-3-(3-hydroxy-4-pivaloyloxybenzyl)-2,5-diketomorpholine as potential prodrug of L-dopa. *Bioorganic Med. Chem. Lett.* 2000, *10*, 1385–1388.
234. Neri-Nani, G., López-Ruiz, M., Estrada-Bellmann, I., Carrasco, H., Enríquez-Coronel, G., González-Usigli, H., Leal-Ortega, R., Otero-Cerdeira, E., Rodríguez, R., Pedro, A.A. Mexican consensus on the diagnosis of Huntington's disease. *Arch. Neurocienc.* 2016, *21*, 64–72.
235. National Institute of Neurological Disorders and Stroke. *Parkinson's Disease: Hope through Research*, National Institute of Neurological Disorders and Stroke: Bethesda, MD, USA, 1994.
236. Sturchio, A., Marsili, L., Mahajan, A., Grimberg, M., Kauffman, M.A., Espay, A.J. How have advances in genetic technology modified movement disorder nosology? *Eur. J. Neurol.* 2020, *27*, 1461–1470.
237. Hachinski, V., Iadecola, C., Petersen, R.C., Breteler, M.M., Nyenhuis, D.L., Black, S.E., Powers, W.J., DeCarli, C., Merino, J.G., Kalaria, R.N. National Institute of Neurological Disorders and Stroke – Canadian Stroke Network Vascular Cognitive Impairment Harmonization Standards. *Stroke* 2006, *37*, 2220–2241.

238. Kappos, L., Gold, R., Miller, D.H., MacManus, D.G., Havrdova, E., Limmroth, V., Polman, C.H., Schmierer, K., Yousry, T.A., Yang, M. Efficacy and safety of oral fumarate in patients with relapsing-remitting multiple sclerosis: A multicentre, randomised, double-blind, placebo-controlled phase IIb study. *Lancet* 2008, *372*, 1463–1472.
239. Salzer, J., Svenningsson, A., Sundström, P. Neurofilament light as a prognostic marker in multiple sclerosis. *Mult. Scler. J.* 2010, *16*, 287–292.
240. Michaeli, M.F., Ahi, G., Ramazani, F., Behnejad, S. The effect of a pain management program in reducing the pain in patients with multiple sclerosis. *J. Res. Health* 2016, *6*, 336–344.
241. Holden, C.A., Yuan, Q., Yeudall, W.A., Lebman, D.A., Yang, H. Surface engineering of macrophages with nanoparticles to generate a cell–nanoparticle hybrid vehicle for hypoxia-targeted drug delivery. *Int. J. Nanomed.* 2010, *5*, 25.
242. Sanai, N., Berger, M.S. Glioma extent of resection and its impact on patient outcome. *Neurosurgery* 2008, *62*, 753–766.
243. Özdemir, Y.G., Pehlivan, S.B., Sekerdag, E. *Nanotechnology Methods for Neurological Diseases and Brain Tumors: Drug Delivery Across the Blood–Brain Barrier*, Academic Press: Cambridge, MA, USA, 2017.
244. Bidros, D.S., Vogelbaum, M.A. Novel drug delivery strategies in neuro-oncology. *Neurotherapeutics* 2009, *6*, 539–546.
245. Leslie-Barbick, J.E., Saik, J.E., Gould, D.J., Dickinson, M.E., West, J.L. The promotion of microvasculature formation in poly (ethylene glycol) diacrylate hydrogels by an immobilized VEGF-mimetic peptide. *Biomaterials* 2011, *32*, 5782–5789.
246. Kuo, Y.-C., Liang, C.-T. Catanionic solid lipid nanoparticles carrying doxorubicin for inhibiting the growth of U87MG cells. *Colloids Surf. B Biointerfaces* 2011, *85*, 131–137.
247. Gonçalves, M., Mignani, S., Rodrigues, J., Tomás, H. A glance over doxorubicin based-nanotherapeutics: From proof-of-concept studies to solutions in the market. *J. Control. Release* 2020, *317*, 347–374.
248. Kuo, Y.-C., Lee, C.-H. Inhibition against growth of glioblastoma multiforme in vitro using etoposide-loaded solid lipid nanoparticles with ρ-Aminophenyl-α-D-mannopyranoside and folic acid. *J. Pharm. Sci.* 2015, *104*, 1804–1814.
249. Kuo, Y.-C., Wang, I.-H. Enhanced delivery of etoposide across the blood–brain barrier to restrain brain tumor growth using melanotransferrin antibody-and tamoxifen-conjugated solid lipid nanoparticles. *J. Drug Target.* 2016, *24*, 645–654.
250. de Mendoza, A.E.-H., Préat, V., Mollinedo, F., Blanco-Prieto, M.J. In vitro and in vivo efficacy of edelfosine-loaded lipid nanoparticles against glioma. *J. Control. Release* 2011, *156*, 421–426.
251. Martins, S., Costa-Lima, S., Carneiro, T., Cordeiro-da-Silva, A., Souto, E., Ferreira, D. Solid lipid nanoparticles as intracellular drug transporters: An investigation of the uptake mechanism and pathway. *Int. J. Pharm.* 2012, *430*, 216–227.
252. Jose, S., Anju, S., Cinu, T., Aleykutty, N., Thomas, S., Souto, E. In vivo pharmacokinetics and biodistribution of resveratrol-loaded solid lipid nanoparticles for brain delivery. *Int. J. Pharm.* 2014, *474*, 6–13.
253. Chirio, D., Gallarate, M., Peira, E., Battaglia, L., Muntoni, E., Riganti, C., Biasibetti, E., Capucchio, M.T., Valazza, A., Panciani, P. Positive-charged solid lipid nanoparticles as paclitaxel drug delivery system in glioblastoma treatment. *Eur. J. Pharm. Biopharm.* 2014, *88*, 746–758.
254. Jabir, N.R., Tabrez, S., Firoz, C., Kashif Zaidi, S., Baeesa, S.S., Hua Gan, S., Shakil, S., Amjad Kamal, M. A synopsis of nano-technological approaches toward

anti-epilepsy therapy: Present and future research implications. *Curr. Drug Metab.* 2015, *16*, 336–345.
255. Bennewitz, M.F., Saltzman, W.M. Nanotechnology for delivery of drugs to the brain for epilepsy. *Neurotherapeutics* 2009, *6*, 323–336.
256. Kohane, D.S., Holmes, G.L., Chau, Y., Zurakowski, D., Langer, R., Cha, B.H. Effectiveness of muscimol-containing microparticles against pilocarpine-induced focal seizures. *Epilepsia* 2002, *43*, 1462–1468.
257. Ali, A., Pillai, K.K., Ahmad, F.J., Dua, Y., Khan, Z.I., Vohora, D. Comparative efficacy of liposome-entrapped amiloride and free amiloride in animal models of seizures and serum potassium in mice. *Eur. Neuropsychopharmacol.* 2007, *17*, 227–229.
258. Lakhan, S.E., Kirchgessner, A., Hofer, M. Inflammatory mechanisms in ischemic stroke: Therapeutic approaches. *J. Transl. Med.* 2009, *7*, 1–11.
259. Sacco, R.L., Kasner, S.E., Broderick, J.P., Caplan, L.R., Connors, J., Culebras, A., Elkind, M.S., George, M.G., Hamdan, A.D., Higashida, R.T. An updated definition of stroke for the 21st century: A statement for healthcare professionals from the American Heart Association/American Stroke Association. *Stroke* 2013, *44*, 2064–2089.
260. Choi, D.W., Rothman, S.M. The role of glutamate neurotoxicity in hypoxic-ischemic neuronal death. *Annu. Rev. Neurosci.* 1990, *13*, 171–182.
261. Rego, A.C., Oliveira, C.R. Mitochondrial dysfunction and reactive oxygen species in excitotoxicity and apoptosis: Implications for the pathogenesis of neurodegenerative diseases. *Neurochem. Res.* 2003, *28*, 1563–1574.
262. Thompson, B.J., Ronaldson, P.T. Drug delivery to the ischemic brain. *Adv. Pharmacol.* 2014, *71*, 165–202.
263. González-Nieto, D., Fernández-Serra, R., Pérez-Rigueiro, J., Panetsos, F., Martinez-Murillo, R., Guinea, G.V. Biomaterials to neuroprotect the stroke brain: A large opportunity for narrow time windows. *Cells* 2020, *9*, 1074.
264. Sarmah, D., Saraf, J., Kaur, H., Pravalika, K., Tekade, R.K., Borah, A., Kalia, K., Dave, K.R., Bhattacharya, P. Stroke management: An emerging role of nanotechnology. *Micromachines* 2017, *8*, 262.
265. Crielaard, B., Lammers, T., Morgan, M., Chaabane, L., Carboni, S., Greco, B., Zaratin, P., Kraneveld, A., Storm, G. Macrophages and liposomes in inflammatory disease: Friends or foes? *Int. J. Pharm.* 2011, *416*, 499–506.
266. Kakkar, V., Muppu, S.K., Chopra, K., Kaur, I.P. Curcumin loaded solid lipid nanoparticles: An efficient formulation approach for cerebral ischemic reperfusion injury in rats. *Eur. J. Pharm. Biopharm.* 2013, *85*, 339–345.
267. Tsai, M.-J., Wu, P.-C., Huang, Y.-B., Chang, J.-S., Lin, C.-L., Tsai, Y.-H., Fang, J.-Y. Baicalein loaded in tocol nanostructured lipid carriers (tocol NLCs) for enhanced stability and brain targeting. *Int. J. Pharm.* 2012, *423*, 461–470.
268. Neves, A.R., Queiroz, J.F., Reis, S. Brain-targeted delivery of resveratrol using solid lipid nanoparticles functionalized with apolipoprotein E. *J. Nanobiotechnology* 2016, *14*, 1–11.
269. Hassanzadeh, P., Arbabi, E., Atyabi, F., Dinarvand, R. Ferulic acid-loaded nanostructured lipid carriers: A promising nanoformulation against the ischemic neural injuries. *Life Sci.* 2018, *193*, 64–76.
270. Moosmann, B., Behl, C. Antioxidants as treatment for neurodegenerative disorders. *Expert Opin. Investig. Drugs* 2002, *11*, 1407–1435.
271. Cacciatore, I., Caccuri, A., Di Stefano, A., Luisi, G., Nalli, M., Pinnen, F., Ricci, G., Sozio, P. Synthesis and activity of novel glutathione analogues containing an urethane backbone linkage. *Il Farm.* 2003, *58*, 787–793.

272. Souto, E., Müller, R., Gohla, S. A novel approach based on lipid nanoparticles (SLN®) for topical delivery of α-lipoic acid. *J. Microencapsul.* 2005, *22*, 581–592.
273. Laserra, S., Basit, A., Sozio, P., Marinelli, L., Fornasari, E., Cacciatore, I., Ciulla, M., Türkez, H., Geyikoglu, F., Di Stefano, A. Solid lipid nanoparticles loaded with lipoyl–memantine codrug: Preparation and characterization. *Int. J. Pharm.* 2015, *485*, 183–191.
274. Duarte, A.M.G. Resveratrol and Grape's Extract-Loaded Solid Lipid Nanoparticles for the Treatment of Parkinson's and Alzheimer's Diseases. Master's Thesis, Faculty of Engineering of University of Porto, Porto, Portugal, 2015.
275. Loureiro, J.A., Andrade, S., Duarte, A., Neves, A.R., Queiroz, J.F., Nunes, C., Sevin, E., Fenart, L., Gosselet, F., Coelho, M.A.N. et al. Resveratrol and grape extract-loaded solid lipid nanoparticles for the treatment of Alzheimer's disease. *Molecules* 2017, *22*, 277.
276. Fernandes, F., Dias-Teixeira, M., Delerue-Matos, C., Grosso, C. Critical review of lipid-based nanoparticles as carriers of neuroprotective drugs and extracts. *Nanomaterials* 2021, *11*, 563.
277. Thi, T.T.H., Suys, E.J., Lee, J.S., Nguyen, D.H., Park, K.D., Truong, N.P. Lipid-based nanoparticles in the clinic and clinical trials: From cancer nanomedicine to COVID-19 vaccines. *Vaccines* 2021, *9*, 359.
278. Mistraletti, G., Paroni, R., Umbrello, M., Moro Salihovic, B., Coppola, S., Froio, S., Finati, E., Gasco, P., Savoca, A., Manca, D. Different routes and formulations of melatonin in critically ill patients. A pharmacokinetic randomized study. *Clin. Endocrinol.* 2019, *91*, 209–218.

Index

Note: Page locators in **bold** and *italics* represents tables and figures, respectively.